World Health Organization Classification of Tumours

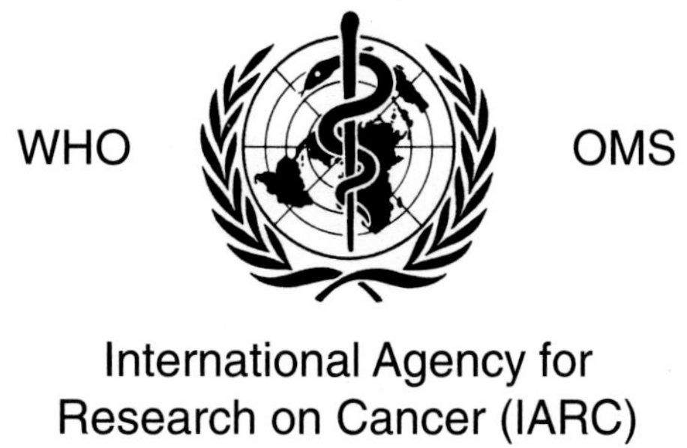

International Agency for
Research on Cancer (IARC)

Pathology and Genetics of Tumours of the Nervous System

Edited by

Paul Kleihues
Webster K. Cavenee

IARC*Press*

Lyon, 2000

World Health Organization Classification of Tumours

Series editors — Paul Kleihues, M.D.
Leslie H. Sobin, M.D.

Pathology and Genetics of Tumours of the Nervous System

Editors	Paul Kleihues, M.D. Webster K. Cavenee Ph.D.
Editoral Assistance	Wojciech Biernat, M.D. Nikolai Napalkov, M.D. Anna Sankila, M.D.
Layout	Katja Mückenhaupt Katarzyna Szymanska
Illustrations	George Mollon
Printed by	Team Rush 69603 Villeurbanne, France
Publisher	IARC*Press* International Agency for Research on Cancer (IARC) 69372, Lyon, France

This volume was produced in collaboration with the

International Society of Neuropathology (ISN)

International Academy of Pathology (IAP)

and

The Preuss Foundation for Brain Tumor Research

The WHO Classification of Tumours of the Nervous System presented in this book reflects the view of a Working Group that convened for an Editorial and Consensus Conference in Lyon, France, July 27-30, 1999.

Members of the Working Group are mentioned in the list of Contibutors on page 255.

Published by IARC Press, International Agency for Research on Cancer,
150 cours Albert Thomas, F-69372 Lyon cedex 08, France

IARC Library Cataloguing in Publication Data
Pathology and genetics of tumours of the nervous system/
editors, P. Kleihues, W. K. Cavenee

1. Central Nervous System Neoplasms - genetics 2. Central Nervous System
2. Neoplasms - pathology I. Kleihues, P. (Paul) II. Cavenee, Webster 1951-. III. Title

ISBN 92 832 2409 4 (NLM Classification: QZ 15)

Contents

WHO Classification of Tumours of the Nervous System

TUMOURS OF NEUROEPITHELIAL TISSUE

Astrocytic tumours

Diffuse astrocytoma	9400/3[1]
Fibrillary astrocytoma	9420/3
Protoplasmic astrocytoma	9410/3
Gemistocytic astrocytoma	9411/3
Anaplastic astrocytoma	9401/3
Glioblastoma	9440/3
Giant cell glioblastoma	9441/3
Gliosarcoma	9442/3
Pilocytic astrocytoma	9421/1
Pleomorphic xanthoastrocytoma	9424/3
Subependymal giant cell astrocytoma	9384/1

Oligodendroglial tumours

Oligodendroglioma	9450/3
Anaplastic oligodendroglioma	9451/3

Mixed gliomas

Oligoastrocytoma	9382/3
Anaplastic oligoastrocytoma	*9382/3*[2]

Ependymal tumours

Ependymoma	9391/3
Cellular	*9391/3*
Papillary	9393/3
Clear cell	*9391/3*
Tanycytic	*9391/3*
Anaplastic ependymoma	9392/3
Myxopapillary ependymoma	9394/1
Subependymoma	9383/1

Choroid plexus tumours

Choroid plexus papilloma	9390/0
Choroid plexus carcinoma	9390/3

Glial tumours of uncertain origin

Astroblastoma	9430/3
Gliomatosis cerebri	9381/3
Chordoid glioma of the 3rd ventricle	*9444/1*

[1] Morphology code of the International Classification of Diseases for Oncology (ICD-O) and the Systematized Nomenclature of Medicine (SNOMED). Behaviour is coded /0 for benign tumours, /1 for low or uncertain malignant potential or borderline malignancy, (/2 for in *situ lesions*) and /3 for malignant tumours.

[2] The italicised numbers are provisional codes proposed for the third edition of ICD-O. They should, for the most part, be incorporated into the next edition of ICD-O, but they are subject to change.

Neuronal and mixed neuronal-glial tumours

Gangliocytoma	9492/0
Dysplastic gangliocytoma of cerebellum (Lhermitte-Duclos)	*9493/0*
Desmoplastic infantile astrocytoma / ganglioglioma	*9412/1*
Dysembryoplastic neuroepithelial tumour	*9413/0*
Ganglioglioma	9505/1
Anaplastic ganglioglioma	*9505/3*
Central neurocytoma	*9506/1*
Cerebellar liponeurocytoma	*9506/1*
Paraganglioma of the filum terminale	8680/1

Neuroblastic tumours

Olfactory neuroblastoma (Aesthesioneuroblastoma)	9522/3
Olfactory neuroepithelioma	9523/3
Neuroblastomas of the adrenal gland and sympathetic nervous system	9500/3

Pineal parenchymal tumours

Pineocytoma	9361/1
Pineoblastoma	9362/3
Pineal parenchymal tumour of intermediate differentiation	*9362/3*

Embryonal tumours

Medulloepithelioma	9501/3
Ependymoblastoma	9392/3
Medulloblastoma	9470/3
Desmoplastic medulloblastoma	9471/3
Large cell medulloblastoma	*9474/3*
Medullomyoblastoma	9472/3
Melanotic medulloblastoma	*9470/3*
Supratentorial primitive neuroectodermal tumour (PNET)	9473/3
Neuroblastoma	9500/3
Ganglioneuroblastoma	9490/3
Atypical teratoid/rhabdoid tumour	9508/3

TUMOURS OF PERIPHERAL NERVES

Schwannoma

(Neurilemmoma, Neurinoma)	9560/0
Cellular	*9560/0*
Plexiform	*9560/0*
Melanotic	*9560/0*

Neurofibroma	9540/0
Plexiform	9550/0
Perineurioma	*9571/0*
Intraneural perineurioma	*9571/0*
Soft tissue perineurioma	*9571/0*
Malignant peripheral nerve sheath tumour (MPNST)	*9540/3*
Epithelioid	*9540/3*
MPNST with divergent mesenchymal and / or epithelial differentiation	*9540/3*
Melanotic	*9540/3*
Melanotic psammomatous	*9540/3*

TUMOURS OF THE MENINGES

Tumours of meningothelial cells	
Meningioma	9530/0
Meningothelial	9531/0
Fibrous (fibroblastic)	9532/0
Transitional (mixed)	9537/0
Psammomatous	9533/0
Angiomatous	9534/0
Microcystic	*9530/0*
Secretory	*9530/0*
Lymphoplasmacyte-rich	*9530/0*
Metaplastic	*9530/0*
Clear cell	*9538/1*
Chordoid	*9538/1*
Atypical	*9539/1*
Papillary	*9538/3*
Rhabdoid	*9538/3*
Anaplastic meningioma	9530/3

Mesenchymal, non-meningothelial tumours	
Lipoma	8850/0
Angiolipoma	8861/0
Hibernoma	8880/0
Liposarcoma (intracranial)	8850/3
Solitary fibrous tumour	*8815/0*
Fibrosarcoma	8810/3
Malignant fibrous histiocytoma	8830/3
Leiomyoma	8890/0
Leiomyosarcoma	8890/3
Rhabdomyoma	8900/0
Rhabdomyosarcoma	8900/3
Chondroma	9220/0
Chondrosarcoma	9220/3
Osteoma	9180/0
Osteosarcoma	9180/3
Osteochondroma	9210/0
Haemangioma	9120/0
Epithelioid haemangioendothelioma	9133/1
Haemangiopericytoma	9150/1
Angiosarcoma	9120/3
Kaposi sarcoma	9140/3

Primary melanocytic lesions	
Diffuse melanocytosis	*8728/0*
Melanocytoma	*8728/1*
Malignant melanoma	8720/3
Meningeal melanomatosis	*8728/3*

Tumours of uncertain histogenesis	
Haemangioblastoma	9161/1

LYMPHOMAS AND HAEMOPOIETIC NEOPLASMS

Malignant lymphomas	9590/3
Plasmacytoma	9731/3
Granulocytic sarcoma	9930/3

GERM CELL TUMOURS

Germinoma	9064/3
Embryonal carcinoma	9070/3
Yolk sac tumour	9071/3
Choriocarcinoma	9100/3
Teratoma	9080/1
Mature	9080/0
Immature	9080/3
Teratoma with malignant transformation	9084/3
Mixed germ cell tumours	9085/3

TUMOURS OF THE SELLAR REGION

Craniopharyngioma	9350/1
Adamantinomatous	*9351/1*
Papillary	*9352/1*
Granular cell tumour	*9582/0*

METASTATIC TUMOURS

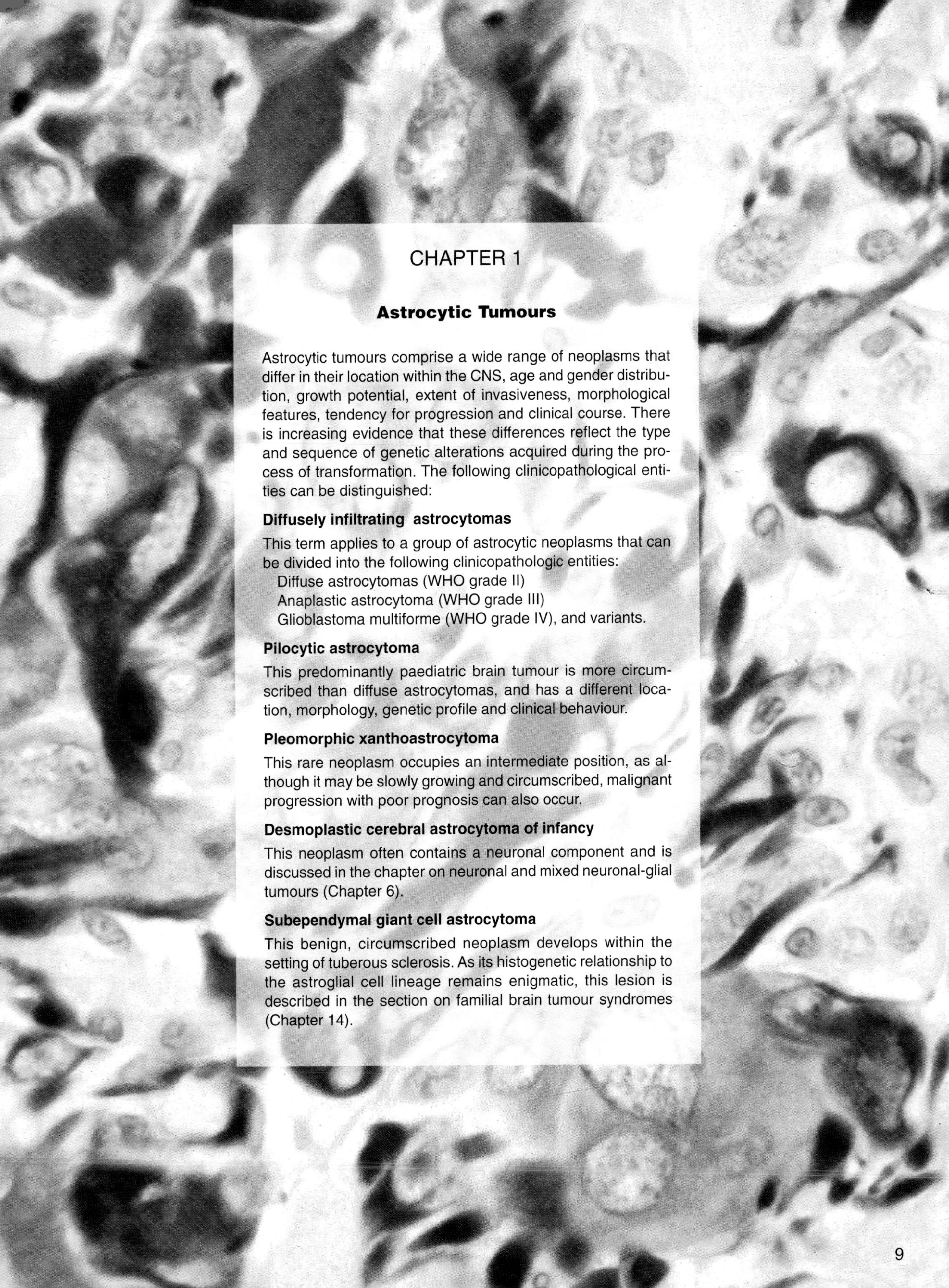

CHAPTER 1

Astrocytic Tumours

Astrocytic tumours comprise a wide range of neoplasms that differ in their location within the CNS, age and gender distribution, growth potential, extent of invasiveness, morphological features, tendency for progression and clinical course. There is increasing evidence that these differences reflect the type and sequence of genetic alterations acquired during the process of transformation. The following clinicopathological entities can be distinguished:

Diffusely infiltrating astrocytomas

This term applies to a group of astrocytic neoplasms that can be divided into the following clinicopathologic entities:

Diffuse astrocytomas (WHO grade II)
Anaplastic astrocytoma (WHO grade III)
Glioblastoma multiforme (WHO grade IV), and variants.

Pilocytic astrocytoma

This predominantly paediatric brain tumour is more circumscribed than diffuse astrocytomas, and has a different location, morphology, genetic profile and clinical behaviour.

Pleomorphic xanthoastrocytoma

This rare neoplasm occupies an intermediate position, as although it may be slowly growing and circumscribed, malignant progression with poor prognosis can also occur.

Desmoplastic cerebral astrocytoma of infancy

This neoplasm often contains a neuronal component and is discussed in the chapter on neuronal and mixed neuronal-glial tumours (Chapter 6).

Subependymal giant cell astrocytoma

This benign, circumscribed neoplasm develops within the setting of tuberous sclerosis. As its histogenetic relationship to the astroglial cell lineage remains enigmatic, this lesion is described in the section on familial brain tumour syndromes (Chapter 14).

Diffusely infiltrating astrocytomas

W.K. Cavenee
F.B. Furnari
M. Nagane
H.-J.S. Huang
E.W. Newcomb
D.D. Bigner
M. Weller
M.E. Berens
K.H. Plate
M.A. Israel
M.D. Noble
P. Kleihues

Definition

Diffusely infiltrating astrocytomas share the following characteristics: (1) they may arise at any site in the CNS, preferentially in the cerebral hemispheres; (2) they usually manifest clinically in adults; (3) they have a wide range of histopathological features and biological behaviour; (4) they show a diffuse infiltration of adjacent and distant brain structures that is largely irrespective of histological grade; (5) they have an inherent tendency for malignant progression, with the glioblastoma as the most malignant phenotypic endpoint.

Synonyms and historical annotation

The term astrocytoma was used as early as the late 19th century by Virchow {1554} but was firmly introduced into histopathological classification in 1926 by Bailey and Cushing {58}. A detailed account of the historical evolution of astrocytoma terminology has been given by Zülch {1684, 1686} and by Russell and Rubinstein {1305, 1306}.

Incidence

Diffusely infiltrating astrocytomas are the most frequent intracranial neoplasms and account for more than 60% of all primary brain tumours. The incidence differs between regions, but is usually in the range of 5–7 new cases per 100'000 population per year.

Grading and patient survival

While neurological symptoms resulting from glioma development depend primarily on the site of tumour within the CNS, the length of the patient's history and chance of a long, recurrence-free survival are more closely associated with the intrinsic biology of the neoplasm. Significant indicators of anaplasia in gliomas include nuclear atypia (*e.g.* coarse nuclear chromatin, nuclear pleomorphism, multinucleation), mitotic activity, cellularity, vascular proliferation, and necrosis. For practical purposes, these histopathological characteristics are condensed into a grading scheme. As a general rule, grading is based on areas showing the highest degree of anaplasia, on the assumption that this tumour cell population eventually determines the course of disease. Historically, grading of astrocytomas according to Kernohan {763} and Ringertz {1260} prevailed, but today the malignancy scale of the WHO classification is more widely accepted {779, 780}. For diffuse astrocytomas, the St Anne/Mayo grading system, based on only four criteria (nuclear atypia, mitosis, microvascular proliferation and/or necrosis) has proved to be both reproducible and predictive of patient survival {304, 772}. A comparison of these two grading schemes is shown in Table 1.1.

Patient survival also depends on a variety of clinical parameters, including: the patient's age {175, 1318, 1434} and condition, as reflected in the Karnofsky performance score {1434}, tumour location and treatment, *e.g.* extent of surgical resection {33, 89, 1062}, radiotherapy {33, 873}, and chemotherapy {881}. Despite these variables, typical ranges of survival are more than 5 years for diffuse astrocytomas WHO grade II, 2–5 years for anaplastic astrocytomas WHO grade III, and less than 1 year for the majority of patients with glioblastoma WHO grade IV {183, 304, 772}.

Aetiology of astrocytic tumors

Analytical epidemiological studies have revealed an increased risk of gliomas in association with a variety of conditions but, with the exception of therapeutic X-irradiation, attempts to unequivocally identify a specific causative exposure or environmental agent have so far been unsuccessful {859}. Children receiving prophylactic irradiation of the CNS for acute lymphocytic leukaemia (ALL) have an increased risk of developing low-grade diffuse and anaplastic astrocytomas, glioblastomas {167, 209, 362, 1319, 1570, 2431} and, less frequently, gliosarcomas {733}. In a retrospective cohort study of 9720 children treated for ALL, there was a 22-fold excess risk of subsequently developing a CNS tumour, the estimated cumulative proportion of affected children being 2.5% {1063}. The risk was even higher in children aged five years or less at the time at which ALL was diagnosed {1063}. After a standard therapeutic dose of 2440 cGy at a mean age of 4.8 years, the interval until manifestation of the brain tumour was 7.6±2.3 years {167}.

Gliomas have also been observed following irradiation of pituitary adenomas {153}, with a 16-fold excess risk {1519}. Similarly, second primary tumours of neuroepithelial origin were observed after irradiation of craniopharyngioma {778}, pineal parenchymal tumours {601}, germinoma {778}, and following brachytherapy of malignant gliomas {1395}. Even low-dose irradiation for the treatment of tinea capitis may subsequently result in the development of gliomas {1435}.

There is accumulating evidence that a significant fraction of human neoplasms in-

Table 1.1
Comparison of the World Health Organization (WHO) and St. Anne/Mayo grading system of astrocytomas.

WHO grade	WHO designation	St. Anne / Mayo Designation	St. Anne / Mayo Histological criteria
I	Pilocytic astrocytoma		
II	Diffuse astrocytoma	Astrocytoma grade 2	One criterion, usually nuclear atypia
III	Anaplastic astrocytoma	Astrocytoma grade 3	Two criteria, usually nuclear atypia and mitotic activity
IV	Glioblastoma multiforme	Astrocytoma grade 4	Three criteria: nuclear atypia, mitoses, endothelial proliferation and/or necrosis

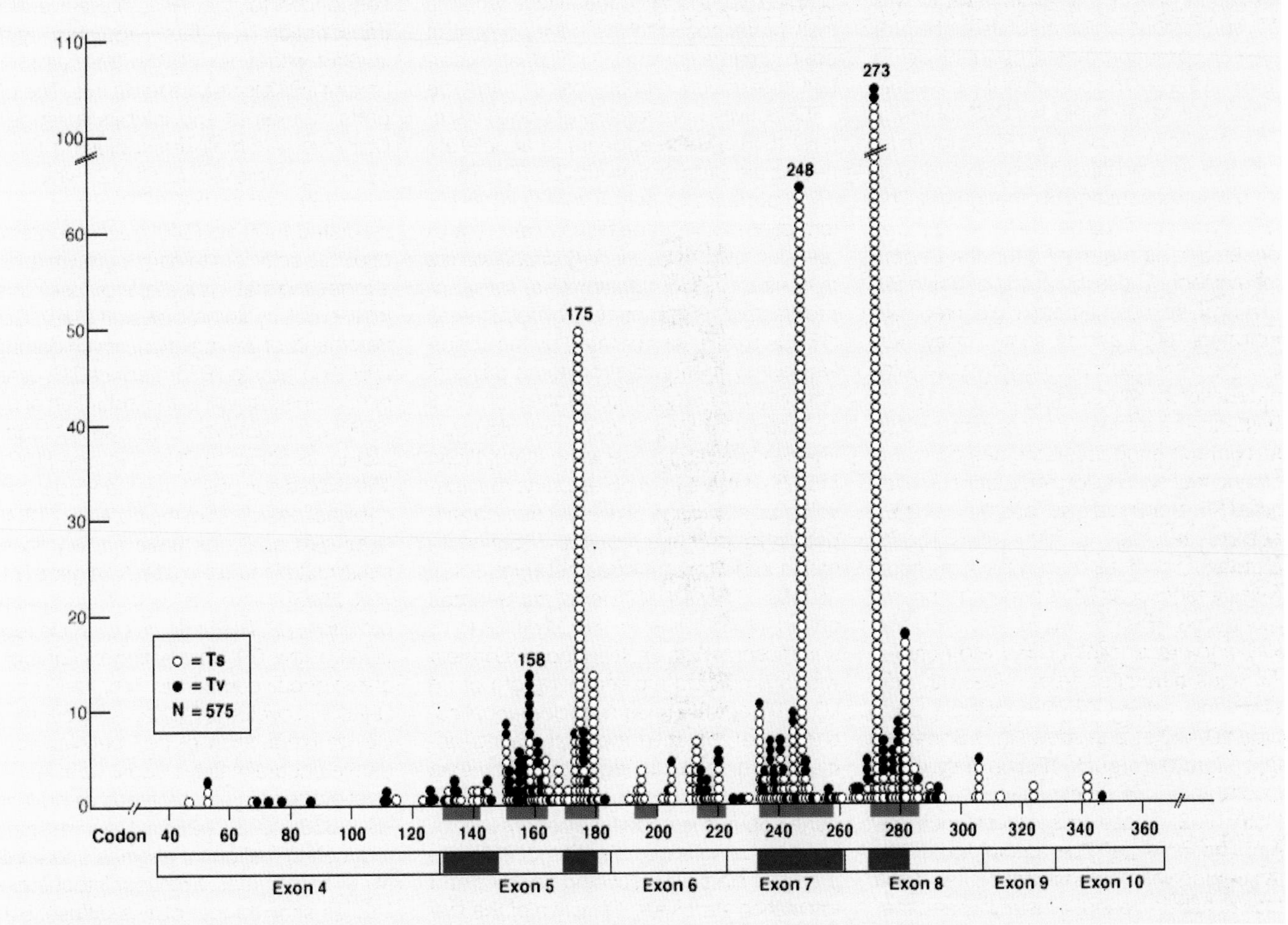

Fig. 1.1 Distribution of mutations within the human *TP53* gene in astrocytomas WHO grades II–IV. Codons 40–360 of a total of 393 codons in exons 4–10 of the *TP53* gene are shown. The vertical columns represent the number of mutations occurring at particular codons. Transition mutations are denoted by open circles, whereas transversion mutations are represented by closed circles. The seven known hotspots for mutation occurring at CpG sites within the *TP53* gene are codons 175, 196, 213, 245, 248, 273 and 282. The open horizontal bar shows exons 4–10 of the *TP53* gene and the blue areas represent regions that are highly conserved. The green boxes below the line representing the *TP53* gene designate the seven recognized hotspot areas for mutations: codons 130–142, 151–164, 171–181, 193–200, 213–223, 234–258 and 276–286. The data represent 575 mutations compiled from the literature.

cluding brain tumours {92} contain DNA sequences identical to SV40 large T antigen {2536}. In astrocytic tumours, this occurs at a frequency of up to 50% {2532, 2231} and appears to be the result of the use of SV40 contaminated polio vaccine during 1955 to 1963. It is currently unclear whether SV40 plays a role in the evolution of certain human cancers. On the basis of available evidence it appears more likely that SV40 constitutes a bystander infection due to an intra-tumoural microenvironment that favours viral replication in humans with latent SV40 infection.

The pattern of *TP53* mutations in human astrocytic tumours is characterized by a high frequency of GC>AT mutations of which more than 50% are located at CpG sites (see Li-Fraumeni syndrome, Chapter 14). This suggest a role of 5-methylcytosine deamination by endogenous processes rather than by exogenous genotoxic carcinogens {2522}.

Genetic susceptibility

Familial clustering of astrocytomas is not uncommon. The association with defined inherited tumour syndromes includes the Li-Fraumeni syndrome, Turcot syndrome, tuberous sclerosis, neurofibromatosis (NF1) and multiple enchondromatosis (Maffucci/Ollier disease) {2469, 2527, 2523} syndrome (see Chapter 14).

Molecular and cytogenetics

The formation of human tumours is a complex process involving the accumulation of genetic lesions in genes that normally regulate the pathways of cell proliferation, differentiation and death required for organ development. As with tumours that occur at other sites, two types of genes have been identified which are the targets for this dysregulation. Dominantly acting oncogenes whose protein products serve to accelerate cell growth are typically altered by increased gene dosage (amplification) or by activating mutations. Tumour suppressor genes whose protein products serve as brakes on cell growth are typically altered by physical elimination or by inactivating mutations.

TheTP53/MDM2/p21 pathway

TP53. The *TP53* gene, located on chromosome 17p13.1, encodes a 53 kDa protein which plays a role in several cellular processes including the cell cycle, response of cells to DNA damage, cell death, cell differentiation, and neovascularization {138}. The gene product has several regions which mediate these processes, perhaps most important being those in the central portion of the molecule which are responsible for DNA binding. This capacity allows the TP53 protein to function as a positive or negative regulator of the transcription of other genes. The regions of the *TP53* gene encoding these protein motifs are most often the targets for mutation. These mutations diminish the ability of the mutant protein to carry out its activities {609} and in some cases can bestow new dominant negative or gain-of-function properties (Fig. 1.1).

Evidence for a causal involvement of *TP53* in glial tumourigenesis comes from the finding that expression of exogenous wild-typeTP53 activity in glioblastoma cell lines suppresses their growth {995, 1537}. Moreover, cortical astrocytes from mice without functional TP53 appear to be immortalized when grown *in vitro* and rapidly acquire a transformed phenotype. Cortical astrocytes from mice with one functional copy of *TP53* resemble wild-type astrocytes and show signs of immortalization and transformation only upon loss of their one functional copy of *TP53* {137, 1652}. Those cells without functional TP53 become markedly aneuploid {1652}, in keeping with the observation that *TP53* loss results in genomic instability and that astrocytomas with mutant *TP53* are often aneuploid {1538}. Interestingly, mice whose *TP53* genes have been removed by homologous recombination do not develop brain tumours. Whether this is due to their early demise from leukemia or lymphoma or suggests that *TP53* mutation is not early enough in progression to be a predisposing factor, remains to be seen.

Loss or mutation of the*TP53* tumour suppressor gene has been detected in many types of glioma and represents an early genetic event in a subset of astrocytomas {437, 1417, 1535, 1559}. Allelic loss of chromosome 17p and *TP53* mutations are observed in approximately one-third of all three grades of adult astrocytomas, suggesting that inactivation of *TP53* is important in the formation of the grade II tumours. Moreover, high-grade astrocytomas with homogeneous *TP53* mutations can evolve clonally from subpopulations of similarly mutated cells present in tumours that are initially low grade {1417}. This implication is further supported by patients with the Li-Fraumeni syndrome, which is caused by germline transmission of some types of *TP53* mutations, who are then predisposed to the development of brain tumours early in life {950}. An important consequence of the loss of wild-type TP53 activity is increased genomic instability {546}, which appears to accelerate neoplastic progression {853, 950}. Thus, *TP53* appears to play a role both in the formation of low-grade disease and in progression towards secondary glioblastoma. In contrast, *TP53* mutations are rare (approximately 10%) in primary glioblastomas {1586}. This is corroborated by the observation that younger astrocytoma patients not only had higher incidences of *TP53* mutation/17p loss {1233}, but also survived longer than those without mutations {1567}. Therefore, glioblastomas may develop by either one of at least two distinct pathways: one that requires *TP53* inactivation and one that does not (Fig. 1.33).

MDM2. The *MDM2* gene (sometimes called *HDM2*) lies in the 12q14.3–q15 chromosomal region. It encodes a protein with a predicted molecular weight of 54 kDa. This protein has a nuclear-localization signal, putative metal-chelating domains and an acidic region, all hallmarks of a transcription factor {1025}. The *MDM2* gene appears to code for at least five proteins by using a combination of different promoter start sites, splicing patterns and translation start sites. Only two of the five forms can interact with TP53 {527, 1104}. The MDM2 protein binds to mutant and wild-type TP53 proteins, thereby inhibiting the ability of wild-type TP53 to activate transcription from minimal promoter sequences {1025, 1102}. Conversely, the transcription of the *MDM2* gene is induced by wild-type TP53 {64, 1672}. In normal cells, this autoregulatory feedback loop regulates both the activity of the TP53 protein and the expression of MDM2 {1171}. In addition, MDM2 promotes the degradation of TP53 {554, 827}. Therefore, amplification or overexpression of *MDM2* is an alternative mechanism for escaping TP53-regulated control of cell growth. Amplification is observed in about 10% of those glioblastomas without *TP53* mutations {1239}, *i.e.* the primary glioblastoma {113}. Overexpression of MDM2 was observed immunohistochemically in more than 50% of primary glioblastomas, but the fraction of immunoreactive cells varied considerably {113}.

p21 (WAF1/CIP1). The *CDKN1A* gene on chromosome 6p encodes a protein of 21 kDa. Its promoter contains recognition sequences for the TP53 protein and its transcription is, in fact, regulated by the level of wild-type TP53 in the cell {369}; mutant TP53 is unable to do this. The p21 protein binds to and inhibits a range of CDK/cyclin complexes, including the G_1 cyclins complexed to CDK2, which are most relevant to the G_1/S-phase arrest mediated by TP53 {540}. Overexpression of p21 is sufficient to cause growth arrest, suggesting that it is a major player in controlling cell cycle progression {540}. Drug treatments or X-irradiation, which damage DNA and lead to TP53-mediated G_1-arrest or apoptosis, result in the induction of p21 {368}; cells that lack TP53 can not induce p21 in response to DNA damage {1001}. The expression of p21 is enhanced in most gliomas regardless of their grade {718} but extensive analyses have shown no somatic mutations in the *CDKN1A* gene {718, 797, 2525}.

p27/kip1. p27/kip1 affects cell cycle regulation at the G1-S transition by inhibition of cyclin-cdk complexes, including cyclin D-CDK4, cyclin E-CDK2, and cyclin A-CDK2. Modulation of p27 cellular abundance occurs mainly at post-translational level by the ubiquitin-proteasome proteolysis {2535, 2533}. p27/kip1 expression is reduced in malignant gliomas and a variety of carcinomas. Immunohistochemical studies showed that p27 is diffusely and strongly expressed in astrocytomas WHO grade II (mean LI, 44%), but much less in anaplastic astrocytomas (LI, 6%) and glioblastomas (LI, 2%). Loss of p27 expression is independent from histological features {2534}.

The p16/p15/CDK4/CDK6/RB pathway

p16/p15. The transition from low-grade to anaplastic astrocytoma is accompanied by allelic losses on chromosomes 9p, 13q and, less frequently, by 12q amplification. As discussed in several reviews {440, 916, 1566}, these abnormalities now appear to converge on one critical cell cycle regulatory complex {1692}.

The genes encoding p16 and p15 – *CDKN2A* and *CDKN2B*, respectively – map to chromosome 9p21, a site that is significantly associated with interstitial and homozygous deletions in high-grade astrocytomas and in two-thirds of glioma cell lines {676, 1103}. The protein products of these genes act as inhibitors of cyclin dependent kinases (CDK, especially CDK4 and CDK6) and of their ability to phosphorylate the RB protein in conjunction with

cyclin D {1388}. This activity is essential for the G_1/S-phase transition of the cell cycle and removal of p16 and p15 activities can allow uncontrolled proliferation.
There is now direct experimental evidence that *CDKN2A* and/or *CDKN2B* represent the tumour suppressor gene(s) targeted by these structural abnormalities. For example, transfection and expression of the *CDKN2A* in glioblastoma cell lines that lack the gene results in growth suppression, while it has no effect in similar non-mutated glioblastoma cells {39}. Although mutational analyses of these genes have shown few mutations involving 9p allelic loss in primary astrocytomas {1525}, some of these ablate the growth-suppressing effects and biochemical properties of p16 {39, 1365}. Moreover, mice in which the *CDKN2A* genes are disrupted by homologous recombination develop spontaneous tumours, although not gliomas, at an early age and are especially sensitive to carcinogens {1389}. While genetic analyses of primary tumour tissues have shown high frequencies of homozygous deletion {696, 1080, 1366}, there are several mechanisms other than mutation/deletion by which p15/p16 function can be overcome. A proportion of malignant gliomas with intact *CDKN2A* genes do not express the protein {1080}, and it has been shown that hypermethylation of the CpG island in the 5' region of the gene causes structural changes of the chromatin, thereby silencing gene transcription {281}. This alternative mechanism for inactivation has also been shown for the *CDKN2B* gene in gliomas {575}.

CDK4 and CDK6. The gene encoding the 33 kDa CDK4 protein maps to chromosome 12q13–14, while that encoding the 38 kDa CDK6 protein maps to chromosome 7q21–22. Both are proteins with catalytic kinase activities, both can form complexes with members of the cyclin D family, and both are inhibited by p16 and p15. Thus overexpression of either CDK might be expected to mimic mutation of the p16/p15 inhibitors and to override their function.
The *CDK4* gene is amplified in nearly 15% of high-grade gliomas {1080, 1241}, particularly in those without *CDKN2A/CDKN2B* alterations. Additionally, a few tumours without *CDKN2A/CDKN2B* mutations or *CDK4* amplification have been shown to have *CDK6* amplification, suggesting that the two proteins can functionally compensate for each other {282}.

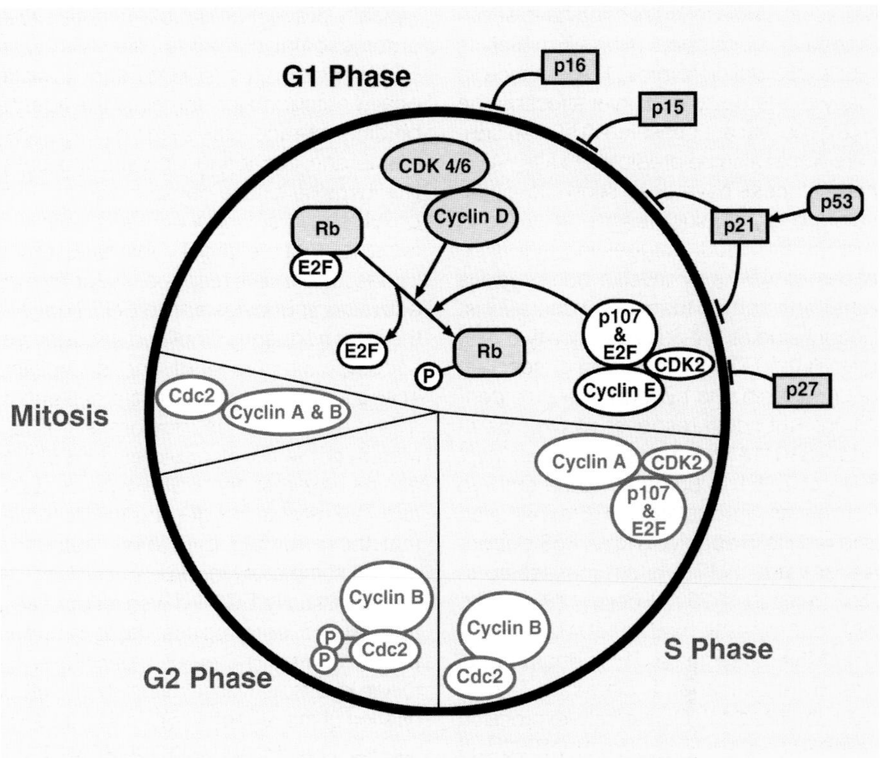

Fig. 1.2 The G1 phase of the cell cycle as a concerted target for the mutations in glioma. The proteins required for orderly traverse of the mitotic cycle are shown within the portion where they exert their effects. Those in circles are checkpoint accelerators or regulators while those in squares are inhibitors. Those which are shaded have been shown to have altered expression or to be mutated in gliomas. Figure modified from Hunter and Pines {1692}.

RB. The ultimate target of the kinase activities of the CDK4/CDK6-cyclin D complexes is the 107 kDa retinoblastoma (RB) protein. Phosphorylation of RB allows the release of the E2F transcription factor it complexes with and this in turn activates genes necessary for cell proliferation {1388}. The *RB1* gene maps to chromosome 13q14, a site which is altered in about one-third of high-grade astrocytic tumours {572, 674}.
As mutations in the *RB1* gene can have the same functional consequences as *CDK4/CDK6* amplification or *CDKN2A/CDKN2B* mutation, and as in astrocytic tumours these events are almost exclusive of one another, it appears that a considerable proportion of anaplastic astrocytomas and nearly all glioblastomas have alterations in one or another component of the pathway {644, 1525, 1693} (Fig. 1.2).
Since the *p16/CDK4/RB/E2F* pathway is disrupted at a high frequency in astrocytic tumours, it may constitute a candidate target for gene therapy strategies. Adenovirus-mediated *p16* gene transfer to *p16*-null glioma cells has been shown to cause growth arrest at the G1 phase of the cell cycle and to suppress invasive activity *in vitro* {1785}. While p16 expression did not induce apoptosis, it resulted in resistance to a variety of cytocidal drugs {1790, 1792}. In contrast, adenovirus-mediated transfer of exogenous E2F-1 induced generalized apoptosis in glioma cells independent of their TP53, p16 or RB status {1789, 1791}, suggesting that gene therapy using specific components of this pathway may allow modulation of chemotherapeutic responses.

$p14^{ARF}$. The human and murine *CDKN2A* loci also contain an alternative reading frame encoding the unrelated proteins, human $p14^{ARF}$ {1787, 1800, 1811} and murine $p19^{ARF}$ {1809}. Ectopic expression of ARF protein suppresses growth of human glioma cells through an RB-independent pathway {1784} and can induce both G_1- and G_2-phase arrest in a variety of cell types {1809, 1812}, which is TP53-dependent {1797} but independent of p16. *ARF*-null mice expressing functional p16 develop tumours early in life, a phenotype similar to that of *CDKN2A/ARF*-disruption {1797, 1389}, thus providing evidence that *ARF* functions as a tumour suppressor.

Moreover, *ARF*-deficient mice have spontaneously developed gliomas, which is rare in *p53*-deficient mice {1795}. Although many of the point mutations affecting the *p16* gene that are observed in human cancers would also be predicted to alter *ARF*, none of these have been shown to inactivate the growth suppressive activities of ARF {1784, 1808}, suggesting that alterations of *ARF* may involve homozygous deletions rather than point mutations. Recent studies provide evidence that ARF modulates TP53 function as a checkpoint of oncogenic and hyperproliferative conditions but not in response to DNA damage {1810, 1812}. Overexpression of Myc, E1A, or E2F1 in primary mouse embryo fibroblasts upregulates ARF expression and results in apoptosis in a TP53-dependent manner, which is not manifested in *ARF*-null and *TP53*-null cells {1786,1815}. ARF can directly bind to MDM2, and inhibit MDM2-mediated TP53 degradation and transactivational silencing {1796, 1806, 1812,1814}. Conversely, expression of ARF is negatively regulated by TP53 and inversely correlates with TP53 function in human tumour cell lines {1812}. Thus the two distinct tumour suppressors, p16 and ARF, encoded by the single genetic *CDKN2A/ARF* locus, regulate the RB and TP53 pathways, respectively, both of which are essential components of cell cycle and apoptosis control.

Epidermal growth factor receptor

The majority of gene amplification events in high-grade astrocytomas involve the gene for the receptor tyrosine kinase, epidermal growth factor receptor (EGFR) {119, 896, 1636}. EGFR is a transmembrane receptor responsible for sensing its extracellular ligands, EGF and transforming growth factor alpha (TGF-α), and for transducing this signal to the cell. EGFR has been associated with cancer for three main reasons: (1) it is the cellular homologue of the *v-erbB* oncogene found in the acutely transforming avian erythroblastosis virus {1529}; (2) when expressed ectopically in cells, it can set up a transforming autocrine loop, so that cellular transformation is ligand-dependent {333}; and (3) it has been shown to be amplified in several tumour types, with an increased copy number that is directly correlated to an increase in the number of receptors on the cell surface.

While the gene encoding EGFR maps to chromosome 7, the amplified genes are typically present as double-minute extrachromosomal elements. The wild-type EGFR protein is 170 kDa, and is composed of four major domains: the ligand-binding extracellular domain; the transmembrane anchoring domain; the catalytic tyrosine kinase domain; and the carboxyl terminus, which contains both five tyrosines that are target substrates for the kinase, and motifs responsible for ligand-activated endocytosis. The *EGFR* gene is the most frequently amplified oncogene in astrocytic tumours {436}, and is amplified in about one third of glioblastomas and in a few anaplastic astrocytomas {1636}. Moreover, there is also evidence {366} that gliomas express the EGFR ligands, EGF and TGF-α thus suggesting the potential that these tumour cells have autocrine growth stimulatory loops.

Mechanistically, EGFR-driven mitogenesis appears to encompass: ligand-driven dimerization of receptor monomers; tyrosine kinase activation; tyrosine phosphorylation of the receptor; signalling through various coupling and adaptor proteins, like Shc and Grb2, to signal transduction pathways driven by either phospholipase-C-gamma, Ras-MAPK or STAT; and finally, receptor-ligand internalization and lysosomal breakdown leading to signal attenuation {1659}.

In about half of glioblastoma cases with receptor amplification, the event is coupled with gene rearrangement. The most common rearrangement results in a variant form called EGFRvIII, delta EGFR, or de2-7EGFR (herein referred to as mutant EGFR). This mutant lacks a portion of the extracellular ligand-binding domain as the result of genomic deletions that precisely eliminate exons 2–7 in the EGFR mRNA {636, 1467, 1637}. The introduction of this mutant truncated receptor into brain tumour cells dramatically enhances their tumorigenicity *in vivo* {1694}. These mutant receptors are expressed on the cell surface {1694, 1813} and are constitutively autophosphorylated, but at a significantly lower level than is wild-type EGFR activated by ligand exposure {366, 1694}. Unlike wild-type EGFR, the constitutively active mutants are not downregulated, suggesting that their altered conformation does not result in exposure of receptor sequence motifs required for endocytosis, lysosomal degradation and signal attenuation. Consequently, mutant receptors are only internalized at the same low rate as unoccupied wild-type EGFR {631}. Mutational analysis showed that the enhanced tumorigenicity conferred by mutant EGFR was strictly dependent on the intrinsic tyrosine kinase activity and was mediated through the carboxyl terminus, in a similar way to wild-type EGFR function. However, in contrast to wild-type receptors, mutation of any single major tyrosine autophosphorylation site abolished its enhanced tumorigenicity. Moreover, recent evidence strongly suggests that the mutant receptors are incapable of forming dimers {249}.

Mutant EGFR constitutively transduces its signals through the Shc-Grb2-Ras pathway in glioma cells {1807}, or through the PI-3 kinase and JNK pathways in NIH3T3 cells {1783, 1801}, and bestows enhanced tumorigenicity through both increased cellular proliferation and reduced apoptosis {1804}. Overexpression of mutant EGFR in glioma cells also confers resistance to chemotherapeutic drugs such as cisplatin through modulation of Bcl-X_L expression and consequent inhibition of induction of apoptosis by the drug treatment {1803}. In addition, EGFR autocrine signalling induces cell scattering and migration in glioma cells *in vitro* {1788}, and glioma cells expressing mutant EGFR show greater invasiveness when implanted in the mouse brain than control cells {1816}.

Several approaches to using this mutant receptor as a therapeutic target are underway. Selective tyrosine kinase inhibitors have been utilized in an attempt to reverse the mutant EGFR-mediated inhibition of apoptosis. One such inhibitor, the tyrophostin AG1478, effectively inhibits autophosphorylation of mutant EGFR {1793}, downregulates Bcl-X_L expression, and synergistically enhances the cytocidal effect of cisplatin in glioblastoma cells expressing mutant EGFR {1803}. A truncated kinase-deficient mutant derived from the ectodomain of erbB2 forms heterodimers with wild-type and the mutant EGFR, inhibits their kinase activity and growth promoting abilities and thereby may serve as a dominant negative receptor {1805}. Monoclonal antibodies to the truncation epitope of mutant EGFR have been produced for potential use for immunotoxin delivery through antibody-mediated internalization of the mutant receptor {1813}. Alternatively, vaccination using the peptide encompassing the fusion junction of mutant EGFR elicits antitumour activity against murine tumour

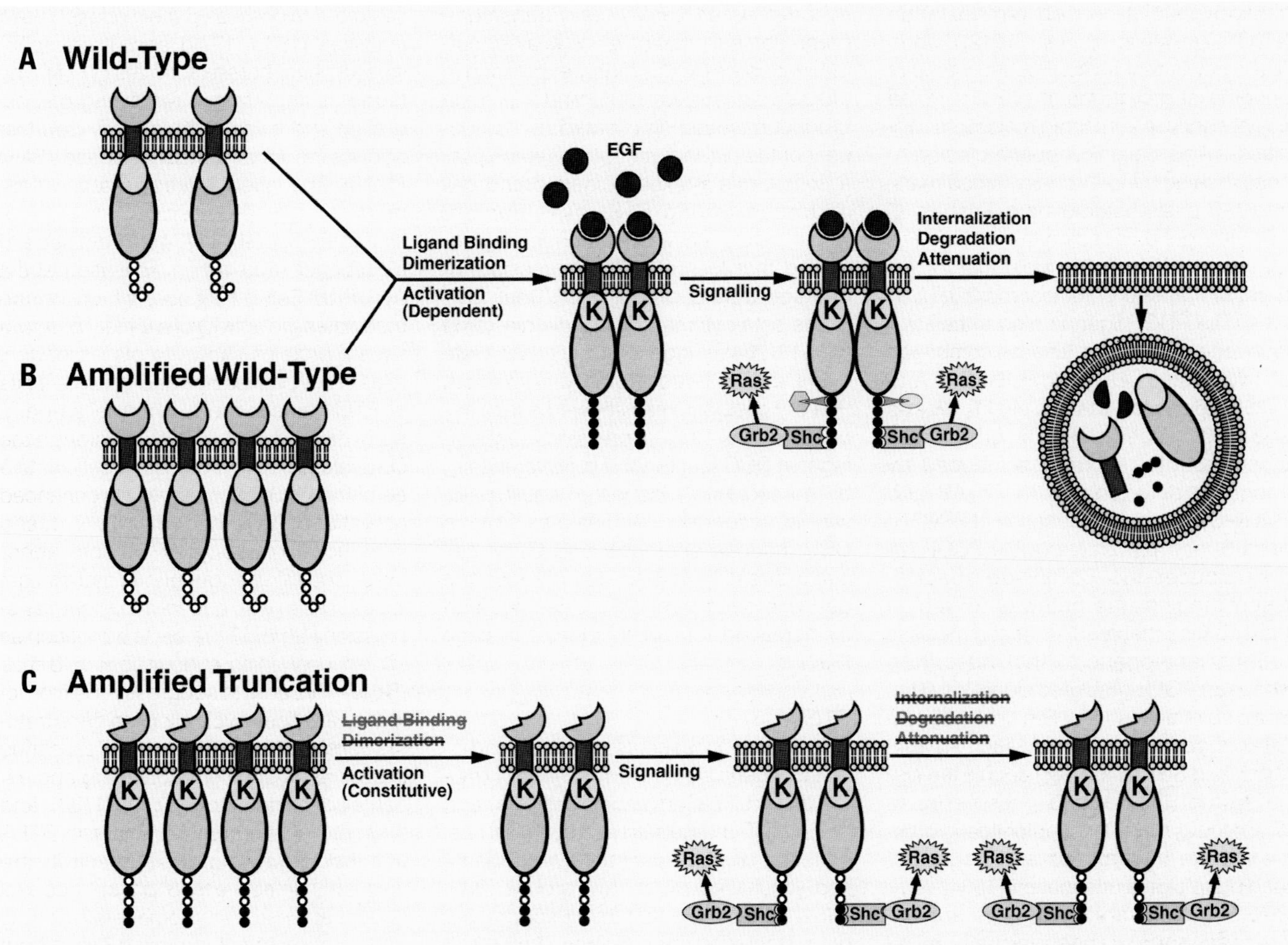

Fig. 1.3 A Wild-type EGF receptors dimerize upon ligand (filled balls) exposure and their kinase activities (capital K) are activated causing carboxylterminal tyrosine residues (small open circles) to become phosphorylated (small filled circles). This modification allows interaction with adaptor molecules like Shc or Grb2 to couple the receptor to various signalling pathways, most notably that involving Ras activation. These interactions expose motifs instructing endocytic internalization, receptor-ligand degradation and signal attenuation. **B** In some gliomas, the number of genes for the wild-type receptor is increased by gene amplification. This leads to an increased number of receptors on the cell surface and increased signalling with the same general characteristics as the pathway described in (**A**). **C** In a sizable proportion of high grade gliomas, gene amplification is accompanied by specific deletion of a proportion of the extracellular domain. These receptors are constitutively active, do not dimerize, chronically signal through coupling molecules similar to those in (**A**) and (**B**) but do not internalize or attenuate their signal.

cells expressing mutant EGFR {1802}. Amplification and overexpression of the *EGFR* gene occurs in approximately one-third of glioblastoma cases {366, 367, 635, 638, 855, 1098, 1233, 1549, 1564, 1636}. Recent studies have shown that this constitutes a hallmark of primary glioblastomas (see Fig. 1.33), more than 60% of which show upregulated *EGFR* expression {1586}. This is in contrast to *TP53* mutations, which are common in secondary glioblastomas that evolved through progression from diffuse astrocytomas or anaplastic astrocytomas {1799, 1245}; thus *TP53* inactivation and *EGFR* amplification are mutually exclusive lesions {1586}. All glioblastomas with *EGFR* amplification show simultaneous loss of chromosome 10 {1564}. However, *EGFR* amplification occurs at similar frequencies among glioblastomas with or without homozygous deletions or mutations of the *PTEN/MMAC1* gene, which is located on chromosome 10q23 {1798}, although about 20% of primary glioblastomas show both *EGFR* amplification and *PTEN* mutations {1754}. In contrast, *EGFR* amplification is typically associated with *CDKN2A* deletions {558, 2443}. A recent study using transgenic and knockout mice provides evidence that supports the importance of these genetic alterations for the development of glioblastoma {1794}. Brain specific expression of a doubly mutant form of EGFR that also lacks the C-terminal regulatory domain induces glioma-like lesions in the mouse brain at high frequencies when the genes involved in the RB pathway, *CDK4* or *CDKN2A*, are also mutated. In this model, *TP53* disruption does not cooperate with the *EGFR* mutation to generate tumours. These results suggest that cells with *EGFR* alterations may require additional alterations associated with cell cycle deregulation through disruption of the RB pathway for tumour formation, and that *EGFR* alterations and *TP53* inactivation may represent distinct molecular pathways leading to gliomagenesis.

Platelet-derived growth factor and its receptors

Many growth factors and their receptors are overexpressed in astrocytomas, including platelet-derived growth factor (PDGF) (reviewed in Ref. {1612}), fibroblast growth factors (FGFs) and vascular endothelial growth factor (VEGF). PDGF activity derives from three molecules: disulfide-linked, cationic, heparin-binding A-chain homodimers; B-chain homodimers; and A-B-chain heterodimers. Each is 30 kDa. The gene encoding the A-chain lies on chromosome 7p22, while that for the B-chain maps to chromosome 22q12.3–13.1. The PDGF ligands bind to cell-surface receptor tyrosine kinases composed of two protein entities, PDGFR-α and PDGFR-β, which map to 4q11–12 and 5q33–35, respectively. Dimerization of these receptor subunits is induced by ligand binding, so that PDGF-AB and PDGF-BB cause the formation of PDGFR-αα, αβ, and ββ dimers, while PDGF-AA only induces the PDGFR-αα species. Upon binding, the pathway for signal transduction that leads to mitogenesis is roughly analogous to that described above for EGFR-mediated signalling. That is, receptor phosphorylation allows attachment of adaptor molecules such as Shc, Grb2, and Sos, which then couple the signal to the Ras-Raf and phospholipase C-γ pathways before receptor-ligand complexes are internalized and degraded leading to signal attenuation {1364}.

PDGF ligands and receptors are expressed approximately equally in all grades of astrocytoma, suggesting that such overexpression is also important in the initial stages of astrocytoma formation. Tumours often overexpress both PDGF ligands and receptors suggesting the establishment of autocrine stimulatory loops {576}. While rare astrocytomas have amplification of the PDGF-α receptor gene, in most cases, the actual transcriptional mechanisms of PDGF overexpression have not been elucidated.

Loss of chromosome 17p in the region of the *TP53* gene is closely correlated with PDGF-α receptor overexpression. This may imply that *TP53* mutations have an oncogenic effect mainly in the presence of overexpression of PDGF-α receptor. This potential interdependence is supported by observations that mouse astrocytes without functional TP53 become transformed only in the presence of specific growth factors {137}.

Deleted in colorectal cancer (DCC) expression

The *DCC* gene on chromosome 18q21 encodes a 1447 amino-acid transmembrane domain protein, which is a cell surface receptor. DCC is highly expressed in the nervous system {395} and the gene product has been implicated as component of the netrin-1 receptor. Netrins play a critical role in axon guidance and cell migration during CNS development {2454}. DCC immunohistochemistry revealed that loss of DCC expression increases during progression from low-grade astrocytoma (7%) to glioblastoma (47%) {1254}, suggesting that this is a late event during astrocytoma progression. Primary glioblastomas showed a less frequent loss of DCC expression, suggesting that DCC inactivation is preferentially, but not exclusively, lost in the genetic pathway to secondary glioblastoma {1254}. DCC induces apoptosis and G2/M cell cycle arrest in tumour cells {2526} but germline deletion of *DCC* does not lead to increased tumour incidence in mice {394}.

PTEN

The *PTEN* (*p*hosphatase and *ten*sin homology) gene also known as *MMAC1* (*mu*tated in *m*ultiple *a*dvanced *c*ancers) and *TEP-1* (*T*GF-β-regulated and *e*pithelial cell-enriched *p*hosphatase) {893}, was identified simultaneously by two groups {893, 1451} as a candidate tumour suppressor gene located at chromosome 10q23.3. It is mutated in 30-44% of high-grade gliomas {1780}, particularly primary glioblastoma {1754} and a variety of extraneural neoplasms, including prostate, endometrial, renal and small cell carcinoma, melanoma, and meningioma {1772, 1451}. Germline *PTEN* mutations have been detected in the autosomal dominant cancer predisposition disorders, Cowden disease, Bannayan-Zonana syndrome and juvenile polyposis syndrome {1769, 895}. These syndromes are notable for harmatomas, benign tumours consisting of normal differentiated cells within highly disorganised tissue architectures (see Chapter 14).

The protein product of the *PTEN* gene contains a central domain with perfect homology to the catalytic region of protein tyrosine phosphatases, and an amino terminal domain with extensive homology to tensin and auxilin, which are cytoplasmic proteins involved in interactions with actin filaments at focal adhesions, and uncoating of clathrin-coated vesicles, respectively. As such, PTEN has been demonstrated to possess protein phosphatase activities {1830, 1778} and 3' phosphoinositol phosphatase activities {1774}. The former is important in regulating cell migration and invasion by directly dephosphorylating focal adhesion kinase (FAK) {1778}. The latter is directed against the product of phosphoinositide 3-kinase (PI3-K), PtdIns-3,4,5-P_3 {1774}, a lipid second messenger required for activation of the AKT/PKB Ser/Thr kinase, which in turn modulates the activity of a variety of downstream proteins shown to play important roles in cell proliferation and survival. Loss of PTEN function in tumour cells and in cells derived from *PTEN* deficient mice correlates with an increase in cellular levels of PtdIns-3,4,5-P_3 leading to enhanced activation of AKT/PKB {1776, 1777, 1782}. Introduction of wild-type *PTEN* into glioma cells containing endogenous mutant alleles causes *in vitro* and *in vivo* growth suppression {1768, 1771}, but is without effect in cells containing endogenous wild-type PTEN. This growth suppression is mediated by a G_1 cell cycle block in glioblastoma cells {1770, 1772}, however sensitivity to anoikis, detachment induced apoptosis, can also be detected {1770, 1776}. Furthermore, although some mutants of PTEN that lack growth-suppressive activity are invariably defective for 3' phosphoinositol phosphatase activity, some retain activity against protein substrates {1770, 1776}, indicating that the lipid phosphatase activity of PTEN is essential for glioma growth control.

Chromosome 10. Loss of one copy of chromosome 10 is a frequent event in glioblastomas, occurring in the great majority, while being rare in lower grades of astrocytic tumours {122, 674}. While PTEN appears to be a bona fide tumour suppressor involved in glioma progression, there is a discrepancy between LOH for the chromosomal region containing *PTEN* (75-95% of glioblastomas) and the mutation frequency of the gene (30-44%) {1779}. It remains to be determined whether other genes on 10q such as *DMBT1* {1775} and *MXI1* {1781} are also involved in gliomagenesis {2484}.

Chromosome 19q. Allelic losses of chromosome 19q occur in 40% of high-grade astrocytic tumours {1558}. While a tumour suppressor gene seems likely to be involved, its identity remains to be identified. Deletion mapping has narrowed the candidate region to the 19q13.3 region between the *D19S*412 and *STD* loci {1283}.

Chromosome 22. Loss of heterozygosity (LOH) of chromosome 22q occurs in 20–30% of gliomas of all grades {438, 674}, suggesting the presence of a tumour suppressor gene that plays a role in the early stages of gliomagenesis. The neurofibromatosis 2 (*NF2*) gene has been mapped to this region, but sequence analysis of *NF2* in astrocytomas of various grades did not reveal any mutations {1297}. Moreover, other cytogenetic and LOH studies have pinpointed 22q loss to regions telomeric to *NF2* {1228}. Thus, this potentially interesting gene remains undefined.

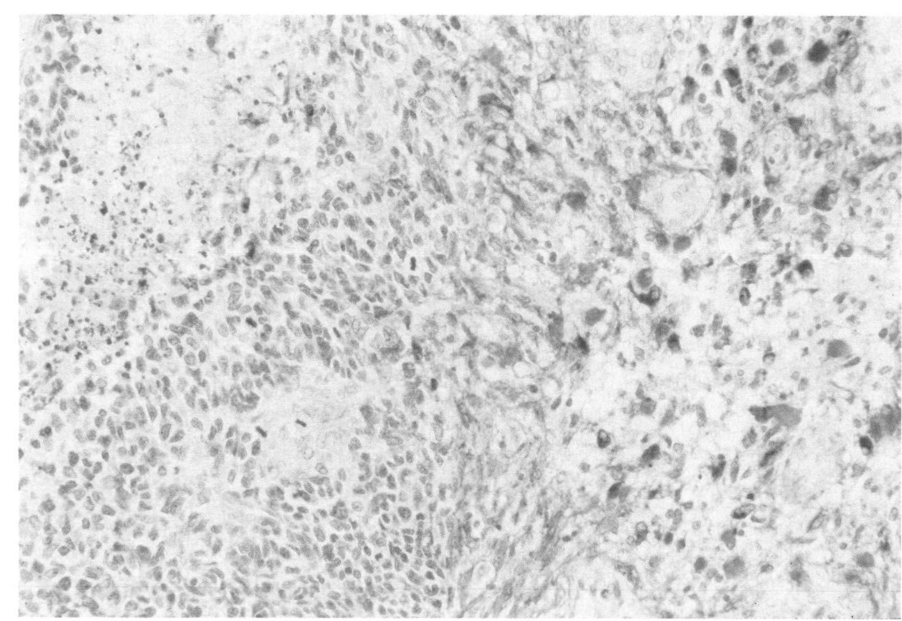

Fig. 1.4 Emergence in a glioblastoma of a well delineated focus of highly anaplastic tumour cells lacking GFAP immunoreactivity, suggesting a new clone with additional genetic alteration(s).

Astrocytoma progression

When patients with diffuse astrocytoma WHO grade II develop a recurrent lesion, the second surgical biopsy often shows histopathological evidence of increased nuclear atypia, hyperchromasia, mitotic activity (anaplastic astrocytoma) and, eventually, microvascular proliferation and/or necrosis, *i.e.* features of the glioblastoma. The acquisition of anaplastic features, though an inherent property of diffusely infiltrating astrocytomas, is largely unpredictable clinically and histopathologically, in particular, as regards the time over which these changes take place. While some astrocytomas show no change in histological grade over more than 10 years following the first operation, others show a rapid transition to malignancy within 1–2 years, the mean interval being 4-5 years {1585, 2449, 2450}. Progression from anaplastic astrocytoma to glioblastoma is more rapid, within approximately 2 years {1585}.

Histopathology

Anaplastic changes are usually diffuse, although it is often possible to distinguish within a surgical biopsy areas with low- and high-grade features. Occasionally, the change in histology is abrupt {1367}. A sharply delineated, often round, focus of anaplastic tumour cells appears, with a high mitotic rate and lack of GFAP expression. In glioblastomas, this may be associated with the acquisition of incipient adenoid features (Fig. 1.4). It is assumed that these foci reflect new clones of neoplastic astrocytes with an additional genetic alteration, e.g. LOH on chromosome 10q {2456}.

Associated genetic alterations

There is increasing evidence that the progression from low-grade to anaplastic astrocytoma and glioblastoma is associated with a cumulative acquisition of multiple genetic alterations {74, 266, 674, 916, 1072, 232, 1098, 1519, 1417}. The sequence of genetic alterations from diffuse astrocytoma WHO grade II to anaplastic astrocytoma and glioblastoma is shown in Fig. 1.33. In diffuse astrocytomas WHO grade II, *TP53* mutations {1585, 1586} and overexpression of PDGFR {254, 566} are the prevailing alterations. Anaplastic astrocytomas may, in addition, show LOH on chromosome 19q, while progression to glioblastoma is typically associated with LOH on chromosome10q and, less frequently, with *PDGFRA* amplification {577}.

Mechanisms of astrocytoma invasion

The wide dissemination of malignant astrocytomas in the brain typically follows anatomical structures of white matter tracts, but cells may also disperse within the cerebrospinal fluid, as well as egress along vascular conduits, or beneath the subdural sheets {1821}. The latter two trajectories include stromal cells that elaborate a basement membrane containing the extracellular matrix (ECM) proteins laminin, collagen type IV, fibronectin, and vitronectin. The route along myelinated fibers is generally considered to be a structure refractory to normal cell permeation, but uniquely vulnerable to, and exploited for, astrocytoma invasion. Evidence supporting the elaboration of a migration-enhancing ECM substrate for invasion by the astrocytoma cells is accumulating {1822}, as is the secretion of proteolytic enzymes by which the environment is rendered permissive for astrocytoma invasion {1817}. Astrocytoma cell locomotion utilizing ligands in the matrix is associated with changes in a variety of receptors, including the ECM and homotypic cell receptors: integrins and DCC; the hyaluronate receptors: CD44, RHAMM, and BEHAB; and the developmentally associated matrix protein, SPARC. Soluble factors evoke both proliferative and migratory responses from astrocytoma cells {1823}. Production of PDGF-AA, PDGF-BB, PDGFRα, PDGFRβ, TGFα, EGFR, and bFGF has been demonstrated in astrocytoma biopsy specimens {1825}. The full extent of the interplay between these different matrix and growth factor receptors, and the aberrations in expression or mutated gene sequences which facilitate astrocytoma invasion, is being recognized as a composite, dynamic consequence of diminished cell-cell adhesion, proteolytic remodelling or synthesis of the ECM, and selective expression and activation of integrins {2419}. At the leading invasive edge where astrocytoma cells penetrate brain parenchyma, tenascin (a migration activating matrix protein) is deposited {1818}, although other matrix proteins may serve similar purposes. Astrocytoma cells modulate their migratory behaviour on ECM proteins depending on the ligand density and the varied expression of different integrins

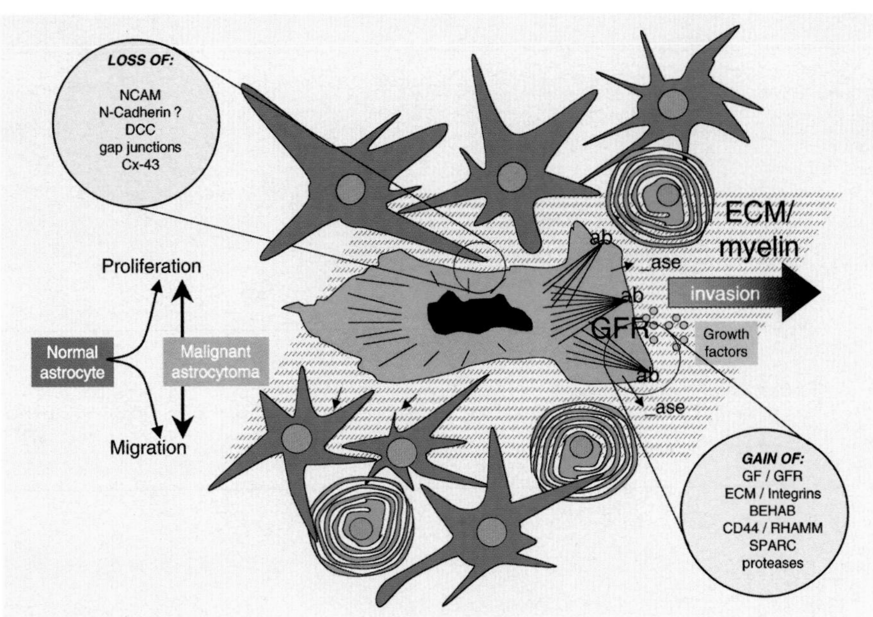

Fig. 1.5 Schematic drawing of cellular and molecular mechanisms oprative in glioma invasion. Modified, from M.E. Berens and A. Giese {2419}.

{1819}. When the migratory phenotype of astrocytoma cells is engaged by permissive substrate, the proliferation rate decreases substantially {1820}, which may have consequences on the geographical and biological vulnerability of these cells to therapy. Such invasive astrocytoma cells reside outside the contrast-enhancing rim of the tumour, thereby escaping surgical resection and evading focused external beam radiation; the diminished proliferation or modulated cell adhesion may also render the cells less responsive to cytotoxic insult {1824}.

Mechanisms of Angiogenesis

Glioma development and progression are accompanied by the formation of a blood vessel system. While the vasculature of low-grade gliomas closely resembles that of normal brain, malignant gliomas show prominent microvascular (*e.g.* smooth muscle/pericyte and endothelial cell) proliferation and often contain areas with a much higher vascular density than low-grade gliomas and normal brain {1183, 1343}. Indeed, glioblastomas are among the best-vascularized tumours in humans. In addition to necrosis, the presence of microvascular proliferations (previously called endothelial cell proliferations) is a histopathological hallmark of glioblastomas. The association of microvascular proliferations with necrosis was noticed by Scherer in 1935 who proposed an "angioplastic" process in gliomas and suggested that glioma cells gain the ability to recruit blood vessels from the neighbouring tissue {1343}.

The pathogenesis of microvascular proliferation in glioblastomas most likely depends on two different pathophysiological mechanisms: (1) angiogenesis, the sprouting of vascular endothelial cells from capillaries pre-existing in the normal surrounding brain, and (2) vascular remodeling through smooth muscle cell/pericyte recruitment. Angiogenesis in gliomas is regulated by a set of endothelial cell receptor tyrosine kinases such as VEGF receptor-1, VEGF receptor-2, Tie-1, Tie-2, PDGF receptor-ß, c-met and integrins such as avß3. Typically, these receptors are not expressed in quiescent endothelium (such as in the normal adult brain) but are upregulated in proliferating tumour vessels, in a way that suggests a role in tumour progression {576, 1182, 1183, 1184, 1186, 553, 1762}. The ligands for these receptors typically are expressed in the tumour cells, arguing in favour of a paracrine (glioma cell-endothelial cell) regulation of tumour angiogenesis {94, 576, 1185}. Current evidence suggests that vascular endothelial growth factor (VEGF) which binds to VEGF receptor-1 and VEGF receptor-2, is the most important regulator of vascular functions in glioma induced-angiogenesis {229,770, 1003, 1317, 1765}. VEGF is a secreted dimeric glycoprotein, which specifically acts on endothelial cells and induces angiogenesis and vascular permeability *in vivo*. During glioma progression, it is upregulated in tumour cells and is particularly highly expressed in glioblastomas, being abundant in the perinecrotic pseudopalisading cells {1183, 1416, 1762}. As VEGF is hypoxia-inducible, a major trigger of angiogenesis in gliomas appears to be cellular hypoxia {645, 1416}. Due to its dual function, VEGF may be responsible for both angiogenesis (microvascular proliferation) and vascular permeability (peritumoural oedema) in malignant gliomas {1183, 1593}. This notion is supported by the observation that dexamethasone, the most widely used drug for the treatment of peritumoural oedema, downregulates the expression of VEGF {565, 1765}.

Vascular remodelling, *e.g.* proliferation and recruitment of smooth muscle cells/pericytes is regulated by a different set of receptors/ligands, including Tie-2, PDGF receptor-ß, and TGF-ß. The Tie-2 receptor is specifically upregulated on endothelial cells during glioma progression. Its agonistic ligand, angiopoietin-1 {1472}, is constitutively expressed in glioma cells, whereas its antagonistic ligand, angiopoietin-2, is specifically upregulated in angiogenic glioma vessels {1767}. Angiopoietin-2 mediated inhibition of tie-2 functions on vascular endothelial cells may therefore be necessary for glioma angiogenesis *in vivo*, presumably by loosening contacts between perivascular support cells and endothelial cells which in turn become accessible for angiogenesis inducers, such as VEGF {1764, 1763}.

Mechanisms of apoptosis and drug resistance

Current concepts of the biology of gliomas include the hypothesis that defects in pathways that regulate susceptibility to apoptosis are both involved in the development and malignant progression of gliomas, and also responsible for their intrinsic resistance to adjuvant chemotherapy. Apoptosis refers to a cell-autonomous type of death with specific morphological features that involves active cellular participation. A few key players have assumed a central role in regulating susceptibility to apoptosis. The Bcl-2 protein family consists of antiapoptotic, *e.g.,* Bcl-2 and Bcl-XL, and proapoptotic, *e.g.,* Bax, members which are thought to control cell death at the level of mitochondrial integrity, by preventing cytochrome c release, and of caspase activation (Fig. 1.8). Caspases are a growing family of enzymes, which constitute the chief execution machinery of apoptosis. Death receptors of the tumour necrosis factor (TNF) family, notably CD95 (Fas/APO-I), and their respective death ligands, *e.g.,* CD95L, seem to be signalling molecules for apoptosis *in vivo*. Subcellularly, TP53 is a key switch for apoptosis in mammalian cells where it enhances the expression of CD95 and Bax but inhibits the expression of Bcl-2, changes predicted to enhance the sensitivity to apoptotic stimuli {1113, 1749} consistent with its common alteration in gliomas. The role of death ligand and receptor expression in gliomas is currently still an area of much controversy. CD95L expression has been detected on tumour cell membranes, whereas CD95 expression was restricted to tumour cells surrounding areas of necrosis {502, 1477}. Clearly, some glioma cells co-express CD95L and CD95, yet fail to undergo suicide or fratricide, suggesting the presence of antiapoptotic protective proteins in these cells {1753}, *e.g.,* Bcl-2 family members {1601} or the recently identified inhibitor-of-apoptosis (IAP) proteins {1759}. The role of TP53 in regulating CD95 expression in human gliomas has remained controversial {1503, 1746}. The detection of multiple genetic alterations in human astrocytomas in pathways thought to modulate susceptibility to apoptosis has also provided a series of candidate genes for the causation of the drug resistance phenotype. Although expression of the Bcl-2 family of proteins in various brain tumours has been studied extensively (*e.g.* refs. {1748, 1587}), no definite biological function in the development or progression of brain tumours could be linked to them. One approach to evaluate the significance of apoptosis-regulatory proteins in gliomas is to assess their expression *in vivo* and to correlate the expression patterns with clinical parameters such as overall survival {1745} or response to chemotherapy {1752}; similar to earlier studies on TP53 status and clinical outcome, these studies have not revealed predictive power for Bcl-2 family proteins in glioblastoma multiforme. The role of specific gene products for resistance to radiochemotherapy may also be assessed in primary glioma cell cultures and in long-term glioma cell lines. In the more relevant primary glioma cell cultures, loss of wild-type TP53 has been associated with increased resistance to chemotherapy {656, 1744}. Moreover, reintroduction of wild-type TP53 by adenoviral transfer restored apoptotic activity {488}. In contrast, ectopic expression of a temperature-sensitive *TP53* transgene in glioma cells increased chemoresistance {1761}, and the TP53 status did not predict sensitivity to drug-induced apoptosis in a large panel of glioma cell lines {1760}. In the latter study, not only TP53 but also p16, CDK4, MDM2, and Bcl-2 family protein expression lacked predictive value for drug sensitivity. Recent studies have implicated the CD95/CD95L system in radiation- and drug-induced apoptosis in nonglial cells {432}. Cytotoxic agents were hypothesised to promote the expression of CD95L and CD95, using both TP53-dependent and TP53-independent pathways, and trigger apoptosis by autocrine suicide or paracrine fratricide. Such a role for CD95/CD95L interactions can probably be excluded as a mediator of drug-induced apoptosis in glioma cells {1743} because ectopic expression of the viral caspase inhibitor, crm-A, blocks apoptosis induced by the cytotoxic cytokines, CD95L, APO2L and TNF-α, but does not affect radiation- or drug-induced cell death. Moreover, neutralizing CD95L antibodies do not modulate drug-induced apoptosis, and glioma cells selected for resistance to CD95L do not acquire cross-resistance to chemotherapeutic drugs. In contrast, caspases, the down-stream effectors of death receptor-mediated apoptosis, are activated in human glioma cells in response to drug treatment in a CD95-independent fashion. However, caspases other than caspases 8 and 3 seem to mediate drug cytotoxicity in human glioma cells {1743}. Importantly, caspase-depen-

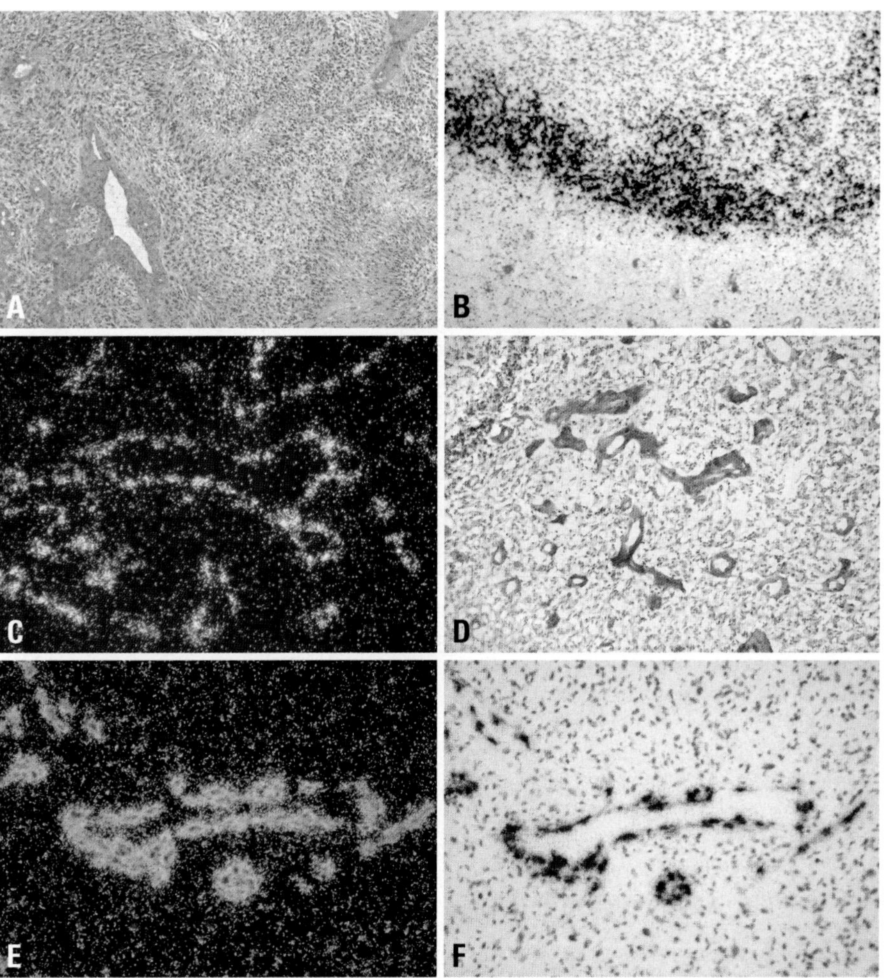

Fig. 1.6 Angiogenesis in glioblastoma. **A** Pseudopalisading necrosis with adjacent microvascular proliferation. **B** VEGF mRNA expression in hypoxic perinecrotic palisading tumour cells. **C** Upregulation of VEGFR-1 in vascular endothelial cells. **D** VEGF immunoreactivity prevails in tumour vessels. Expression of PDGFR-β in endothelial and smooth muscle cells (microvascular proliferation), demonstrated by in situ hybridization in **(E)** dark-field and **(F)** conventional illumination.

		Normal brain capillary	Astrocytoma vessels	Glioblastoma vessels
Astrocytes / astrocytoma cells	VEGF	→	↑	↑
	Ang-1	→	→	→
	PDGF-A	→	↑	↑
	PDGF-B	→	↑	↑
	HGF / SF	→	↑	↑
Endothelial cells (EC)	VEGFR-1	→	↑	↑
	VEGFR-2	↓	→	↑
	TIE-1	↓	↑	↑
	TIE-2	→	↑	↑
	Ang-2	↓	→	↑
	C-met	↓	→	→
Smooth muscle cells / Pericytes (SMC)	PDGFR-β	↓	→	↑
	TGF-β	→	→	→

Fig. 1.7 Modulation of gene expression associated with angiogenesis.

dent pathways of apoptosis mediate acute cytotoxic cell death that evolves within 1-3 days after drug exposure and which requires exposure to drug concentrations unlikely to be achieved *in vivo* {1760}. Conversely, clonogenic cell death measured by the ability to form colonies from individual cells post-treatment, the mode of cell death that is probably responsible for the moderate effects of current radiochemotherapy *in vivo*, seems to evolve entirely death receptor- and caspase-independent in human gliomas. Thus, one may speculate that the overall failure to trigger suicidal/fratricidal death ligand/receptor interactions and to activate caspases in response to clinically achievable drug concentrations may be key reasons for the resistance to chemotherapy in human malignant gliomas. Consistent with this hypothesis, direct targeting of this killing cascade, either at the level of CD95/TRAIL-R death receptor activation {1753, 1751, 1750} or at the level of signalling using the adaptor protein, FADD {1742} or down-stream at the level of caspase activation {1747}, can overcome resistance to apoptosis in human glioblastoma cells.

Drug resistance of gliomas has also been linked to the DNA repair protein, O^6-alkylguanine-DNA alkyltransferase (AGT) which effectively removes O^6-alkylguanines from tumour DNA. These adducts are typically produced by treatment with nitrosoureas, including the cross-linking agents, 1,3-bis-(2-chloroethyl)-1-nitrosourea (BCNU), 1-(2-chloroethyl)-3-cyclohexyl-1-nitrosourea (CCNU), 3-[(4-amino-2-methyl-5-pyrimidinyl)methyl]-1-(2-chloroethyl)-1-nitrosourea hydrochloride (ACNU). The therapeutic efficacy of these drugs can be enhanced by depletion of the AGT by O^6-benzylguanine in vitro and in-patients {2531, 2530). Restoration of susceptibility to chloroethylnitrosoureas is also possible through AGT depletion by alkylating agents that are themselves used in chemotherapy, e.g. dacarbacin and temozolomide. It remains to be shown to which extent drug resistance can be overcome by AGT depletion in human cancers {2529, 2528}.

Radiosensitivity

Radiation therapy is the most important adjuvant treatment for brain tumours, although tumours arising in glia are widely regarded as being relatively radiation resistant. The molecular mechanisms of resistance to irradiation are not understood, although correlates of resistance have been defined including tumour cell hypoxia, the ability of tumour cells to repair sublethal or potentially lethal DNA damage, and the re-population of tumour between doses of fractionated radiation. DNA is the primary target of therapeutic radiation. Cell death following radiation-induced DNA damage occurs by apoptosis and so-called mitotic cell death that occurs when cells are unable to continue dividing, even if still alive. Apoptosis following DNA damage is, in most cell types, mediated by TP53, although in cell lines derived from astrocytic tumours, extensive

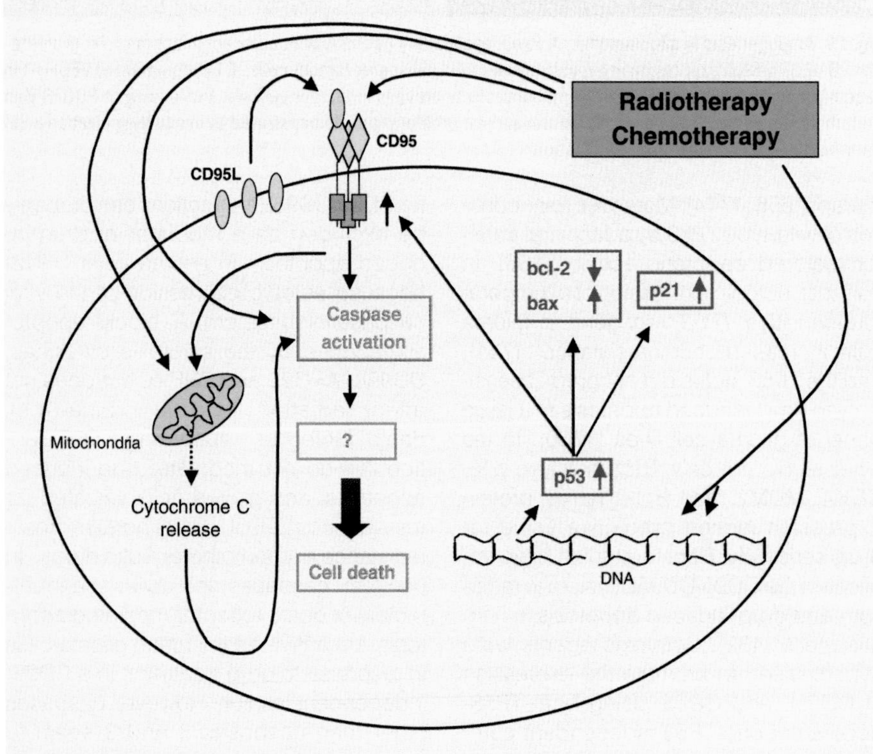

Fig. 1.8 Molecular targets of radio- and chemotherapy-induced apoptosis.

TP53-mediated apoptosis does not occur whether an otherwise functional TP53 is present or not {1826}. Resistance to apoptosis may be a major component of the therapeutic resistance of these tumour types {1827}. Medulloblastoma undergoes extensive TP53 mediated apoptosis following DNA damage and is clinically regarded as a much more radiosensitive tumour than astrocytic tumours {1829}.

Histogenesis

Integration of the increasing understanding of the multiple lineages that contribute to the development of the brain and spinal cord with our understanding of brain tumours presents an important challenge for neuropathology. Multiple precursor cell populations, each of which could give rise to different kinds of tumours, have been identified in studies on CNS development. Most of these studies have been conducted in the rat, and the study of analogous human cells is still in its infancy.

The best studied of the CNS precursor cells is the bipotential oligodendrocyte-type-2 astrocyte progenitor (O-2A) cell, which can give rise *in vitro* to oligodendrocytes and a particular astrocyte population (type-2 astrocytes). At least two distinct O-2A progenitor cell populations exist during development and in the adult animal, and these populations differ in such basic properties as their cell cycle length, migratory rate and ability to undergo continued self-renewal {2089}. The O-2A lineage has been claimed to be the cell of origin of a subset of glioblastomas {1087}.

Developmentally earlier in its appearance than the O-2A progenitor cell is a tripotential glial-restricted precursor (GRP) cell that has been isolated from the embryonic rat spinal cord {2196}. GRP cells differ from O-2A progenitor cells in their survival requirements, response to mitogens and in their differentiation potential, for these precursor cells are able to make oligodendrocytes and two distinct astrocyte populations. The appearance of GRP cells appears to represent the first lineage restriction that occurs in CNS development, and is paralleled by the appearance of neuron-restricted precursor (NRP) cells, a population able to generate several kinds of neurons but no glial cell types {2197}. It is not yet known whether either of these precursor cell populations can be isolated from older animals.

Still broader in its developmental potential is the totipotent neuroepithelial (NEP) stem cell, which can give rise to all of the major cell types of the brain and spinal cord. NEP cells can be isolated from all regions of the developing CNS, and from several different regions of the adult CNS. At least two different NEP cell populations exist, one of which responds to epidermal growth factor as a mitogen and a second that divides in response to fibroblast growth factor {2197, 2198}.

With the exception of NRP cells, all of the CNS precursor cells can give rise to astrocytes, and there may also be still other precursor cells that give rise only to astrocytes {2198, 2196, 2199, 2200}. The current pace of discovery in CNS precursor cell biology suggests that we may be far from identifying all of the different lineages and cell types involved in the development of the CNS.

Diffuse astrocytoma

P. Kleihues
R.L. Davis
H. Ohgaki
P.C. Burger
M.M. Westphal
W.K. Cavenee

Definition

An astrocytic neoplasm characterized by a high degree of cellular differentiation, slow growth, and diffuse infiltration of neighbouring brain structures. These lesions typically affect young adults and have an intrinsic tendency for malignant progression to anaplastic astrocytoma and, ultimately, glioblastoma.

ICD-O code: 9400/3

Grading

Diffuse astrocytomas correspond to WHO grade II {779}.

Synonyms and historical annotation

The term diffuse astrocytoma, if not otherwise specified, refers to low-grade (WHO grade II) diffuse astrocytomas of adults {779}. In previous editions of the WHO classification, the term 'astrocytoma' was used {1685, 779}. Some authors prefer the term 'well-differentiated astrocytoma' or 'fibrillary astrocytoma' {180}, but this latter designation is more commonly used for the respective histological subtype of low-grade diffuse astrocytomas. Diffuse astrocytomas must be strictly separated from the pilocytic astrocytoma, which is usually more circumscribed, with a different age distribution, location and biology.

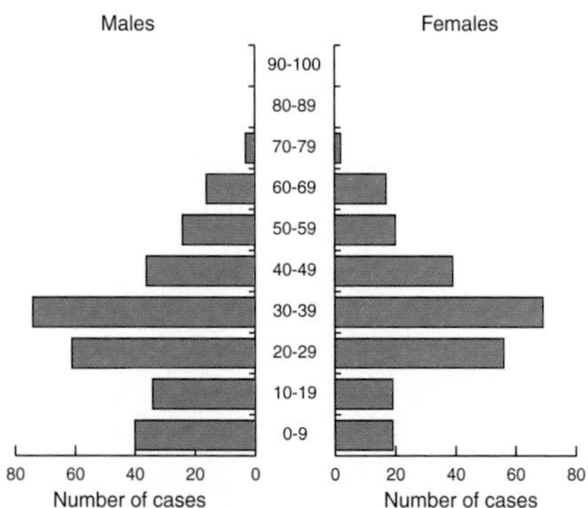

Fig. 1.9 Age distribution of diffuse astrocytomas WHO grade II, based on biopsies of 529 patients from the Tumor Registry of the University of California, San Francisco (courtesy of Ms. Nancy Drungilas) and the Institute of Neuropathology, University Hospital Zurich.

Incidence

Diffuse astrocytomas represent 10-15% of all astrocytic brain tumours, with an incidence of approximately 1.4 new cases per 1 million population and year {2477}. Epidemiological data suggest that in several Scandinavian countries and in North America the incidence of astrocytomas in children has increased during the past three decades {2465, 2464, 2477, 2462}.

Age and sex distribution

The age distribution of diffuse astrocytomas is shown in Fig. 1.9. The peak incidence is in young adults between age 30 and 40 (25% of all cases). Approximately 10% occur below the age of 20, 60% between 20-45 years of age, and about 30% over 45 years. The mean age of occurrence is 34 years. There is predominance for males (M:F ratio, 1.18:1).

Localization

Diffuse astrocytomas may be located in any region of the CNS but most commonly, they develop supratentorially in the cerebrum in both children and adults, the frontal and temporal lobes being most frequently affected (one third of cases each). The brain stem and spinal cord are the next most frequently affected sites, while diffuse astrocytomas are distinctly uncommon in the cerebellum.

Clinical features

Symptoms and signs

Seizures are a common presenting manifestation of the tumour, although with retrospect it may be seen that subtle abnormalities, such as speech difficulties, changes in sensation, vision, or some motor change may have been present earlier. With frontal lobe tumours, changes in behaviour or personality may be the presenting feature. Any such change may have been present for months before diagnosis, but symptoms may also be very abrupt in onset.

Neuroimaging

Like clinical features, the results of neuroimaging studies can be extremely variable. On CT scans, diffuse astrocytomas most often present as ill-defined, homogeneous masses of low density without contrast enhancement. However, calcification, cystic change and even varying degrees of enhancement may be present early. MRI studies usually show hypodensity on T1-weighted images and hyperintensity on T2-weighted images with enlargement of the areas involved early in the evolution of the tumour. Gadolinium enhancement is not common in low-grade diffuse astrocytomas, but tends to appear during tumour progression.

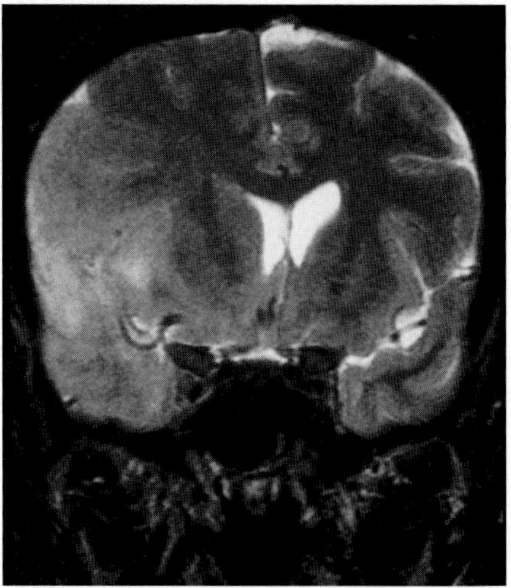

Fig. 1.10 T2-weighted MRI of a diffuse astrocytoma involving the fronto-temporal region with considerable mass effect. In the affected brain region, the cortex is enlarged but still recognizable.

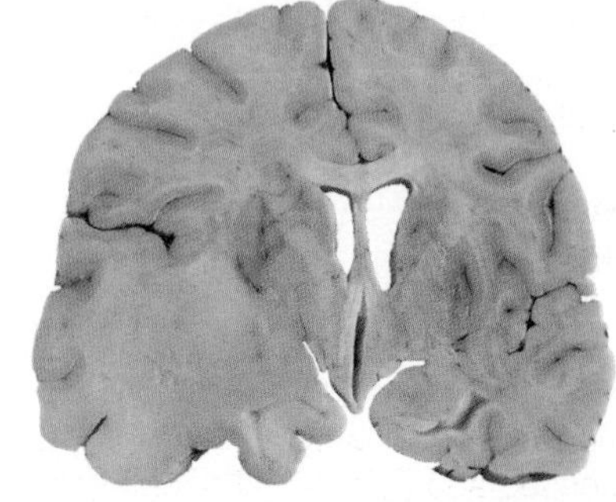

Fig. 1.11 Large fibrillary astrocytoma occupying the left temporal lobe, with extension to the Sylvian fissure. Note the homogenous surface and the enlargement of local anatomical structures.

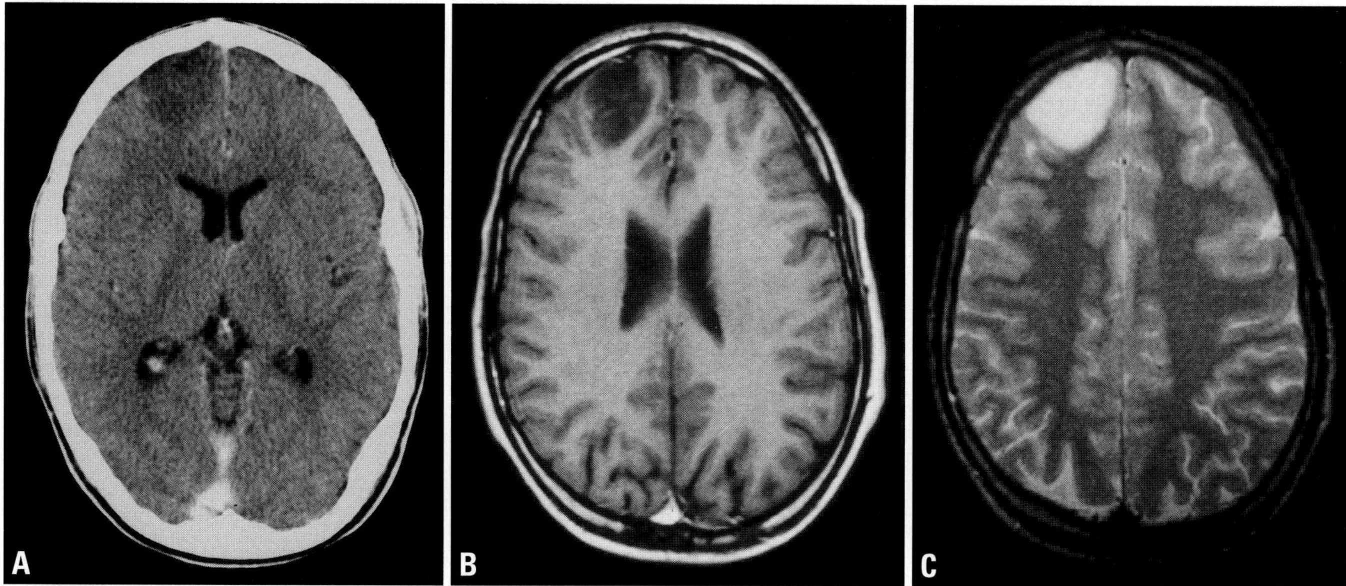

Fig. 1.12 Diffuse astrocytoma WHO grade II, presenting as (**A**) hypodense frontal lesion on contrast enhanced CT, as (**B**) hypointense focus on gadolinium enhanced MRI, and (**C**) as well-delineated hyperintense lesion on T2-weighted MRI.

Macroscopy

Because of their infiltrative nature, these tumours usually show blurring of the gross anatomical boundaries. There is enlargement and distortion, but not destruction, of the invaded anatomical structures, *e.g.* cortex and compact myelinated pathways. Local mass lesions may be present in either grey or yellow-white matter, but they have indistinct boundaries, and changes such as smaller or larger cysts, granular areas and zones of firmness or softening may be seen. Cystic change most commonly appears as a focal spongy area, with multiple cysts of varying size. Extensive microcyst formation may cause a gelatinous appearance. Occasionally, a single large cyst filled with clear fluid may be present. Tumours with prominent gemistocytes sometimes have single large smooth-walled cysts. Focal calcification may also be present, and a more diffuse grittiness may be observed. Extension into contralateral structures, particularly in the frontal lobes, is often observed.

Histopathology

Diffuse astrocytomas are composed of well differentiated fibrillary or gemistocytic neoplastic astrocytes on the background of a loosely structured, often microcystic tumour matrix. Cellularity is moderately increased and occasional nuclear atypia is a typical feature. Mitotic activity is generally absent but a single mitosis does not yet allow the diagnosis of anaplastic astrocytoma. The presence of necrosis or microvascular proliferation is incompatible with the diagnosis of diffuse astrocytoma.

Phenotypically, neoplastic astrocytes may vary considerably with respect to their size, the prominence and disposition of cell processes, and the abundance of cytoplasmic glial filaments. The pattern may vary markedly in different regions of the neoplasm.

Histological recognition of neoplastic astrocytes using H&E staining on sectioned material depends mainly on nuclear characteristics. The normal astrocytic nucleus is oval-to-elongate, but on sectioning, occasional round cross-sections are seen. It is typically vesicular, with intermediate-sized masses of chromatin and often with a distinct nucleolus. Normal human astrocytes show no stainable cytoplasm that is distinct from the background feltwork. Reactive astrocytes are defined by enlarged nuclei and the presence of stain

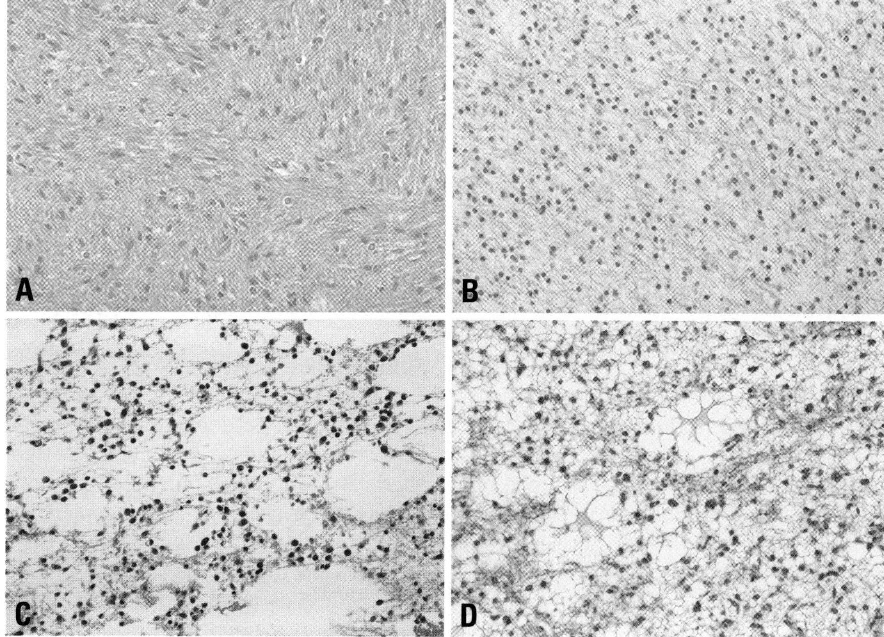

Fig. 1.13 Fibrillary astrocytoma. **A** Low cellularity with minimal nuclear atypia. **B** Neoplastic fibrillary astrocytes on the background of a loosely structured tumour matrix. **C** Extensive microcyst formation with (**D**) variable, diffuse GFAP expression.

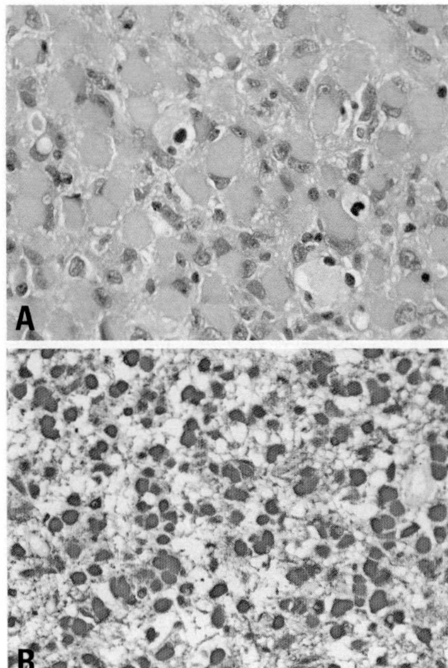

Fig. 1.14 Gemistocytic astrocytoma. **A** Tumour cells have a large slightly eosinophilic cytoplasm with nuclei displaced to the periphery and (**B**) strong, consistent GFAP expression.

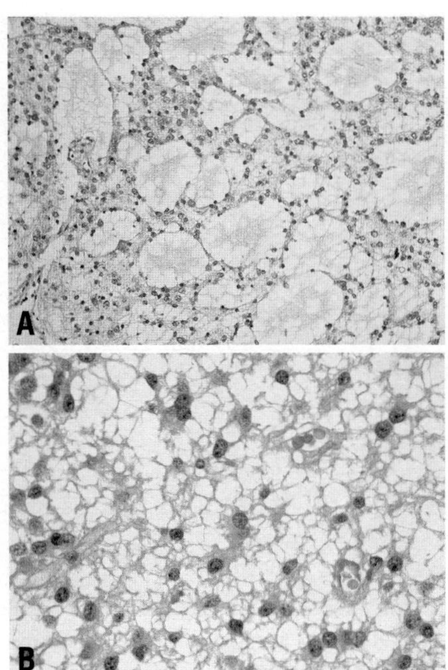

Fig. 1.15 Protoplasmic astrocytoma showing (**A**) extensive mucoid degeneration. **B** Tumour cells have few, flaccid processes on the background of microcystic degeneration.

able defined cytoplasm, culminating in the gemistocyte, which has a mass of eosinophilic cytoplasm, and often has an eccentric nucleus, and with a cytoplasm that extends into fine processes.

The diffuse astrocytomas contain astrocytes that are increased in number and also usually in size, but are otherwise difficult to distinguish on an individual basis from the normal or reactive cells. In minor degrees of anaplasia, it is their number and most commonly the monotony of their morphology that is most helpful in recognizing their neoplastic nature. Reactive astrocytes are rarely all in the same stage of reactivity at one time, so reactions reveal mixtures of astrocytes; some with enlarged nuclei, others with varying amounts of cytoplasm, most often on a somewhat rarified background. With diffuse astrocytomas, almost all of the nuclei appear identical, and the background is at least of normal density, or shows increased numbers of cellular processes. Microcystic change may be present, but again most cells look like one another, without the admixture of gemistocytes more often seen as reaction to injury. Preexisting cell types, *e.g.* neurons, are often entrapped. Mitoses are very rare or absent.

The smear or 'squash' technique is often used during stereotaxic biopsies and yields similar findings, although estimating cellularity with this method is highly unreliable. Many histological features are exaggerated and amplified, e.g. nuclear folds, abnormal chromatin pattern and astrocytic processes. On reducing the light by removing the top lens of the condenser, astrocytic processes are often emphasized. The presence of many round-to-oval nuclei with smooth chromatin can herald the presence of a mixed oligodendroglial component or, if the nuclei are less prominent, the background white matter.

Histologically, there may be great variation, certainly between tumours, and not rarely within the same lesion. According to the prevailing cell type, three major variants can be distinguished, but often, a clear subclassification is not feasible.

Fibrillary astrocytoma

This most frequent histological variant of astrocytoma is predominantly composed of fibrillary neoplastic astrocytes. Nuclear atypia is a diagnostic criterion but mitotic activity, necrosis and microvascular proliferation are absent. A single mitosis does not yet allow the diagnosis of anaplastic astrocytoma The occasional or regional occurrence of gemistocytic neoplastic cells is compatible with the diagnosis of fibrillary astrocytoma.

Cell density is low to moderate. The cytoplasm is often scant and barely discernible, creating the appearance of 'naked nuclei'. Nuclear atypia, *i.e.* enlarged, cigar-shaped, or irregular hyperchromatic nuclei, is a histological hallmark distinguishing tumour cells from normal and reactive astrocytes. Even prominent nuclear atypia is compatible with the diagnosis of diffuse astrocytoma WHO grade II so long as mitoses are very rare or absent. In more cellular lesions, neoplastic cell processes form a loose fibrillary matrix. Microcysts containing mucinous fluid are a characteristic feature and often dominate the histological picture. Cartilage formation is very rare {760, 969}.

Immunohistochemistry. Glial fibrillary acidic protein (GFAP) is consistently expressed, although to a variable degree and not by all tumour cells; in particular, small round cells with scanty cytoplasm and processes tend not to express GFAP. Often, GFAP immunoreactivity is restricted to a small perinuclear rim. The fibrillary matrix, which consists of a network of neoplastic cell processes (and entrapped reactive astrocytes), forms a diffuse GFAP-positive background {781}. Vimentin, a 57 kDa intermediate filament protein originally thought to be expressed only in mesenchymal cells, shows a pattern of immunoreactivity similar to that of GFAP, although it has been noted that vimentin immunoreactivity has a tendency to be seen mainly in the perinuclear region while GFAP is also expressed intensively in the cellular processes {579}. Vimentin-positive cells may lack GFAP expression. As vimentin is expressed early in astrogliogenesis, its presence in astrocytomas could indicate a lower degree of differentiation. There is indeed a tendency for vimentin to be expressed more consistently in high-grade astrocytomas {1035}. Tumour cells usually show immunoreactivity to S-100 protein in the nucleus and in cell processes, but this feature has no diagnostic relevance {774, 781}. This is also true for expression of αB-crystallin {735}.

Electron microscopy. Fibrillary neoplastic astrocytes are characterized by the presence in the perikaryon and cell processes of intermediate filaments ranging in diameter from 7–11 nm. However, these and other ultrastructural features are of limited diagnostic significance. In particular, they do not allow a distinction between tumour cells and reactive astrocytes.

Proliferation. Mitotic activity is typically absent in diffuse astrocytomas. Accordingly, the growth fraction, as determined by the Ki67/MIB-1 labelling index, is usually less than 4%, with a mean value of 2.5 {1584}.

Gemistocytic astrocytoma

This variant of astrocytoma is characterized by the presence of a conspicuous though variable fraction of gemistocytic neoplastic astrocytes. Gemistocytes should amount to more than approximately 20% of all tumour cells; the occasional occurrence of gemistocytes in a diffuse astrocytoma does not justify the diagnosis of gemistocytic astrocytoma.

The mean size of the fraction of gemistocytes is approximately 35% {1755}. The cut-off value of 20% proposed by Krouwer *et al.* {826} is somewhat arbitrary but a useful criterion in borderline cases. The histopathological picture of gemistocytes is dominated by plump, glassy, eosinophilic cell bodies of angular shape. Stout, randomly oriented, processes form a coarse fibrillary network. The gemistocytic neoplastic astrocytes consistently express GFAP in their perikarya and cell processes. Nuclei are usually eccentric, with small nucleoli. Perivascular lymphocyte cuffing is frequent {183}. Electron microscopical analysis confirms the presence of abundant, compact glial filaments in the cytoplasm and in cell processes. Enlarged mitochondria have also been noted {354}.

Proliferation. The growth fraction, as determined by the Ki67/MIB-1 labeling index, is usually less than 4%. However, the gemistocytic neoplastic astrocytes show a significantly lower rate of proliferation than the intermingled small-cell component {621, 826, 1107, 1584, 1587}.

Although the gemistocytic variant appears to be particularly prone to progress to anaplastic astrocytoma and glioblastoma {826, 1306, 1353}, this does not justify a general classification of the gemistocytic astrocytoma as anaplastic astrocytoma {180, 1353}.

Protoplasmic astrocytoma

This rare variant is predominantly composed of neoplastic astrocytes showing a small cell body with few, flaccid processes with a low content of glial filaments and scant GFAP expression. Cellularity is low and mitotic activity absent. Mucoid degeneration and microcyst formation are common and characteristic features.

Nuclei are uniformly round to oval. GFAP immunostaining is variable and generally

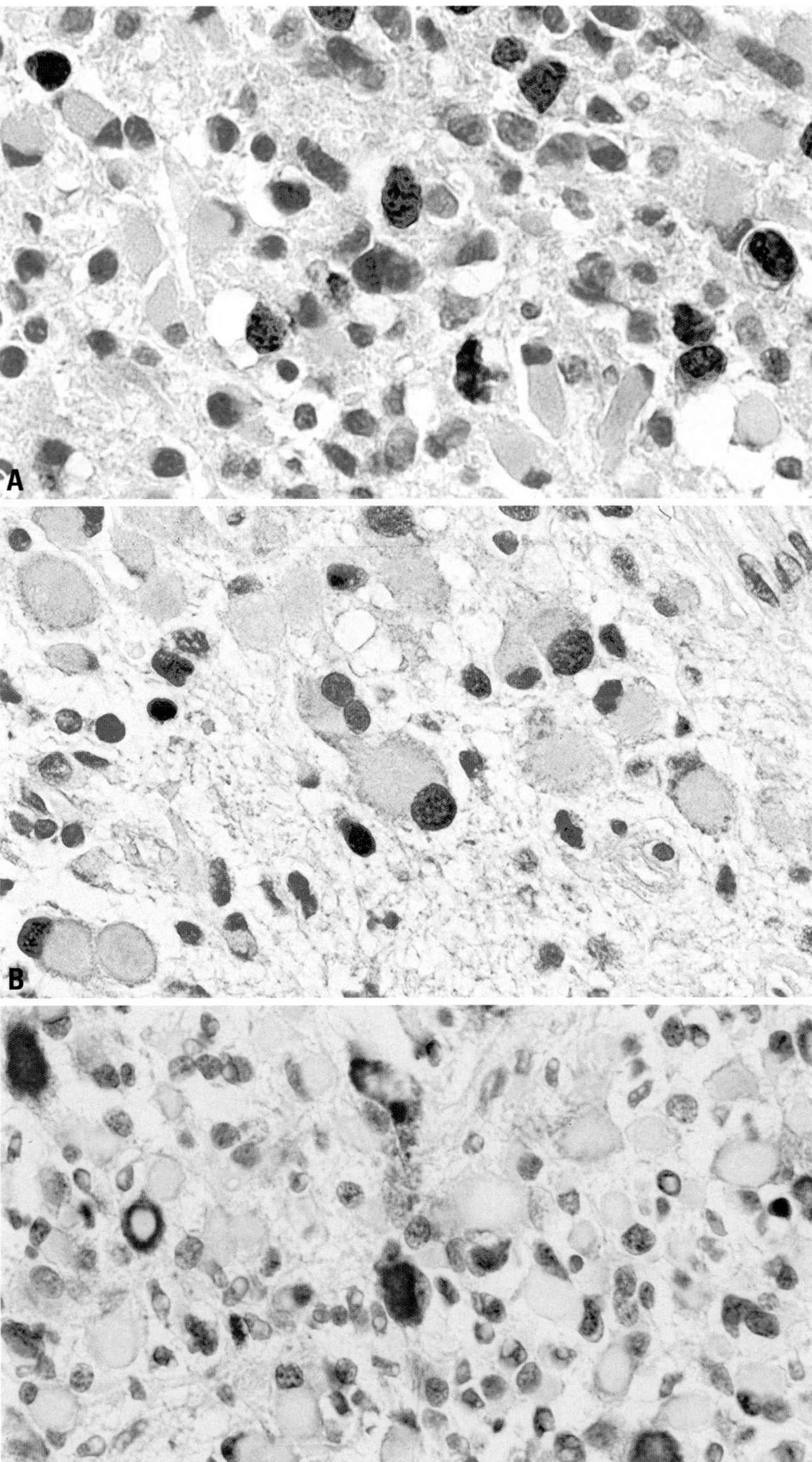

Fig. 1.16 Immunoreactivity of gemistocytes in diffuse astrocytomas WHO grade II. **A** Labelling with MIB-1 is largely restricted to tumour cells with a small rim of cytoplasm, whereas gemistocytes have a low proliferative potential. **B** TP53 accumulation is marked in nuclei of small and gemistocytic tumour cells. **C** Expression of BCL-2 occurs almost exclusively in gemistocytes, suggesting that these cells may escape apoptosis. Reprinted from Watanabe *et al.* {1587}.

low. A clinico-pathological study indicates that protoplasmic astrocytomas manifest after a mean history of 6 yr. of seizures and that they are preferentially located in the fronto-temporal region {1203}. The mean size of the growth fraction as determined by the MIB-1 labeling index was <1% {2475}. This lesion is not well defined and is considered by some authors as an occasional histopathological feature rather than a reproducibly identifiable variant. When occurring in children, this neoplasm may be difficult to separate from pilocytic juvenile astrocytomas {1203, 1306}.

Genetic susceptibility

Diffuse astrocytomas may occur in patients with inherited *TP53* germline mutations (see Chapter 14) although affected family members more frequently develop anaplastic astrocytoma and glioblastomas. More recently, low-grade astrocytomas have been diagnosed in patients with inherited multiple enchondromatosis type 1 (Ollier disease; MIM 225795) which also predisposes to chondrosarcoma {2474, 2469}.

Molecular genetics

TP53. In low-grade diffuse astrocytomas progressing to glioblastoma, mutation frequencies >60% have been reported {1585, 1245}. In the gemistocytic variant, >80% of cases contained a *TP53* mutation {1755}. TP53 protein accumulation is similarly frequent but does not always reflect the presence of a mutation (concordance in 74% of cases) {1585}.

During malignant progression of low-grade astrocytomas, the frequency of *TP53* mutations does not significantly increase, indicating that this genetic change is an early event and in 90% of positive cases already present in the first biopsy {1417, 1585, 1586, 1559}. If they were the initial 'gatekeeper' event {2473} one would expect that patients with inherited *TP53* germline mutations would also develop brain tumours preferentially of astrocytic lineage and this is indeed the case (see ref. {784} and Chapter 14). Further, if low-grade diffuse astrocytomas are of monoclonal origin {1833} and if *TP53* mutations are indeed the initial genetic event, they should be present in all tumour cells. However, a clonal assay of cells from low-grade diffuse astrocytoma showed that the fraction of mutated cells is lower than in recurrent lesions with a higher degree of malignancy from the same patient {1417}, indicating clonal expansion of a small fraction of mutated cells within a pre-existing low-grade diffuse astrocytoma.

PDGFRα. Increased mRNA expression of the platelet-derived growth factor receptor alpha was observed in astrocytic tumors of all stages but gene amplification was only detected in a small subset of glioblastomas {576}.

Other genetic changes. Since approximately 25% of diffuse astrocytomas WHO grade II do not contain a *TP53* mutation, other genetic alterations are likely to be involved. Comparative genomic hybridisation (CGH) analyses showed as most frequent genomic imbalance a gain of chromosome 7q and amplification of 8q {2470, 2471}. A recent study indicates that LOH on 10p occurs in a subset of diffuse astrocytomas WHO grade II {2484}. LOH on 22q has been reported to be present at a frequency of 17% {2517} and chromosome 6 deletions in 14% of cases {2542}.

Predictive factors

The mean survival time after surgical intervention is in the range of 6-8 years, with marked individual variation. The total length of disease is mainly influenced by the dynamics of malignant progression to glioblastoma which tends to occur after a mean time interval of 4-5 years {1585, 2449, 2450, 2467}. Even in the presence of a *TP53* mutation in the first biopsy, long-term survival is possible in the absence of additional genetic alterations, e.g. LOH on 10, and 19q {2448}.

Clinical prognostic factors. Young age {2416} and gross total tumour resection {2466} are considered predictive of delayed recurrence and progression.

TP53. Neoplasms with *TP53* mutations appear to progress more frequently, but the evidence for this correlation is still circumstantial {655, 807, 1233}. The time interval until progression appears to be shorter in patients with low-grade diffuse astrocytomas carrying a *TP53* mutation {1585}. In the study by Choziek *et al.* {245}, immunoreactivity for TP53 protein in diffuse astrocytomas was associated with shorter patient survival, but other studies showed that the presence of *TP53* mutations or TP53 accumulation had no effect on clinical outcome {13, 807,1362, 2463}.

Proliferation and histopathology. Analysis of a wide range of astrocytic tumours showed a gross correlation of proliferation with clinical outcome {618, 1200}. A Ki-67 labelling index (LI) >7.5% was associated with higher histological grade and poorer survival, and this value was a more significant factor statistically than histological grading {1027}. In another study, a Ki-67 LI of >5% was found to constitute a threshold value for predicting shorter survival {683}. Some studies suggest that in diffuse astrocytomas WHO grade II, the proliferative potential correlates inversely with survival and time to recurrence but this finding is inconsistent and in individual cases, the size of the growth fraction as determined by the MIB-1 labelling index cannot be regarded of being prognostic {620, 649, 1027, 1353, 2463}.

The presence of numerous *microcysts* appears to be associated with a somewhat better prognosis {1353}. Some studies indicate that *perivascular lymphocyte cuffing* carries a somewhat more favourable prognosis {162, 1125}, while others failed to note a correlation with patient survival {184, 649}.

It is generally acknowledged that diffuse astrocytomas WHO grade II with a significant fraction of *gemistocytes* tend to undergo malignant progression more rapidly than the ordinary fibrillary astrocytoma {826, 1306, 1353, 2466}, despite the fact that the majority of neoplastic gemistocytes are in a non-proliferative state (G_0 phase of the cell cycle) suggestive of terminal differentiation {1587}.

Anaplastic astrocytoma

P. Kleihues
R.L. Davis
S.W. Coons
P.C. Burger

Definition

A diffusely infiltrating astrocytoma with focal or dispersed anaplasia, and a marked proliferative potential. Anaplastic astrocytomas arise from low-grade astrocytomas, but are also diagnosed at first biopsy, without indication of a less malignant precursor lesion. They have an intrinsic tendency for malignant progression to glioblastoma.

ICD-O code: 9401/3

Grading

Anaplastic astrocytoma corresponds to WHO grade III {779, 780}.

Synonyms

These neoplasms are also referred to as 'malignant astrocytoma' and 'high-grade astrocytoma', but these terms are somewhat ambiguous as they are also occasionally applied to the glioblastoma.

Age and sex distribution

The age distribution of anaplastic astrocytomas is shown in Fig. 1.17. In the Zurich series, the mean age at biopsy is approximately 41 years, *i.e.* higher than that of patients with diffuse low-grade astrocytoma (mean, 34 yr.) but significantly lower than that of glioblastoma patients (mean, 53 yr.). Males are more frequently affected (M:F ratio, 1.8:1).

Localization

Localization of anaplastic astrocytomas largely corresponds to that of other diffusely infiltrating astrocytomas, with a preference for the cerebral hemispheres.

Clinical features

Symptoms and signs

Symptoms are similar to those of patients with diffuse astrocytoma WHO grade II. Typical are signs of a recurrent glioma (increasing neurological deficit, seizures, intracranial pressure), following initial resection of a diffuse low-grade astrocytoma. Not infrequently, patients with anaplastic astrocytoma present after a history of few months, without evidence of a preceding diffuse astrocytoma WHO grade II.

Neuroimaging

Anaplastic astrocytoma presents as an ill-defined mass of low density. In contrast to diffuse astrocytomas WHO grade II, partial contrast enhancement is usually observed but the typical ring enhancement of glioblastomas is absent. The more rapid tumour growth with development of a perifocal oedema may lead to mass shifts and increased intracranial pressure.

Macroscopy

Frequently, it is not possible to grossly distinguish between an anaplastic and a diffuse astrocytoma WHO grade II. On a cut surface, the higher cellularity of the anaplastic astrocytoma produces a discernible tumour mass with sometimes more clear distinction from surrounding brain structures than seen in diffuse astrocytomas WHO grade II. As in the latter, there is a tendency to infiltrate without frank tissue destruction. This often leads to a marked enlargement of invaded structures, e.g. adjacent gyri and basal ganglia. Macroscopic cysts are uncommon, but frequently there are areas of granularity, opacity and a softer consistency.

Histopathology

The principal histopathological features are those of a diffusely infiltrating astrocytoma with increased cellularity, distinct nuclear atypia and marked mitotic activity. The presence of microvascular glomerula or festoons and of necrotic foci reflects progression to glioblastoma and is incompatible with the diagnosis of anaplastic astrocytoma.

Regional or diffuse hypercellularity is an important diagnostic criterion. With progressive anaplasia, the nuclear morphology becomes more complex, with increasing variations in nuclear size, shape, coarseness or dispersion of chromatin, increasing nucleolar prominence and number. Additional signs of anaplasia are nuclear inclusions, multinucleated tumour cells and abnormal mitoses. Cytoplasmic variability may also increase. Gemistocytic tumour cells are often present, but rarely to an extent that would allow the diagnosis of an anaplastic gemistocytic astrocytoma. Capillaries are lined with a single layer of endothelial cells. Microvascular proliferation and necrosis are absent. Occasionally, VEGF expression and incipient microvascular proliferation are observed, but limited to occasional tumour vessels. Immunoreactivity for GFAP is a consistent feature although not in all tumour cells. The expression of S-100 protein, vimentin and αB-crystallin is more uniform but of limited diagnostic significance.

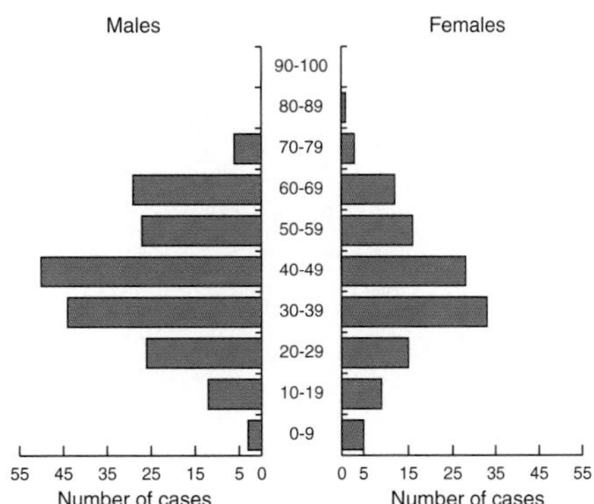

Fig. 1.17 Age distribution of anaplastic astrocytomas, based on biopsies of 319 patients treated at the University Hospital, Zurich.

Proliferation

In contrast to diffuse astrocytomas WHO grade II, anaplastic astrocytomas typically display mitotic activity. Growth fraction, as determined by the antibodies Ki-67/MIB-1, is usually in the range 5–10%, but may overlap with values for low-grade diffuse astrocytomas on one side and for glioblastoma on the other {272, 683, 728, 1220}.

Molecular genetics

From a clinical, morphological and genetic point of view, the anaplastic astrocytoma constitutes an intermediate stage on the route of progression to glioblastoma (Fig. 1.33). It has a high frequency of *TP53* mutations, similar to that of diffuse astrocytomas WHO grade II. Studies on patients with multiple biopsies showed that in >90% of cases with a mutation, the *TP53* gene alteration is already present in the preceding low-grade astrocytoma {1585}.

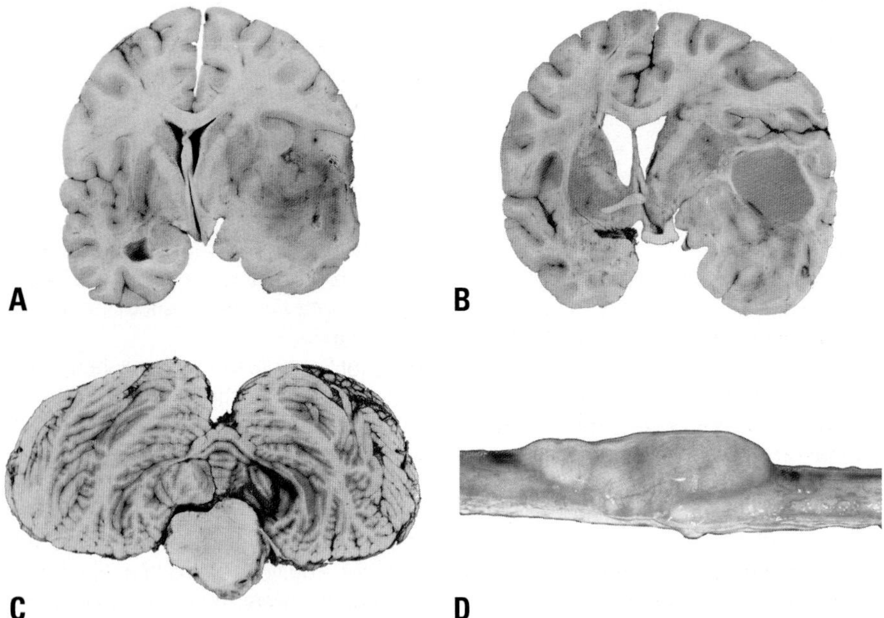

Fig. 1.18 Macroscopic appearance of anaplastic astrocytomas (**A**) in the right fronto-temporal region. Note the ill-defined borders with the adjacent brain structures. **B** Another lesion in a similar location contains a large cyst but no macroscopically discernable necrocis. **C** Anaplastic astrocytoma of the medulla with gross enlargement of local structures. **D** Anaplastic astrocytoma of the spinal cord with exophytic growth into the subarachnoid space.

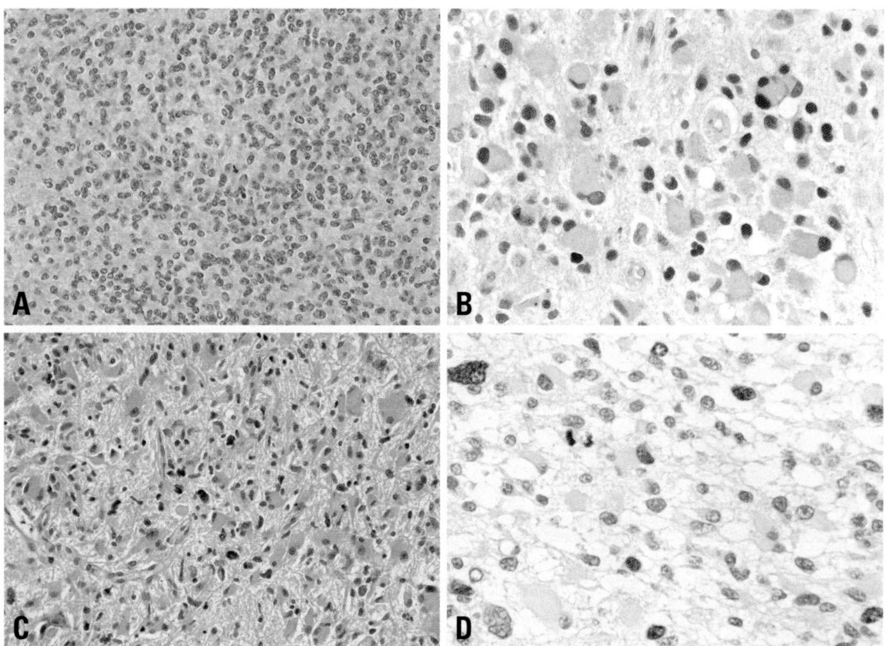

Fig. 1.19 Anaplastic astrocytoma with (**A**) high cellularity, and (**B**) nuclear accumulation of TP53 protein in a large fraction of tumour cells. **C** Marked nuclear atypia and mitotic activity in a tumour area with fibrillary and gemistocytic neoplastic astrocytes. **D** Several tumour cells show immunoreactivity for the proliferation marker MIB-1, including a cell in mitosis.

Additional genetic changes reflecting the higher degree of malignancy affect cell cycle regulatory genes including *p16* deletion (approx. 30% of cases), *RB* alterations (25%), *p19^{ARF}* deletion (15%), and *CDK4* amplification (10%). *PTEN/MMAC1* mutations and LOH on chromosome 10q have been reported in 15% and 30%, respectively. Loss of heterozygosity is also observed on chromosome 19q in approx. 40% {1558}, and on on 22q in approx. 30% of cases {2517}. *EGFR* amplification is rarely observed (<10% of cases). One recent study using 53 microsatellite markers on 53 cases of anaplastic astrocytoma reported a >60% frequency of LOH on chromosome 10 {2484}. Deletion of chromosome 6 occurs in approximately one third of cases {2542}.

Histogenesis and pathogenesis

Anaplastic astrocytomas are assumed to be derived from differentiated astrocytes or precursor cells committed to astrocytic differentiation. Their evolution from diffuse astrocytomas WHO grade II and their progression to glioblastoma is morphologically well defined and is supported by molecular genetic findings (Fig. 1.33). Less clear is, whether *all* anaplastic astrocytomas develop from diffuse astrocytomas WHO grade II, *i.e.* including those which present clinically *de novo* without identifiable precursor lesion. The pattern of genetic changes, in particular the high frequency (> 70%) of *TP53* mutations {1585} would be compatible with the assumption that such tumours progressed rapidly from diffuse astrocytomas WHO grade II. The very rare occurrence of *EGFR* and *MDM2* amplification strongly suggest that the anaplastic astrocytoma can only in exceptional cases be considered a precursor lesion of the primary glioblastoma.

Predictive factors

The progression of anaplastic astrocytomas to glioblastoma is a key prognostic factor. The time interval (time till progression) varies considerably, with a mean of 2 years {1585} and a total length of disease of 3 years {2250}. The presence of an oligodendroglial component is associated with a significant increase in survival (>7yr.) Factors predicting the clinical outcome have often been analyzed in conjunction with those for glioblastoma patients and showed increased survival in younger patients, high preoperative Karnofsky score, and gross total resection.

Glioblastoma

P. Kleihues
P.C. Burger
V.P. Collins
E.W. Newcomb
H. Ohgaki
W.K. Cavenee

Definition

Glioblastoma is the most malignant astrocytic tumour, composed of poorly differentiated neoplastic astrocytes. Histopathological features include cellular polymorphism, nuclear atypia, brisk mitotic activity, vascular thrombosis, microvascular proliferation and necrosis. Glioblastoma typically affects adults and is preferentially located in the cerebral hemispheres. Glioblastomas may develop from diffuse astrocytomas WHO grade II or anaplastic astrocytomas ('secondary glioblastoma'), but more frequently, they manifest after a short clinical history *de novo*, without evidence of a less malignant precursor lesion ('primary glioblastoma').

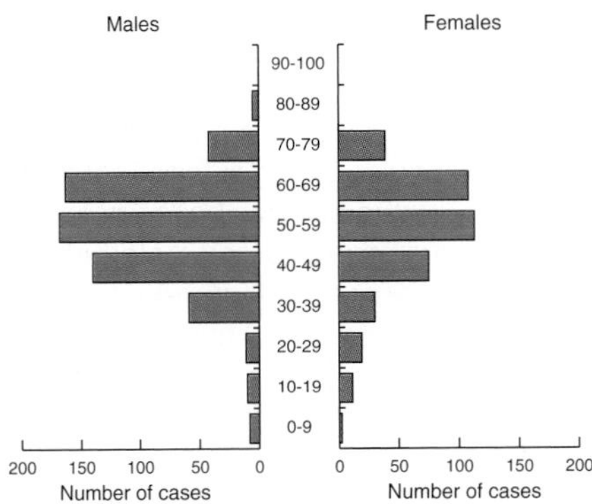

Fig. 1.20 Age distribution of glioblastomas, based on biopsies of 1003 patients treated at the University Hospital, Zurich.

ICD-O code: 9440/3

Grading

The glioblastoma and its variants correspond to WHO grade IV.

Synonyms and historical annotation

Identified in 1863 by Virchow as a tumour of glial origin {1554}, the first comprehensive description of this lesion was given by Strauss and Globus {481}. In 1926, Bailey and Cushing changed the name from spongioblastoma multiforme to glioblastoma multiforme {58}, a term first used by Mallory in 1914 {951}. A more detailed historical account has been given by Zülch {1686} and by Russell and Rubinstein {1306}. Today, the term glioblastoma is used synonymously with glioblastoma multiforme. Scherer {1340} and Kernohan {763} were instrumental in developing the concept that glioblastoma is a malignant astrocytoma that sometimes develops by progression from a lower grade lesion. This view has received strong support from molecular genetic studies showing that there is a characteristic sequential accumulation of genetic alterations from diffuse astrocytomas WHO grade II to the glioblastoma (Fig. 1.33).

Incidence

The glioblastoma is the most frequent brain tumour, accounting for approximately 12–15% of all intracranial neoplasms {1686} and 50–60% of all astrocytic tumours. In most European and North American countries, the incidence is in the range of 2–3 new cases per 100'000 population per year {859}.

Age and sex distribution

Glioblastoma may manifest at any age, but preferentially affects adults, with a peak incidence between 45 and 70 years. In a review of 1003 glioblastoma biopsies from the University Hospital Zurich, two-thirds (70%) of patients fell into this age group. The mean age at biopsy was 53 years and males were significantly more frequently affected (M:F ratio, 1.5:1). Similar data have been reported by others {1686}. In a series of 488 cases, Dohrman {341} reported that 8.8% of glioblastomas occur in children. Congenital cases of glioblastoma are rare {2410}. Ultrasonograpic *in utero* diagnosis of malignant glioma {2406, 2407, 2408} has revealed that prenatal manifestation of glioblastoma may occur as early as at 29 weeks of gestation {2408}.

Localization

Glioblastomas occur most often in the subcortical white matter of the cerebral hemispheres. In a series of 987 glioblastomas from the University Hospital Zurich, the most frequently affected sites were the temporal (31%), parietal (24%), frontal

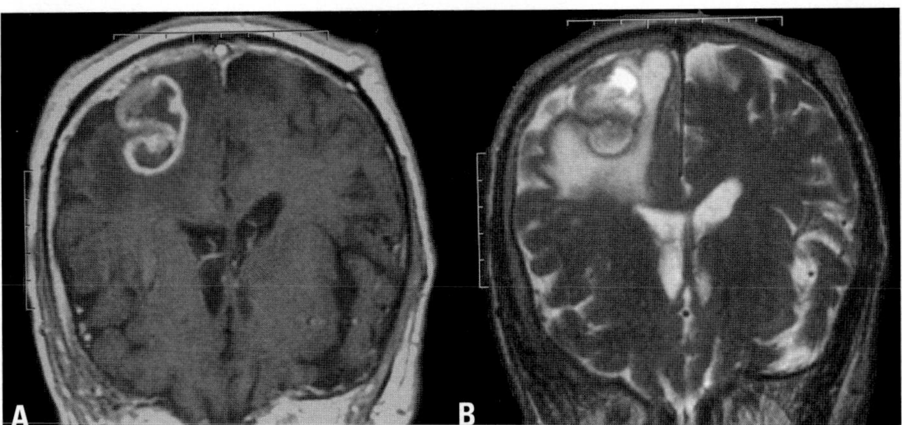

Fig. 1.21 Glioblastoma. **A** T1-weighted MRI with marked gadolinium enhancement, indicating neovascularization and vascular permeability. **B** T2-weighted MRI reveals extensive perifocal oedema.

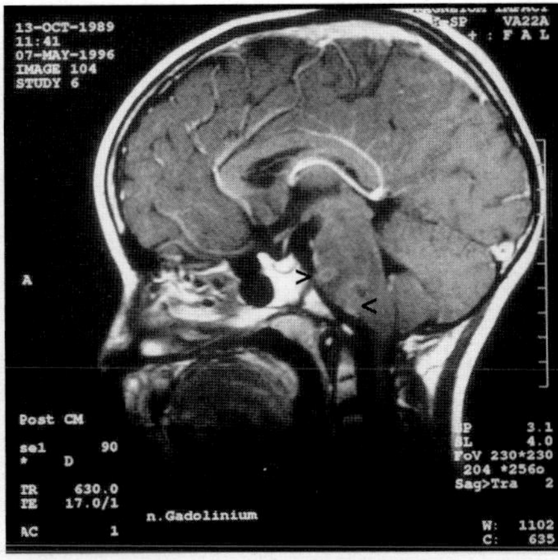

Fig. 1.22 Malignant brainstem glioblastoma MRI of a 6 year-old child. Arrows indicate foci of necrosis.

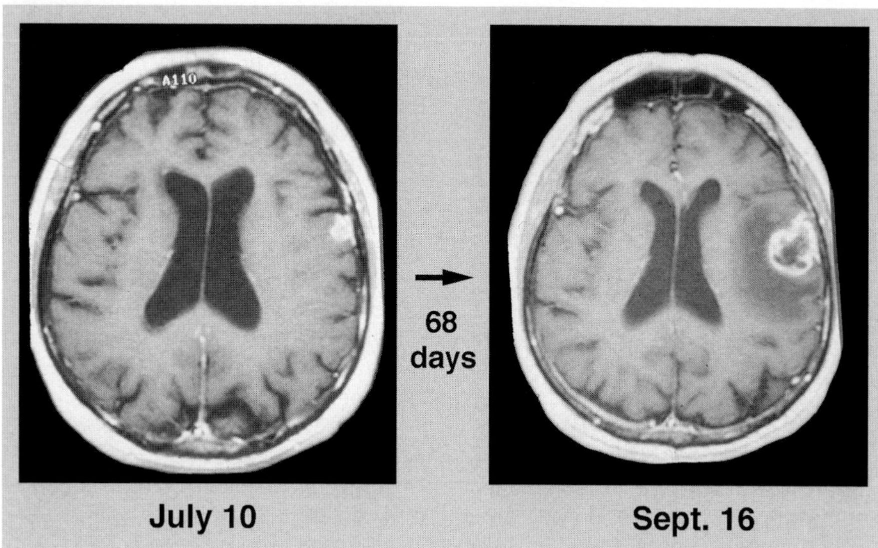

Fig. 1.23 Rapid evolution of a primary glioblastoma in a 79 year-old patient. MRI shows a small cortical lesion that within 68 days developed into a full-blown glioblastoma with perifocal oedema and central necrosis.

(23%) and occipital lobes (16%). Combined fronto-temporal location is particularly typical. Tumour infiltration often extends into the adjacent cortex, the basal ganglia and the contralateral hemisphere. Intraventricular glioblastomas (Fig. 1.24G) are exceptional {2409}. Glioblastomas of the brainstem ('malignant brainstem glioma') are infrequent and often affect children {341}, while cerebellum and spinal cord are rare sites for this neoplasm.

Clinical features

Symptoms and signs

The clinical history of the disease is usually short (less than 3 months in more than 50% of cases), unless the neoplasm has developed from diffuse astrocytoma WHO grade II or anaplastic astrocytoma (secondary glioblastoma). Patients often present after an epileptic seizure with non-specific neurological symptoms, headache and personality changes, but the most threatening aspect is the rapid development of increased intracranial pressure.

Neuroimaging

On CT scans, glioblastomas typically present as irregularly shaped lesions with a peripheral, ring-like zone of contrast enhancement around a dark, central area of necrosis that is usually hypodense. On T1-weighted MRI images, the contrast-enhanced ring structure corresponds to the cellular and highly vascularised peripheral area of the neoplasm. Analysis of untreated glioblastomas in whole brain sections clearly showed that this ring structure does not represent the outer tumour border, as infiltrating glioma cells can be easily identified within, and occasionally beyond, a 2 cm margin {176, 2411}. In T2-weighted images this zone is broader, less well defined and overlaps with the surrounding vasogenic oedema. On PET scans, regional glucose consumption closely correlates with cellularity {574} and reduced survival {1140}.

Macroscopy

Glioblastomas are poorly delineated, the cut surface showing a variable colour with peripheral greyish tumour masses, yellowish necrosis from myelin breakdown and stippled with the red and brown of recent and remote haemorrhages. The central necrosis may occupy as much as 80% of the total tumour mass. Macroscopic cysts, when present, contain a turbid fluid and represent liquefied necrotic tumour tissue, quite in contrast to the well-delineated retention cysts in diffuse astrocytomas WHO grade II. However, extensive haemorrhages may occur and evoke stroke-like symptoms, which are sometimes the first clinical sign of the tumour. The lesion is usually unilateral, but those in the brainstem and corpus callosum can be bilaterally symmetrical.

Most glioblastomas of the cerebral hemispheres are clearly intraparenchymal with an epicenter in the white matter, but some are largely superficial and in contact with the leptomeninges and dura. As these latter neoplasms are frequently rich in collagen, they may be interpreted by the surgeon or neuroradiologist as metastatic carcinoma, or as an extra-axial lesion such as meningioma.

Despite the short duration of symptoms in many cases of glioblastoma, the tumours are often surprisingly large at the time of presentation, and may occupy much of a lobe. Surrounding the central necrotic area is a hypercellular zone which, when fully formed, is visible as a soft, grey rim. In some lesions, this area forms an obvious grey band of tissue; in others, necrotic tissue may abut directly on normal brain without any neoplasm being macroscopically detectable. Cortical infiltration may produce a preserved gyriform rim of thickened grey cortex overlying a necrotic zone in the white matter.

Spread and metastasis

Although infiltrative spread is a common feature of all diffuse astrocytic tumours, glioblastomas are particularly notorious for their rapid invasion of neighbouring brain structures {176}. A very common feature is extension of the tumour through the corpus callosum into the contralateral hemisphere, creating the image of a bilateral, symmetrical lesion ('butterfly glioma'). Similarly, rapid spread is observed in the internal capsule, fornix, anterior commissure and optic radiation. These structures may become enlarged and distorted but continue to serve as a 'highway', allowing the formation of new tumour masses at their opposite projection site, thus leading to the neuroradiological image of a multifocal glioblastoma.

Despite its rapid, infiltrative growth, the glioblastoma tends not to invade the subarachnoidal space and, consequently, rarely metastasizes via the cerebrospinal fluid {473}. Extension within and along perivascular spaces is another typical mode of infiltration, but invasion of the vessel lumen seems to occur infrequently {97, 2413}. Haematogeneous spread to extraneural tissues is very rare in patients without previous surgical intervention {36, 602, 634, 1137, 1138}. Peritoneal metastasis via ventriculoperitoneal shunt has been observed {2414}. Penetration of the dura, venous sinus and bone is exceptional {37, 852, 1163, 1195, 1414}.

Multifocal glioblastomas

The question of whether true multiple independent gliomas occur outside the setting of inherited neoplastic syndromes is controversial. This is because even care-

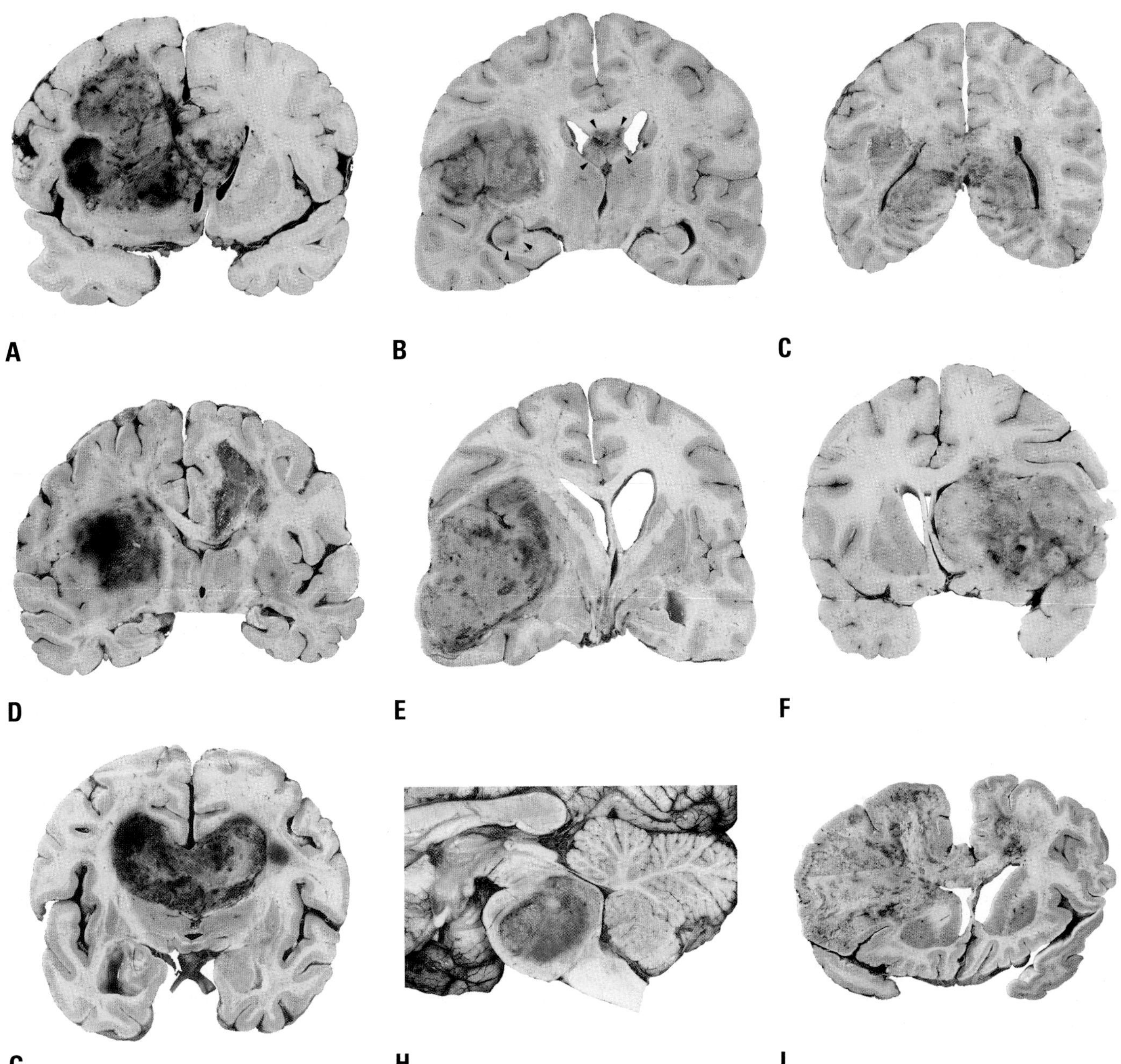

Fig. 1.24 Macroscopic features of glioblastoma multiforme (GBM). **A** Large GBM in the left frontal lobe extending into the corpus callosum and the contralateral white matter. **B, C** GBM of the left frontotemporal region with invasion of the fornices (arrows), spread to the lower horn of the left ventricle (arrow) and (**C**) extension to the corpus callosum and adjacent parieto–occipital structures. **D** GBM of the left basal ganglia and spread into the right hemisphere with formation of a cystic necrosis. **E, I** Glioblastomas of the left hemisphere with extensive necrosis occupying most of the tumour mass. **F** Right fronto–temporal GBM with mass shifting and subfalcial herniation. **G** GBM with unusual intraventricular location. **H** Malignant brainstem GBM in a child.

ful post-mortem studies on whole brain sections may not always reveal a connection between apparently multifocal gliomas, as the cells infiltrating along myelinated pathways are often small, polar and largely undifferentiated. In a careful histological analysis, Batzdorf & Malamud {75} concluded that 2.4% of glioblastomas are truly multiple independent tumours, a value similar to that reported by Russell & Rubinstein (2.3%; ref. {1306}). In a post-mortem study, Barnard & Geddes {68} found that 7.5% of gliomas (including oligodendrogliomas) are multiple independent tumours and that in approximately 3% of these, tumour foci vary in their histological appearance. True multifocal glioblastomas are most likely polyclonal if they occur infra- and supratentorially, *i.e.* outside easily accessible routes like the cerebrospinal fluid pathways or the median commissures {2415}. Multiple independently arising gliomas would, by definition, be of polyclonal origin and their existence can only be proven by application of molecular markers which, in informative cases, allow a distinction between tumours of common or independent origin {93, 112, 808}.

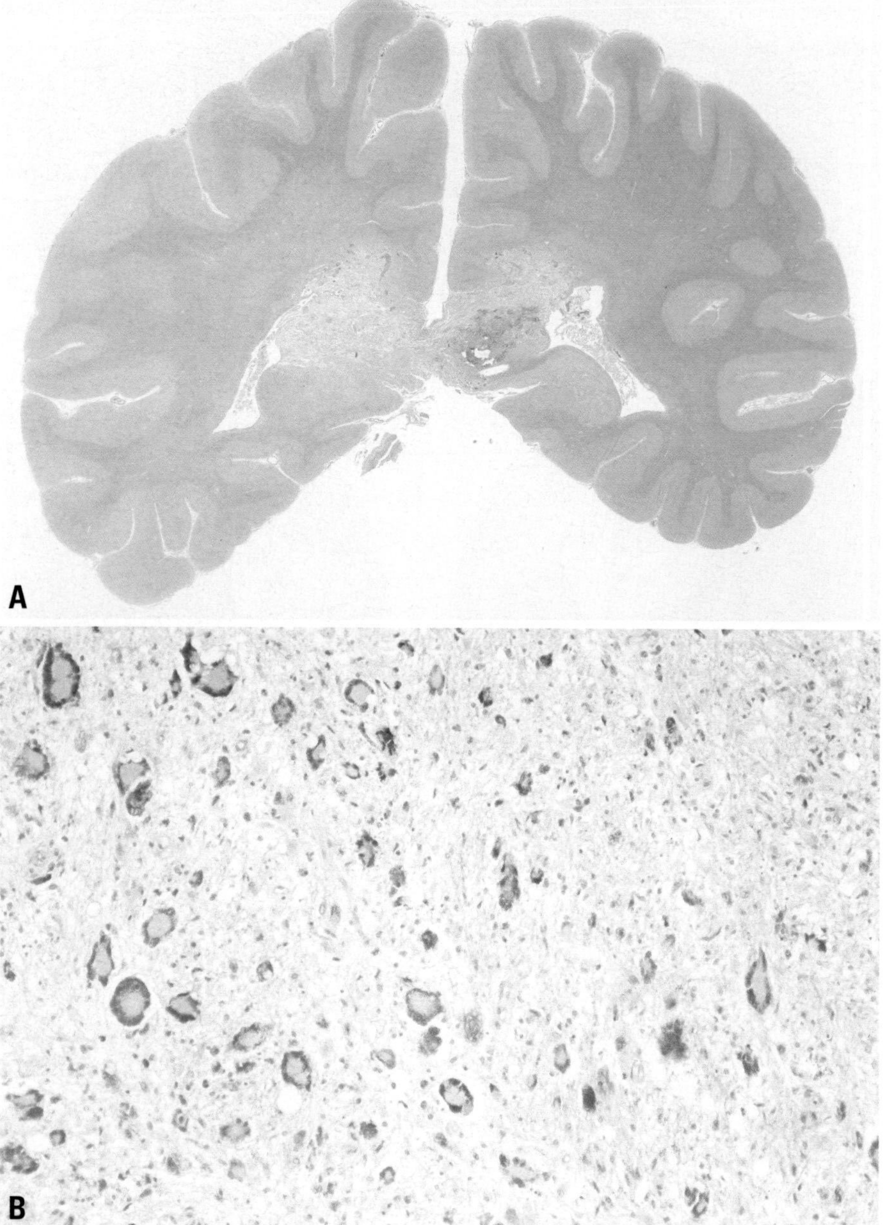

Fig. 1.25 Glioblastoma that has spread into the corpus callosum and to adjacent occipital lobes (**A**). Histopathology of the same case reveals numerous multinucleated giant cells (**B**).

Primary and secondary glioblastoma

The terms primary and secondary glioblastoma were first used by Scherer in 1940 who noted: 'From a biological and clinical point of view, the secondary glioblastomas developing in astrocytomas must be distinguished from 'primary' glioblastomas; they are probably responsible for most of the glioblastomas of long clinical duration' {1340}.

Primary glioblastomas account for the vast majority of cases in older people (mean, 55 years). After a short clinical history, usually of less than 3 months, they manifest *de novo*, *i.e.* without clinical or histopathological evidence of a pre-existing, less malignant precursor lesion. In selected cases with sequential MRI-imaging, it was shown that within 3 months, a primary glioblastoma may develop truly *de novo*, *i.e.* without demonstrable precursor lesion or from a small cortical lesion of ~1cm diameter (Fig. 1.23).

Secondary glioblastomas typically develop in younger patients (<45 yr.) through malignant progression from diffuse astrocytoma WHO grade II or anaplastic astrocytoma. The time for progression from diffuse astrocytoma WHO grade II to glioblastoma varies considerably, with time intervals ranging from less than 1 year to more than 10 years {2448}, the mean interval being 4-5 years {1585, 2449, 2450}. The time till progression appears to be shorter in patients older than 45 year {2416}. It is still a matter of controversy, whether the prognosis of patients with secondary glioblastoma is better than {1625} or similar to {2417}, that of patients with primary (*de novo*) lesions.

There is increasing evidence that primary and secondary glioblastomas constitute distinct disease entities, that evolve through different genetic pathways (Fig. 1.33), affect patients at different ages, and are likely to differ in response to therapy {2434}.

Histopathology

An anaplastic, cellular glioma composed of poorly differentiated, often pleomorphic astrocytic tumour cells with marked nuclear atypia and brisk mytotic activity. Prominent microvascular poliferation and/or necrosis are essential diagnostic features.

As the term glioblastoma multiforme suggests, the histopathology of this tumour is extremely variable. While some lesions show a high degree of cellular and nuclear polymorphism with numerous multinucleated giant cells, others are highly cellular, but rather monotonous. The astrocytic nature of the neoplasms may be easily identifiable, at least focally, in some tumours, but difficult to recognize in others, owing to the high degree of anaplasia. The regional heterogeneity of glioblastomas is remarkable and poses a serious challenge where the histopathological diagnosis is based solely on stereotaxic needle biopsies {177}.

Tissue patterns

The diagnosis of glioblastoma is typically based on the tissue pattern rather than on the identification of certain cell types. The presence of highly anaplastic glial cells, mitotic activity, vascular proliferation and/or necrosis is required. The distribution of these key elements within the tumour is variable but large necrotic areas usually occupy the tumour centre, while viable tumour cells tend to accumulate in the periphery. Vascular proliferation is seen throughout the lesion, with a certain tendency towards being found around necrotic foci and in the peripheral infiltration zone.

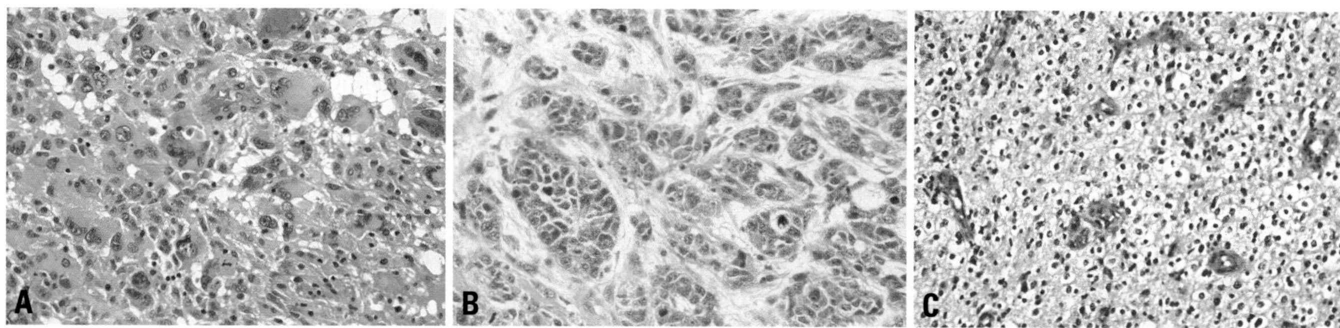

Fig. 1.26 **A** Glioblastoma with high degree of anaplasia. **B** Adenoid GBM with formation of glandular structures. **C** Oligodendroglial component in a GBM.

Secondary structures

The migratory capacity of glioblastoma cells within the CNS becomes readily apparent when they reach borders that constitute a barrier: tumour cells line up and accumulate in the subpial zone of the cortex, in the subependymal region and around neurons ('satellitosis'). Such patterns are called 'secondary structures' {1341}. They result from the interaction of glioma cells with host brain structures, and are highly diagnostic. This concept also extends to the adaptation of tumour cells to myelinated pathways, where they often acquire a fusiform, polar shape. The unequivocal identification of neoplastic astrocytes in the perifocal oedema and at more distant sites poses a challenge for the pathologist, in particular, when dealing with stereotaxic biopsies {306}. A feature of many glioblastomas, especially the small cell variants, is the extensive involvement of the cerebral cortex. A series of so-called 'secondary structures' may be noted, as in other highly infiltrative gliomas such as gliomatosis cerebri and oligodendroglioma {1339, 1341}. These formations are seen as aggregation of cells in the subpial zone, the immediate perineuronal regions or the perivascular regions. Frequently, in the terminal stages of disease, the subependymal region is also diffusely infiltrated. Secondary structures and most of the apparently multifocal glioblastomas reflect the pathways of migration of glioma cells in the CNS {2447}.

Epithelial structures

Occasionally, glioblastomas contain foci with glandular and ribbon-like epithelial structures {1284}. These elements have a large oval nucleus, prominent nucleolus and round, well-defined cytoplasms. They are also referred to as 'adenoid' glioblastoma. Expression of GFAP in these areas may be reduced, but the astrocytic nature of these structures can usually be established unequivocally. Small cells with even more epithelial features and cohesiveness are less common {756}. A mucinous background and a 'mesenchymal' component (gliosarcoma) are not uncommon in such neoplasms.

Cellular composition

Few human neoplasms are as heterogeneous in composition as are glioblastomas. While poorly differentiated, fusiform, round or pleomorphic cells may prevail, more differentiated neoplastic astrocytes are usually discernible, at least focally {177}. This is particularly true of glioblastomas resulting from the progression of diffuse astrocytomas WHO grade II. The transition between areas that still have recognisable astrocytic differentiation and highly anaplastic cells may be continuous or abrupt. A sudden change in morphology may reflect the emergence of a new tumour phenotype through the acquisition of one or more additional genetic alterations {2455}.

Cellular pleomorphism includes the formation of small, undifferentiated, lipidized, granular and giant cells. In addition, there are often areas where bipolar, fusiform cells form intersecting bundles and fascicles prevail. The accumulation of highly polymorphic tumour cells with well-delineated plasma membranes and a lack of cell processes may mimic metastatic carcinomas or melanomas.

Multinucleated giant cells

Large, multinucleated tumour cells are often considered a hallmark of glioblastomas and occur with a spectrum of increasing size and pleomorphism. The presence

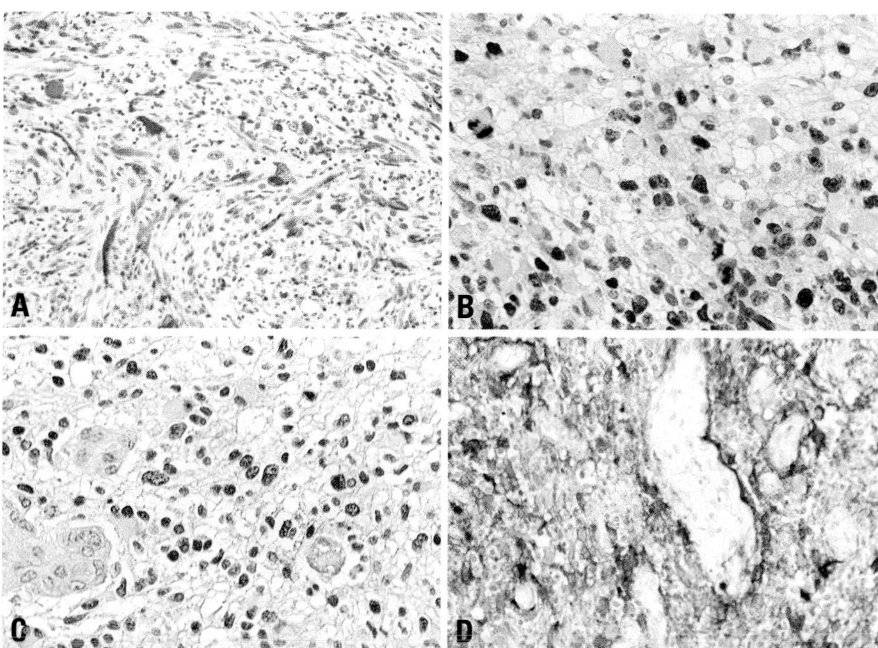

Fig. 1.27 Glioblastomas with **(A)** variable degree of GFAP expression, **(B)** high proliferative activity (immunoreactivity to MIB-1), **(C)** nuclear accumulation of TP53 protein in tumour cells but not endothelial cells, **(D)** overexpression of the EGF receptor in the plasma membrane of glioma cells.

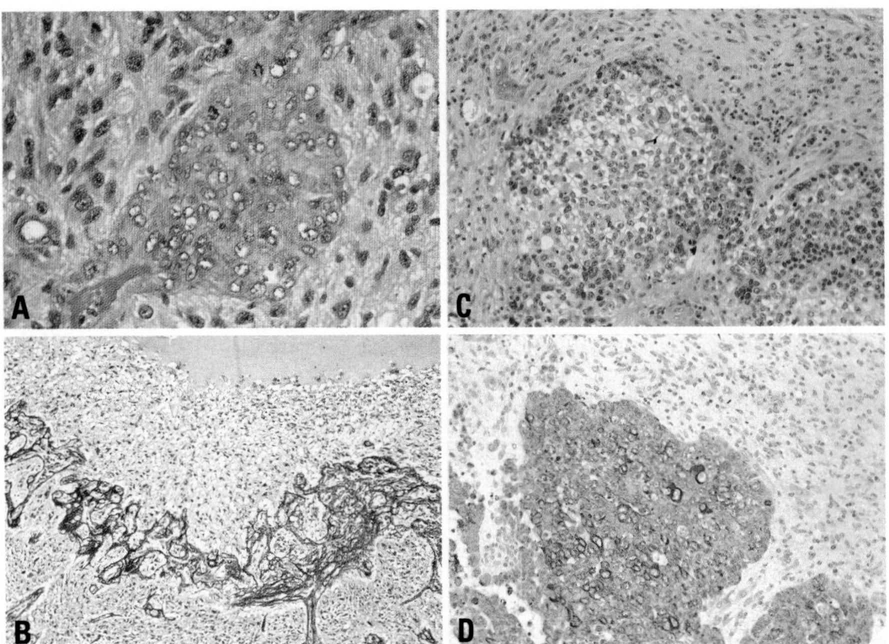

Fig. 1.28 A,B Microvascular proliferation in a glioblastoma with **(A)** formation of a multilayerd 'glomeroid tuft' and **(B)** reticulin stain showing a 'fenton' of proliferated glioma vessels. **C** Squamous cell metaplasia in a glioblastoma with **(D)** marked cytokeratin expression.

of multinucleated giant cells is typical of glioblastoma, but is neither an obligatory feature nor associated with a more malignant clinical course {175}.
Despite their malignant appearance, these cells are regarded as a type of regressive change. If multinucleated giant cells dominate the histopathological picture, the designation 'giant cell glioblastoma' is justified (see below).

Gemistocytes
At the other extreme of glioblastoma differentiation are 'gemistocytes' and the related 'fibrillary astrocyte', recognizing that transition forms connect these two types. Gemistocytes have copious, glassy, nonfibrillary cytoplasm that appears to displace the dark, angulated nucleus to the periphery of the cell. Processes radiate from the cytoplasm, but are stubby and not long-reaching. GFAP staining is largely confined to the periphery of the cell, with the central hyalin organelle-rich zone remaining largely unstained. Perivascular lymphocytes frequently populate gemistocytic regions while often avoiding other regions in the same neoplasm. Immunohistochemical studies have emphasised the low proliferation index of the neoplastic gemistocyte itself, despite the tendency of gemistocytic astrocytoma WHO grade II or III lesions to rapidly progress to glioblastoma {1587}. When present in large numbers, particularly in a patient known to have a pre-existing glioma, these cells may represent a lower-grade precursor lesion within a 'secondary glioblastoma'. Better-differentiated areas can sometimes be identified radiographically as a non-contrast-enhancing peripheral region and, in whole brain sections, as grade II to III astrocytomas clearly distinct from foci of glioblastoma {177, 1339}.

Granular cells
Large cells with a granular, periodic acid-Schiff (PAS) positive cytoplasm may occur scattered within glioblastomas. In rare cases, they may dominate and create the impression of a granular cell tumour indistinguishable from that of the pituitary stalk or other tissues {327, 541}, where they are thought to be myogenic or Schwann-cell-derived (see chapter 15). GFAP expression may be absent, but transitional forms between granular cells and neoplastic astrocytes can be identified. There have been reports of rare cases of malignant cerebral granular cell tumours without any apparent link to a glioblastoma {22, 253, 744}. The immunohistochemical profile varies, but the consistent PAS-positivity and the frequent immunoreactivity for alpha-1-antichymotrypsin and MB2 suggest a histiocytic origin. However, in these cases, GFAP immunoreactivity is also present in some tumour cells. On the basis of both these and additional, recently reported findings {459}, it is most likely that the granular cells represent glioma cells with a distinct degenerative pathway.

Lipidized cells
Cells with a foamy cytoplasm are another feature occasionally observed in glioblastomas. In rare cases, they predominate, and the respective lesion has been designated 'malignant glioma with heavily lipidized (foamy) tumour cells' {752, 758, 1284, 1483}. The lipidized cells may be grossly enlarged {463}. If such lesions are superficially located in young people, the diagnosis of pleomorphic xanthoastrocytoma should be considered, particularly if the xanthomatous cells are surrounded by basement membranes positive on reticulin staining {753}.

Perivascular lymphocytes
Perivascular lymphocyte cuffing occurs in the majority of glioblastomas. Most typically, lymphocytic infiltration is present in areas with a marked gemistocytic component. They have been phenotypically characterized on the basis of their immunoreactivity. CD8+ T-lymphocytes, which are MHC-class-I-restricted, prevail and occur in approximately 75% of tumours. CD4+ lymphocytes appear to be present in smaller numbers {134, 1286} while B-lymphocytes are detectable in less then 10% of cases {1286}. Expression of CD44 and ICAM-1 is observed in glioma cells, but not in tumour-infiltrating lymphocytes {838}. Whether perivascular lymphocyte infiltration influences tumour growth is still a matter of dispute: while some studies indicate a beneficial effect {162, 1125}, others failed to note a correlation with patient survival {184, 649}. In addition to haematogeneous lymphocytes, there are perivascular cells that are supposedly resident in the CNS; they express MHC class II antigens and immunoreactivity to PGM1 antibody, and may have a scavenger role {767}.

Metaplasia
In general, this term refers to the reversible acquisition by a differentiated cell of morphological features typical of another differentiated cell type, and is most frequently observed as a preneoplastic lesion of epithelial tissues. However, the term is also used to designate aberrant differentiation in neoplasms. In glioblastomas, this is exemplified by foci displaying fea-

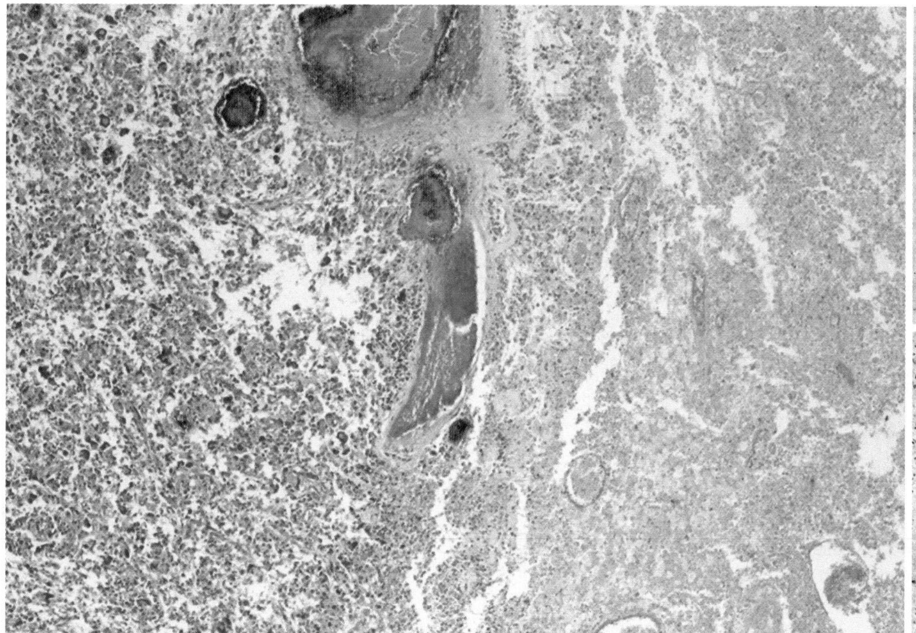

Fig. 1.29 Necrogenesis in glioblastoma. Large ischaemic necrosis (right). Also note several large, thrombosed tumour vessels.

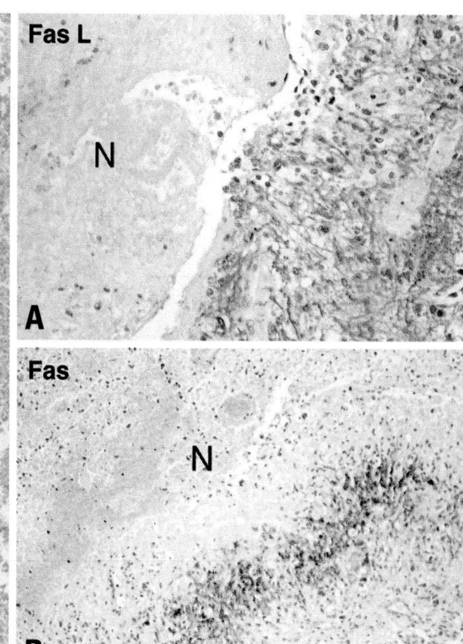

Fig.1.31 Necrosis (N) in glioblastoma. Constitutive, diffuse expression of Fas ligand vs selective induction of Fas in perinecrotic tumour cells. Reprinted from Gratas *et al.* {502}.

tures of squamous epithelial cells, *i.e.* epithelial whorls with keratin pearls and cytokeratin expression {180, 1039}. On the cellular level, immunoreactivity for GFAP and cytokeratins are mutually exclusive {1039}. Adenoid and squamous epithelial metaplasia is more common in gliosarcomas than in the ordinary glioblastoma {756, 1039}. This is similarly true for the formation of bone and cartilage, which prevails in gliosarcomas (see below) and in a variety of childhood CNS neoplasms {969}.

Microvascular proliferation

In addition to necroses, the presence of microvascular proliferations (previously called endothelial cell proliferations) is a histopathological hallmark of glioblastomas. On light microscopy, microvascular proliferations typically appear as 'glomeruloid tufts', which are most commonly located in the vicinity of necrosis. Histologically, microvascular proliferations in glioblastoma typically consist of multilayered, mitotically active endothelial cells together with smooth muscle cells/ pericytes {522, 1051, 1609}. Morphologically inconspicuous vessels have an MIB-1 labelling index of 2-4% while proliferated tumour vessels have an index of >10% {1584}. Vascular thrombosis often occurs, and this may play a role in the pathogenesis of ischaemic tumour necrosis.

Necrosis and apoptosis

Two major types of necrosis can be distinguished. Those seen macroscopically and by neuroimaging as non-enhancing core are large areas of destroyed tumour tissue and may comprise more than 80% of the total tumour mass. Microscopically, they appear as a yellow or white granular coagulum {173} in which necrotic glioma cells can still vaguely be identified, as well as the faded images of large, dilated necrotic tumour vessels. These areas of necrosis do not generally attract a large number of phagocytes. Occasionally, preserved tumour vessels with a corona of viable tumour cells are seen within extensive areas of necrosis. It is assumed that these large necroses are due to insufficient blood supply and are therefore ischaemic in nature. Large ischaemic necroses are a hallmark of the primary glioblastoma {1340, 1503} and are associated with poor prognosis {65, 175, 1065}. Although the Fas receptor is preferentially expressed in glioma cells surrounding such areas of necrosis, apoptosis is not a common fea-

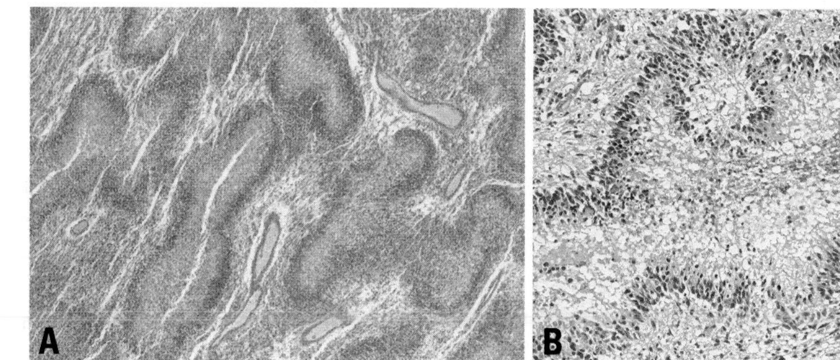

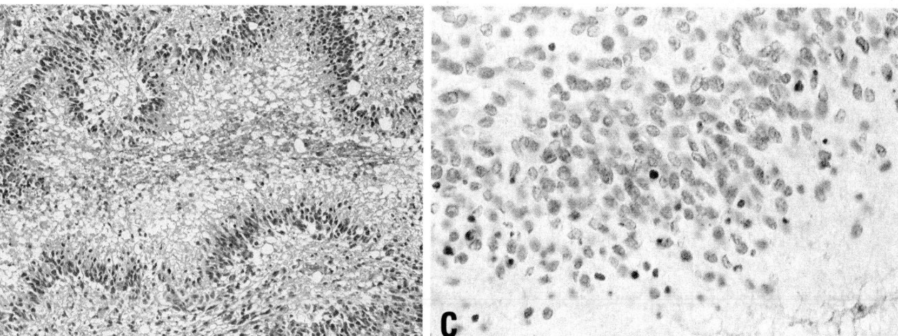

Fig. 1.30 Necrogenesis in glioblastoma. **A** Multiple serpentine pseudopalisading necroses. **B** Higher magnification showing peripheral accumulation and pseudopalisading of tumour cells, many of which undergo apoptosis, as demonstrated by TUNEL immunohistochemistry (**C**).

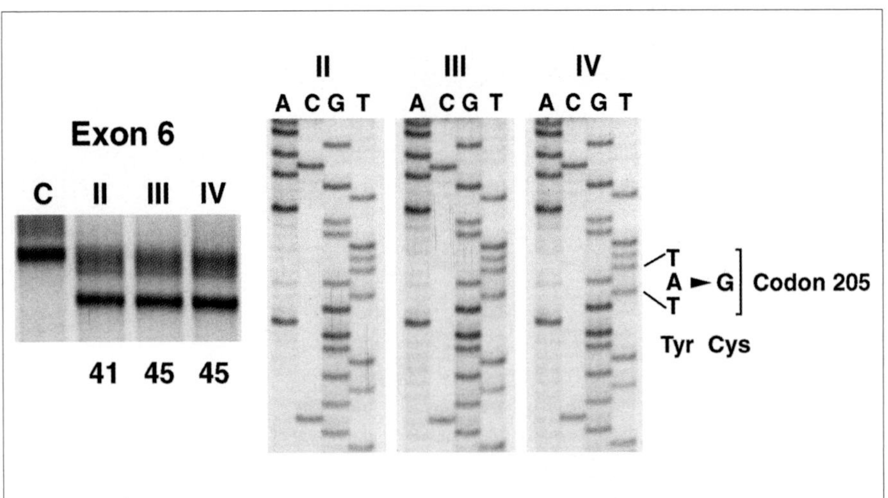

Fig. 1.32 SSCP analysis and DNA sequencing autoradiographs of exon 6 of the *TP53* gene in a patient who had subsequent biopsies for low-grade (WHO grade II), anaplastic astrocytoma (WHO grade III) and glioblastoma (WHO grade IV) at the age of 41 and 45 years. Mobility shift (left) and TAT->TGT point mutation (right) were present from the first biopsy. Reprinted from Watanabe *et al.* {1585}.

ture {1477}. Another pathway potentially important in regulating death of glioma cells involves APO2L/TRAIL and its receptors {2446}. APO2L is consistently expressed in astrocytic tumours largely irrespective of their degree of malignancy.
A second type of necrosis consists of multiple, small, irregularly-shaped band-like {1686} or serpiginous {180} foci, surrounded by radially orientated, densely packed, small, fusiform glioma cells in a 'pseudopalisading' pattern, a histological hallmark of the glioblastoma {859}. The central area of such foci often consists of a fine fibrillary network in which neither viable nor necrotic glioma cells are identified. Instead, pseudopalisading glioma cells frequently undergo apoptosis, suggesting that this unique tissue pattern results from programmed cell death at lower degrees of focal hypoxia. These pseudopalisading necroses are equally frequent in primary and secondary glioblastomas {1503}. The pseudopalisading cells strongly express VEGF. This upregulation is induced by hypoxia {1185,1416} and is considered responsible for microvascular proliferation. Although many aspects of necrogenesis remain to be elucidated, the histology of glioblastomas is compatible with a sequence starting from small clusters of apoptotic cells, which then enlarge into pseudopalisading necrosis and, eventually, large areas of ischaemic necrosis.

Immunohistochemistry

The degree and geographic extent of GFAP reactivity is highly variable in glioblastomas. Generally, astrocyte-like tumour cells, in particular gemistocytes, are strongly positive, while small, undifferentiated cells tend to be negative or stain only weakly. Multinucleated giant cells stain variably, with marked differences in GFAP expression even between neighbouring cells. Although large portions of a glioblastoma may lack GFAP expression, wider sampling usually reveals at least occasional tumour cells that are immunoreactive for this marker. Although GFAP expression tends to decrease during glioma progression, there is no indication that its extent is a prognostic factor. On occasion, sharply delineated, round, GFAP-negative foci arise on the background of a more differentiated lesion {1367, 1368}, suggesting the emergence of a new tumour clone through the acquisition of an additional genetic alteration {2455}. Vimentin expression is common. Less consistent is immunoreactivity for αB-crystallin and ubiquitin {735}.
Several transformation-associated genes are frequently upregulated in glioblastomas, including *EGFR, MDM2*, and *PDGF* receptor alpha and this can be assessed immunohistochemically. Similarly, loss of expression (*CDKN2A, RB, p27*) or amplification (*CDK4*) of genes involved in cell cycle regulation has been analyzed on a cellular level but this cannot generally replace molecular genetic analyses {2340}. Expression of the gap junction protein connexin43 is reduced in glioblastomas, reflecting an impairment of cell to cell interaction {2452}; transfection of cx43 into glioblastoma cells was shown to reverse the neoplastic phenotype {2453}. Hepatocyte growth factor/scatter factor (HGF/SF) modulates mitogenesis, and glioma motility and may act as a chemokine for microglia {2441}. The co-expression of HGF/SF and its receptor c-Met is greatly enhanced in glioblastomas, as shown by fluorescence staining {2451} and immunohistochemistry {2442}.

Ultrastructure

The polymorphic nature of the glioblastoma is also evident from electron microscopic studies. The number of intermediate filaments present depends on the degree of differentiation. Enlarged mitochondria containing atypical christae have been noted, as have undulation of the plasma membrane and frequent intranuclear cytoplasmic invaginations. Tonofilament bundles are often lacking and intercellular contacts are poorly developed {1306}. None of these features is of diagnostic relevance.

Proliferation

Proliferative activity is usually prominent, with numerous typical and atypical mitoses. The growth fraction, as determined by the antibodies Ki67/MIB-1, shows great regional variation. Mean values of 15–20% have been reported {182, 324, 683, 728, 1374}. Small, undifferentiated, fusiform cells often show marked proliferative activity, in contrast to neoplastic gemistocytes, which typically have a lesser degree of proliferation {1587}.

Molecular genetics

Malignant transformation of neuroepithelial cells is a multistep process driven by the sequential acquisition of genetic alterations. One would, therefore expect that of all astrocytic neoplasms, the glioblastoma should contain the greatest number of genetic changes and this is indeed the case.
On the basis of the different combinations of *TP53* mutations, loss of heterozygosity on chromosomes 17p and *EGFR* amplification the presence of subsets of glioblastomas with distinct genetic alterations was postulated {855, 1567}. A study by von Deimling *et al.* {1567} showed that *EGFR* amplification occurs significantly more often in elderly patients, without LOH on chromosome 17p. Lang *et al.* {855} characterized *de novo* glioblastomas as tumours without *TP53* mutations but with

amplification of *EGFR* and LOH of chromosome 10 {855}, and glioblastomas that progressed from astrocytoma as neoplasms with *TP53* mutations and LOH of chromosome 17p.

Primary vs. secondary glioblastoma
Over the past five years, the concept of different genetic pathways leading to the glioblastoma as the common phenotypic endpoint has gained general acceptance. As shown in Fig. 1.33, these pathways show little overlapping, indicating that genetically, primary and secondary glioblastomas constitute different disease entities. However, most of the data generated so far are based on cohorts of patients carefully selected on the basis of clinical and histopathological criteria {1586, 2434} and additional pathways to glioblastoma may exist {1799}. This has already been shown for two histopathological variants, the giant cell glioblastoma and the gliosarcoma (see next chapters).

EGFR. The epidermal growth factor receptor (*EGFR*) gene is involved in the control of cell proliferation and is amplified and overexpressed in more than one third of glioblastoma cases, sometimes in a truncated and rearranged form {896, 367, 1637}. Glioblastomas with *EGFR* amplification typically show a simultaneous loss of chromosome 10 {1564, 855}. In unselected series of glioblastomas, *EGFR* amplification has been reported to occur at a frequency of approximately 30-40% {1799, 1098}. In a study by Tohma *et al.*, *EGFR* amplification was present in 11/28 (39%) of primary, but in none of 22 secondary glioblastomas {1754}. Immunoreactivity for the EGFR also prevailed in primary glioblastomas (>60% of cases) vs. 10% in secondary glioblastomas {1586}. All primary glioblastomas with *EGFR* amplification showed EGFR overexpression and 11 of 15 (73%) of those with EGFR overexpression showed *EGFR* amplification {1754}. Only one out of 49 glioblastomas showed EGFR overexpression and a *TP53* mutation {1586}. This indicates that overexpression of EGFR and mutations of the *TP53* tumour suppressor gene are mutually exclusive events in the evolution of primary and secondary glioblastoma, respectively {1586}.

TP53. *TP53* mutations were among the first genetic alterations identified in astrocytic brain tumours {2460}. In unselected series of glioblastomas, the reported frequency varies considerably, with a mean of 25-30% {915, 1098}. A different picture emerges if primary and secondary glioblastomas are analysed separately. *TP53* mutations are less common in primary (*de novo*) glioblastomas (~10%) while secondary glioblastomas have a high incidence of *TP53* mutations (>65%), of which >90% are already present in the first biopsy {1585, 1586, 2448, 558}. The frequency of TP53 protein accumulation is higher than that of *TP53* mutations {855, 2386, 1072, 1585} but is also significantly higher in secondary (>90%) than in primary glioblastomas (<35%) {1586}. The percentage of glioma cells with TP53 protein accumulation appears to increase from the first biopsy to recurrent tumours {1245, 1585} and one study suggests that this reflects the clonal expansion of glioma cells carrying a *TP53* mutation {1417}.

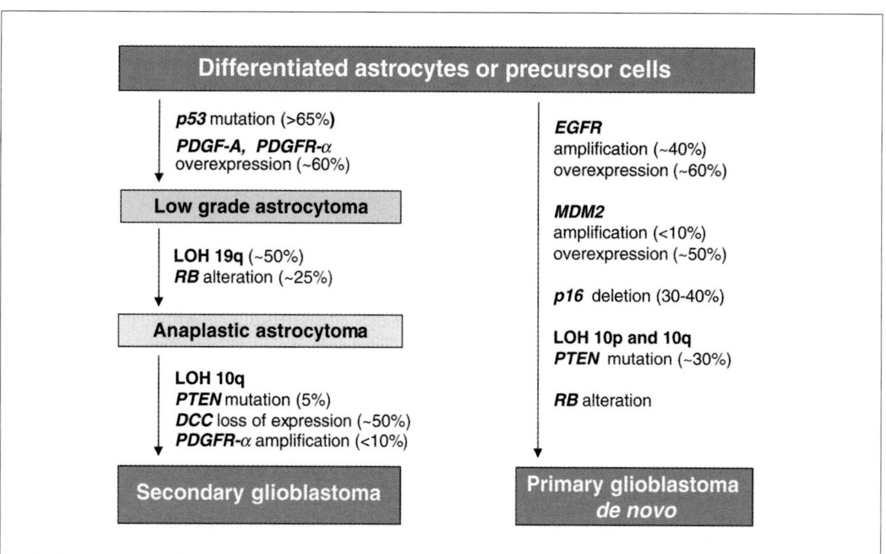

Fig. 1.33 Genetic pathways operative in the evolution of primary and secondary glioblastoma. Modified, from Kleihues and Ohgaki {2434}.

MDM2. The MDM2 protein forms a complex with TP53, thereby abolishing its transcriptional activity {1672}. Thus, MDM2 amplification/overexpression constitutes an alternative mechanism to escape from TP53-regulated control of cell growth. Amplification of *MDM2* is present in ~8% of glioblastomas {1239} and all of these appear to be primary glioblastomas which lack a *TP53* mutation {1239, 113}. Overexpression of MDM2 is observed immunohistochemically in more than 50% of primary glioblastomas, but the fraction of immunoreactive cells varies considerably {113, 2351, 1745}. In contrast, less than 10% of secondary glioblastomas show overexpression of *MDM2*. Thus, overexpression of *MDM2*, with and without gene amplification, is a genetic hallmark of the primary glioblastoma that typically lacks a *TP53* mutation.

It has been reported that the majority of glioblastomas (22 of 32; 69%) contains short forms of alternatively spliced *MDM2* transcripts which lack a region that includes the TP53 binding domain {2459}. The biological significance of these splice variants is still unclear. A recent study suggests, that wild-type TP53 stabilisation occurs in the presence of an *MDM2* splice variant and that this could explain wilde-type TP53 protein accumulation in glioblastoma cells even in the presence of *MDM2* gene amplification {2445}.

CDKN2A and MDM2. The *CDKN2A* locus codes for two gene products (p16 and $p14^{ARF}$) through differences in the first exon and alternative reading frames located in the common second exon {2440}. The putative tumour suppressor $p14^{ARF}$ blocks MDM2-induced degradation and transactivational silencing of TP53 by blocking nucleo-cytoplasmic shuttling of the *MDM2* gene product {2444}.

CDKN2A, CDK4, and RB pathway. The p16 tumour suppressor is also encoded by *CDKN2A* and exerts growth control by inhibition of the cyclin-dependent kinases CDK4 and CDK6, which reduces their capacity to phosphorylate, in conjunction with cyclin D, the RB protein, and thereby allowing G_1/S phase transition of the cell cycle. Thus, loss of cell cycle control may result from altered expression of any of these genes, *i.e.* loss of *p16* expression, overexpression/amplification of CDKs or loss of RB function. In unselected and selected series of glioblastomas, *p16* deletion and RB alterations were found to be mutually exclusive {1525, 1693, 2340}. Inactivation of genes in this pathway is common in both primary and secondary glioblastomas {1693} at an overall frequency of 40-50%. There was no difference in the frequency of loss of RB expression or *CDK4* amplification, but *p16* deletions were significantly more frequent in primary (36%) than in secondary glioblastomas (4%) {1693}. The majority of glioblastomas with *EGFR* amplification shows a *p16* deletion {2443, 558}. This corroborates data showing that homozygous deletion of *p16* occurs in one third of primary glioblastomas but is rarely observed in secondary glioblastomas {1693}. One-third of glioblastomas with normal p16 expression showed accumulation of MDM2 protein ($P<0.05$) {1745}.

PDGFR. Platelet derived growth factor (PDGF), a major mitogen for connective tissue cells and glia, is a dimer composed of combinations of A and B chains. The ligands are recognized by two types of cell surface receptors, PDGFR-α and PDGFR-β, which belong to the tyrosine kinase family of receptors {254, 566}. PDGFR-α overexpression was found in both low- and high-grade astrocytomas, suggesting that PDGFR-α is involved in tumour cell proliferation in both early and late stages of glioma development. In contrast, amplification of the PDGFR-α gene was detected only in a small fraction (16%) of glioblastomas {577}. Comparison of *in situ* hybridisation for PDGFR-α with genetic alterations in the same tumour showed a significant correlation between high expression levels of PDGFR-α and loss of heterozygosity on chromosome 17p {577}. This suggests that amplification and overexpression of PDGFR-α is typical in the pathway leading to secondary glioblastomas.

LOH on chromosome 10, PTEN (MMAC1) and DMBT1. Loss of heterozygosity (LOH) on large regions at 10p, 10q23, and 10q25-26 loci or loss of an entire copy of chromosome 10 are the most frequent genetic alterations in glioblastomas {1567, 855, 2458}.

The tumour suppressor gene *PTEN* (*MMAC1*) on chromosome 10q23.3 {1451, 893} is mutated in approximately 30% of unselected glioblastomas {2339, 2155, 1910, 2375}. Mutations are absent in diffuse astrocytomas WHO grade II and rare in anaplastic astrocytomas, they were initially considered a late event during astrocytoma progression. However, a recent study showed that *PTEN* mutations occur almost exclusively in primary (*de novo*) glioblastomas (32%) and rarely (4%) in secondary glioblastomas {1754}.

The gene Deleted in Malignant Brain Tumours 1 (*DMBT1*) on chromosome 10q25-26 is considered a candidate tumour suppressor {1775}. It is homozygously deleted in 23 to 38% of glioblastomas {1775, 2368}. The genomic structure of *DMBT1* has recently been elucidated and points to a possible role of this gene in the evolution of chromosomal instability {2457}.

There is evidence that loss of chromosome 10 is a determining factor in the evolution of the glioblastoma phenotype. The formation of foci of histologically abrupt transition from diffuse astrocytoma WHO grade II or anaplastic astrocytoma to glioblastoma (Fig. 1.4) is frequently associated with LOH on 10q {2455}. Primary glioblastomas with LOH10 usually show loss of the entire chromosome while in secondary glioblastomas LOH is usually restricted to chromosome 10q {2456}.

LOH #19q. LOH on chromosome 19q was reported to occur in 44% of anaplastic astrocytomas and 21-24% of glioblastomas {1565, 2461}. The somewhat lower frequency in unselected glioblastomas may suggest that this change is typical for the pathway leading to secondary glioblastomas. This was confirmed by microsatellite analyses showing that LOH on 19q is more frequent in secondary (54% of cases) than in primary (6%) glioblastomas {2478}.

Adult vs. paediatric glioblastomas

Glioblastomas in children have a pattern of genetic alterations different from that in glioblastomas of adult patients. Among glioblastomas analyzed to date, approximately 40% show *TP53* gene mutations and a similar frequency for LOH 17p. This frequency is somewhat lower than that of secondary glioblastomas although paediatric glioblastomas usually develop *de novo*. An exception are malignant brainstem glioblastomas of children in which *TP53* mutations occur at a frequency of >50%. The genetic pathway leading to primary (*de novo*) glioblastoma of elderly patients (>45 years) appears to be very rarely involved in children, as reflected by the low frequency of *EGFR* amplification (6%), *CDKN2A* deletion (19%) and the absence of *MDM2* amplification {2519, 2520}. LOH on chromosome 10 occurs at a high frequency (> 50%) in paediatric and adult glioblastomas, supporting the view that LOH 10 is instrumental in the evolution of the glioblastoma phenotype.

Predictive factors

Despite extensive clinical trials, individual prediction of clinical outcome has remained an elusive goal. These attempts should be judged in view of the fact that glioblastomas are among the most malignant human neoplasm with a mean total length of disease of patients with primary glioblastoma of less than one year and the depressing observation that after exclusion of malignant oligodendrogliomas and irrespective of aggressive radio- and chemotherapy, only 5 out of 279 patients (1,8%) survived more than 3 years {2438}.

Necrosis. Several studies suggest that the presence and extent of necrosis in glioblastomas correlates with poor clinical outcome {65, 175, 1065, 2439}. The area of necrosis was usually smaller in young adults, reflecting their overall more favourable prognosis.

Clinical prognostic factors. Evaluation of the extent of resection as prognostic factor has been controversial, but there is some evidence that complete resection favours longer survival {14, 332, 1625, 1639}. In one study using magnetic resonance imaging, individuals with malignant gliomas for which residual tumour visualised postoperatively had a significantly higher (6.6 fold) risk of death (shorter survival time) than those in whom all of the contrast-enhancing tumour had been removed {14}. Not all studies show a significant survival difference for lesions with a greater extent of resection {809}.

Age. Young patients (below 45 years) have a considerably better prognosis than the elderly {175, 1318, 1434}. This may in part be explained by the higher frequency of secondary glioblastomas in younger patients {175, 1586} but some data suggest an intrinsically more rapid malignant progression in elderly patients {2416}.

Proliferation. There is general agreement that the proliferative potential of diffusely infiltrating astrocytomas correlates with histological grade {182, 469, 728, 1027, 1106, 1220}. In glioblastomas, tumour volume depends on the balance between proliferation and necrosis. While some studies suggest that glioblastomas can be subdivided on the basis of their proliferative activity {518, 1509, 1574}, others have failed to detect significant differences {1175}. There is general consensus that the MIB1 labelling index and related proliferation markers do not allow a prognosis in individual patients. A hypertriploid DNA profile appears to correlate with prolonged survival {1318}, and this correlates with the observation that the presence of multinucleated giant cells in glioblastomas is associated with a slightly better outcome {175}.

Genetic alterations. While some studies have reported that amplification and overexpression of the *EGFR* gene in anaplastic astrocytomas and glioblastomas is associated with poor prognosis {380, 587, 638, 1509}, other investigators have not confirmed this finding {117, 2437}. Similarly, TP53 immunostaining showed no prognostic significance {2437} An extensive study on 80 adult patients with glioblastoma showed that survival is not correlated with altered expression of *CDKN2A*, *TP53*, *EGFR*, *MDM2* or *Bcl-2* genes. However, high levels of expression of PTEN/MMAC1 {2436} were found to be associated with longer survival while high levels of expression of cathepsin B was a predictor of poor prognosis {2435}.

Giant cell glioblastoma

H. Ohgaki
A. Peraud
Y. Nakazato
K. Watanabe
A. von Deimling

Definition

A histological variant of glioblastoma with a predominance of bizarre, multinucleated giant cells, an occasionally abundant stromal reticulin network and a high frequency of *TP53* mutations.

ICD-O code: 9441/3

Grading

Giant cell glioblastoma corresponds histologically to WHO grade IV.

Synonyms and historical annotation

Because of the often prominent stromal reticulin network, the giant cell glioblastoma was originally termed monstrocellular sarcoma {1685, 1686} but the consistent expression of GFAP has firmly established its astrocytic nature {682, 1306, 779}.

Incidence

The giant cell glioblastoma (WHO grade IV) is a rare variant, which accounts for less than 1% of all brain tumours and up to 5% of glioblastomas {1124}.

Age and sex distribution

In a series of 35 cases, the mean age at clinical manifestation was 42 years, but the age distribution of this tumour covers a wider range than other diffuse astrocytomas and includes children {1000, 1165}. Males are more frequently affected (M/F ratio, 1.6).

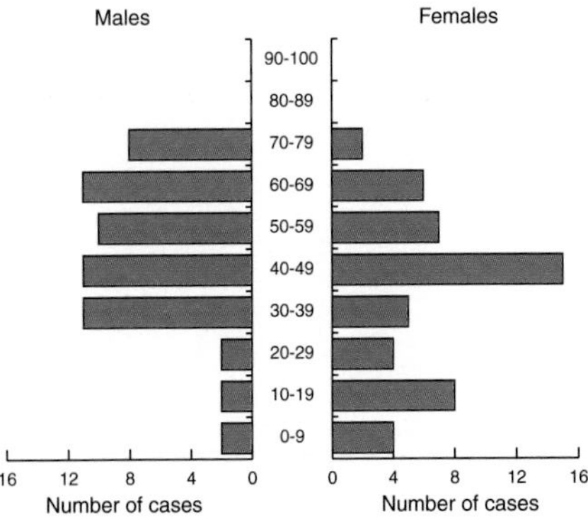

Fig. 1.34 Age distribution of giant cell glioblastoma, based on 108 published cases.

Clinical features

Symptoms and signs

Giant cell glioblastomas develop *de novo* after a short preoperative history and without clinical or radiological evidence of a less malignant precursor lesion. Symptoms are similar to those of the ordinary glioblastoma.

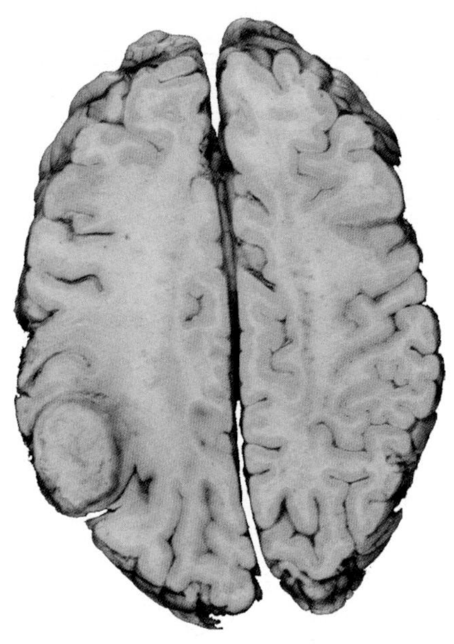

Fig. 1.35 Well-circumscribed, superficially located giant cell glioblastoma in the left parietal lobe.

Neuroimaging, localization and macroscopy

Giant cell glioblastomas are distinctive because of their circumscription and firmness caused by the marked production of tumour stroma. They are often located subcortically in the temporal and parietal lobes. On CT and MRI, they may mimic a metastasis.

Histopathology

A glioblastoma with numerous multinucleated giant cells, small fusiform syncytial cells and, to a varying extent, a reticulin network.

The giant cells are often extremely bizarre and may measure more than 500 µm in diameter. The number of nuclei ranges from a few to more than 20. They are often angulated, may contain prominent nucleoli and, on occasion, have cytoplasmic inclusions. Both pseudopalisading and large ischaemic necrosis are observed. Atypical mitoses are frequent, but the overall proliferation rate is similar to that of ordinary glioblastomas. GFAP expression is highly variable. Occasionally, perivascular lymphocyte cuffing is noted. A typical, although not invariable, feature is the perivascular accumulation of tumour cells with the formation of a pseudorosette-like pattern. Cases with *TP53* mutations typically show a marked nuclear accumulation of the gene product.

Table 1.2
Clinical and genetic profile of the giant cell glioblastoma, in comparison with primary and secondary glioblastoma. Modified, from Peraud *et al.* {2112}.

	Primary GBM	Giant cell GBM	Secondary GBM
Clinical onset	de novo	de novo	secondary
Preoperative history	1.7 mo.	1.6 mo.	>25 mo.
Age at GBM diagnosis	55 years	42 years	39 years
M/F ratio	1.4	1.6	0.8
PTEN mutation	32%	33%	4%
EGFR amplification	39%	5%	0%
TP53 mutation	11%	84%	67%
p16 (CDKN2A) deletion	36%	0%	4%

Genetics

Giant cell glioblastomas are characterized by frequent *TP53* mutations (75–90% of cases) and *PTEN* mutations (33%), but typically lack *EGFR* amplification/ overexpression and homozygous *p16* deletion {1000, 1165, 2112}. These results indicate that giant cell glioblastomas occupy a hybrid position, sharing with primary *(de novo)* glioblastomas a short clinical history, the absence of a less malignant precursor lesion and frequent *PTEN* mutations. With secondary glioblastomas that develop through progression from low-grade astrocytomas, they have in common a younger patient age at manifestation and a high frequency of *TP53* mutations {2112}.

Prognosis

Most giant cell glioblastomas carry a poor prognosis {2517} but some reports indicate that the clinical outcome is somewhat better than that of the ordinary glioblastoma {80, 184, 959, 2518}, possibly because of a less infiltrative behaviour.

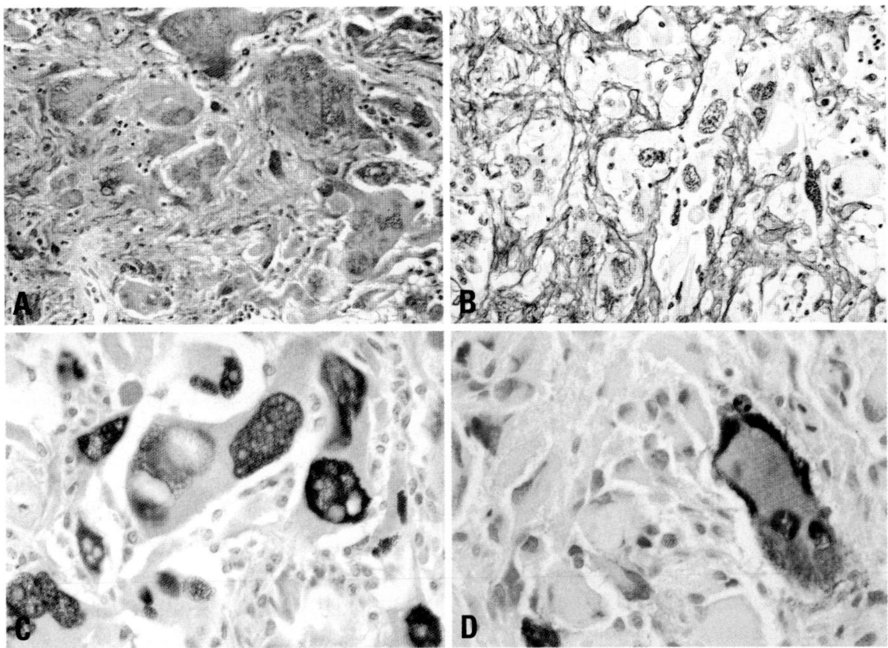

Fig. 1.37 Giant cell glioblastoma. **A** Most but not all tumour cells express GFAP. **B** Marked stromal reaction (Bodian silver stain). **C** Accumulation of TP53 protein in giant cell nuclei. **D** Occasional giant cells express EGFR, in the plasma membrane.

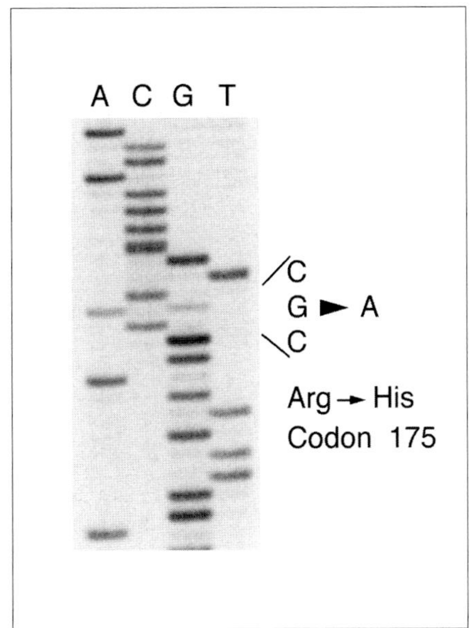

Fig. 1.36 GC->AT transition mutation in codon 175 of the *TP53* gene in a giant cell glioblastoma. Reprinted from Peraud *et al.* {1165}.

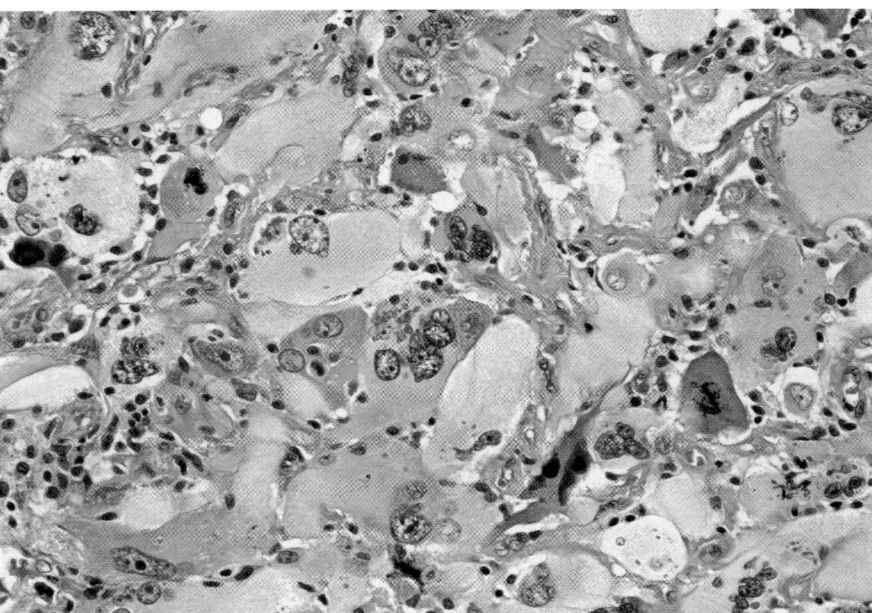

Fig. 1.38 Giant cell glioblastoma with typical bizarre monstrous multinucleated tumour cells. Nuclei vary in size and some cells show irregularly shaped chromatin fragments.

Gliosarcoma

H. Ohgaki
W. Biernat
R. Reis
M. Hegi
P. Kleihues

Definition

A glioblastoma variant characterized by a biphasic tissue pattern with alternating areas displaying glial and mesenchymal differentiation.

ICD-O code: 9442/3

Grading

Gliosarcomas correspond histologically to WHO grade IV.

Synonyms and historical annotation

The term gliosarcoma was introduced in 1898 by Stroebe {1463}. Feigin & Gross {397} defined the gliosarcoma as a glioblastoma in which proliferating tumour vessels had acquired the features of a sarcoma, but this view is not supported by recent genetic analysis which point to a monoclonal origin.

Incidence, age and sex distribution

It has been estimated that gliosarcomas constitute approximately 2% of all glioblastomas {399, 988}. The age distribution of 136 published cases is similar to that of the primary glioblastoma, with preferential manifestation between ages 40 and 60 (mean, 53 years). Males are more frequently affected (M:F ratio, 1.8:1).

Localization

Gliosarcomas are usually located in the cerebrum, involving the temporal, frontal, parietal and occipital lobes in decreasing order of frequency.

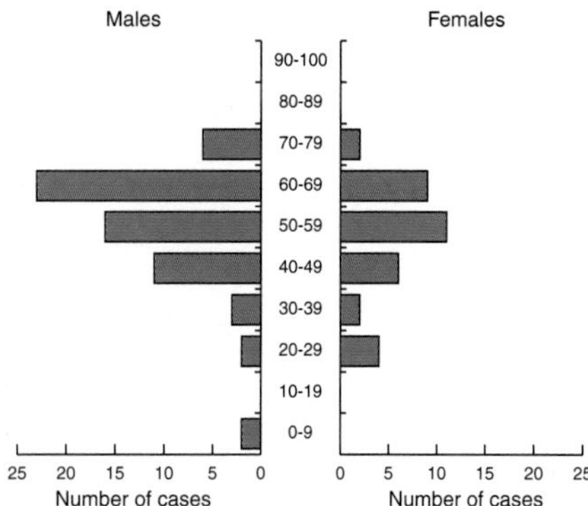

Fig. 1.39 Age distribution of gliosarcomas, based on 97 published cases.

Clinical features

Symptoms and signs

The symptoms reflect the location of the tumour and increased intracranial pressure. The clinical history is usually short; most patients present with seizures and paresis.

Neuroimaging

At angiography, some gliosarcomas reveal mixed dural and pial vascular supply {665}. CT scans often show the features of a diffusely infiltrating glioblastoma {947, 1457}. In cases with a predominant sarcomatous component, the tumour appears as a well-demarcated hyperdense mass with homogeneous contrast-enhancement {556, 947} which may mimic a meningioma.

Macroscopy

The sarcomatous component produces a firm, often superficial, rather discrete mass in a lesion that may elsewhere have typical features of glioblastoma.

Histopathology

A biphasic tissue pattern with areas displaying gliomatous or mesenchymal differentiation is essential for the diagnosis of the gliosarcoma. The occurrence of spindle cells within a glioblastoma does not justify the diagnosis of gliosarcoma; it is necessary to identify unequivocally areas with neoplastic mesenchymal appearance and reticulin formation.

The glial portion usually shows the typical features of a glioblastoma, with a varying degree of anaplasia and GFAP expression. The sarcomatous areas often show the typical herringbone pattern of fibrosarcomas, with densely packed long bundles of spindle cells. Occasionally, the histology resembles features of a malignant fibrous histiocytoma {988,1075}. The sarcomatous part also shows signs of malignant transformation, *e.g.* nuclear atypia, mitotic activity and necrosis. It forms a reticulin network, which shows that the sarcomatous areas are usually well-demarcated from the glial tumour portion. For diagnostic purposes, the demonstration of reticulin in the sarcomatous component and GFAP in the gliomatous portion is important {987}.

Gliosarcomas may show a variety of additional lines of mesenchymal differentiation, e.g. the formation of cartilage {63}, bone {969}, osteoid-chondral tissue {556, 1479}, and smooth and striated muscle {67, 523}. Furthermore, epithelial metaplasia with clusters of keratinizing stratified epithelia {1039} and adenoid formations {756} have been noted.

Genetics

Gliosarcomas show genetic aberrations similar to those occurring in glioblastomas, *i.e.* gain of chromosome 7, loss of chromosome 10 and 17, deletions of the short arm of chromosome 9, alterations of chromosome 3, and mutations of the *TP53* tumour suppressor gene {112, 135, 427, 1146, 2130} and the *PTEN* gene {2130}.

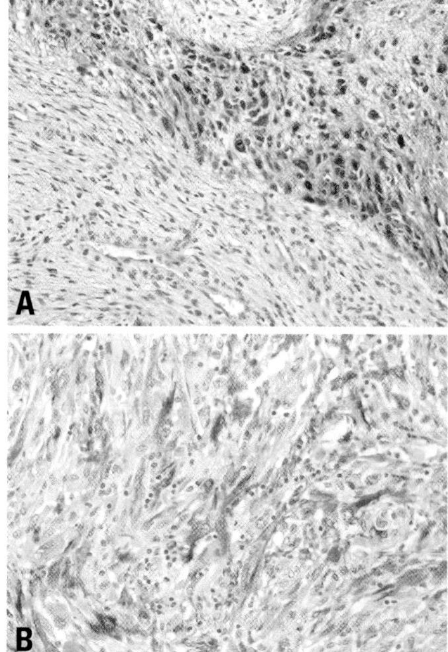

Fig. 1.40 Gliosarcoma. The gliomatous component shows strong GFAP expression and may be (**A**) geographically separated from or (**B**) intermingled with, the sarcomatous tumour cells.

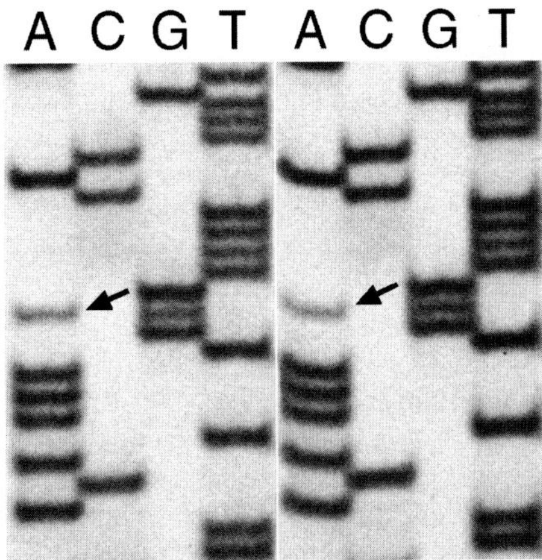

Fig. 1.41 Gliosarcoma. Glial and sarcomatous areas were microdissected. DNA sequencing revealed an identical G to A mutation (arrows) in codon 274 of the *PTEN* gene, suggesting a monoclonal origin of both tumour components. From Reis *et al.* {2130}.

Homozygous *p16 (CDKN2A)* deletion was detected by differential PCR in 7 (37%) gliosarcomas {2130}. The overall incidence of alterations in RB pathway (*p16* deletion, *CDK4* amplification, or loss of pRb immunoreactivity) was 53%, and these changes were mutually exclusive {2130}. None of the gliosarcomas showed *EGFR* amplification or overexpression {2130}. These data show that gliosarcomas have a distinct profile, similar to that of primary glioblastomas, except for the absence of overexpression or amplification of the *EGF* receptor. Similar genetic alterations have been found in the gliomatous and sarcomatous components, indicating a monoclonal origin (see below).

Histogenesis

As vascular proliferation is a hallmark of glioblastomas, the assumption that the sarcomatous component is of vascular origin seemed plausible biologically and was widely accepted. Several immunohistochemical studies seemed to support this concept by demonstrating immunoreactivity to factor-VIII-related antigen {1357}, *Ulex europaeus* I agglutinin (UEA-I) {1429}, and monohistiocytic markers {500, 501, 791}. Some studies suggested that the sarcomatous portion results from advanced glioma progression with loss of GFAP expression and acquisition of a sarcomatous phenotype {706, 987}. In a study using fluorescent *in situ* hybridisation, two of three gliosarcomas showed identical numerical aberrations of chromosomes 10 and 17 in the glial and

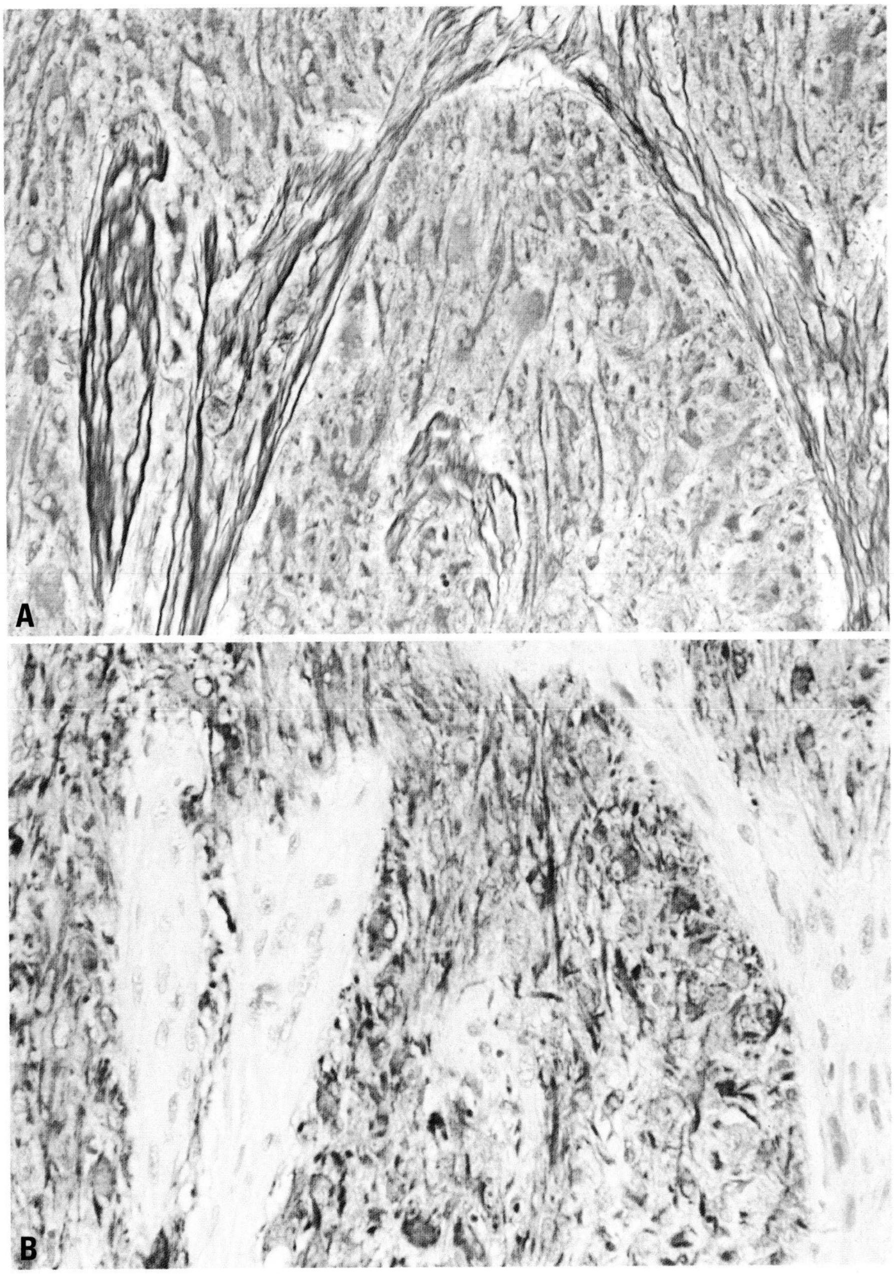

Fig. 1.42 Gliosarcoma. **A** Areas with a dense reticulin network are (**B**) largely devoid of tumour cells with glial phenotype and GFAP expression.

Table 1.3
Genetic and clinical profile of the gliosarcoma. Modified, from Reis *et al.* {2130}.

	Primary glioblastoma	Gliosarcoma
Preoperative clinical history	1.7 months	2 months
Sex ratio M/F	1.4	1.65
Age of diagnosis	55 yr	56 yr
TP53 mutation	1/19 (11%)	8/35 (23%)
PTEN mutation	9/28 (32%)	8/21 (38%)
p16 (CDKN2A) deletion	10/28 (36%)	7/19 (37%)
MDM2 amplification	8/104 (8%)	1/19 (5%)
EGFR amplification	11/28 (39%)	0/19 (0%)

mesenchymal components, whereas in a third case, trisomy X was restricted to the chondrosarcomatous element {1146}. Similar cytogenetic patterns were also observed in both glial and mesenchymal components in a study using fluorescent *in situ* hybridisation, comparative genomic hybridisation (CGH) and microsatellite allelic imbalance and cytogenetic analysis {135}. These results suggested that both were derived from neoplastic glial cells. This view has further been supported by the observation of TP53 immunoreactivity in both tumour components {17}. Biernat *et al.* {112} provided proof of a monoclonal origin by demonstrating that in two cases of gliosarcoma the gliomatous and sarcomatous components contained an identical *TP53* mutation. More recently, identical *PTEN* mutations, *p16 (CDKN2A)* deletions, and co-amplification of *MDM2* and *CDK4* were detected in the gliomatous and sarcomatous tumor components {2130}, strongly supporting the view that the sarcomatous areas represent a phenotypic change of glioblastoma cells, rather than constituting a separate, additional neoplasm.

Gliofibroma

Little is known about the histogenesis of the gliofibroma, an astrocytic neoplasm of young people that shows marked, ubiquitous deposition of a reticulin-positive collagenous matrix around glioma cells {1687}. In contrast to the gliosarcoma, the 'marbled' appearance of two tissue components is lacking. In some gliofibromas, collagen is produced by the glioma cells themselves ('desmoplastic astrocytoma') {1688}, whereas in others it appears to be deposited by mesenchymal cells (mixed glioma/fibroma) {1689}.

Prognostic factors

It has been suggested that gliosarcomas carry a somewhat more favourable prognosis {947} than ordinary glioblastomas, but large clinical trials have failed to reveal significant differences in outcome {988, 2113, 2114}.

Pilocytic astrocytoma

P.C. Burger
B.W. Scheithauer
W. Paulus
J. Szymas
C. Giannini
P. Kleihues

Definition
A generally circumscribed, slowly growing, often cystic astrocytoma occurring in children and young adults, histologically characterized by a biphasic pattern with varying proportion of compacted bipolar cells with Rosenthal fibers and loose textured multipolar cells with microcysts and granular bodies.

ICD-O code: 9421/1

Grading
Pilocytic astrocytomas correspond to WHO grade I.

Incidence
Pilocytic astrocytoma, the most common glioma in children, represents 10% of cerebral and 85% of cerebellar astrocytomas.

Age and sex distribution
Pilocytic astrocytomas typically present in the first two decades show, with no clear gender predilection; thereafter, the incidence decreases, with only few examples manifesting in patients older than 50 years.

Localization
Pilocytic astrocytomas arise throughout the neuraxis. Preferred sites include: (1) optic nerve ('optic nerve glioma') {624}, (2) optic chiasm/hypothalamus {1269}, (3) thalamus and basal ganglia {975}, (4) cerebral hemispheres {256, 423, 741, 1126, 1190}, (5) cerebellum ('cerebellar astrocytoma') {293, 559}, and (6) brainstem (dorsal exophytic brainstem glioma) {171, 172, 764, 1192}. Pilocytic astrocytomas of the spinal cord are less frequent but not uncommon {1015, 1234, 1287}. Large hypothalamic, thalamic, and brainstem lesions may be predominantly intraventricular, their site of origin being difficult to define.

Clinical features
Signs and symptoms
Pilocytic astrocytomas produce focal neurological deficits or nonlocalizing signs *e.g.*, macrocephaly, headache, endocrinopathy, or increased intracranial pressure due to mass effect or ventricular obstruction. Seizures are uncommon since the lesions infrequently involve the cerebral cortex {256, 423}. Given their slow rate of growth, the clinical presentation of pilocytic tumours is generally not that of a rapidly evolving lesion.
Pilocytic astrocytomas of the optic pathways often produce visual loss. Proptosis may be seen with intraorbital examples. Early, radiologically detected lesions may be unassociated with visual symptoms or ophthalmologic deficits {624, 902}. Hypothalamic/pituitary dysfunction, including obesity and diabetes insipidus, is often but not invariably apparent in large hypothalamic examples {1269}. Some hypothalamic-chiasmatic lesions of young children have been associated with leptomeningeal seeding and a poor outcome {2077}. It is unclear whether such tumours constitute a distinct entity {284, 2078}.
Pilocytic astrocytomas of the thalamus generally present with signs of CSF obstruction or neurological deficits, such as hemiparesis, due to internal capsule compression.
Cerebellar pilocytic astrocytomas usually present in the first two decades with clumsiness, increased headache, nausea, and vomiting. Brainstem examples often cause hydrocephalus or signs of brainstem dysfunction. In contrast to diffuse astrocytoma of the pons, which produces symmetric "pontine hypertrophy", pilocytic tumours of the brainstem are usually dorsal and exophytic. Spinal cord examples produce non-specific signs of an expanding mass {1015, 1234, 1287}.

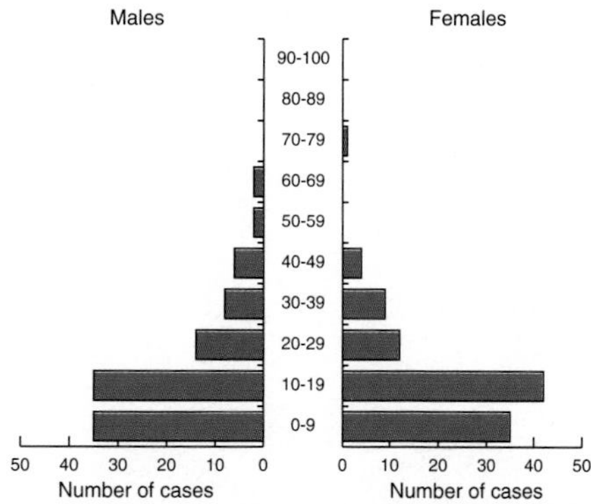

Fig. 1.43 Age and sex distribution of pilocytic astrocytoma, based on biopsies from 205 patients treated at the University Hospital, Zurich.

Neuroimaging
By either computerized tomography or magnetic resonance imaging, pilocytic astrocytomas are well circumscribed and contrast-enhancing {435, 869}. Only a minority are calcified. Those in the optic nerve are somewhat restrained in their outward expansion by the optic nerve sheath, growing along the course of the nerve to produce a fusiform mass. Optic pathway lesions have only a limited capacity to spread posteriorly, for example, from optic nerve to chiasm or from chiasm to optic tracts. Although sensitive neuroimaging may suggest extensive infiltration, the relative contribution of neoplasm, oedema, and Wallerian degeneration to T2 hyperintensity is unclear.
Pilocytic astrocytomas are found at all levels of the brainstem, are relatively discrete, often exophytic and are contrast enhancing {172, 764, 1192}. Cyst formation is common. Relative circumscription and enhancement distinguish them from diffuse astrocytomas WHO grade II of the basal pons which only show contrast enhancement after progression to anaplastic astrocytoma.
A diagnostically important feature suggesting pilocytic astrocytoma or some other WHO grade I lesion, is cyst association {1126}, a common feature of cerebellar, spinal cord and cerebral hemispheric examples. Cysts may be either solitary and massive, the tumour being a mural nodule, or multiple, smaller with intratumoural lacunae.

Macroscopy
Most pilocytic astrocytomas are soft, grey and rather discrete. Intra- or paratumoural cyst formation is common. A syrinx formation may be conspicuous in spinal cord

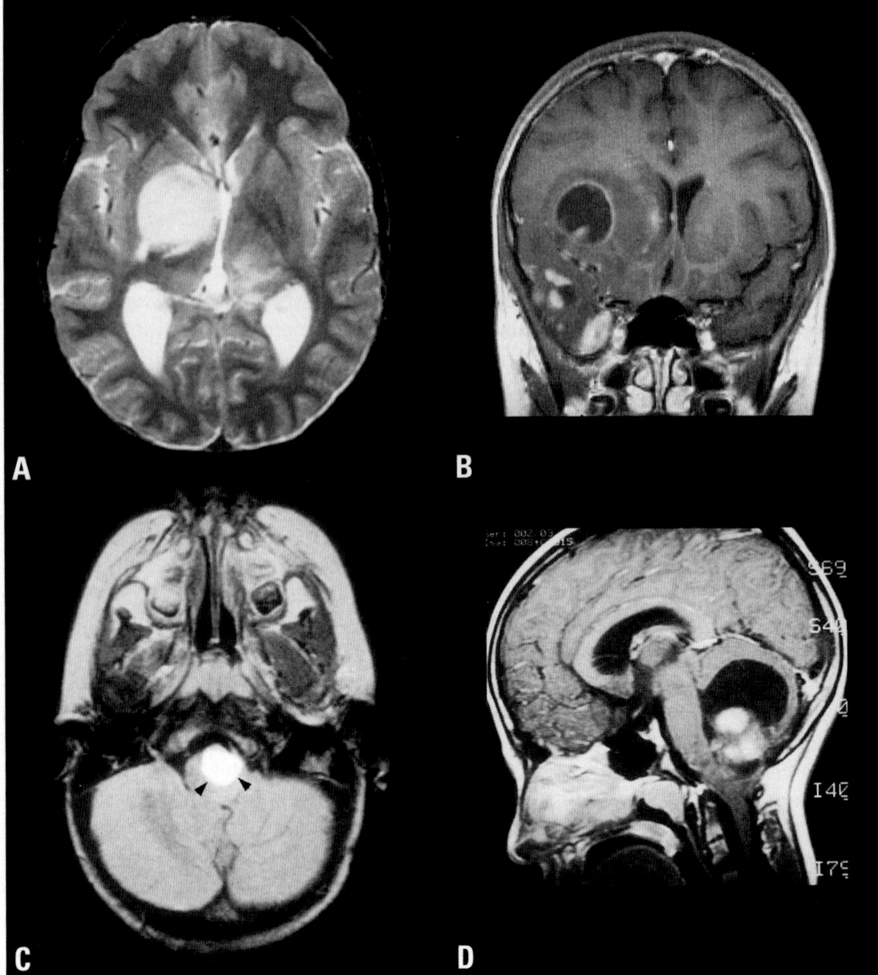

Fig. 1.44 Neuroimaging of pilocytic astrocytoma. **A** Solid, well-circumscribed hyperintense hemispheric lesion in a T2-weighted image. **B** Pilocytic astrocytoma of the frontal lobe presenting on T1 MRI as a hyperintense mural nodule with a large cyst. **C** Discrete pilocytic astrocytoma in the medulla (T1 MRI). **D** Cystic cerebellar lesion with a contrast-enhancing mural nodule.

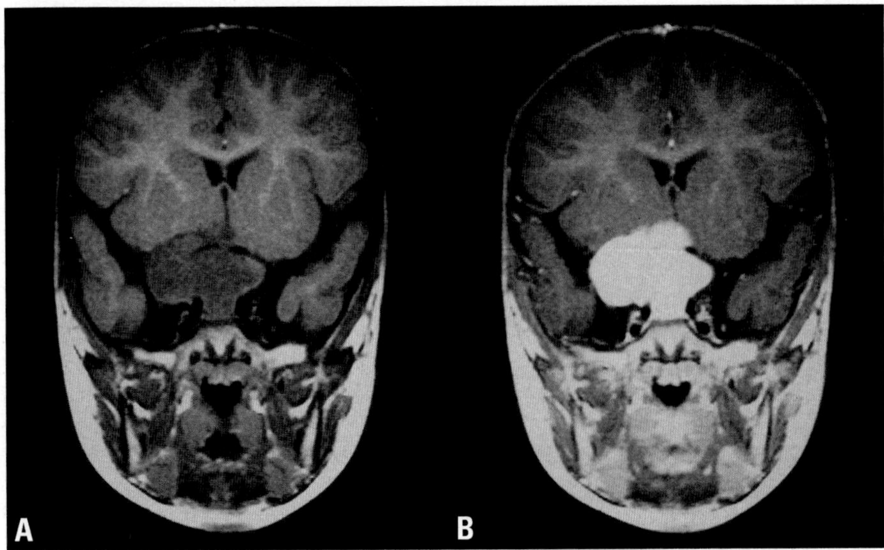

Fig. 1.45 Pilocytic astrocytoma of the optic nerve and chiasm. **A** Coronal T1 weighted MRI shows a well-demarcated lesion with (**B**) intense gadolinium (Gd) enhancement. The tumour causes a compression and shift of the adjacent fronto-basal brain structures.

and can extend over many segments {1234, 1015}. Chronic lesions may contain calcium or haemosiderin deposits. Optic nerve tumours often show collar-like involvement of the subarachnoid space {1459}.

Histopathology

An astrocytic tumour of low cellularity exhibiting a biphasic pattern with varying proportions of compacted bipolar cells with Rosenthal fibers and loose textured multipolar cells with microcysts and granular bodies. Rare mitosis, occasional hyperchromatic nuclei, microvascular proliferation and infiltration of the meninges are compatible with the diagnosis of pilocytic astrocytoma and not a sign of malignancy.

Due to heterogeneity of histologic features and tissue patterns, pilocytic astrocytomas show considerable cytological variation in smear preparations. Two basic cytologies are seen, often in combination. Derived from compact portions of the tumour, bipolar piloid cells exhibit long hair-like processes that often extend without interception across a microscopic field. These are frequently Rosenthal fiber-associated. The nuclei of piloid cells are typically elongate and cytologically bland. Highly fibrillated, these cells are glial fibrillary acidic protein (GFAP) immunopositive.

Cells derived from loose textured microcystic areas are often termed protoplasmic astrocytes. Such cells possess round to oval nuclei, a small cell body and relatively short, cobweb-like processes. Unlike the piloid cells, these are fibril-poor and only weakly GFAP-positive. Their nuclei are cytologically bland. It is this growth pattern that is particularly associated with eosinophilic granular bodies.

Other less frequently seen cells include ones that closely resemble oligodendrocytes. Cells indistinguishable from those of diffuse astrocytoma WHO grade II may also be seen.

While many pilocytic astrocytomas are benign, some tumours show considerable hyperchromasia and pleomorphism. Rare mitoses are seen in up to 30%. In occasional, often cerebellar tumours a diffuse growth pattern overshadows the more typical compact and microcystic ones. In such cases, finding hyperchromatic nuclei can cause confusion with high-grade diffuse astrocytoma. Less worrisome is obvious degenerative atypia with pleomorphism, smudgy chromatin and nuclear cytoplasmic pseudoinclusions.

These are frequently seen in longstanding lesions, especially of the cerebellum or cerebral hemispheres. The designation 'pennies on a plate' has been utilized to describe circumferential orientation of multiple nuclei in giant cells {559}. Hyalinized and glomeruloid vessels are prominent features of pilocytic astrocytoma. Perivascular lymphocytes may also be seen.

Since pilocytic astrocytomas to some extent overrun normal tissue, preexisting neurons are sometimes trapped. Such tumours should be distinguished from ganglioglioma, the glial component of which is often pilocytic in appearance (see Chapter 6).

Rosenthal fibers

These are tapered corkscrew-shaped, brightly eosinophilic, hyaline masses the intracytoplasmic location of which is best seen on smear. Rosenthal fibers are most common in compact, piloid tissue. They appear bright blue on a luxol fast blue (LFB) stain. Although helpful in diagnosis, Rosenthal fibers are by no means a requisite feature. Many pilocytic astrocytomas lack these distinctive structures. Lastly, Rosenthal fibers are not specific for pilocytic astrocytoma, or for that matter, for neoplasia. They are a common finding in chronic reactive gliosis (see Histogenesis). Densely fibrillar, paucicellular lesions containing a myriad of Rosenthal fibers are as likely to be reactive gliosis as a pilocytic astrocytoma. Ultrastructurally, Rosenthal fibers lie within astrocytic processes and consist of an amorphous electron-dense mass surrounded by intermediate (glial) filaments {338, 848}. Being composed of αB crystallin {486}, they often lack GFAP immunoreactivity.

Eosinophilic granular bodies (EGB)

EGBs form globular aggregates within astrocytic processes. Best seen in smear preparations, the intracellular localization is usually not discernible in tissue sections. They are an important diagnostic feature of several neoplasms, including ganglion cell tumours, pilocytic astrocytoma and pleomorphic xanthoastrocytoma, but are not indicative of neoplasia. Brightly eosinophilic in H&E-stained sections and PAS-positive, they show alpha-1-antichymotrypsin and alpha-1-antitrypsin immunoreactivity {740}.

Vasculature

Pilocytic astrocytomas are highly vascular, as is evidenced by their contrast enhancement {435,869}. Although generally obvious in H&E stained sections, it is accentuated in *Ulex europeus* preparations or on immunostains for basement membrane (collagen IV, laminin) or endothelial cells (CD31, CD34). Such glomeruloid vasculature should not prompt tumour misclassification or over-grading. Glomeruloid vasculature is common in pilocytic astrocytoma, not only within the tumour, but in accompanying cyst walls and occasionally at a distance from the lesion.

Regressive changes

Given the indolent nature and often slow clinical evolution of pilocytic astrocytomas, it is not surprising that regressive changes are seen. Thus, they are common in longstanding lesions, as in those of cerebellum and cerebral hemisphere. Markedly hyalinized, sometimes telangiectatic vessels are one such feature. When neoplastic cells are scant, it can even be difficult to distinguish the tumour from cavernous angioma with accompanying piloid gliosis. Evidence of previous haemorrhage (haemosiderin) further augments the likeness. Whereas evidence of old haemorrhage is common, presentation with acute haemorrhage is an infrequent event. Calcification, necrosis, and lymphocytic infiltrates are additional examples of regressive changes {2076}. On balance, calcification is an infrequent finding, only rarely seen in optic nerve or hypothalamic/thalamic examples.

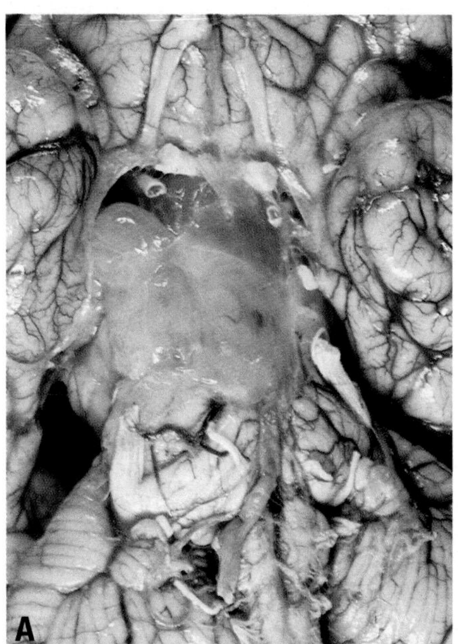

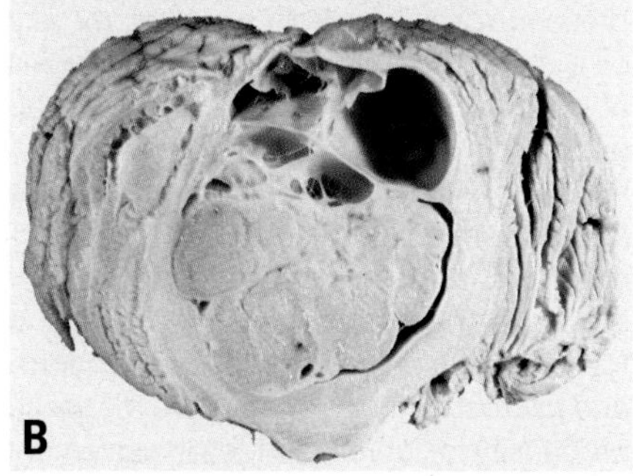

Fig. 1.46 A Large pilocytic astrocytoma extending into the basal cisterns. **B** Large, multilobular cystic cerebellar lesion with projection into the fourth ventricle and compression of the brain stem.

Cysts are a common feature of pilocytic astrocytoma, especially in locations specified above (see Fig. 1.44). Single or multiple, their fluid content is apparently rich in factors capable of stimulating vascular proliferation. Such neovascularity often lines cyst walls, thus explaining the narrow band of intense contrast enhancement seen at the circumference of some cysts. External to this vascular layer, one frequently sees dense piloid tissue with accompanying Rosenthal fibers. When this layer is narrow and well defined from surrounding normal tissue, it may be considered reactive in nature. In other instances the glial zone is more prominent, less well demarcated, and resembles tumour. Surgeons generally assume that the walls of large cysts are non-neoplastic or at least do not require resection.

Necrosis is occasionally seen in otherwise well-differentiated pilocytic astrocytomas. It more often resembles infarction than spontaneous tumour necrosis, in that pseudopalisading of neoplastic cells and apoptosis are lacking. Necrosis is of no prognostic significance.

Tissue patterns

Although most pilocytic astrocytomas represent a clearly defined clinical, radiologic, and pathologic entity, they include a wide range of tissue patterns, several of which may be found within the same lesion {180}. This difficulty stems in part from lack of specific immunohistochemical, cytogenetic, or molecular markers. Some pathologists accept a wide range of patterns, whereas others are less accepting of what to them are unproven variants. Tumours with distinctive palisades, clusters, or organoid cell aggregates are examples of contentious lesions. The same is true of mucin-rich spindle cell neoplasms. Although astrocytomas in children are usually assigned to either the pilocytic or fibrillary type, in reality there are many which do not fit clearly into either category. In some instances, small biopsy size contributes to difficulties in classification.

The classic lesion consists of often alternating compact tissue composed of piloid cells and microcystic tissue rich in so-called protoplasmic astrocytes. This biphasic pattern is best seen in cerebellar tumours. Microcysts contain often peripherally vacuolated colloid. EGBs occur mainly in microcystic tissue, whereas Rosenthal fibers populate compact regions. A variant of the compact, piloid pattern occurs when the elongate cells are less compact but separated by mucin. In such cases, individual cell processes can be visualized and cell shape varies to include more full bodied and pleomorphic, less obviously piloid cells. A distinctive lobular pattern results when leptomeningeal involvement engenders a desmoplastic reaction. At this site, tissue texture varies but Rosenthal fibers are usually abundant.

Oligodendroglioma-like cells may be seen in pilocytic astrocytomas, especially in cerebellar examples. Arranged in sheets or dispersed within parenchyma, the overall appearance is that of an oligodendroglioma, particularly in a limited sample. It is the finding of foci of classic pilocytic astrocytoma that usually permits the correct classification of these lesions. A striking feature in some pilocytic astrocytomas is alignment of cells in prominent, regimented palisades. Such enfilades resemble those of the primitive polar spongioblastoma, which is thought to be more a tissue pattern than a defined tumour entity and therefore no longer contained in the WHO classification {1355}.

Pilocytic astrocytoma in infants. A newly described entity, as yet of uncertain relation to the pilocytic group, occurs among suprasellar tumours {2078, 284}. Most present during the first two or three years of life. Their similarity to pilocytic lesions is created by a mucinous background and general cellular elongation. Features atypical for pilocytic astrocytomas are relative frequency of mitoses and lack of a biphasic architecture and often of Rosenthal fibers as well as EGBs. In many but not all cases, this lesion is noted for aggressive behaviour. Some patients have survived for years after the diagnosis.

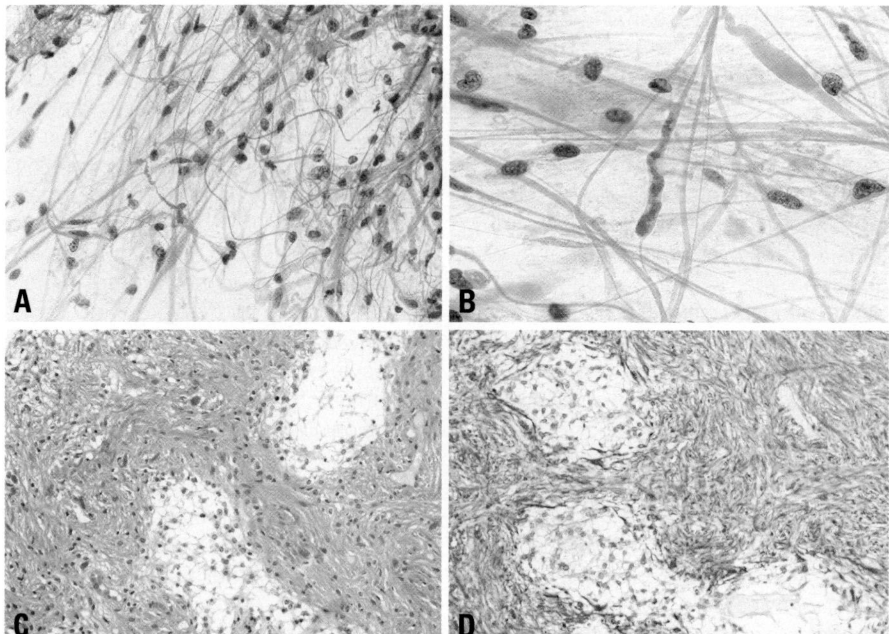

Fig. 1.47 Intraoperative squash preparations of pilocytic astrocytoma showing (**A**) long, bipolar tumour cells and (**B**) a Rosenthal fiber. **C, D** Typical biphasic pattern of compact, fiber-rich, GFAP-expressing areas and hypocellular areas with microcysts, lacking GFAP immunoreactivity.

Growth pattern

As a rule, pilocytic astrocytomas are macroscopically discrete. Thus, when regional anatomy permits, many can be removed *in toto, e.g.* cerebellum or cerebral hemispheres {293, 423, 559, 1126, 1190}. Microscopically, however, many lesions are not well defined with respect to surrounding brain. Typical lesions permeate parenchyma for a distance of several millimetres. As a result, neurons may be entrapped within the tumour. Nevertheless, as compared to diffuse gliomas, pilocytic astrocytomas are relatively solid and do not aggressively overrun surrounding tissue. This property is of diagnostic value in the study of small specimens. If only neoplastic tissue and no underlying normal brain is seen, especially in the presence of cellular elongation, microcysts or a mucinous background, a diagnosis of pilocytic astrocytoma should be entertained.

Pilocytic astrocytomas of the optic nerve and chiasm differ somewhat in their macroscopic and microscopic pattern of growth, being less well circumscribed and therefore difficult to stage, both macro- and microscopically. They share the same propensity for leptomeningeal involvement as seen in pilocytic tumours at other sites, but are somewhat more diffuse relative to the optic nerve. This is evident when pathologists attempt to stage a lesion by analysis of sequential nerve margins. Microscopically, the lesion can be followed to a point beyond which it becomes less cellular, but has no clearly defined termination.

There has been considerable discussion regarding a "diffuse" variant of pilocytic astrocytoma {477, 559, 1127}. Although some are simply classic pilocytic tumours in which the infiltrative edge is somewhat broader than expected or an artifact of plane of section, there are occasional, distinctly infiltrative lesions that mimic diffuse fibrillary astrocytoma. In two large studies, outcomes for children with "diffuse" pilocytic astrocytoma of the cerebellum were excellent, thus confirming the notion that such tumours belong to the spectrum of pilocytic astrocytoma {1127, 559}. Regarding cerebellar astrocytic tumours in NF1, the relative incidence of diffuse vs pilocytic examples and their natural history and prognosis, we refer the reader to Chapter 14. *Bona fide* infiltrating, diffuse astrocytomas represent up to 15% of astrocytic tumours of the cerebellum but are usually high grade tumours with significant nuclear atypia, mitotic activity {559}. As a rule, the distinction of pilocytic from diffuse astrocytomas is based on the focal presence of typical pilocytic features, *i.e.*, compact and microcystic elements, Rosenthal fibers, and EBGs.

Infiltration of the meninges
Involvement of the subarachnoid space is a cardinal feature of pilocytic astrocytoma, often seen in cerebellar examples in which tumour fills sulci and cements adjacent folia. This is not an expression of aggressive or malignant behaviour, but a characteristic, even diagnostically helpful feature. It does not portend subarachnoid dissemination. In cytological and histological terms, the tumour here is no different than that which is in parenchyma.
Similar leptomeningeal invasion occurs at other sites, particularly in the optic nerve (see above under Macroscopy and Growth pattern). In this setting, more so than in the cerebellum, the leptomeningeal component is reticulin-rich. Another typical pattern of tumour growth is extension into and filling of perivascular spaces.

Distant spread and metastasis
Surprisingly, otherwise typical pilocytic astrocytomas occasionally seed the neuraxis, sometimes even before the primary lesion is detected {446, 952, 1017, 1193, 1550, 2077}. The proliferation index in such cases varies but can be low {1017}. The hypothalamus is the usual primary site. Even this finding is not necessarily an indicator of future aggressive growth, since both the primary lesion and the implants may grow only slowly {446, 1017, 1161, 1193}. Indeed, the implants may be asymptomatic and long-term survival is possible, even without adjuvant treatment {1193}. With the possible exception of a lesion arising in the suprasellar/ hypothalamic region (see below), this atypical behaviour of pilocytic astrocytoma cannot be predicted {284, 2078}.

Malignant transformation
As a group, pilocytic astrocytomas are remarkable in maintaining their WHO grade I status over years and even decades. As a rule, alterations are in the direction of regressive change rather than of anaplasia. One large study found the acquisition of atypia, particularly of increased cellularity, nuclear abnormalities and occasional mitoses to be of no prognostic significance {1508}. There have, however, been rare examples of pilocytic astrocytoma undergoing malignant transformation {27, 96, 339, 1082, 1508}. These lesions often feature multiple mitoses per single high power field, microvascular proliferation and palisading necrosis. Such tumours should not be designated glioblastoma. Since their prognosis is not uniformly grim, the designation anaplastic (malignant) pilocytic astrocytoma is preferred. Since most such tumours had undergone prior radiotherapy, radiation may be a factor promoting malignant change {339, 1508}.

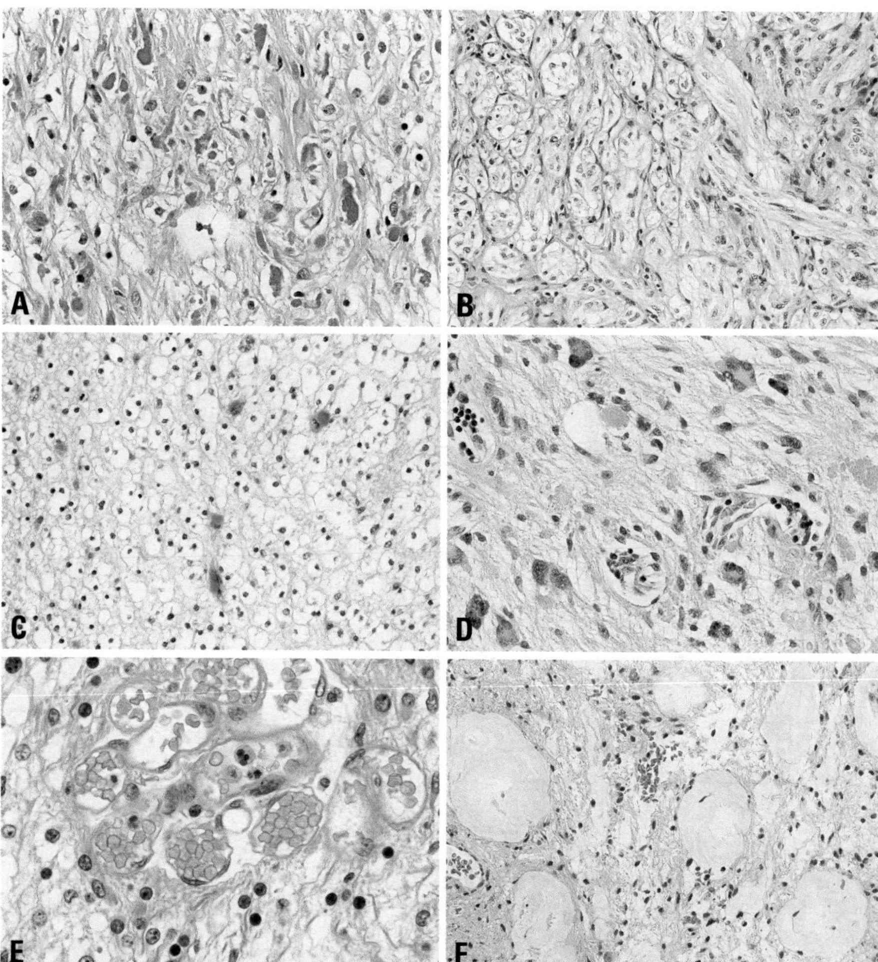

Fig. 1.49 Histological features of pilocytic astrocytoma. **A** Focal accumulation of Rosenthal fibers. **B** Lobular tissue pattern. **C** Tumour area with honeycomb cells resembling oligodendroglioma. **D** Marked nucear atypia is not a sign of malignancy. Note the numerous eosinophilic granular bodies. **E** Vascular wickerwork pattern typically encountered in cerebellar lesions. **F** Tumour vessels with extensive hyalinization.

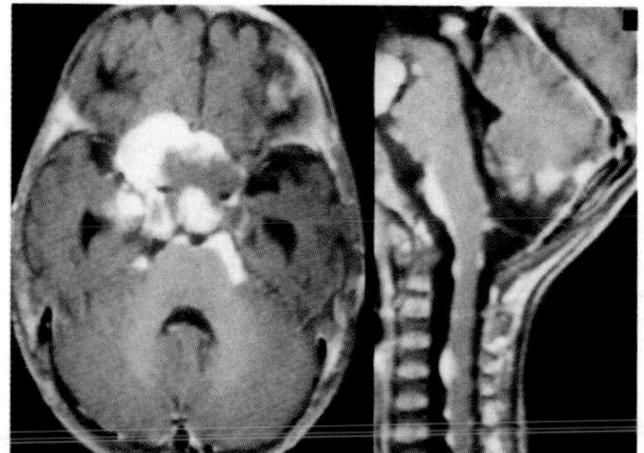
Fig. 1.48 Diencephalic pilocytic astrocytoma with leptomeningeal spread.

Proliferation
Studies using the DNA S-phase marker bromodeoxyuridine have documented a generally low labelling index, often less than one percent and only occasionally higher. In one study this index was of little predictive value relative to outcome {651}. The same study noted generally higher labelling in tumours of young patents as well as a tendency to reduced labelling in subsequently obtained specimens. Indeed, tumour growth appeared to slow by about age 20. A more recent study of proliferative activity in both pilocytic and diffuse astrocytomas showed mitoses to vary from 0 to an exceptional 4 per 10 high power fields, and MIB-1 labelling indices to range from 0 to 3.9% (mean 1.1%) in pilocytic tumours {2075}. The latter values overlapped with those of diffuse astrocytoma WHO grade II (mean 2.3). Thus, despite a significant difference in labelling

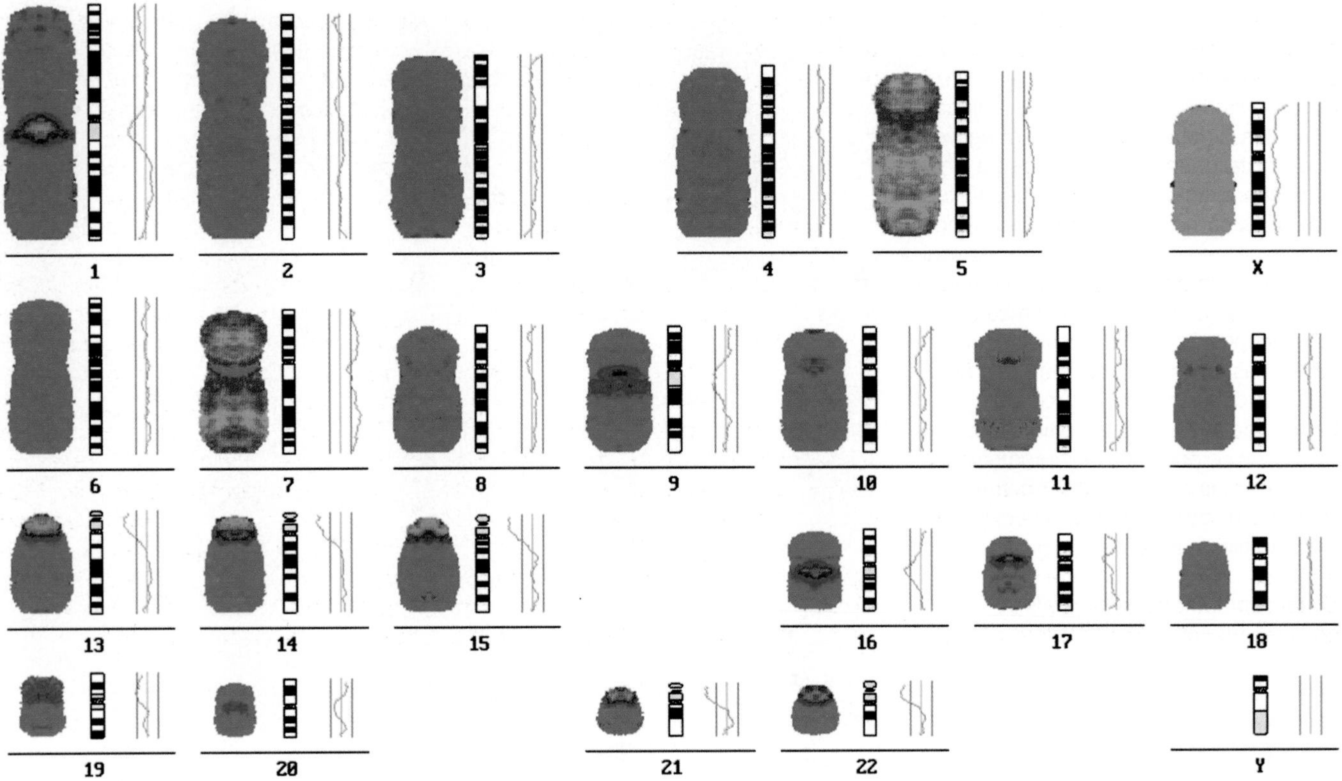

Fig. 1.50 Comparative genomic hybridization (CGH) of a pilocytic astrocytoma. Deletions are depicted in red, amplifications in green and equilibrium between the tumour and normal DNA in blue. The sum karyogram shows losses on chromosomes 9q,13q, 14q, 19p and gains on chromosomes 1q, 2q, 3p, 4q, 7p, 7q, 8q, 9p, 10p, 10q, 11q, 13q and 15q. The red curves depict the average ratio profiles.

of the two tumour types, MIB-1 labeling indices were of limited use in differential diagnosis. These observations are in keeping with the facts that growth of the solid component of pilocytic astrocytomas is an infrequent cause of death and that such tumours show little tendency to progression and almost none to malignant transformation {1508}.

Genetic susceptibility

Pilocytic astrocytomas are the principal central nervous system neoplasm of neurofibromatosis type 1 (NF1). Optic nerve involvement, especially when bilateral, is the classic finding, but other anatomic sites, sometimes multiple, may also be affected. Approximately 15% of patients with neurofibromatosis type 1 develop pilocytic astrocytomas {887}, particularly of the optic nerve. Conversely, up to one-third of patients with a pilocytic astrocytoma at this location have NF1 {455}.

Cytogenetics

Cytogenetic analyses of pilocytic astrocytomas have revealed either a normal karyotype or a variety of aberrations. No distinct pattern suggesting the loss of a particular tumour suppressor gene has been reported {7, 675, 697, 731, 1228, 1499}. Fluorescence *in situ* hybridisation has shown gains of chromosomes 7 and 8 in a third of pilocytic astrocytomas {1615}. Comparative genomic hybridization (CGH) showed considerable variety in chromosomal imbalances {2577}, with gains and deletions on chromosomes 19 and gains on chromosome 22 being most frequently observed (Fig. 1.50).

Molecular genetics

In contrast to the diffuse astrocytomas, mutational inactivation of the *TP53* gene does not seem to play a role in the evolution of pilocytic astrocytoma {1096}. Of a large number of tumours investigated in various laboratories, missense *TP53* mutations were either absent or very rare {856, 1141, 1096}. Increased levels of the TP53 protein have been observed {856} but are not indicative of a gene mutation. Occasionally, sporadic pilocytic astrocytomas may show a loss of chromosome 17q, which includes the region encoding the *NF1* gene {1563}. Since the *NF1* gene has tumour suppressor functions, loss of expression of *NF1* could play a role in the evolution of various neoplasms associated with this familial cancer syndrome, including pilocytic astrocytomas. To date, however, screening of *NF1* coding sequences, including the critical GRD region, has failed to detect mutations {1187}. Neurofibromin, the *NF1* gene product, contains a four-hundred-amino-acid region corresponding to the GTP-ase activating proteins. Immunohistochemically, neurofibromin has been found to be overexpressed in pilocytic astrocytomas {1187}. Splice variations of the *NF1* gene lead to a variety of transcript isoforms. In pilocytic astrocytomas there was a conspicuous overexpression of transcripts containing exon 23a and a lack of expression of exon 9br {1187}. These isoforms have been shown to be expressed in normal, reactive {476} and neoplastic astrocytes {516}. Thus, current evidence does not support a role of the tumour suppressor gene *NF1* in the genesis of pilocytic astrocytomas.

Histogenesis

Having the capacity to form Rosenthal fibers, the hair-like, piloid cells of pilocytic astrocytomas are remarkably similar to reactive astrocytes surrounding various chronic lesions of the hypothalamus, cerebellum, and spinal cord. Similar cells are also found in the glial stroma of the normal pineal gland. Their histologic and cytologic resemblance makes such cells prime candidates as precursors. Obviously this simple notion does not take protoplasmic astrocytes and microcystic tumours rich in EGBs into consideration.

Predictive features

As a group, pilocytic astrocytomas are slowly growing masses which at any point in their evolution may stabilize or even regress. Stability in terms of grade and differentiation may be maintained for decades {1121}. Although, the lesion is uncommonly fatal, there are only few long-term studies documenting the ultimate outcome of patients with this distinctive tumour. Recurrent hypothalamic and brainstem lesions can be lethal, but usually only after a prolonged clinical course marked by multiple recurrences {1269, 172, 764, 1193, 559, 423, 1015}. Clinical "recurrence" is more often a reflection of cyst reformation than of enlargement of the solid tumour component. As a general rule, neurofibromatosis-associated tumours remain stable or grow only slowly, especially those of the optic nerve {624, 902, 1269}. The biologic behaviour of cerebellar astrocytic tumours in NF1 might be more aggressive {2076}, but a clear distinction of pilocytic and diffuse tumours is not always as readily achieved in this disorder (see chapter 14); occasional tumours even regress {874}.

The definition and prognostic significance of lesions sometimes designated as atypical and malignant have been addressed {1508}. Such lesions often occur in the cerebellum. It is the varied presence of increased cellularity, mitotic activity, microvascular proliferation and necrosis that generates concern. The solitary mitosis (1-2/50 HPF) occurs in approximately 30% of pilocytic astrocytomas {2075}. When seen in conjunction with nuclear atypia and increased cellularity, the designation atypical pilocytic astrocytoma has been applied, but was found to be of no clinical significance {1508}. At present, there are no proven criteria of atypical pilocytic astrocytoma. Only when mitotic activity can be expressed in terms of mitoses per single HPF and is associated with microvascular proliferation and/or necrosis, can the designation anaplastic (malignant) pilocytic astrocytoma be applied {1508}. Most are associated with growth and aggressive behaviour, but others are cured by surgical excision with or without adjunctive radio- or chemotherapy.

Pleomorphic xanthoastrocytoma

J.J. Kepes
D.N. Louis
C. Giannini
W. Paulus

Definition

An astrocytic neoplasm with a relatively favourable prognosis, typically encountered in children and young adults, with superficial location in the cerebral hemispheres and involvement of the meninges. Characteristic histological features include pleomorphic and lipidized cells expressing GFAP and often surrounded by a reticulin network as well as eosinophilic granular bodies.

ICD-O code: 9424/3

Grading

Pleomorphic xanthoastrocytomas correspond histologically to WHO grade II. For lesions with significant mitotic activity (5 or more mitoses per 10 HPF) and/or with areas of necrosis, the designation "pleomorphic xanthoastrocytoma with anaplastic features" may be used {2159}. At present, the term "anaplastic pleomorphic xanthoastrocytoma (WHO grade III)" is not recommended.

Synonyms and historical annotation

Before the introduction of immunostaining, pleomorphic xanthoastrocytomas were thought to represent mesenchymal neoplasms of the meninges and brain, partly because the lipidized neoplastic glial cells resemble 'xanthoma' cells, and partly because many tumour cells produce a basement membrane. However, GFAP immunostaining has clearly shown that the tumour cells are neoplastic astrocytes {761} and the earlier suggestion that the tumour represented fibrous xanthomas of the meninges {757, 1153} has been dismissed.

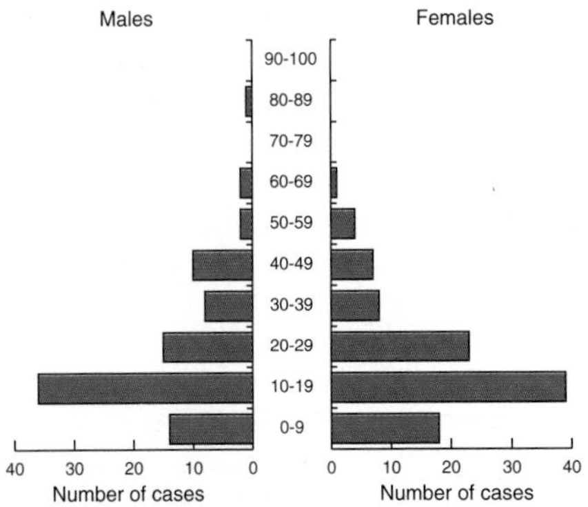

Fig. 1.51 Age distribution of patients with pleomorphic xanthoastrocytoma.

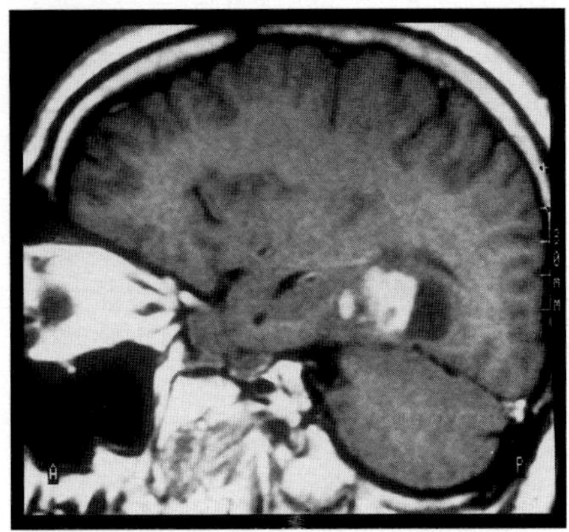

Fig. 1.52 T1 MRI of a pleomorphic xanthoastrocytoma of the temporal lobe presenting as hyperintense mural nodule with a large cyst.

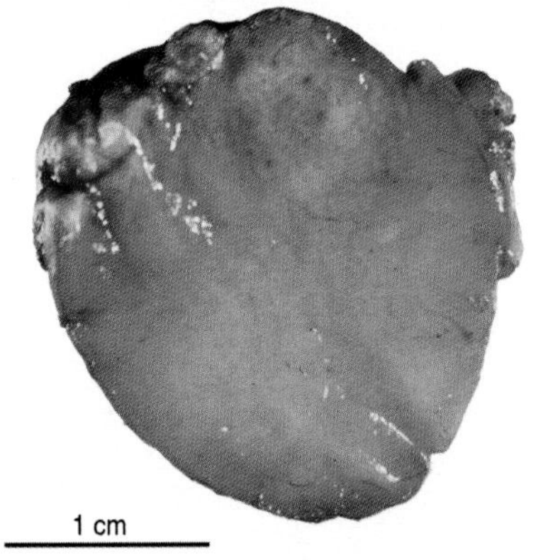

Fig. 1.53 Typical macroscopic appearance of a pleomorphic xanthoastrocytoma. The yellow areas correspond to xanthomatous parts of the tumour.

Incidence

Pleomorphic xanthoastrocytomas account for less than 1% of all astrocytic neoplasms. Since the initial description of 12 cases {761}, approximately 180 additional cases have been reported {471, 2159}.

Age and sex distribution

This neoplasm typically develops in children and young adults, without a significant gender bias. Two-thirds of patients are less than 18 years old {471}, but manifestation in older patients, *e.g.* 62 and 82 years old {2159, 2160} have also been reported.

Localization

A superficial location, involving the meninges and cerebrum ("meningocerebral") is typical of this neoplasm. Ninety-eight percent occur supratentorially, in particular the temporal lobe {2159, 761}. Cases involving the cerebellum and spinal cord are also on record {580, 1581}, and recently two children with primary pleomorphic xanthoastrocytoma of the retina were reported {2163}.

Clinical features

Symptoms and signs

Because of the superficial cerebral location of the lesion, many patients present with a fairly long history of seizures. Cerebellar and spinal cord cases have symptoms that reflect the sites of involvement.

Neuroimaging

CT and MRI scans usually outline the tumour mass and/or its cyst. Perifocal oedema is usually not pronounced, owing to the slow growth of the tumour.

Macroscopy

Pleomorphic xanthoastrocytomas are attached to the meninges and are frequently accompanied by a cyst, sometimes forming a mural nodule within the cyst wall. Invasion of the dura is exceptional, but a case of recurrent pleomorphic xanthoastrocytoma invading the tentorium and falx cerebri is on record {316}. Diffuse leptomeningeal spread (with positive spinal fluid cytology) from a pleomorphic xanthoastrocytoma initially involving the left Sylvian fissure has been reported {2164}.

Histopathology

A pleomorphic tumour composed of fibrillary and giant, often multinucleated neoplastic astrocytes. Diagnostic hallmarks are large xanthomatous cells expressing GFAP, a dense intercellular reticulin network, and lymphocytic infiltrates.

The key histopathological features of the pleomorphic xanthoastrocytoma are now well established {753, 825}. The adjective 'pleomorphic' refers to the variable histological appearance of the tumour, in which spindly elements are intermingled with mono- or multinucleated giant cells, the nuclei of which show great variation in size and staining. In some cases, the neoplastic astrocytes are closely packed and assume an 'epithelioid' pattern {657}. The term 'xanthoastrocytoma' refers to the fact that many cells in this neoplasm show intracellular accumulation of lipids. This is usually in the form of droplets, and quite often occupies much of the cell body, pushing to the periphery the usual cytoplasmic structures (including glial filaments) that by conventional stains or immunohistochemical methods generally make the astrocytic character easy to recognize. Eosinophilic granular bodies, similar to those seen in pilocytic astrocytomas and ganglion cell tumours, are also frequently encountered, as are focal collections of benign reactive lymphocytes, occasionally with plasma cells.

The third histological hallmark of pleomorphic xanthoastrocytoma is the sometimes striking density of reticulin fibers seen when the tumour is examined using silver impregnations. Not only reactive changes in the meninges result in the presence of reticulin fibers; the individual tumour cells may be surrounded by basement membranes that stain positively for reticulin and these can be recognized ultrastructurally as pericellular basal laminae.

Rarely, pleomorphic xanthoastrocytomas are part of a combination tumour in which they form the glioma portion of a ganglioglioma {2510}. Occasional neuronal differentiation of the tumour cells themselves has been suggested {1199}. Some highly vascularized forms have been denoted as 'angiomatous' {1468}.

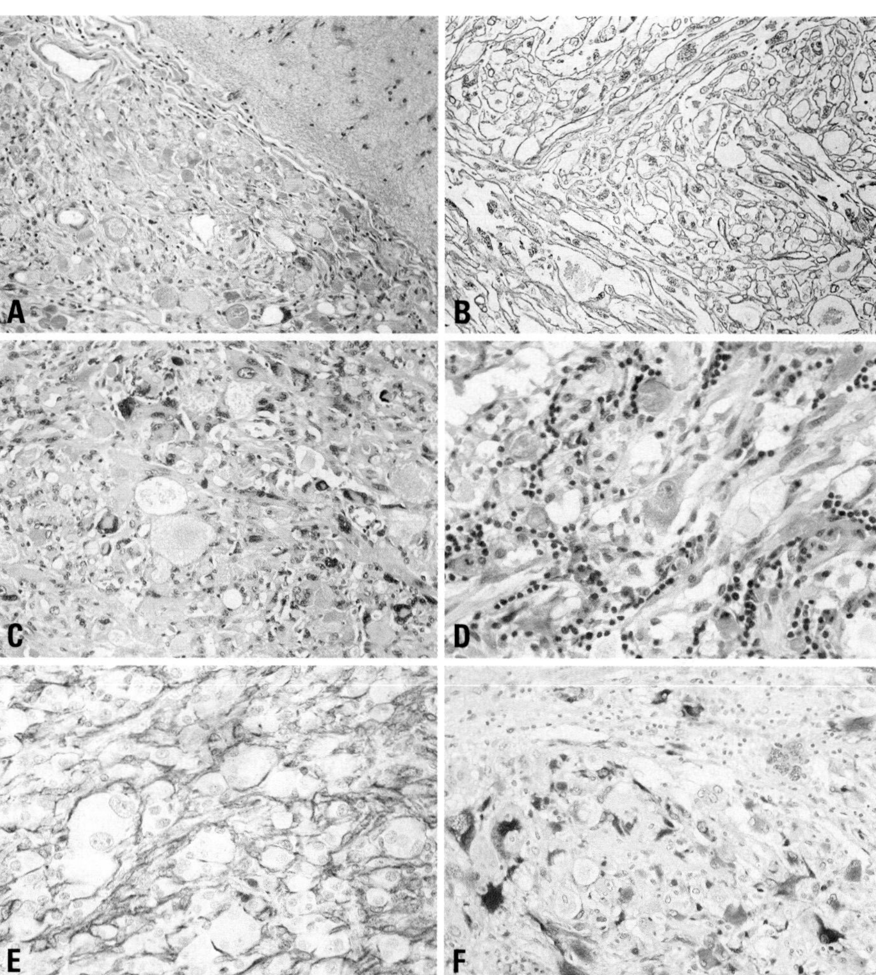

Fig. 1.54 Histological features of pleomorphic xanthoastrocytoma (PXA). **A** Leptomeningeal PXA, sharply delineated from the cerebral cortex. **B** Reticulin network surrounding individual tumour cells. **C** Tumour cells showing nuclear and cytoplasmic pleomorphism and xanthomatous change. **D** Mature ganglion cell and lymphocytic infiltrates in a PXA (from Kros *et al.*, ref. 825). **E** Spindle-shaped tumour cells forming a GFAP-positive network. **F** GFAP immunostaining of large pleomorphic tumour cells.

Tumour progression

With some notable exceptions {759, 1599, 1617}, pleomorphic xanthoastrocytomas behave in a less malignant fashion than might be suggested by their highly pleomorphic histology {761}. Cases with survival as long as 40 years after surgery have been published soon after the original description of this tumour {2583}. In many instances, pleomorphic xanthoastrocytomas show slow evolution with long symptom-free periods, even after incomplete resection. Recurrences may show a histological pattern analogous to the original tumour, but increasing anaplasia may also set in, in some cases histologically being indistinguishable from glioblastoma and featuring both necrosis and endothelial hyperplasia. Pleomorphism may cease to be a feature and closely packed smaller cells may come to dominate the tumour. In addition, with increasing malignancy, the rich reticulin network may become fragmented or disappear completely. Necrosis usually occurs in these more anaplastic recurrences {759}.

Proliferation

In most cases, mitotic figures are rare or absent {2159}. MIB-1/Ki67 and PCNA labelling indices are generally lower than 1% {26, 846, 930, 1581, 2159}. S-phase fractions, as determined by flow cytometry, are also low {622, 1581}.

Aetiology

No specific aetiologies have been implicated in the evolution of pleomorphic xanthoastrocytomas. The types of *TP*53 mutations encountered do not suggest particular carcinogenic insults {1151}. The occasional association with cortical dysplasia or with ganglionic lesions has suggested that their formation may be facilitated in malformative states {846}.

Genetic susceptibility

There are no distinct associations with hereditary tumour syndromes, with the exception of rare reports of pleomorphic xanthoastrocytomas in NF1 patients {828, 1114}. Given the well-known association of NF1 with many different forms of astrocytomas, occasional cases are not surprising. Familial clustering of pleomorphic xanthoastrocytomas has not been reported.

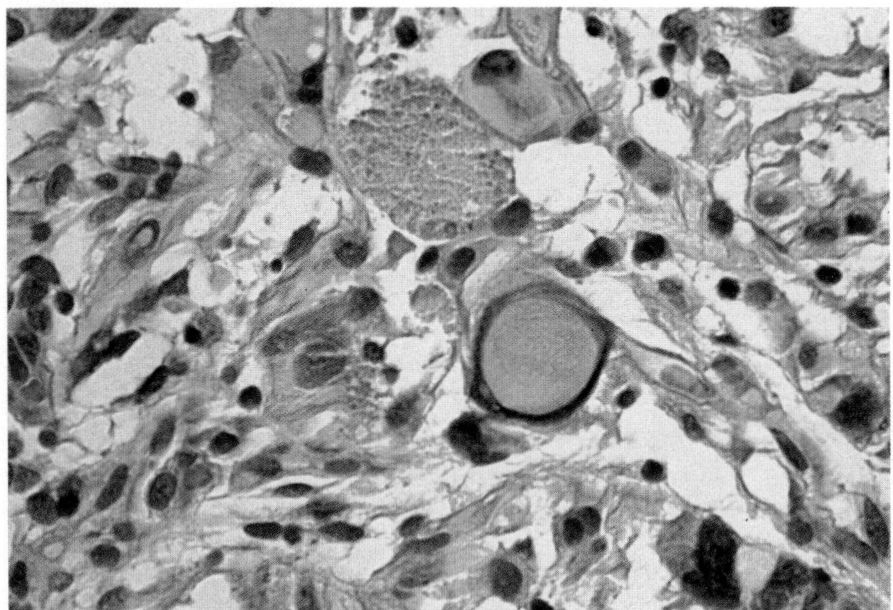

Fig. 1.55 Pleomorphic xanthoastrocytoma. The cytoplasm of a tumour cell is filled with eosinophilic granules. The cell below exhibits a large intranuclear cytoplasmic inclusion.

Cytogenetics

Complex karyotypes have been documented, with gains of chromosomes 3 and 7, as well as alterations of the long arm of chromosome 1 {894, 1331, 1333}. These cytogenetic changes, however, have also been reported in other types of astrocytoma. The tumours appear to be predominantly diploid {622, 1581}, occasionally with polyploid populations {622}, possibly due to subgroups of particularly bizarre, multinucleated tumour cells.

Molecular genetics

In two series of a total of 14 pleomorphic xanthoastrocytomas (4 of which underwent subsequent malignant progression), a *TP*53 missense mutation at codons 220, 273 and 292 was identified in three tumours, including a non-recurring lesion, a grade II recurrence (the primary tumour being non-mutant) and a tumour that later underwent malignant transformation {1047, 1151}. Amplification of the *EGFR* gene was observed only in the second higher-grade recurrence of an initial grade II pleomorphic xanthoastrocytoma, while no loss of heterozygosity on chromosomes 10q and 19q was reported {1151}. These data suggest that the timing of genetic alterations may differ from that typically encountered in diffuse astrocytomas.

Histogenesis

It has been postulated, but not yet proven, that these neoplasms originate from subpial astrocytes. Subpial astrocytes of the human cortex are invested by basal laminae that appear to be a product of the astrocytes themselves and not that of the pial elements {1225, 842}. The recent demonstration of synaptophysin and neurofilament protein in some pleomorphic xanthoastrocytomas has been taken as evidence for neuronal differentiation and suggests a more complex histogenesis {1199}, although it remains under discussion whether synaptophysin immunoreactivity alone is evidence of neuronal differentiation {2159, 2025}.

Predictive factors

A series of 71 patients reported *recurrence-free survival* of 72% at 5 years and 61% at 10 years {2159}. Recurrence-free survival curves, based on a review of previously published cases (n=121), are similar. The extent of the resection of the original tumour mass appears to be the most significant predictive factor, followed by a low mitotic index {2159}. Both factors are independently predictive of recurrence-free survival.

Overall survival has been estimated as 81 % at 5 years and 70 % at 10 years {2159}. Mitotic activity (more than 5 per HPF) is the only independent predictor of survival. Necrosis, although significantly associated with survival (p=0.04), was not an independent predictor. A review of the previously published cases has also shown a significant association of necrosis with survival (p= 0.008) {2159, 1122}.

No reliable correlation between *TP53* mutation and malignant progression or recurrence has been established in the few cases analyzed to date {1047, 1151}.

CHAPTER 2

Oligodendroglial Tumours

Oligodendroglial tumours are well characterized clinico-pathological entities. Their origin from differentiated oligodendrocytes or progenitor cells committed to oligodendroglial differentiation is difficult to prove, owing to a lack of reliable immunohistochemical markers. Genetic alterations in oligodendrogliomas differ significantly from those commonly found in diffuse astrocytomas. The following lesions are distinguished:

Oligodendroglioma (WHO grade II)

These slowly growing neoplasms often manifest after several years of preoperative epileptic seizures and have a favourable prognosis regarding the time till recurrence.

Anaplastic oligodendroglioma (WHO grade III)

This neoplasm often responds favourably to chemotherapy but the criteria for the grading of oligodendrogliomas are less defined than those indicating progression of astrocytomas. Some tumours may develop histological features commonly found in glioblastomas.

Mixed Gliomas

The diagnosis of mixed gliomas requires the identification of at least two unequivocally neoplastic components resembling different macroglial lineages, i.e. astrocytic, oligodendroglial and/or ependymal differentiation.

Oligoastrocytoma (WHO grade II)

This is by far the most frequent type of mixed glioma. Recent studies suggest at least two distinct genetic pathways, but no indication of a polyclonal origin.

Anaplastic oligoastrocytoma (WHO grade III)

This malignant variant displays histological features of anaplasia and mitotic activity. The prognosis is generally poor although some lesions respond well to chemotherapy.

Oligodendroglioma

G. Reifenberger
J.M. Kros
P.C. Burger
D.N. Louis
V.P. Collins

Definition

A well-differentiated, diffusely infiltrating tumour of adults, typically located in the cerebral hemispheres and composed predominantly of cells morphologically resembling oligodendroglia.

ICD-O code: 9450/3

Grading

Oligodendroglioma corresponds histologically to WHO grade II.

Histologically, oligodendroglial tumours comprise a continuous spectrum ranging from well-differentiated neoplasms to frankly malignant tumours. The WHO grading system recognizes two malignancy grades for oligodendroglial tumours: WHO grade II for well-differentiated tumours, and WHO grade III for anaplastic oligodendroglioma (see following pages). Grading of oligodendroglial tumours according to WHO criteria has been shown to be a significant predictor of survival {2229, 2242, 2584}.

Several other systems have been used for the histological grading of oligodendroglial tumours, including the four-tiered Kernohan {763} and St Anne/Mayo systems {1398} (both originally designed for astrocytic tumors), the Smith grading system {1431}, as well as three-tiered systems, such as the Ringertz system {1260} and a three-tiered modification of the Smith scheme {820, 821}. In addition, a two-tiered system based on morphological and imaging criteria has been proposed {2491}. Each of these grading systems is capable of distinguishing subsets of oligodendroglial tumours, but most studies suggest that there are basically two groups that differ prognostically {1079, 1398, 1469, 2491}, which is in line with the two-tiered WHO system.

Historical annotation

The first description of an oligodendroglioma was published by Bailey & Cushing {58} followed by the classic paper of Bailey & Bucy {55} on 'oligodendrogliomas of the brain'.

Incidence

The central brain tumour registry of the United States of America reported in 1995 {214} an annual incidence for all oligodendroglial tumours (including anaplastic forms) of 0.3 per 100'000 individuals. In a 25-year survey of the Norwegian Cancer Registry, oligodendroglial tumours accounted for 4.2% of all primary brain tumours {1037}. In other studies, these tumours represented between 5% and 18% of all intracranial gliomas {1306, 1347, 1686}.

Age and sex distribution

The majority of oligodendrogliomas arise in adults with a peak incidence in the fifth and sixth decade {820, 1037, 1398, 1686}. In a series from the Department of Neuropathology, University of Düsseldorf, Germany, the mean age at operation for 64 patients with WHO grade II oligodendrogliomas was 42.6 years. About 6% of oligodendrogliomas arise during infancy and childhood {1037} with mean ages at operation of about 10 years for supratentorial cases and 7.5 years for infratentorial cases {1118, 1502}. Males appear to be affected slightly more frequently than females, with ratios between 2:1 {233, 1398} and 3:2 {1037} reported. In the Düsseldorf series, the male:female ratio was 1.1:1.

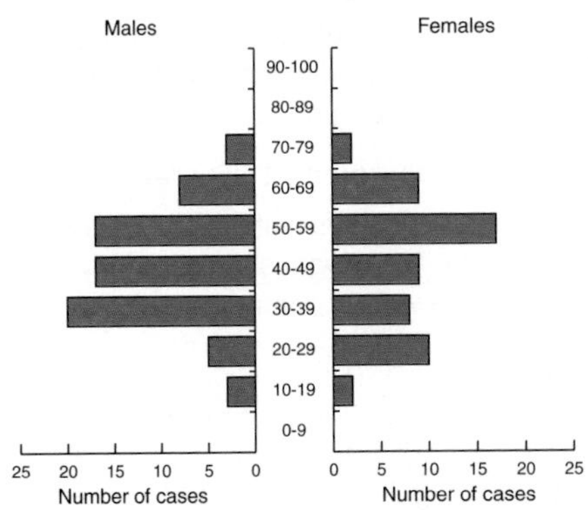

Fig. 2.1 Age distribution of 130 patients with oligodendroglioma and anaplastic oligodendroglioma. Based on combined biopsy series from the Universities of Düsseldorf (Germany) and Zurich (Switzerland).

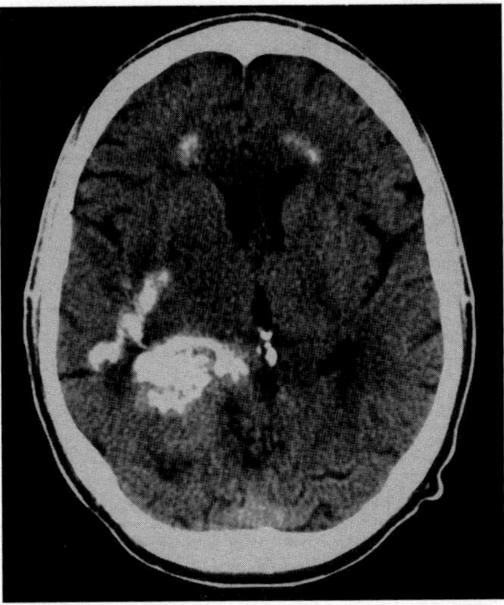

Fig. 2.2 CT scan showing an extensively calcifying oligodendroglioma in the right temporo-occipital region. The enhancement in front of both anterior horns represents tumour spread.

Localization

Oligodendrogliomas arise preferentially in the cortex and white matter of the cerebral hemispheres. The frontal lobe is involved in 50–65% of the patients {820, 1079, 1398}. The temporal, parietal and occipital lobes are affected with decreasing frequencies. Patients with cerebellar, brain stem, spinal cord, and primary leptomeningeal oligodendrogliomas have also been reported {29, 227, 425, 1118, 1180, 1275, 2590}.

Clinical features

Symptoms and signs

Patients may present with a long pre-operative history of neurological signs and symptoms. Reported intervals of more than 5 years are not uncommon {233, 1079}. The most common signs are epileptic seizures and headache {233, 926, 1079, 1398}. The particularly high incidence of seizures in patients with oligodendrogliomas may be related to the tendency of these tumours to diffusely infiltrate the cerebral cortex.

Neuroimaging

The tumour mass can be readily demon-

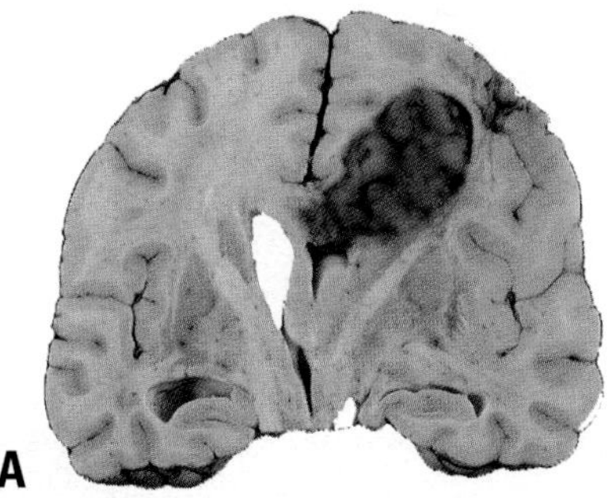

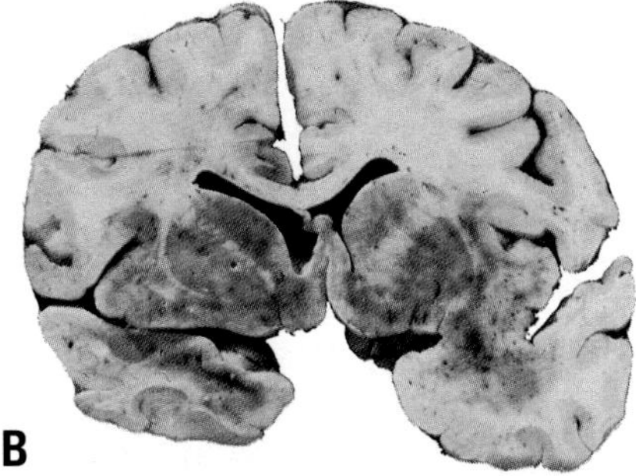

Fig. 2.3 A Well-circumscribed, partly haemorrhagic oligodendroglioma of the left frontal lobe. **B** Recurrent oligodendroglioma with bilateral, diffuse infiltration of the frontal and temporal lobes.

strated by CT and MRI. On CT, the tumours usually appear as hypo- or isodense, well-demarcated mass lesions, usually located in the cortex and subcortical white matter. Calcification is common but not diagnostic. MRI studies typically demonstrate a hypointense lesion in T1-weighted images and a hyperintense lesion in T2-weighted images which appears well-demarcated and shows little perifocal oedema {868}. Some tumours may demonstrate heterogeneous images of variable intensities due to intratumoral haemorrhages and/or areas of cystic degeneration.

Macroscopy

Oligodendrogliomas usually appear as well-defined soft masses of greyish-pink colour. Cases with extensive mucoid degeneration may appear gelatinous. The tumour is typically located in the cortex and white matter, and infiltration of the overlying leptomeninges may be seen. Calcification is frequent, in particular, in the tumour periphery and the adjacent cortex. Zones of cystic degeneration, as well as intratumoral haemorrhages, may be seen.

Histopathology

Oligodendrogliomas are moderately cellular and composed of tumour cells with rounded, homogeneous nuclei and, on paraffin sections, a swollen, clear cytoplasm ('honeycomb' appearance). Additional features include microcalcifications, mucoid/cystic degeneration and a dense network of branching capillaries. Marked nuclear atypia and an occasional mitosis are compatible with the diagnosis of WHO grade II oligodendroglioma but significant mitotic activity, prominent microvascular proliferation or conspicuous necrosis indicate progression to anaplastic oligodendroglioma WHO grade III.

Cellular composition

Oligodendrogliomas are monomorphous gliomas of moderate cellularity, although some small biopsies may show only scattered oligodendroglioma cells, identifiable by their characteristic nuclei, infiltrating the brain parenchyma. Areas of increased cellularity, often in the form of circumscribed nodules, may occur in some otherwise well-differentiated tumours. The tumour cells have uniformly round nuclei which are slightly larger than those of normal oligodendrocytes and show an increase in chromatin density. Mitotic activity is either absent or low. In routinely formalin-fixed and paraffin-embedded material, the tendency of the tumour cells to undergo degeneration by acute swelling results in an enlarged rounded cell with a well-defined cell membrane and clear cytoplasm around a central spherical nucleus. This creates the typical honeycomb appearance which, although artefactual, is a helpful diagnostic feature when present. This artefact is seen neither in smear preparations nor in frozen sections, and may also be absent in rapidly fixed tissue and in paraffin sections made from frozen material.

Some oligodendrogliomas contain tumour cells with the appearance of small gemistocytes, *i.e.*, they have a somewhat larger, often eccentric cytoplasm that is positive for glial fibrillary acidic protein (GFAP). These cells have been referred to as minigemistocytes or microgemistocytes (see below). In rare tumours, GFAP-negative mucocytes or even signet-ring cells may be seen {1306}. Rare cases of oligodendroglioma consisting largely of signet-ring cells (signet ring cell oligodendroglioma) have been described {822}. Eosinophilic granular cells may also occur in some oligodendrogliomas {1482}.

Oligodendrogliomas typically show a dense network of branching capillaries resembling the pattern of chicken-wire. In some cases, the capillary stroma tends to subdivide the tumour into lobules. The tumours have a tendency for intratumoral haemorrhages.

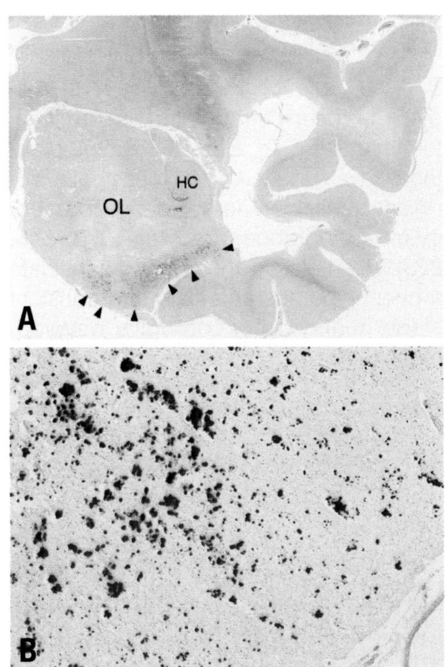

Fig. 2.4 Oligodendroglioma (OL) of the temporal lobe with infiltration of the hippocampus (HC). Note the zone of calcification (arrows) at the periphery of the lesion and below at higher magnification.

Calcifications

An important histological feature is the presence of microcalcifications, sometimes associated with blood vessels, within the tumour tissue proper as well as in the invaded brain. However, this feature is not specific for oligodendroglial tumours and, due to the generally incomplete tumour sampling, may sometimes not be found in the available tissue sections even if clearly demonstrated neuroradiologically. Areas characterized by extracellular mucin deposition and/or microcyst formation are frequent.

Growth pattern

Oligodendrogliomas grow diffusely in the cortex and white matter. Within the cortex, tumour cells form secondary structures such as perineuronal satellitosis, perivascular aggregations, and subpial accumulations. Circumscribed leptomeningeal infiltration may induce a marked desmoplastic reaction. A rare growth pattern is the formation of parallel rows of tumour cells with somewhat elongated nuclei forming palisades. Occasionally, perivascular

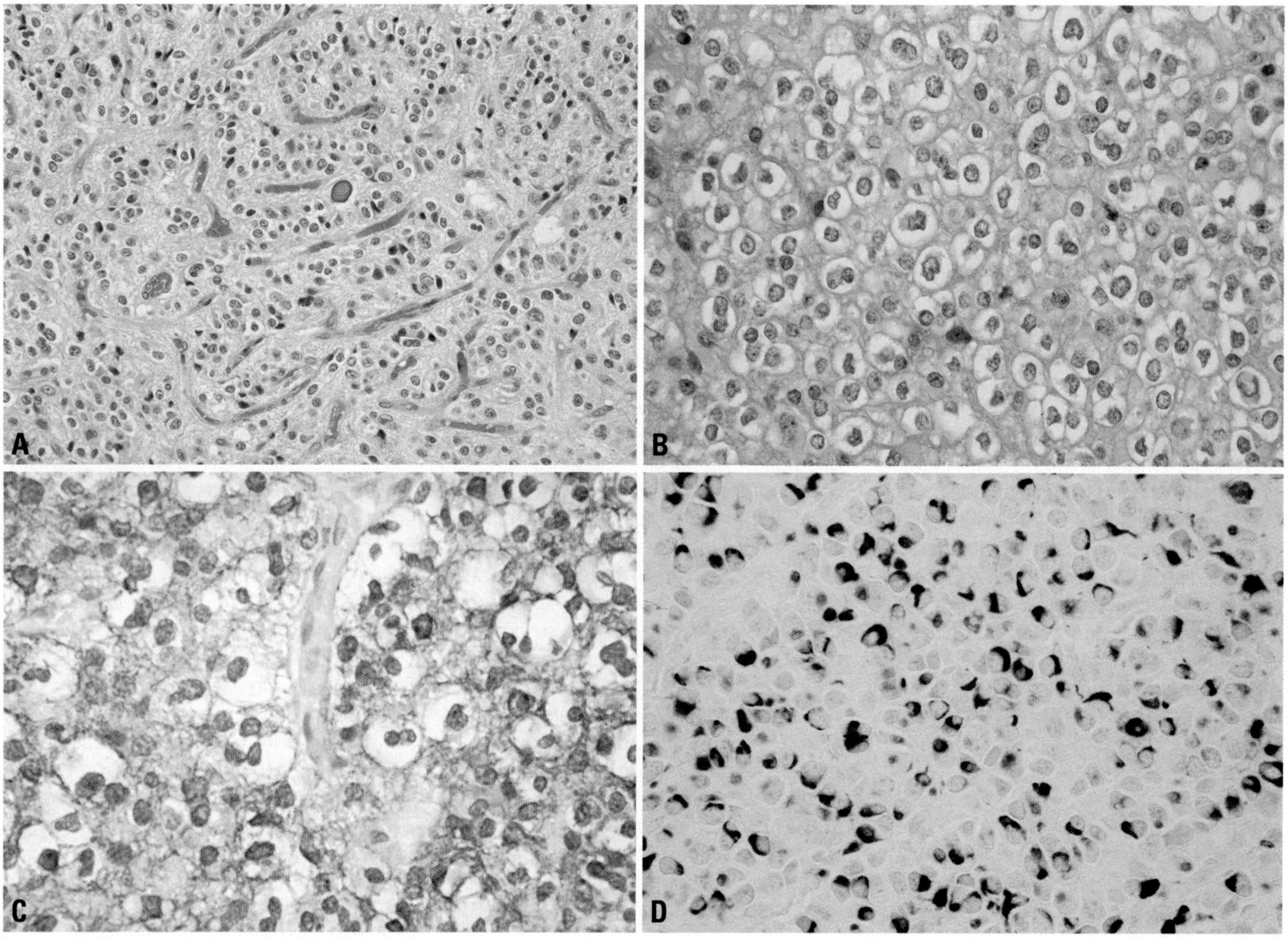

Fig. 2.5 Oligodendroglioma showing (A) the typical dense network of branching capillaries and (B) tumour cells with clear cytoplasm and well defined plasma membrane. C EGFR expression by neoplastic oligodendrocytes. From Reifenberger *et al.* {1691}. D Mini-gemistocytes with marked perinuclear immunoreativity for GFAP.

pseudorosettes may be seen. These patterns are generally present only in some parts of a tumour.

Immunohistochemistry

There is no immunocytochemical marker available that would allow the specific and sensitive recognition of human oligodendroglial tumour cells. Oligodendrogliomas share with many other neuroectodermal tumours the expression of S-100 protein and the carbohydrate epitope recognized by the monoclonal antibody anti-Leu-7 (HNK1, CD57) {1043, 1053, 1243}. Immunoreactivity for gamma-enolase is also frequent {1238}. Glial fibrillary acidic protein (GFAP) may be present not only in intermingled reactive astrocytes but also in neoplastic oligodendroglial cells such as minigemistocytes and gliofibrillary oligodendrocytes {578, 823, 1053, 1243, 1324}. The presence of GFAP in minigemistocytes and gliofibrillary oligodendrocytes has been corroborated by ultrastructural studies {578, 816, 1635}. Some authors have suggested that these cells represent transitional forms between astrocytes and oligodendrocytes {578, 816, 823}. Alternatively, they may recapitulate a phenotype characteristic of a transient stage during oligodendroglial development {237,670}. The presence of minigemistocytes and/or gliofibrillary oligodendrocytes is not correlated to patient survival {823}. Vimentin may be expressed in oligodendrogliomas {291, 1238} while cytokeratins are absent {1238}. However, certain antibodies to cytokeratins, such as AE1/AE3, may cross-react with other intermediate filament proteins, including GFAP, and thus give false positive staining {813}. A number of differentiation antigens that are specifically expressed by normal oligodendrocytes *in vivo* or *in vitro* have been identified. These include myelin basic protein (MBP), proteolipid protein (PLP) and myelin-associated glycoprotein (MAG), galactolipids like galactocerebroside (GC) and galactosulphatide, and a number of gangliosides, as well as several enzymes such as carbonic anhydrase C, 2'-3'-cyclic nucleotide-3'-phosphatase (CNP), glycerol-3-phosphate dehydrogenase and lactate dehydrogenase (LDH). However, so far, none of these antigens has gained

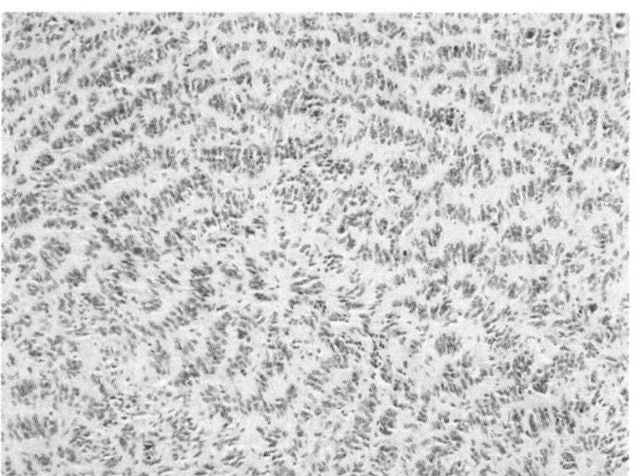

Fig. 2.6 Oligodendroglioma with a striking pattern of nuclear palisading

significance as a diagnostically useful marker for oligodendrogliomas. They either are no longer expressed by neoplastic oligodendrocytes, *e.g.* MBP {1053, 1238}, or they are expressed only in a minority of cases, *e.g.* MAG {1053}, GC {748, 1470}, PLP and CNP {1470}, or their expression is not restricted to oligodendroglial tumour cells, *e.g.* carbonic anhydrase C {1054}.

Proliferation

Mitotic activity is typically absent in WHO grade II oligodendrogliomas and labeling indices for proliferation markers are accordingly low. The Ki67/MIB-1 index is usually below 5% (see predictive factors). Minigemistocytes are reported to be mostly Ki67 (MIB-1) negative and thus non-proliferative, whereas gliofibrillary oligodendrocytes proliferate {818}.

Differential Diagnosis

The differential diagnosis of oligodendroglial tumours includes certain glial and neuronal tumours, such as clear cell ependymoma (see Chapter 3), central neurocytoma (Chapter 6), and dysembryoplastic neuroepithelial tumour (DNT) (Chapter 6). All these entities share with oligodendrogliomas the presence of neoplastic cells with a uniform, round nucleus and clear cytoplasm, collectively referred to as oligodendroglial-like cells (OLC); these cells can readily be differentiated on the basis of their ultrastructural features {212}. Immunocytochemistry for neuronal markers, in particular, synaptophysin, may also be helpful for distinguishing central neurocytoma from oligodendroglioma {465}. However, the interpretation of synaptophysin staining needs care. Residual immunoreactivity from the neuropil in an oligodendroglioma diffusely infiltrating grey matter should not be confused with true expression of synaptophysin by neoplastic cells. Furthermore, several recent studies reported on focal immunoreactivity of tumour cells for neuronal markers, including synaptophysin and neurofilament proteins, in a fraction of otherwise typical oligodendrogliomas {1838, 2229, 2240}. This focal immunoreactivity, however, was not as intense and widespread as in neurocytomas and was not associated with a difference in prognosis {2229, 2240}.

A rare differential diagnosis of oligodendroglioma is clear cell meningioma (see Chapter 11). These tumours can readily

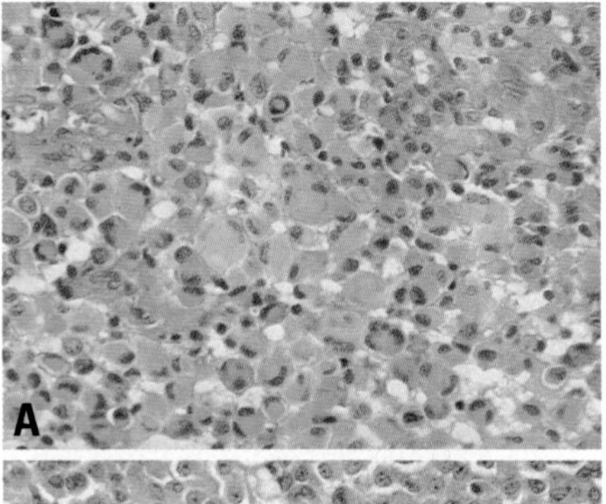

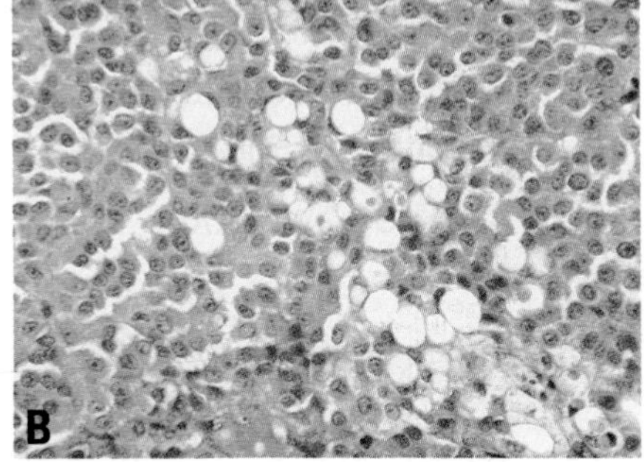

Fig. 2.7 **A** Signet ring cells in an anaplastic oligodendroglioma (WHO grade III). **B** Eosinophilic granular cells in an oligodendroglioma grade II.

be differentiated by abundant diastase-sensitive PAS positivity and immunoreactivity for EMA. Individual anaplastic oligodendrogliomas may superficially resemble metastatic (clear cell) carcinoma. In contrast to oligodendrogliomas, metastatic carcinomas have sharply defined tumour borders and show immunoreactivity for epithelial markers, such as cytokeratins and EMA.

Aetiology

Although oligodendrogliomas and oligoastrocytomas are among the most frequent types of CNS tumours to be induced experimentally in rats by chemical carcinogens such as ethylnitrosourea and methylnitrosourea {1591}, there is no convincing evidence of an aetiological role for these substances in human gliomas. Individual cases of oligodendrogliomas in patients previously irradiated for other reasons have been documented {277, 630}, but these account for only a very small fraction of all oligodendroglial tumours. A recent study reported the presence of sequences from SV40 virus in 3 of 12 oligodendrogliomas {2231}. In addition, 2 of 12 oligodendrogliomas were positive for BK and JC virus sequences. However, other authors failed to detect any JC virus sequences in primary oligodendrogliomas and astrocytomas {2230}. Thus, the role of viral infections in the aetiology of human oligodendroglial tumours is unclear at present.

Genetic susceptibility

Occasional cases of familial clustering have been reported, affecting two brothers {1134}, mother and daughter {1278}, twin sisters {1270} and father and son {403}. The occurrence of polymorphous oligodendrogliomas in a brother and sister has been published by Kros *et al.* {819}. Only occasional patients with an oligodendroglial tumour have been reported in families with hereditary cancer syndromes. In a survey of 47 families from Southern Sweden with hereditary breast and ovarian cancer, one patient with an oligodendroglioma was reported {704}. One patient with Turcot syndrome, who carried a germline mutation in exon 5 of the *hPMS2* mismatch repair gene, developed two metachronous glioblastomas showing histological features of oligodendroglial differentiation {2238}. One of these tumours was shown to have lost alleles on the long

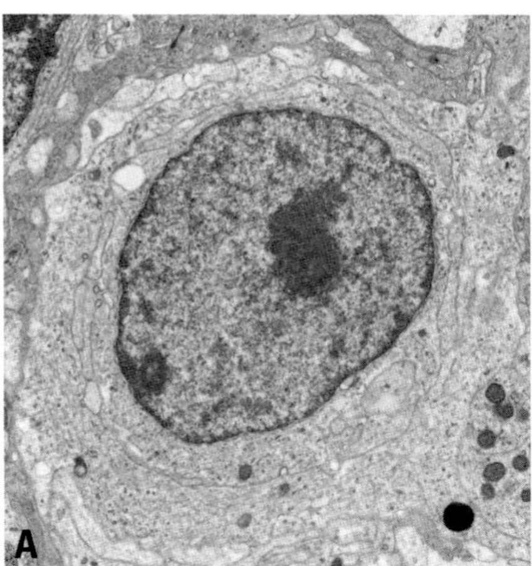

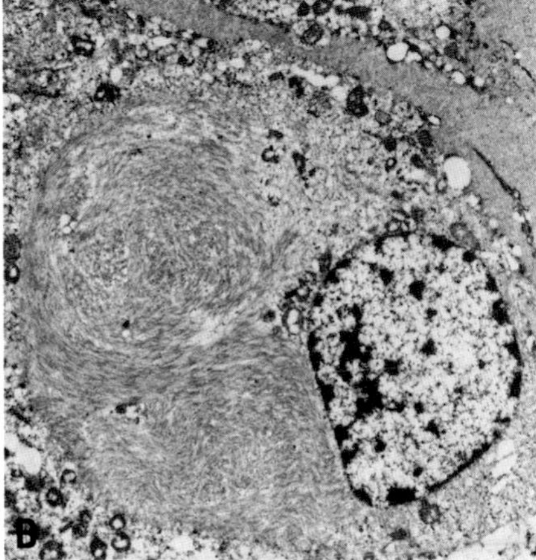

Fig. 2.8 Ultratructure of a typical oligodendroglioma cell (**A**) and of a micro-gemistocytic cell (**B**) with whirls of intermediate filaments.

Oligodendrocytes or precursor cells

LOH 1p LOH 19q LOH 4q	EGFR PDGF/PDGFR overexpression

Oligodendroglioma WHO Grade II

CDKN2A deletion *CDKN2C* mut./del. LOH 9p and 10q	*CDK4, EGFR, MYC* amplification (rare) VEGF overexpression

Anaplastic oligodendroglioma WHO Grade III

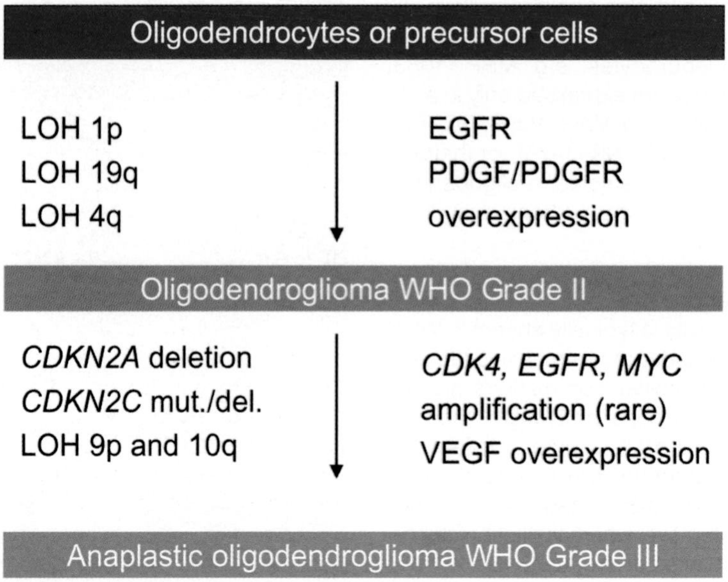

Fig. 2.9 Flow chart showing molecular alterations identified in oligodendrogliomas and anaplastic oligoden-

arm of chromosome 19. The patient's sister also had a glioblastoma with oligodendroglial features, which showed allelic loss on 19q {2238}. So far, oligodendrogliomas were not reported in patients carrying a *TP53* germline mutation (see Chapter 14).

Cytogenetics

G-banded karyotypes of more than 60 oligodendrogliomas have been published {508, 697, 938, 1209, 1228, 1230, 1251, 1499}. The vast majority showed normal or non-clonal karyotypes. A minor subset demonstrated simple clonal abnormalities, while occasional tumours had complex clonal karyotypes. Numerical aberrations reported include loss of one sex chromosome, loss of chromosome 22 and gain of chromosome 7. Structural chromosomal abnormalities, including translocations and deletions, most commonly involve the short arm of chromosome 1. In addition, deletions of 9p are reported at more than random frequency, while structural abnormalities of 19q are only rarely detected.

Molecular genetics

Chromosome 19. The most frequent genetic alteration in oligodendroglial tumours, as determined by loss of heterozygosity (LOH) analysis, is LOH on the long arm of chromosome 19. The incidence of LOH on 19q varies between different studies, ranging from 50% to more than 80% of cases {83, 808, 1244, 1565}. In the majority of oligodendrogliomas, the loss involves all informative loci on 19q, suggesting that all, or almost all, of the chromosome arm had been deleted. However, individual cases demonstrating partial or interstitial LOH have been reported and such cases have been used to narrow down the location of the oligodendroglioma-associated tumour suppressor gene suspected on 19q. Smith *et al.* {2247} recently reported on a region of common deletion on 19q which maps to a 1.5 megabase area between the genetic markers *D19S412* and *D19S596* at 19q13.3. This segment overlaps with the region suspected to carry an astrocytoma-progression associated gene, which has been mapped to an approximately 900 kb segment of 19q13.3–q13.4 between the markers *D19S412* and *STD* {1283}.

Chromosome 1. The second most frequent genetic alteration in oligodendroglial neoplasms is LOH on the short arm of chromosome 1. In one series, LOH was found in 67% (14/21) of tumours {1244}, while other studies reported incidences ranging from 40% (6/15) {808} to 92% (11/12) {85}. Virtually all oligodendrogliomas with loss of heterozygosity on 1p have also lost alleles on 19q, a finding suggesting a synergistic effect of both alterations in conferring a selective growth advantage {83, 808, 1244}. Recent studies indicated that more than a single tumour suppressor gene from 1p may be involved in the pathogenesis of oligodendrogliomas. Deletion mapping of 1p using multiple highly polymorphic microsatellite markers identified at least two distinct putative tumour suppressor gene regions located between *D1S76* and *D1S253* at 1p36.3, and between *D1S482* and *D1S2743* at 1p34-p35 {2244}. The proximal candidate region overlaps with the region of common loss mapped to 1p36 (between *D1S468* and *D1S1612*) by Smith *et al.* {2247}. Other authors have found additional 1p regions demonstrating frequent loss in oligodendrogliomas, with loci located between *D1S252* and *D1S228* (1p13-p36.1) being most commonly affected by LOH {2241}. A small fraction of oligodendroglial tumours has been shown to carry either mutations or homozygous deletions of the cyclin dependent kinase inhibitor gene *CDKN2C* (*$p18^{INK4c}$*) at 1p32 {2244, 2246}. Mutational analysis of the *p73* gene at 1p36.3, which codes for a homologue of the TP53 tumour suppressor protein {2232}, did not detect any alterations in oligodendrogliomas {2233}.

Other chromosomes. In addition to loss of genetic material from 19q and 1p, WHO grade II oligodendrogliomas may show abnormalities of other chromosomes, which most frequently include loss of genetic information from chromosomes 4, 6, 11p, 14, and 22q {1244, 1590, 2241, 2243, 2245}. Chromosomes 9 and 10 are infrequently affected by losses in WHO grade II oligodendrogliomas {1244, 2243, 2245}. One study reported on deletions involving 10q25-q26 in individual low-grade oligodendrogliomas {2225}

TP53. In contrast to astrocytic tumours, loss of 17p is rare (<10%) in oligodendroglial tumours {945, 1244, 2243}. Mutations in the *TP53* gene are limited to about 10–15% of cases {945, 1097, 1245}. However, immunoreactivity for TP53 protein has been reported in a higher percentage of tumours {817,1158}, suggesting accumulation of the wild-type protein.

Growth factors and receptors

About half of both WHO grade II and anaplastic oligodendrogliomas show strong expression of epidermal growth factor receptor (EGFR) mRNA and protein in the absence of EGFR gene amplification {1691}. The molecular mechanisms responsible for the increased transcription of the *EGFR* gene in these tumours are as yet unknown. The simultaneous expression of the mRNAs for the pre-pro-forms of EGF and/or TGFa indicates the possibility of auto-, juxta-, or paracrine growth stimulation via the EGFR system {366}. Several other growth factors, including basic FGF, PDGFs,TGFb, IGF1, and NGF, have been reported to be involved in the regulation of proliferation and or maturation of oligodendroglial cells {186, 510, 977, 1410, 1612}. Platelet-derived growth factors A and B, as well as the corresponding receptors (PDGFR-a and PDGFR-b) are co-expressed in virtually all oligodendrogliomas {2237}.

Several studies have reported on the expression of vascular endothelial growth factor (VEGF) and its receptors in oligodendroglial tumours {2236, 2227, 2224, 2235}. Probably due to the use of different anti-VEGF antibodies, the percentages of tumours demonstrating VEGF immunoreactivity, as well as the distribution of immunoreactivity within the tumour tissue (tumour cells *versus* endothelial cells), varied between these studies. Nevertheless, the available data indicate that VEGF plays an important role as angiogenic factor in oligodendroglial tumours, in particular in anaplastic oligodendrogliomas.

Histogenesis

Although the designation of CNS neoplasms with the morphological characteristics described above as oligodendroglial tumours implies a histogenesis from cells of the oligodendroglial lineage, evidence for this assumption is circumstantial and is based mainly on morphological similarities of the neoplastic cells in these tumours to normal oligodendrocytes. It is also not known whether human oligodendrogliomas arise from neoplastic transformation of mature oligodendrocytes or immature glial precursors. Experimental studies suggest that in developing CNS tissues of rodents, one source of oligodendroglial cells is a bipotential progenitor cell (designated O2-A progenitor), which may differentiate either into oligodendrocytes or type 2 astrocytes (for a review, see ref. {1087}). However, the hypothesis that oligodendrogliomas and oligoastrocytomas are derived from neoplastic transformation of a common precursor cell, *i.e.* a putative human counterpart of the rodent O-2A progenitors, is currently unproven.

Prognosis

Median post-operative survival times ranging from 3 to 5 years have been reported for patients with oligodendroglial tumours of all histological grades {170, 211, 926, 1037}. A study of 32 oligodendrogliomas of WHO grade II reported a mean survival time of 4.4 years and 5- and 10-year survival rates of 38% and 19%, respectively {563}. Dehghani *et al.* {2229} followed up 65 patients with WHO grade II oligodendrogliomas and found a median survival time of 3.5 years and a 5-year survival rate of 76%. Other studies calculated 5- and 10-year survival rates of 47.1% and 30.9% {1469}, as well as 43% and 21% {2242}. Shaw *et al.* {1398} reported a median survival time of 9.8 years and 5- and 10-year survival rates of 75% and 59%, respectively, for patients with oligodendrogliomas of Kernohan grade 1 and 2 {763}. Oligodendrogliomas generally recur locally. Malignant progression on recurrence is not uncommon, although it is considered less frequent than in diffuse astrocytomas.

Predictive factors

Clinical factors. Features associated with more favourable outcome include younger age at operation {1356,1398,1408}, frontal location {820}, post-operative Karnofsky score {1356}, lack of contrast enhancement on neuro-imaging {307}, macroscopically complete surgical removal {211, 1398, 2229}, and irradiation after partial tumour resection {233, 452, 1356, 1398, 1408}.

Histopathology. Parameters that have been shown to be associated with worse prognosis include necrosis, high mitotic activity, increased cellularity, nuclear atypia, cellular pleomorphism, and microvascular proliferation {178, 1036, 1398, 1431, 2229}.

Proliferation. A number of studies have evaluated the prognostic significance of the Ki-67 (MIB-1) index for patients with oligodendroglial tumours {563, 818, 2228, 2229, 2242}. In a study of 32 WHO grade II oligodendrogliomas, Heegaard *et al.* {563} found that Ki-67 labelling indices of higher than 3% were indicative of a worse prognosis. In a study of 89 oligodendroglioma patients, the 5-year survival rate was 83% for patients whose oligodendrogliomas had a MIB-1 labelling index of less than 5% but only 24% for patients with tumours displaying more than 5% MIB-1 positive cells {2229}. Similar data were reported by Coons *et al.* {2228}, who could also discriminate two groups of patients with significantly different survival times when using a cut-off value of 5% MIB-1 positive cells. In line with these data, Kros *et al.* {818} found the Ki-67 labelling index being of prognostic significance independent of patient age, tumour site, and histological grade. In contrast, Wharton *et al.* {2242} found no significant correlation between MIB-1 staining and survival in a series of 32 oligodendroglioma patients. According to Cairncross *et al.* {2226}, response to chemotherapy with procarbazine, CCNU, and vincristine (PCV) of anaplastic oligodendrogliomas was independent from the MIB-1 index. Nevertheless, higher fractions of MIB-1 positive tumour cells were associated with decreased survival {2226}.

Tumour suppressor gene expression. Miettinen *et al.* {2234} reported that patients with oligodendrogliomas lacking nuclear p16 immunoreactivity have poor survival as compared to patients whose tumours have retained p16 expression. Two studies indicated that the immunocytochemical demonstration of TP53 protein in tumour cells correlates with reduced patient survival {817,1158}. However, in the group of anaplastic oligodendrogliomas, *TP53* mutation and p53 expression were not of prognostic significance {2226}. Results obtained by flow cytometry showed that the fraction of tumour cells in S-phase correlates to survival {273}, whereas DNA ploidy was not helpful {273,824}. Evaluation of the apoptotic index has not been shown to be of prognostic significance {1356,2242}.

Anaplastic oligodendroglioma

G. Reifenberger
J.M. Kros
P.C. Burger
D.N. Louis
V.P. Collins

Definition
An oligodendroglioma with focal or diffuse histological features of malignancy and a less favourable prognosis.

ICD-O code: 9451/3

Grading
Anaplastic oligodendroglioma corresponds histologically to WHO grade III.

Incidence
Estimations of the incidence of anaplastic oligodendrogliomas are difficult because many studies do not clearly differentiate between WHO grade II oligodendrogliomas and anaplastic oligodendrogliomas. In one series of 285 consecutive adult supratentorial malignant gliomas, 10 tumours were classified as anaplastic oligodendroglioma (3.5%) {1625}. The percentage of anaplastic tumours (according to WHO criteria) among all oligodendroglial tumours varies between 20% {211, 1079} and 51% (Düsseldorf series). In the series of Shaw *et al.* {1398} anaplastic tumours (Kernohan grade 3 and 4) accounted for 54% of the oligodendroglial tumours.

Age and sex distribution
Anaplastic oligodendrogliomas manifest preferentially in adults. In the Düsseldorf series, the mean age of 66 patients at operation was 48.7 years. Thus, these patients were older on average than the patients with WHO grade II oligodendrogliomas. A correlation between age and histological grade was also reported in other series {820, 926, 2229}. Anaplastic oligodendrogliomas show a slight male predominance. The male:female ratio in the Düsseldorf series was 1.5:1.

Localization
Anaplastic oligodendrogliomas share with WHO grade II oligodendrogliomas a preference for the frontal lobe (60% in the Düsseldorf series), followed by the temporal lobe (33% in the Düsseldorf series).

Clinical features
Symptoms and signs
There are no specific clinical symptoms and signs that allow the anaplastic oligodendroglioma to be distinguished from other anaplastic gliomas. The pre-operative history is often short. However, some patients may present with long-standing signs, suggesting a pre-existing tumour of lower grade.

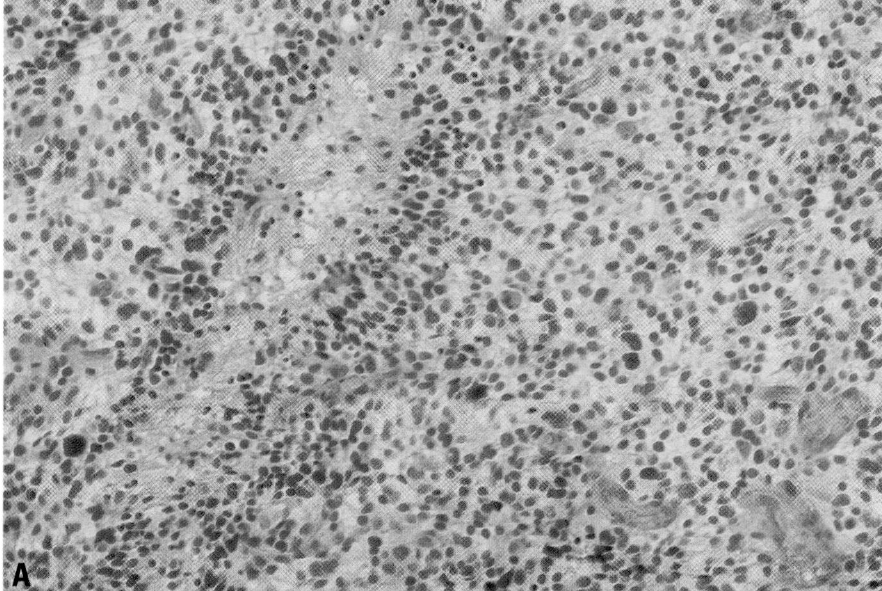

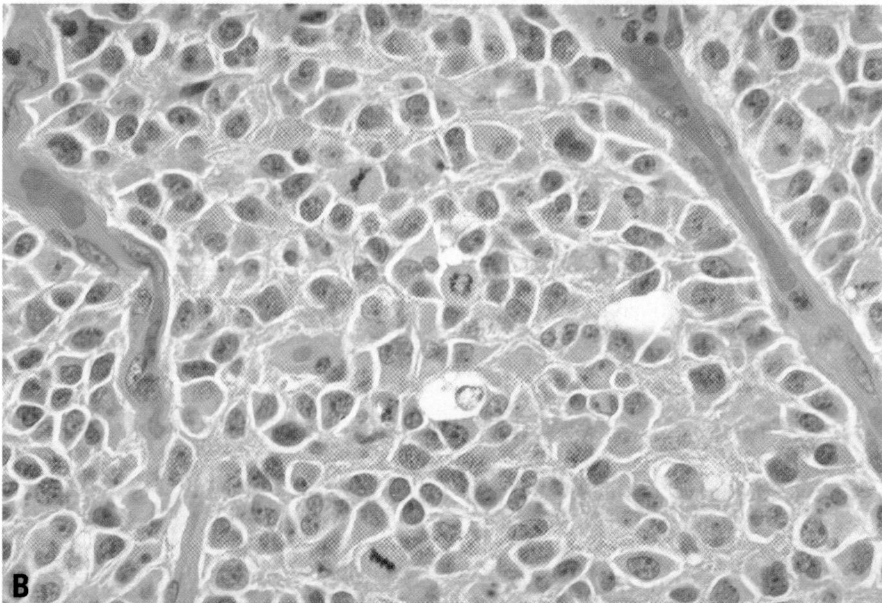

Fig. 2.10 Anaplastic oligodendroglioma showing (**A**) pseudopalisading necrosis, marked nuclear atypia, and incipient microvascular proliferation. **B** Highly anaplastic tumour cells with brisk mitotic activity.

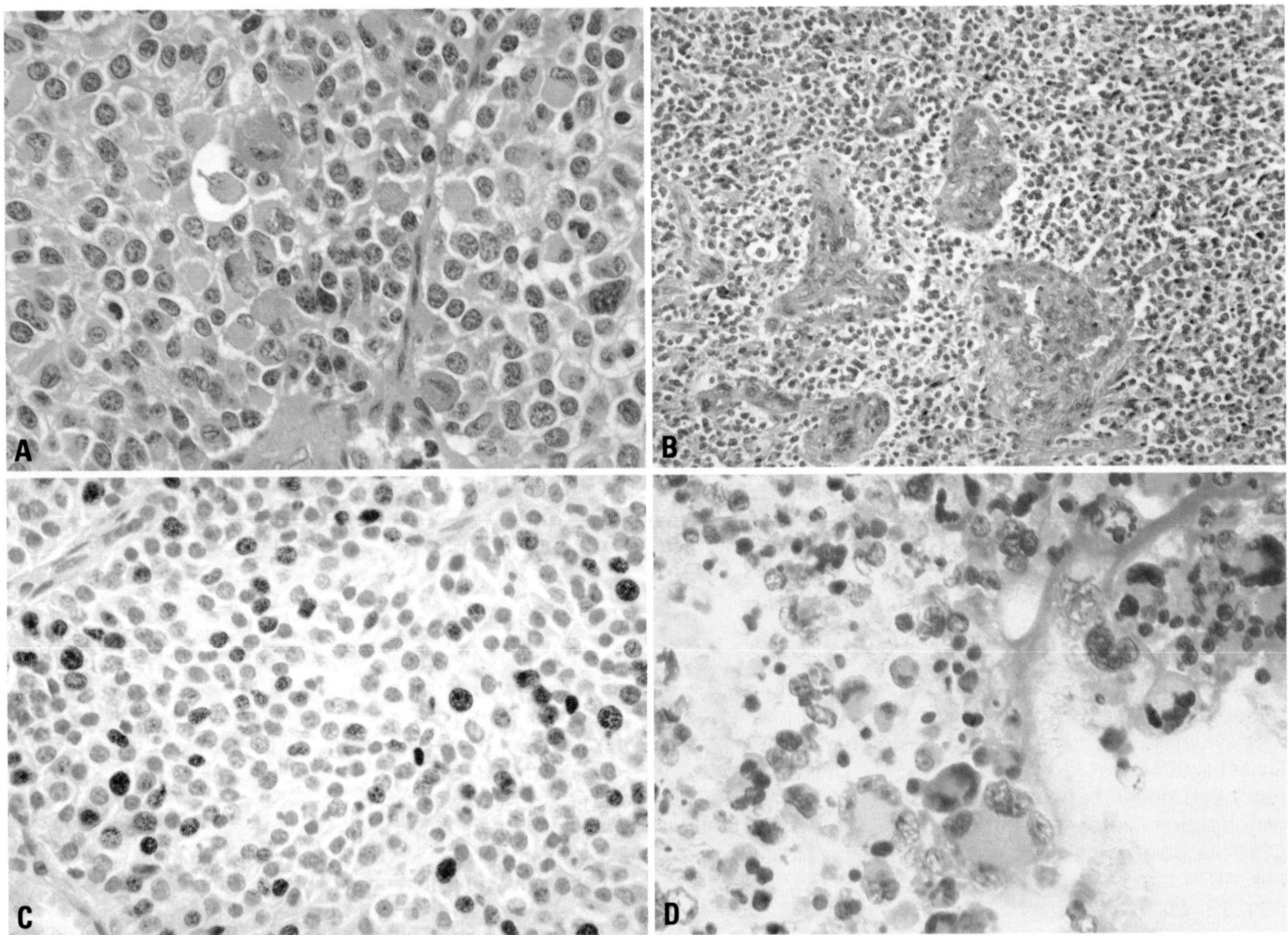

Fig. 2.11 Anaplastic oligodendroglioma. **A** Nuclear atypia and brisk mitotic acivity. **B** Marked microvascular proliferation. **C** High proliferative activity (MIB-1). **D** Intraoperative squash preparation of a highly anaplastic oligodendroglioma.

Neuroimaging

Anaplastic oligodendrogliomas may show heterogeneous patterns, owing to the variable presence of necrosis, cystic degeneration, intratumoral haemorrhages, and calcification. Contrast enhancement on CT and MRI is usual and may be patchy or homogeneous. Ring-enhancement is uncommon and, when present, heralds a poor prognosis {2226}.

Macroscopy

In addition to the macroscopic features described above for WHO grade II oligodendrogliomas, anaplastic oligodendrogliomas may demonstrate areas of tumour necrosis.

Histopathology

An oligodendroglioma with focal or diffuse histological features of malignancy, such as increased cellularity, marked cytological atypia, and high mitotic activity. Microvascular proliferation and necrosis may be present.

Anaplastic oligodendrogliomas are cellular, diffusely infiltrating gliomas that may show considerable morphological variation. The majority of tumour cells demonstrate morphological features that are reminiscent of oligodendroglial cells, *i.e.* rounded hyperchromatic nuclei, perinuclear halos, and few cellular processes. Mitotic activity is usually obvious. Occasional tumours are characterized by marked cellular pleomorphism with multinucleated giant cells (polymorphic variant of Zülch {1686}), or have a conspicuous spindle-cell appearance. Gliofibrillary oligodendrocytes and minigemistocytes are frequent in anaplastic oligodendrogliomas; they do not argue against the diagnosis and are not of prognostic significance {823}. Anaplastic oligodendrogliomas may also feature microvascular proliferation and necrosis with or without pseudopalisading; these features should not prompt the diagnosis of glioblastoma. The correlation between various features of malignancy and patient prognosis remains to be established, as does the validity of subdividing anaplastic oligodendrogliomas into grades III and IV. If the astrocytic component in an anaplastic oligodendroglioma constitutes a significant proportion of the tumour, classification as anaplastic oligoastrocytoma is more appropriate (see following pages). Occasionally, sarcoma-like tumour areas have been observed in oligodendroglial tumours {397, 1135}.

Cytogenetics

In addition to the karyotypic changes described in the section on oligodendrogliomas, occasional cases of anaplastic oligodendrogliomas contain double minute chromosomes, a cytogenetic hallmark of gene amplification {1499}.

Molecular genetics

Although the typical genetic alterations encountered in oligodendroglial tumours, *i.e.* deletions on 1p and 19q, differ significantly from those in astrocytomas, malignant progression appears to be mediated by common molecular mechanisms. This assumption is based on the finding that anaplastic oligodendrogliomas share with low-grade oligodendrogliomas the frequent loss of alleles on 1p and 19q, but additionally show an increased incidence of deletions on the short arm of chromosome 9 and/or on chromosome 10 {1244, 1647, 2226, 2245, 2248}. The latter two alterations are also frequent progression-associated changes in malignant astrocytic tumours. Furthermore, the *CDKN2A* tumour suppressor gene at 9p21 has been shown to be homozygously deleted in about 25% of anaplastic oligodendrogliomas, including tumours with and without allelic loss on 1p and/or 19q {2226, 2243}. Thus, the incidence of homozygous *CDKN2A* deletions in anaplastic oligodendrogliomas is similar to that in anaplastic astrocytomas {644}. Homozygopus deletion of the CDNK2/p18INK4C gene at 1p32 has beeb observed in two anaplastic oligodendrogliomas that did not have CDKN2A deletions {2246}. Mutations of the *PTEN* tumour suppressor gene at 10q23.3, which are common in glioblastomas (see Chapter 1), have been detected in only a small fraction of anaplastic oligodendrogliomas {2155}. Anaplastic oligodendrogliomas with loss of chromosome 10 and gain of chromosome 7 usually lack deletions on 1p and 19q. It has been speculated that these tumours represent a subgroup of anaplastic oligodendrogliomas that is genetically related to glioblastoma and may prognostically differ from lesions with 1p and 19q loss {2248}. In addition to losses on 9p and 10, anaplastic oligodendroglial tumours show an increased frequency of multiple deletions involving chromosomes 4, 6, 11, 15, and 18 {1244, 2241, 2243, 2245}. Thus, the average number of chromosomes involved is higher in anaplastic oligodendrogliomas than in WHO grade II oligodendrogliomas {1244, 1590, 2243, 2248, 2245}, a finding in line with the hypothesis that malignant progression is associated with the acquisition of multiple genetic abnormalities. A small subset (<10%) of anaplastic oligodendrogliomas may demonstrate amplification of proto-oncogenes, including *EGFR, MYC,* MYCN, *CDK4, SAS, GLI and* the renin gene *REN* (for review, see Ref. {1242}).

Prognosis

Shaw *et al.* {1398} reported a median survival time of 3.9 years and 5- and 10-year survival rates of 41% and 20% respectively, for 44 patients with anaplastic oligodendrogliomas (Kernohan grade 3 and 4). Dehghani *et al.* {2229} evaluated 24 patients with anaplastic oligodendroglioma (WHO grade III), which demonstrated a considerably lower median survival time of 0.875 years and a 5-year survival rate of 23%. Current therapies (see below), however, may improve these survival data considerably {2226}. Most patients die from local tumour recurrence. Occasionally, patients may develop metastases via the CSF, or even systemic metastases {934, 1306}. A rare complication of both oligodendroglioma and anaplastic oligodendroglioma is leptomeningeal 'oligodendrogliomatosis' {425, 1180, 1306}.

Predictive factors

The presence of ring enhancement on initial neuroimaging has been reported to correlate with a lack of response to procarbazine, CCNU and vincristine (PCV) treatment and poor prognosis {2226} but there is recent evidence that molecular genetic analysis may provide a more powerful means of separating anaplastic oligodendrogliomas into therapeutically and prognostically significant subgroups. Those anaplastic oligodendrogliomas that have allelic loss on the short arm of chromosome 1, or combined allelic losses on 1p and 19q, are typically sensitive to PCV chemotherapy, with about half of such tumours showing complete neuroradiological responses to PCV {2226}. On the other hand, only 25% of tumours that lack these genetic changes respond to PCV, with only rare complete responses. These genetic differences also affect survival: patients whose anaplastic oligodendrogliomas have LOH on 1p or combined LOH on 1p and 19q have substantially prolonged survival (mean, approximately 10 years) compared with those patients whose tumours lack these genetic changes (mean survival of about 2 years) {2226}. Homozygous deletions of the *CDKN2A* gene were primarily detected in those anaplastic oligodendrogliomas that lacked 1p and 19q losses {2226}. Patients whose tumours had *CDKN2A* deletions generally had shorter survivals {2226}. Thus, there appear to be at least two biologically distinct types of anaplastic oligodendrogliomas, with markedly different clinical behaviour. Whether such powerful molecular predictors apply also to low-grade oligodendrogliomas and mixed oligoastrocytomas remains to be shown.

Oligoastrocytoma

G. Reifenberger
J.M. Kros
P.C. Burger
D.N. Louis
V.P. Collins

Definition

A tumour composed of a conspicuous mixture of two distinct neoplastic cell types morphologically resembling the tumour cells in oligodendroglioma and diffuse astrocytoma of WHO grade II.

Grading

Oligoastrocytoma corresponds histologically to WHO grade II.

ICD-O code: 9382/3

Historical annotation

Mixed oligoastrocytomas were first recognized as an entity by Cooper in 1935 {275}.

Incidence

Because of the high variability of the morphological criteria used for the classification of oligoastrocytomas, estimates of their incidence vary and must be interpreted with caution. Among 4859 patients with intracranial gliomas registered by the Norwegian Cancer Registry between 1956 and 1984, mixed gliomas accounted for 9.2 % of the tumours {568}. Another study reported an incidence between 10 and 19% of supratentorial low-grade gliomas {684}. In contrast, among 5216 gliomas registered from 1990–1992 by the central brain tumour registry of the United States of America, only 96 tumours were listed under the diagnosis mixed glioma (1.8%). The annual incidence was estimated as 0.1 per 100'000 individuals.

Age and sex distribution

Males are affected slightly more frequently than females, with a ratio of 1.2:1 in the Düsseldorf series of 26 patients with WHO grade II oligoastrocytomas and 1.7:1 in another series of 20 low-grade and 10 anaplastic oligoastrocytomas {2249}. Two studies reported on a median age at operation between 35 and 45 years in the Düsseldorf series and the series of Jaskòlski *et al.* {684}

Localization

Oligoastrocytomas arise preferentially in the cerebral hemispheres. The frontal lobes are most commonly affected, followed by the temporal lobes {545, 684, 1397, 2249}. In the Düsseldorf series, 18 of 26 (65%) oligoastrocytomas were located frontally and 5 of 26 (19%) involved the temporal lobe.

Clinical features

Symptoms and signs

Clinically, oligoastrocytomas present with symptoms and signs similar to those described for astrocytomas and oligodendrogliomas, most commonly epileptic seizures, paresis, personality changes, and signs of increased intracranial pressure {684, 1397, 2249}.

Neuroimaging

Neuroradiologically, oligoastrocytomas demonstrate no special features that would allow a reliable distinction from WHO grade II oligodendrogliomas. In the series of Shaw *et al.* {1397}, calcifications were demonstrable in 14% of the tumours. About half of the oligoastrocytomas (12/23) evaluated by CT scanning showed contrast enhancement {1397}.

Macroscopy

The macroscopical appearance of oligoastrocytomas does not usually allow their distinction from other WHO grade II gliomas. Only occasionally are there regional differences in colour and consistency reflecting areas of distinct cellular differentiation.

Histopathology

The diagnosis of oligoastrocytomas requires the recognition of two different glial components both of which must be unequivocally neoplastic.

Oligoastrocytomas are mild to moderately cellular neoplasms with no or low mitotic activity. Microcalcifications and microcystic degeneration may be present but necrosis and microvascular proliferation are absent.

Oligoastrocytomas may be divided into biphasic ("compact") and intermingled ("diffuse") variants {545}. In the biphasic variant, distinct areas of oligodendroglial and astrocytic differentiation are juxtaposed, while in the intermingled variant both components are intimately admixed.

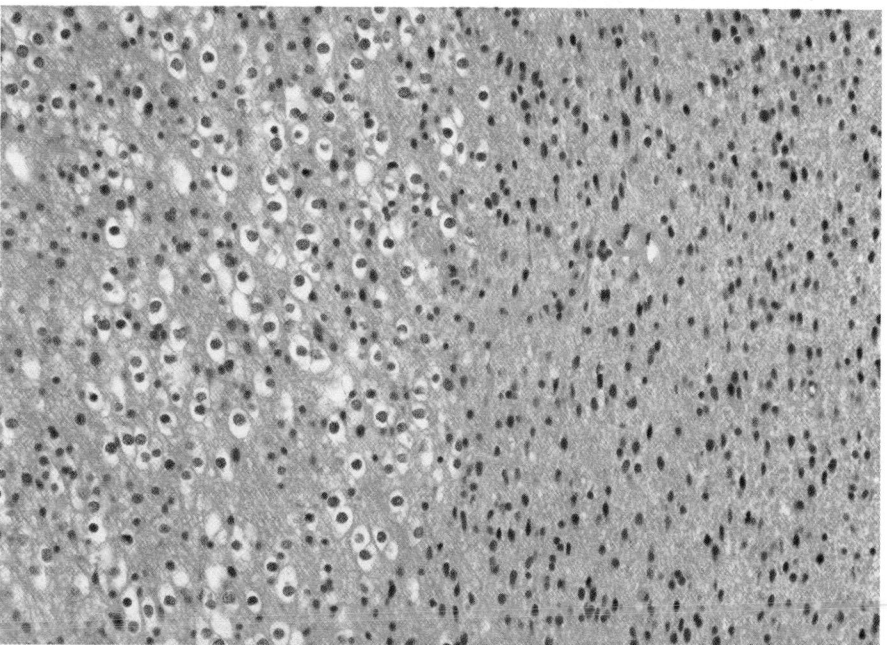

Fig. 2.12 Oligoastrocytoma with distinct components displaying oligodendroglial (left) and astrocytic (right) differentiation.

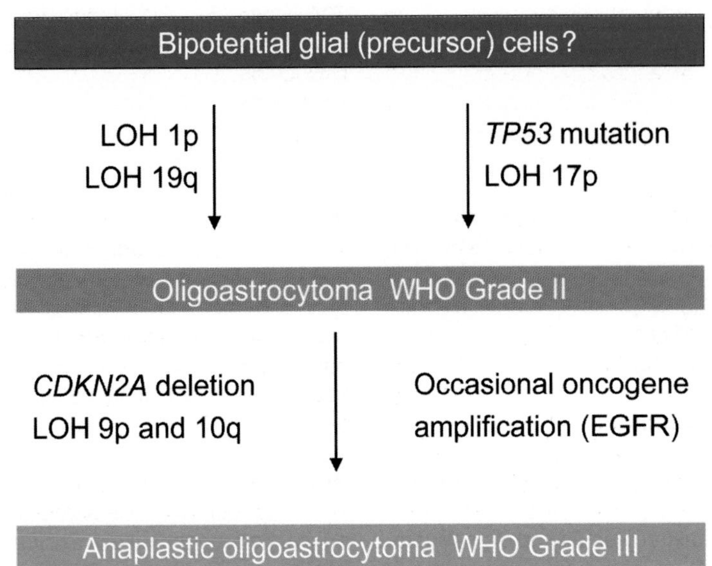

Fig. 2.13 Flow chart showing genetic alterations involved in the development of oligoastrocytoma and anaplastic oligoastrocytoma.

Classification of the intermingled variant is more difficult. In particular, a diffuse admixture in oligodendrogliomas of GFAP-positive minigemistocytes and gliofibrillary oligodendrocytes should not prompt a shift in diagnosis from oligodendroglioma to oligoastrocytoma. Only tumours in which a clear fibrillary, protoplasmic or classic gemistocytic astroglial component is evident in addition to the oligodendroglial cells qualify for the diagnosis of oligoastrocytoma. At the same time, in the presence of numerous minigemistocytes a careful search for an astrocytic component should be performed.

The pronounced phenotypic heterogeneity of the astroglial and oligodendroglial cell lineages and a lack of reliable markers make it difficult to define precise diagnostic criteria. It has been recommended to assess the fractions of the two components but opinions diverge, with the proposed minimum astroglial component ranging from 1% {771}, 25% {1036}, 30% {638}, to approximately 50% {545}. In most instances the precise extent of each component is difficult to determine since tumour cells may not always be easily recognized as either oligodendroglial or astrocytic, *i.e.* they may have features of both lineages. Coons *et al.* {274} suggested that the presence of at least one 100x field which, when considered alone, would warrant a diagnosis of oligodendroglioma, is sufficient for shifting the diagnosis from astrocytoma to oligoastrocytoma. This approach resulted in an improved interobserver concordance and permitted the identification of a prognostically more favourable subgroup of tumours previously included in the anaplastic astrocytoma group {274}. However, it is possible that such a small oligodendroglial area may be missed due to incomplete tissue sampling. Furthermore, it remains to be seen whether gliomas with only a minute oligodendroglial component do in fact respond better to PCV therapy than "pure" astrocytomas.

From a clinical viewpoint, it has become increasingly important to differentiate between oligoastrocytomas and "pure" astroglial tumours because oligoastrocytomas, like oligodendroglial tumours, appear to respond favourably to chemotherapy such as PCV {479, 771, 845}.

Further subclassification of oligoastrocytomas into oligodendroglioma-predominant, astrocytoma-predominant, and tumours with approximately equal oligodendroglial and astroglial components has been suggested {545}. However, prognosis and response to therapy have not been found to be significantly different for these subtypes {545, 771, 1397}.

Immunohistochemistry

The oligodendroglial and astroglial components in oligoastrocytomas show the same immunoreactivity patterns as 'pure' oligodendrogliomas and astrocytomas, respectively. There is no specific immunocytochemical marker which could be used for the reliable distinction of both components. GFAP and vimentin expression are more consistently found in the astroglial component, compared with a more variable expression in the oligodendroglial tumour cells. In support of this immunohistochemical data, analysis of GFAP and its fragments by two-dimensional gel electrophoresis and Western blot analysis has allowed a discrimination of astrocytoma from oligodendroglioma {2251}. However, these techniques are not suitable as routine diagnostic methods and cannot be applied to oligoastrocytomas with a diffuse mixture of both cell types. One study reported that immunoreactivity for the neurotrophin receptors TrkA, B, and C is exclusively found in normal, reactive, and neoplastic astrocytes but not in normal and neoplastic oligodendrocytes {2253}. It remains to be shown whether immunohistochemistry for Trk receptors provides a reliable and routinely applicable method for distinguishing astroglial and oligodendroglial tumour cells in oligoastrocytomas.

Proliferation

Immunocytochemistry for the Ki67 proliferation-associated nuclear antigen generally reveals low labelling indices in oligoastrocytomas, with an average value of less than 6% reported in a series of 20 tumours {1407}. In contrast, the fraction of Ki67-positive tumour cells is usually higher in anaplastic oligoastrocytomas, with a mean value of 14% {324}.

Aetiology

DNA sequences similar to those of JC virus, the etiologic agent of progressive multifocal leukoencephalopathy, have been detected in a human oligoastrocytoma and viral antigen was found to be expressed in the tumour cells {1248}. The authors suggested a possible role of JC virus in the development of some glial neoplasms but this requires further corroboration.

Genetic susceptibility

A clustering has been reported with two family members having cerebral low-grade diffuse astrocytomas and another a cerebellar oligoastrocytoma {219}. Further, oligoastrocytomas were observed in identical twins {388}. Another study reported on two siblings with glioblastoma multiforme and mixed oligoastrocytoma, respectively {2252}. No data are available on germline mutations in cases of familial clustering of oligoastrocytoma.

Molecular genetics

The molecular genetic alterations underlying the oncogenesis and progression of oligoastrocytomas appear to be more heterogeneous than those characteristically associated with "pure" oligodendrogliomas. No consistent genetic abnormalities have been detected that would indicate that oligoastrocytomas are genetically distinct from oligodendrogliomas on the one hand and astrocytomas on the other {1244}. About 30–50% of oligoastrocytomas are characterized by loss of genetic information on chromosomes 19q and 1p {808, 945, 1244}. Kraus *et al.* {808} have microdissected oligodendroglial and astrocytic tumour parts in three oligoastrocytomas and found common genetic alterations, *i.e.* loss of alleles on 1p and 19q, in both components in all three cases. This strongly suggests that oligoastrocytomas are monoclonal neoplasms originating from a single precursor cell rather than representing composition tumours that had developed concurrently.

About 30% of oligoastrocytomas carry genetic aberrations frequently found in astrocytic gliomas, *i.e.* mutations of the *TP53* gene and/or loss of heterozygosity on 17p {945,1244}. Interestingly, those oligoastrocytomas with *TP53* mutations and/or 17p loss do not have LOH on 1p and 19q, and vice versa {945,1244}. Furthermore, the subset of oligoastrocytomas with 1p and 19q loss has been found to be more often oligodendroglioma-predominant, whereas those tumours with *TP53* mutations were more often astrocytoma-predominant {945}. Taken together, these data indicate that tumours morphologically classified as oligoastrocytoma are genetically heterogeneous. One subset appears to be genetically related to oligodendroglial tumours, while another is genetically related to diffuse astrocytomas. The biological basis of the presence of two distinct glial phenotypes in each of these tumours remains to be elucidated.

Histogenesis

The histogenesis of oligoastrocytomas is largely unresolved (see histogenesis of astrocytomas and oligodendrogliomas).

Prognosis

A median survival time of 6.3 years and 5- and 10-year survival rates of 58% and 32%, respectively, have been reported in a study of 60 patients with low-grade (Kernohan grade 1 and 2) oligoastrocytomas {1397}. Somewhat shorter mean survival times of 3.9 years and 3.0 years have been reported by Hart *et al.* {545} and Jaskólsky *et al.* {684}, respectively. Factors associated with longer survival include younger age at operation (less than 37 years), gross total tumour resection, and postoperative radiation therapy {1397}. When comparing biphasic versus intermingled variants, one study found no significant survival differences {545}, while other authors reported a lower Ki-67 proliferation index and longer median survival time for biphasic oligoastrocytomas {1407}. It remains to be seen whether this trend holds true when evaluating larger series of patients.

Anaplastic oligoastrocytoma

G. Reifenberger
J.M. Kros
P.C. Burger
D.N. Louis
V.P. Collins

Definition
An oligoastrocytoma with histological features of malignancy, such as increased cellularity, nuclear atypia, pleomorphism, and increased mitotic activity.

ICD-O code:
The provisional code proposed for the third edition of ICD-O is 9832/32

Grading
Anaplastic oligoastrocytoma corresponds histologically to WHO grade III.

Incidence
No precise epidemiological data on the incidence of anaplastic oligoastrocytomas are available. In a series of 285 supratentorial anaplastic gliomas in adults, anaplastic oligoastrocytomas accounted for 11 tumours (4%) {1625}.

Age and sex distribution
In the Düsseldorf series of 42 patients with anaplastic oligoastrocytomas, the male: female ratio was 1.3:1; the mean age at operation was 45 years.

Localization
Anaplastic oligoastrocytomas are predominantly hemispheric tumours. In the Düsseldorf series, 53% of the anaplastic oligoastrocytomas involved the frontal lobes and 38% the temporal lobes.

Clinical features
Symptoms and signs
The clinical history of patients with anaplastic oligoastrocytomas is usually short. However, a preoperative history of several years may occasionally be encountered,

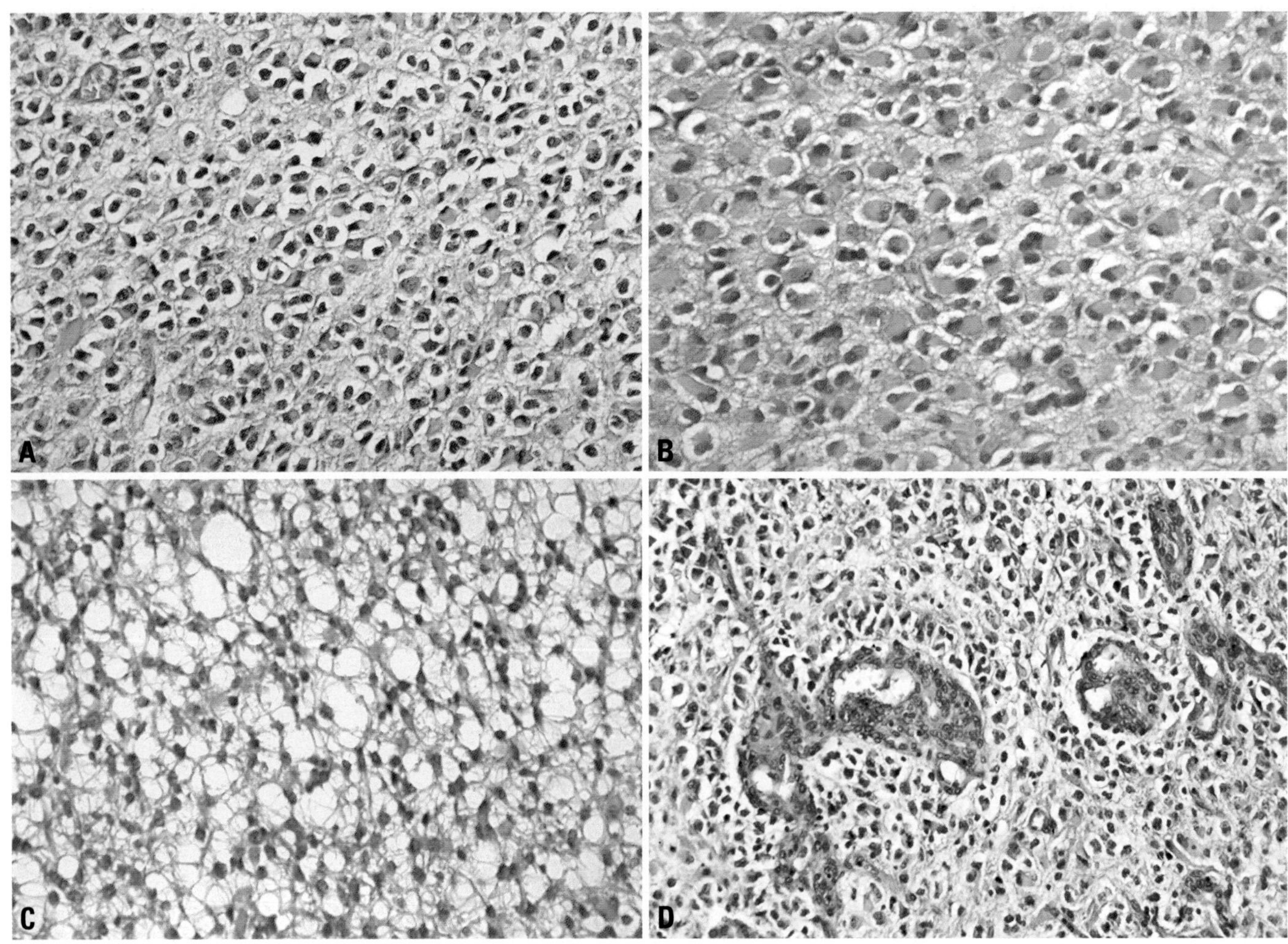

Fig. 2.14 Patterns of differentiation in an anaplastic oligoastrocytoma **A** Tumour area showing the typical morphology of an oligodendroglioma with little evidence of anaplasia. **B** Region with marked nuclear atypia and numerous minigemistocytes. **C** Another area of the same tumour showing fibrillary astrocytic differentiation. **D** Marked microvascular proliferation in the same tumour.

suggesting a pre-existing low-grade glioma.

Neuroimaging

Anaplastic oligoastrocytomas usually show contrast enhancement on CT and MRI.

Macroscopy

There are no consistent features that would allow the macroscopic distinction of anaplastic oligoastrocytoma from other anaplastic glioma types. Foci of necrosis and intratumoral haemorrhages, as well as areas of cystic degeneration and calcifications, may be seen.

Histopathology

Anaplastic oligoastrocytomas are oligoastrocytomas with histological features of anaplasia, including nuclear atypia, cellular pleomorphism, high cellularity, and high mitotic activity. In addition, microvascular proliferation and necrosis may be present. Signs of histological malignancy may be present in the oligodendroglial, the astroglial, or in both components.

The differential diagnosis of anaplastic oligoastrocytoma primarily includes anaplastic oligodendroglioma, anaplastic astrocytoma and glioblastoma. The distinction from anaplastic astrocytoma is straightforward if a definite oligodendroglioma component is identified.

However, as discussed above (see oligoastrocytoma), the definition of an oligodendroglioma component has remained controversial. The identification of an astrocytoma component can be particularly challenging in a high-grade oligodendroglioma with considerable pleomorphism or in the presence of many gemistocytic cells, often in transition from minigemistocytes to classical gemistocytes.

Perhaps most difficult is the differential diagnosis *versus* glioblastoma, since it is increasingly recognized that oligodendroglioma-like foci may be present in glioblastomas. The appropriate terminology for such cases remains unclear; "glioblastoma with oligodendroglioma component" is proposed as a compromise term for such lesions. The key clinical issue is whether the distinction of such tumours from classical glioblastomas identifies a subset of patients who will respond more favourably to PCV chemotherapy and/or has a generally better prognosis. It will also be of particular interest to clarify the role of molecular genetic alterations, such as allelic loss on the short arm of chromosome 1, as predictors of chemosensitivity and/or prognostic factors for patients with anaplastic oligoastrocytoma, anaplastic astrocytoma, and glioblastoma.

Molecular genetics

With respect to progression-associated genetic abnormalities, anaplastic oligoastrocytomas have been found to share many alterations that are also implicated in the progression of astrocytomas and oligodendrogliomas, including LOH on 9p and homozygous deletion of *CDKN2A*, as well as allelic loss on chromosomes 10 and 11p {1244}. Individual cases of anaplastic oligoastrocytomas with amplification of the *EGFR* gene have been reported {1244}.

Prognosis

The prognosis of patients with anaplastic oligoastrocytomas is relatively poor, although still considerably better than for patients with classical glioblastoma.

A median survival time of 2.8 years and 5- and 10-year survival rates of 36% and 9%, respectively, have been reported by Shaw *et al.* {1397} in a study of 11 patients treated by operation and postoperative radiation therapy. A study on 19 patients with anaplastic oligoastrocytoma of WHO grade III treated by operation, irradiation, and PCV chemotherapy reported a median survival time of 49.8 months {771}. In this study, seven patients with anaplastic oligodendroglioma treated in the same way showed a considerably longer median survival time of 76 months. In contrast, another study reported that patients with anaplastic oligoastrocytomas survived longer on average than patients with anaplastic oligodendrogliomas {845}. Donahue and co-workers {2250} found that patients with anaplastic oligoastrocytomas had a better prognosis than patients with "pure" anaplastic astrocytomas. The same authors also reported evidence that "glioblastomas with an oligodendroglial component" are associated with longer survival than classical glioblastomas.

Other mixed gliomas

In a series of 102 mixed gliomas, Hart *et al.* {545} reported 16 tumours to be composed of oligodendroglioma and ependymoma but this frequency appears to be in excess of that of current experience which suggests that such tumours are very rare. The occasional presence of perivascular pseudorosettes in otherwise typical oligodendrogliomas is not sufficient for the diagnosis of oligoependymoma, but should raise the differential diagnosis of clear-cell ependymoma. Only individual examples of mixed gliomas composed of distinct astrocytic and ependymal elements have been described, including one tumour derived from a medulloblastoma {396}, a mixed ependymoma-astrocytoma of the cerebellopontine angle {1004}, and a tumour of the cerebral cortex with morphological and ultrastructural features reminiscent of subependymoma, but without geographical relation to the ventricles {796}.

CHAPTER 3

Ependymal Tumours

This group of neoplasms arises from the ependymal lining of the cerebral ventricles and from the remnants of the central canal of the spinal cord. Ependymomas manifest predominantly in children and young adults and their morphological features and biological behaviour vary considerably. The following entities can be delineated:

Ependymoma (WHO grade II)

This most common ependymal neoplasm is usually located intraventricularly and often causes clinical symptoms by blocking CSF pathways.

Anaplastic ependymoma (WHO grade III)

Anaplastic ependymomas may develop through malignant progression from low-grade ependymoma but typically, this lesion shows anaplastic features at first biopsy.

Myxopapillary ependymoma (WHO grade I)

This ependymoma variant is particularly noteworthy since it occurs almost exclusively in the conus-cauda-filum terminale region, with a generally favourable prognosis.

Subependymoma (WHO grade I)

This benign, slowly growing intraventricular neoplasm is often detected incidentally and has a very favourable prognosis. Some lesions show the histological features of both subependymoma and ependymoma.

Ependymoma

O.D. Wiestler
D. Schiffer
S.W. Coons
R.A. Prayson
M.K. Rosenblum

Definition

A slowly growing tumour of children and young adults, originating from the wall of the cerebral ventricles or from the spinal canal and composed of neoplastic ependymal cells.

ICD-O code: 9391/3

Provisional codes proposed for the third edition of the ICD-O are:

Cellular ependymoma *9391/3*
Papillary ependymoma *9393/3*
Clear cell ependymoma *9391/3*
Tanycytic ependymoma *9391/3*

Grading

Ependymoma corresponds histologically to WHO grade II.

Incidence

Ependymomas account for 3–9% of all neuroepithelial tumours. They amount to 6–12% of all intracranial tumours in children, and to 30% of those in children younger than 3 years {359}. In the spinal cord, ependymomas are the most common neuroepithelial neoplasms, comprising 50–60% of spinal gliomas {1347}.

Age and sex distribution

In principle, ependymomas may develop in all age groups, with a range from 1 month to 81 years {417, 810, 1686, 2151}. Infratentorial ependymomas predominate in children with a mean age at clinical manifestation of 6.4 years and a range of 2 months to 16 years {1663}. A second age peak at 30–40 years has been reported for spinal tumours. Supratentorial ependymomas affect paediatric as well as adult patients. In a large Japanese series {832}, clinical and follow-up data were reported on 23 cases manifesting in the first year of life. Ependymomas appear equally distributed between the two sexes {569, 1061, 1354}.

Localization

These tumours occur at any site along the ventricular system and in the spinal canal. They most commonly develop in the posterior fossa and in the spinal cord, followed by the lateral ventricles and the third ventricle. A recent clinicopathologic study on 61 ependymoma patients with an age range from 1.5 to 74 years confirmed the spinal cord and the fourth ventricle as predominant locations {2151}. In a series of 298 cases, an infratentorial: supratentorial ratio of 101:72 (58/42%) was reported {1354}. In adult patients, infratentorial and spinal ependymomas arise with almost equal frequency, whereas infratentorial ependymomas clearly predominate in young children {832}. In the spinal cord, cervical and cervico-thoracic segments appear to represent primary sites whereas the myxopapillary variant of ependymoma predominantly affects the conus-cauda equina region. Supratentorial parenchymal ependymomas may occur outside the ventricular system, particularly in children; it was hypothesised that these tumours originate from embryonic ependymal remnants in the brain parenchyma. Rare extraneural ependymomas have been observed in the ovaries, soft tissues, mediastinum and the sacrococcygeal area {1028}.

Clinical features

Symptoms and signs

Clinical manifestations are localization-dependent. Signs of hydrocephalus and increased intracranial pressure, such as headache, nausea, vomiting and dizziness predominate in infratentorial ependymomas. Involvement of posterior fossa structures may cause cerebellar ataxia, visual disturbance, dizziness, and paresis. Patients with supratentorial ependymomas show focal neurological deficits, seizures and features of intracranial hypertension {359}. Head enlargement can be encountered in children below the age of two years. Motor and sensory deficits represent the major manifestations in spinal ependymomas.

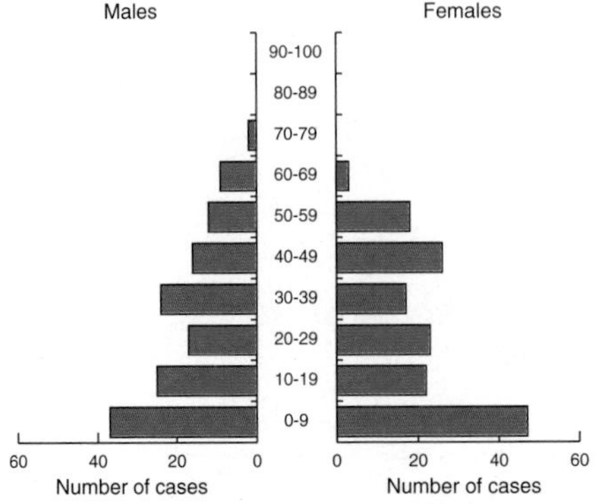

Fig. 3.1 Age and sex distribution of ependymomas, based on 298 cases. Data from Schiffer *et al.* {1354}.

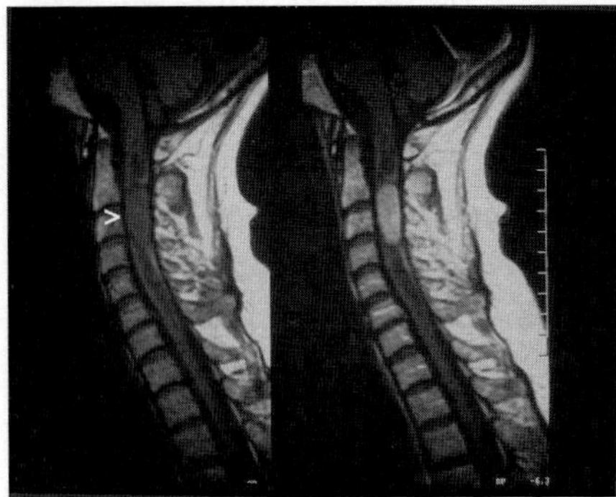

Fig. 3.2 Sagittal MRI showing an ependymoma in the upper cervical spinal cord (left, arrow) with marked gadolinium enhancement (right), delineated on both sides by a typical cyst.

Neuroimaging

Gadolinium-enhanced MRI scans demonstrate a rather well circumscribed lesion with varying degrees of contrast enhancement. Ventricular or brain stem displacement and hydrocephalus are frequent accompanying features. Supratentorial tumours may exhibit cystic components. Intratumoral haemorrhage and extensive calcification are occasionally observed. Gross infiltration of adjacent brain structures and oedema are infrequent. However, in supratentorial parenchymal ependymomas, the neuroradiological distinction from other glioma entities constitutes a diagnostic challenge. MRI appears particularly useful for determining the relationship to surrounding structures and invasion along the CSF pathway. Intramedullary ependymoma is often associated with syrinx formation.

Macroscopy

Macroscopic features of ependymomas vary according to the anatomic location and the size of the tumour. In the posterior fossa, ependymomas originate from the floor or from the roof of the IV ventricle and develop into the ventricular lumen. Tumour tissue may extend into the pontocerebellar angle, protrude into the cisterna magna and extend along the surface of the brain stem and through the foramen magnum. Ependymomas appear generally well demarcated. Occasionally, ependymal tumours may invade adjacent brain parenchyma. Ependymomas are soft, greyish-red tumours, some of which exhibit a cystic element, necrotic foci or haemorrhage. In the spinal cord, they can involve several segments and tend to present as circumscribed intramedullary masses.

Histopathology

Ependymomas are well-delineated, moderately cellular gliomas with a monomorphic nuclear morphology. Key histological features are perivascular pseudorosettes and ependymal rosettes. Mitoses are rare or absent. Occasional non-palisading foci of necrosis are compatible with the diagnosis of ependymoma WHO grade II.

The tumour/parenchymal interface is typically sharp {2145}. Two morphological forms of rosettes can be distinguished. Perivascular pseudorosettes originate from tumour cells arranged radially around blood vessels and occur in the great majority of these neoplasms. True ependymal rosettes and ependymal canals are composed of columnar cells arranged around a central lumen. These are diagnostic for ependymoma but develop only in a minority of cases. Fibrillary elements are frequently encountered. Regressive changes include areas of myxoid degeneration, intratumoral haemorrhage, calcifications and, occasionally, foci of cartilage and bone formation. Marked hyalinization of tumour vessels is not uncommon and may precede calcification. The following histopathological variants of ependymoma can be distinguished:

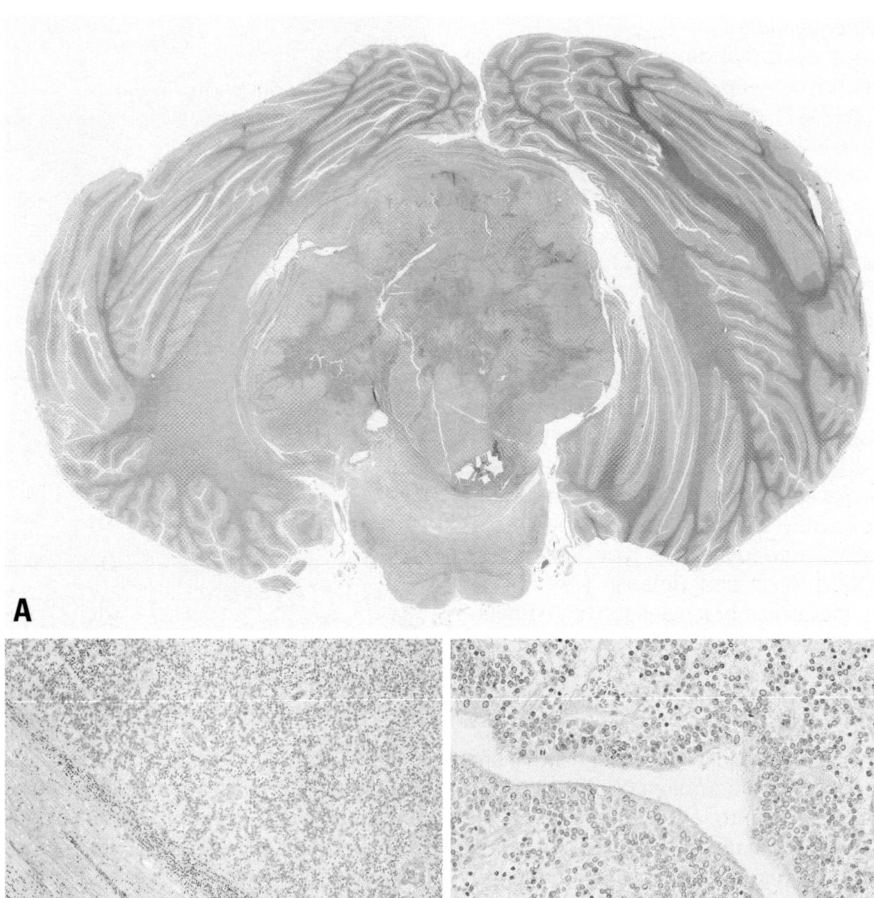

Fig. 3.3 A Ependymoma in a child, filling the entire lumen of the fourth ventricle. Note the displacement of the medulla, **(B)** the relatively clear demarcation from the cerebellar parenchyma and **(C)** the involvement of the ependymal lining in the neoplastic process.

Cellular ependymoma

This variant shows conspicuous cellularity without a significant increase in mitotic rate. Pseudorosettes may be inconspicuous and true ependymal rosettes may be absent. Such tumours have been designated cellular ependymoma. They lack additional properties of anaplastic ependymomas and are, therefore, classified as WHO grade II tumours.

Papillary ependymoma

A rare variant of ependymoma characterized by well formed papillae, in which tumour vessels are covered by a smooth layer of tumour cells. Tumour cell processes abutting capillaries are usually GFAP-positive. The differential diagnosis of papillary ependymoma includes choroid plexus papilloma, papillary meningioma and metastatic papillary carcinomas. Immunohistochemistry for glial, meningothelial and epithelial antigens can be helpful for the distinction of these entities.

Clear cell ependymoma

Tumour cells display an oligodendroglia-like appearance with a clear perinuclear halo. This variant appears to be preferentially located in the supratentorial compartment of young patients {2138}. Clear cell ependymomas need to be distinguished from oligodendroglioma, central neurocytoma, clear cell carcinoma and haemangioblastoma. Ependymal and perivascular rosettes, immunoreactivity for GFAP and EM studies can be helpful to establish the differential diagnosis. The clear cell ependymoma subtype previously classified as Foramen Monro ependymoma {1684} is now recognised as central neurocytoma in most instances (Chapter 6).

Tanycytic ependymoma

Tumour cells are arranged in fascicles of variable width and cell density. The term tanycytic ependymoma has been chosen since its spindly, bipolar elements resemble tanycytes - paraventricular cells with elongated cytoplasmic processes that extend to ependymal surfaces. The term is derived from the Greek word *tanyos,* meaning to stretch {2503}. As ependymal rosettes are typically absent and pseudorosettes only vaguely delineated, the lesion may be misconstrued as astrocytic. Its EM characteristics, however, are ependymal. Tanycytic ependymomas exhibit a decided predilection for the spinal cord.

Other variants

Rare ependymoma variants include ependymoma with lipomatous differentiation {2147}, giant cell ependymoma of the filum terminale {2150}, ependymoma with extensive tumour cell vacuolation {2134}, melanotic ependymoma {2501}, signet ring cell ependymoma {2502} and ovarian ependymoma {2332, 2333, 2334}.

Immunohistochemistry

The great majority of ependymomas display GFAP immunoreactivity. A prominent reaction for GFAP is usually observed in pseudorosettes. Immunoreactivity is more variable in the ependymal rosettes, ependymal canals and papillae, where positive cells may alternate with unlabeled elements. Ependymomas typically express S100 protein and vimentin {774, 1476}. Epithelial membrane antigen (EMA) immunoreactivity has been reported in a high percentage of ependymomas WHO grade II with a prominent signal along the luminal surface of ependymal rosettes. Dot-like immunoreactivity representing microrosettes may be observed. Focal immunoreactivity to cytokeratins can be seen in some cases {955}. Expression of nestin, a neuro-developmental intermediate filament protein, has been noted in ependymomas. Ependymomas do not express neuronal antigens such as synaptophysin.

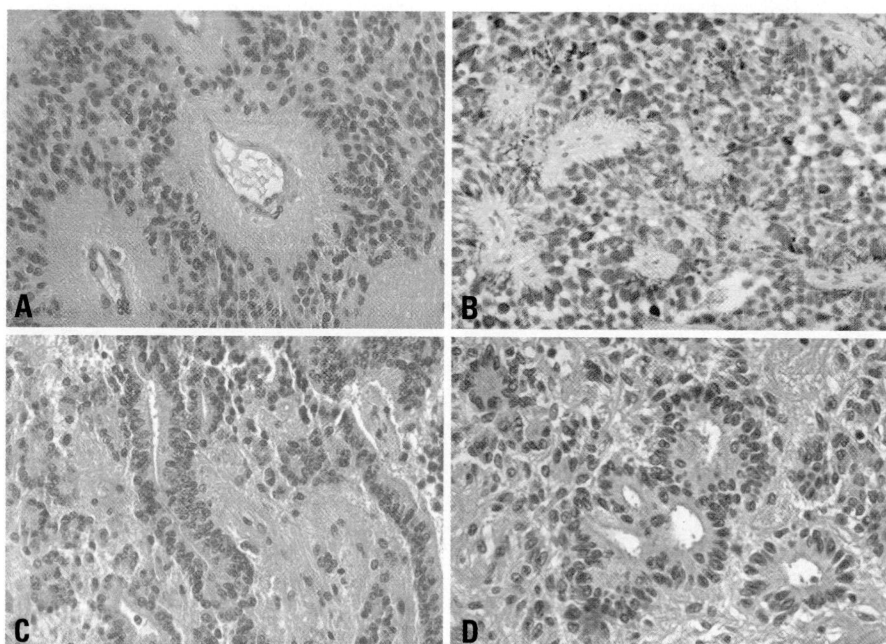

Fig. 3.5 Histological features of ependymoma **A** Perivascular pseudorosettes. **B** GFAP immunoreactivity predominantly around tumour vessels. **C** Ependymal canals and (**D**) rosettes.

Electron microscopy

Ependymomas maintain characteristic ultrastructural properties of ependymal cells such as cilia in a 9+2 arrangement, blepharoblasts and microvilli located at the luminal surface, junctional complexes at the lateral surface and lack of a basement membrane at the internal surface {588}. Cells may form microrosettes into which microvilli and cilia project {483}. Junctional complexes (zonulae adherentes), irregularly linked by zonulae occludentes or gap junctions and cell processes filled with intermediate filaments, may also be encountered {1347}. Intermediate filaments positive for GFAP can be demonstrated in tumour cells by colloidal gold immuno-electron microscopy. A basal lamina may be present at the interface between tumour cells and vascularized stroma. Neurosecretory granules cannot be found.

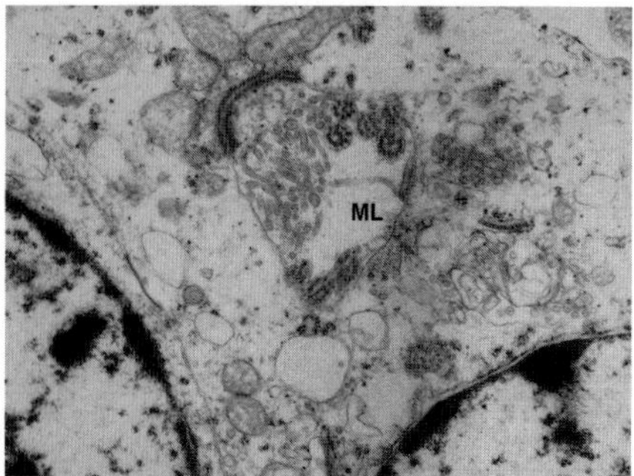

Fig. 3.4 Ultrastructural features of ependymal differentiation: intercellular microlumen (ML) containing microvilli and cilia, bordered by an elongate intercellular junction.

Growth pattern and invasion

Tumour expansion with formation of a clear-cut edge toward the adjacent nervous tissue is characteristic. From the fourth ventricle, ependymomas typically extend into the cerebellopontine angle and protrude into the cisterna magna. Sometimes, isolated tumour cells can be found in the adjacent tissue. Infrequently, there is spread via the CSF, particularly from infratentorial lesions {1173, 1610}. Several case reports describe extraneural metastases, mostly to the lungs.

Proliferation

Using antibodies to Ki-67, a mean growth fraction of 2.6 ± 2.6 % was reported for ependymomas {728, 917}. Other investigators noticed an inverse relationship between Ki-67 indices and the age of ependymoma patients {2143}. MIB-1 labelling and cyclin D1 expression showed a positive correlation in a comparative immunohistochemical analysis of 41 ependymomas {2139}. The prognostic significance of the proliferation index has not yet been firmly established in these tumours.

Aetiology

The identification of SV40 virus large T antigen-related DNA sequences in a significant proportion of human choroid plexus papillomas and ependymomas has received considerable attention since it may reflect latent infection following widespread use of SV 40-contaminated polio vaccines during 1955-1962 {92, 2231}. More recently, natural SV40 strains have been identified in human ependymomas {866}. However, other investigators have not been able to confirm these findings {2153} and it remains to be shown whether SV40 plays a significant role in the pathogenesis of ependymomas.

Genetic susceptibility

Spinal ependymomas are a major manifestation of neurofibromatosis type 2 (NF2) indicating a role for the *NF2* tumour suppressor gene in these neoplasms. Other hereditary forms of ependymoma are uncommon. Two patients with Turcot syndrome and ependymomas have been reported {1510}. In a single instance, a spinal ependymoma was observed in association with multiple endocrine neoplasia syndrome type 1 (MEN1) {734}. A case of

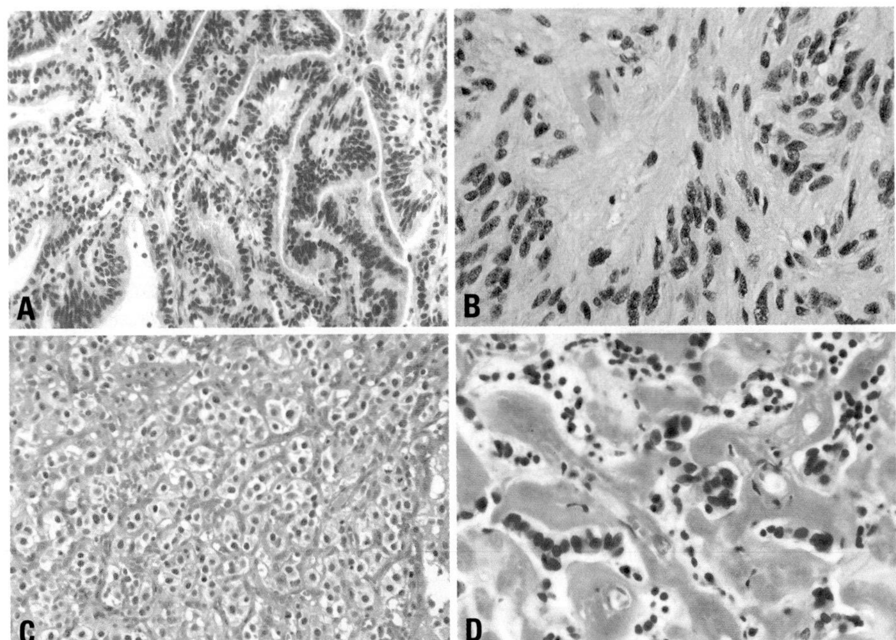

Fig. 3.6 Histopathology of ependymoma, showing **(A)** papillary and **(B)** tanycytic differentiation. **C** Clear cell ependymoma. **D** Ependymoma with extensive vessel hyalinization which often precedes calcification.

anaplastic ependymoma has been recognized in association with a *TP53* germline mutation {999}.

Cytogenetics

Cytogenetic changes have been found in a significant fraction of ependymomas, with a 30% incidence of aberrations involving chromosome 22 as the most frequent change (for review see ref. {532}). Monosomy 22 as well as deletions or translocations involving 22q appear to prevail. Less frequent are abnormalities of 9q, 10, 17 and 13. Gains of chromosome 7 have occasionally been reported {1332, 1427}. Monosomy 10 has been identified in eight cases, but only in three anaplastic ependymomas was loss of chromosome 10 associated with LOH of 17p {1273}. Monosomy 13 was reported in eight cases, half of which occurred in paediatric patients {1462}. Of five cases with monosomy of chromosome 9 or deletions involving 9p, three were anaplastic {1462}. Monosomy 17 has been found in ten cases {1228}. Most of these also showed monosomy 22. Six ependymomas with monosomy 11 have been reported {1608}. A constitutional t(1;22)(p22;q11.2) translocation has been described in a young patient with anaplastic ependymoma. The genes involved at the breakpoints remain to be discovered {2142}.
In a series of 22 childhood ependymomas, loss of chromosome 22 was observed in 2 cases, deletion of chromosome 17 in 2 cases and rearrangements or deletions of chromosome 6 in 5 tumours {2136}.

Molecular genetics

At the molecular genetic level, ependymomas appear clearly distinct from astrocytic gliomas and oligodendrogliomas. A study of 14 ependymomas by Sato and colleagues {1327} failed to detect mutations or deletions of the tumour suppressor genes *CDKN2A* and *CDKN2B*, or amplification of *CDK4* or *CCND1*. In a series of 17 ependymomas, there was no evidence for *EGFR* amplification {125}. Mutations of the *TP53* tumour suppressor gene have only occasionally been observed in ependymomas {409, 1096, 1505}. Von Haken *et al.* {1568} reported a 50% incidence of allelic losses on the short arm of chromosome 17 in 18 paediatric ependymomas. As *TP53* was largely ruled out as a candidate, the responsible gene has yet to be identified. A similar chromosomal region shows frequent loss of heterozygosity (LOH) in medulloblastomas (see Chapter 8).
Due to the increased incidence of ependymomas in neurofibromatosis type 2, *NF2* represents an obvious candidate gene in ependymal neoplasms but initial studies yielded conflicting results. Some investigators have presented evidence for mutations of the *NF2* suppressor gene at 22q12 {127}, whereas others have been unable to identify such mutations in a significant fraction of ependymomas {1297, 1568}. Recent data provide a solution to this puzzle and strongly indicate that ependymomas may occur as genetically distinct subtypes. An analysis of 62 ependymal tumours for LOH 22q, LOH 10q, and for mutations of the *NF2* and *PTEN* tumour suppressor genes revealed 6 cases with mutant *NF2*, all of which were localized in the spinal cord {2152}. The authors conclude from these findings that spinal ependymomas constitute a distinct molecular variant characterized by an altered *NF2* gene on chromosome 22. Genes involved in cerebral ependymomas remain to be uncovered.

Predictive factors

The identification of parameters with prognostic value in ependymomas remains an important, but controversial issue {2148}. This applies in particular to the significance of histopathological properties. The following factors have to be considered in order of importance:
Age and extent of resection. Generally, clinical outcome in children with ependymomas appears to be significantly worse than in adults. To some extent, this difference may reflect the more common posterior fossa location in paediatric patients. In addition, tumours with frank histopathological anaplasia may occur at a higher incidence in this age group. A multi-institutional retrospective analysis of 83 paediatric ependymoma patients revealed age below 3 yr., anaplastic histopathological features and incomplete tumour resection as indicators of a poor outcome {2135}. The Children's Cancer Group recently reported a 5-year progression-free survival of 50% in children with intracranial ependymomas {2144}. Children affected during the first two years of life carry a particularly dismal prognosis {832, 1173}.
In a series on adult patients, survival at 5 and 10 years was 57.1% and 45%, respectively. Complete or near complete resection emerged as an independent prognostic factor {1191}. This has been confirmed by other investigators {687}.
Localization. Supratentorial ependymomas are associated with better survival rates compared to posterior fossa neoplasms {2500}. Spinal ependymomas show a significantly better outcome compared to cerebral lesions. Cerebrospinal dissemination indicates a poor prognosis.

Histopathological grading. In a series of 31 patients, 12 with classic and 19 with anaplastic ependymoma, the 5 and 10 year progression-free survivals were 60% and 48% for ependymoma WHO grade II, 55 % and 26% for anaplastic tumours {802}. In a study on 298 cases, survival of patients with the anaplastic variant, recognised by classic histological criteria {1354}, did not markedly differ from those with ordinary (low-grade) ependymoma. Another study of intracranial ependymomas that excluded localization-linked operative mortality found a median progression-free survival of 7.5 years for grade II ependymomas, but only 1.5 years for anaplastic variants {2499}. Histological progression can occur {2504}. A major and not completely resolved problem relates to the definition of reliable histopathological indicators of anaplasia {2140}. Of the features usually associated with anaplastic change in gliomas (*i.e.* increased mitotic and/or proliferative activity, increased cellularity, vascular endothelial proliferation and tumour necrosis) only mitotic index, proliferation and foci of hypercellular, less differentiated tumour cells appear to correlate with poor outcome in ependymomas {2148}. Marked vascular endothelial proliferation and necrosis are frequently encountered in anaplastic variants; however, they do not appear to qualify as independent variables for the definition of anaplasia.

Proliferation and apoptosis. In a recent survey, a MIB-1 labelling index exceeding 4 % emerged as an independent prognostic criterion for the distinction of ependymoma and anaplastic ependymoma {2151}. Evaluation of tumour cell apoptosis has not yielded prognostically relevant information {1349}.

Anaplastic ependymoma

O.D. Wiestler
D. Schiffer
S.W. Coons
R.A. Prayson
M.K. Rosenblum

Definition

A malignant glioma of ependymal origin with accelerated growth and unfavourable clinical outcome, particularly in children. Anaplastic ependymomas exhibit high mitotic activity, often accompanied by microvascular proliferation and pseudopalisading necrosis.

ICD-O code: 9392/3

Grading

Anaplastic ependymomas correspond histologically to WHO grade III.

Incidence

Incidence data vary considerably, due to the uncertainty regarding histological criteria of malignancy. Anaplastic changes are far more frequent in intracranial ependymomas, particularly posterior fossa examples, than in those of the spinal cord.

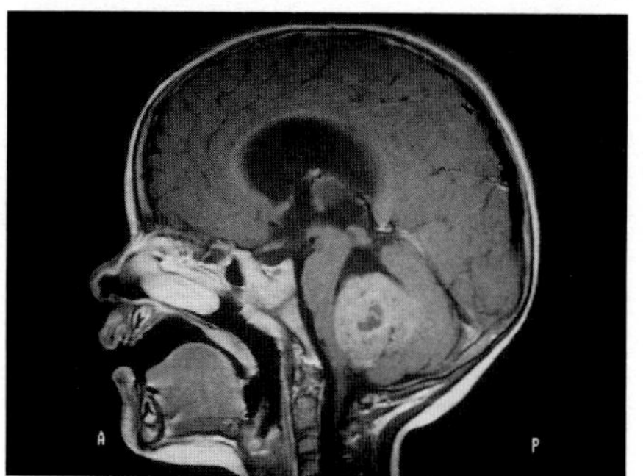

Fig. 3.7 Sagittal, gadolinium enhanced, T1 weighted MRI of an anaplastic ependymoma of the fourth ventricle.

Clinical features

Signs and symptoms are similar to those of ependymomas WHO grade II but ususally develop more rapidly and may cause increased inrtacranial pressure at an early stage of the disease. MRI images typically show contrast enhancement.

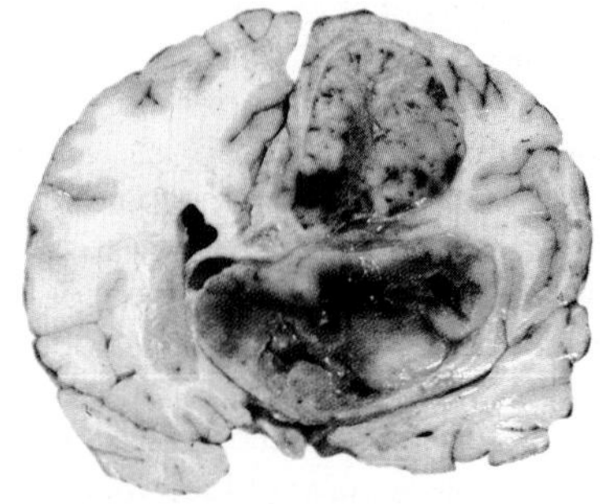

Fig. 3.8 Anaplastic ependymoma of the lateral ventricle in a four-year-old boy with extensive invasion of the right frontal lobe.

Histopathology

Anaplastic ependymomas show increased cellularity and brisk mitotic activity, often associated with microvascular proliferation and pseudopalisading necrosis. Perivascular rosettes are a histological hallmark but ependymal rosettes are rare or absent.

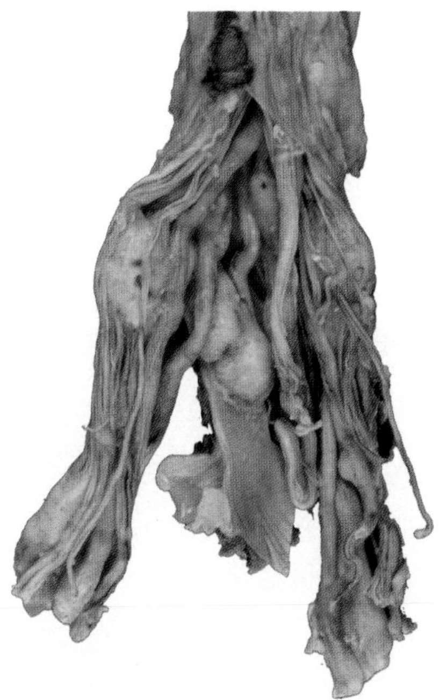

Fig. 3.9 Multiple metastases in the cauda equina of an anaplastic ependymoma.

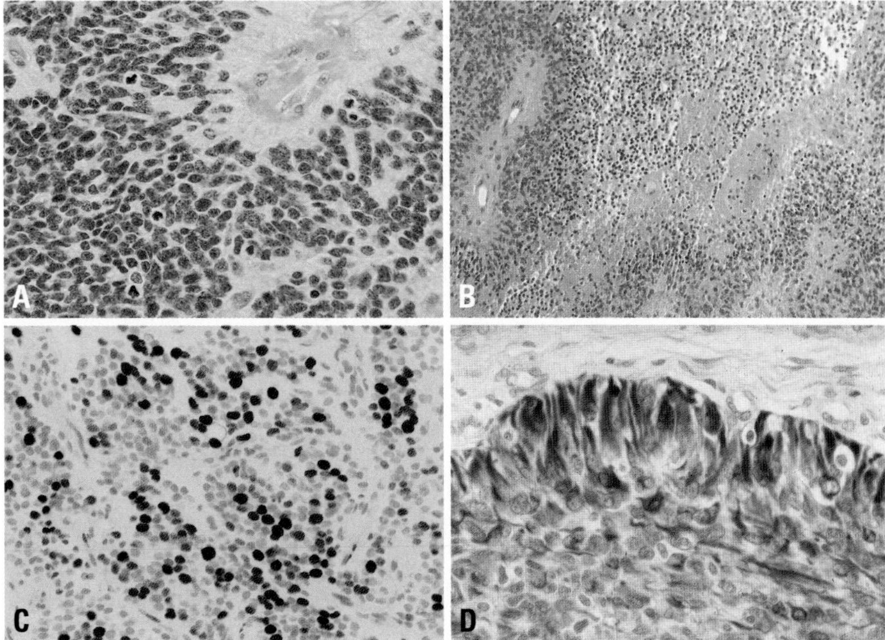

Fig. 3.10 Histological features of anaplastic ependymoma. **A** Poorly differentiated tumour cells with brisk mitotic activity. **B** Large foci of geographic necrosis. **C** High MIB-1 labeling index. **D** Strong GFAP expression in an anaplastic ependymoma invading adjacent brain structures.

Anaplastic ependymomas tend to remain well demarcated, but are occasionally frankly invasive. They often appear highly cellular and poorly differentiated, with pseudorosettes of narrow width and little tendency to form true rosettes. Mitoses are readily identified, some examples exhibiting microvascular proliferation and necrosis with palisading. In the absence of palisading, tumour necrosis (a particularly common phenomenon in posterior fossa ependymomas) should not prompt the diagnosis of anaplasia {2145}. Poorly differentiated examples may be difficult to identify as ependymal in the absence of supporting EM evidence. By definition, embryonal components and ependymoblastic rosettes are not present (see Chapter 8).

Immunohistochemistry

The immunoprofiles of anaplastic ependymomas resemble those of conventional ependymoma, but GFAP expression may be reduced.

Cytogenetics and molecular genetics

Genetic alterations specifically encountered in anaplastic ependymomas are largely unknown. Although some lesions may develop through malignant progression from WHO grade II ependymomas, no underlying sequence of genetic events has been identified. Evidence for the involvement of a putative tumour suppressor gene on chromosome 22 was presented in a study on familial anaplastic ependymomas {2146}. A recent analysis of 23 anaplastic ependymomas for LOH 10q, LOH 22q and mutations of the *NF2* and *PTEN* genes revealed LOH 10q in 4 cases {2152}. The significance of this finding must be confirmed in future experiments.

Predictive factors

An inconstant relationship between histology and outcome has emerged from the clinical studies published to date {1045, 1052, 1352, 1443, 2145, 2499, 2500, 2504, 2505}. In a series of 298 cases, no correlation between the survival of the patients and classical histopathological signs of malignancy could be observed. A relationship with survival became only evident when high cell density and brisk mitotic activity were considered as independent variables {1352}. Age below 3 yr., anaplastic histopathological features, incomplete tumour resection and evidence for CSF metastases have been proposed as indicators of an adverse outcome in children {2135}.

Myxopapillary ependymoma

O.D. Wiestler
D. Schiffer
S.W. Coons
R.A. Prayson
M.K. Rosenblum

Definition
Myxopapillary ependymomas are slowly growing gliomas with preferential manifestation in young adults and are almost exclusively located in the conus-cauda-filum terminale region of the spinal cord. They are histologically characterized by tumour cells arranged in a papillary manner around vascularized mucoid stromal cores.

ICD-O code: 9394/1

Grading
These slowly growing tumours have a favourable prognosis and correspond to WHO grade I. Anaplastic variants are virtually unknown.

Historical annotation
In his original description of 1932, Kernohan defined the distinct morphological properties and preferential location of this entity {2206}.

Incidence
In a series of 298 ependymomas, 13% were found to be of the myxopapillary type {1354}. In the conus/cauda equina segment, myxopapillary ependymomas constitute the most common intramedullary neoplasm.

Age and sex distribution
An average age at manifestation of 36.4 years has been determined, with a broad range between 6 and 82 years. In a study of 271 tumours of the filum terminale, 83% were of the myxopapillary type, with a male: female ratio of 2.2:1 [210}.

Clinical findings and neuroimaging
Myxopapillary ependymomas are typically associated with back pain, often of long duration. MRI usually reveals a sharply circumscribed lesion with enhancement that is often very bright. Extensive cystic change and haemorrhage may be apparent. Some examples evidence local seeding in the caudal spinal canal at presentation.

Localization
Myxopapillary ependymomas occur almost exclusively in the conus-cauda-filum terminale region. They presumably originate from ependymal glia of the filum terminale, involve the cauda equina, and only rarely invade nerve roots or erode sacral bone. Myxopapillary ependymomas can occasionally be observed at other locations, such as the cervical-thoracic spinal cord {1439}, the lateral ventricle {1325}, or the brain parenchyma {242, 905, 1580}. Subcutaneous sacrococcygeal or presacral myxopapillary ependymomas represent a distinct subgroup. They appear to originate from ectopic ependymal remnants {2202}. Intrasacral variants may masquerade clinically as chordoma.

Macroscopy
At the macroscopic level, myxopapillary ependymomas display a lobulated, soft and greyish appearance. They are often encapsulated and do not usually exhibit grossly infiltrative properties.

Histopathology
Myxopapillary ependymomas are characterized by GFAP-expressing, cuboidal to elongated tumour cells radially arranged in a papillary manner around vascularized stromal cores. A mucoid matrix material accumulates between tumour cells and blood vessels, also collecting in microcysts. Mitotic activity is very low or absent.

Immunohistochemical reactions for GFAP, S-100 and vimentin are positive whereas immunoreactivity for cytokeratins is typically absent. Results of nucleolar organizing region staining indicate a low proliferation index in the order of 0.4-1.6% {2203}. Tumour entities to be distinguished from myxopapillary ependymomas include chordoma, myxoid chondrosarcoma, paraganglioma, mesothelioma and papillary adenocarcinoma. Immunoreactivity for GFAP and lack of cytokeratin expression confirm the diagnosis {2201}.

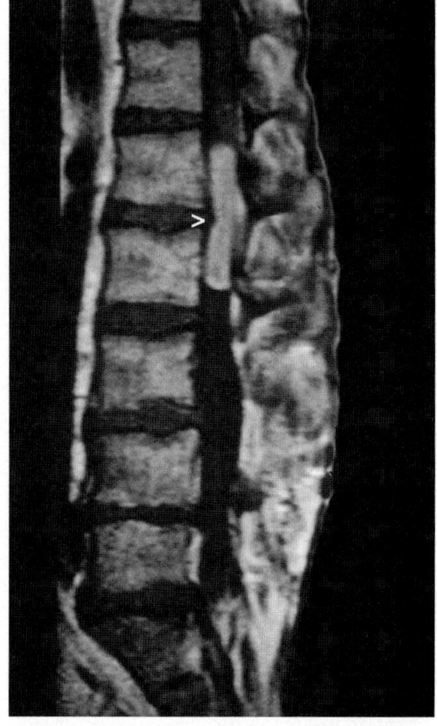

Fig. 3.11 MRI of a myxopapillary ependymoma of the filum terminale (arrow) presenting as a hyperintense spinal mass.

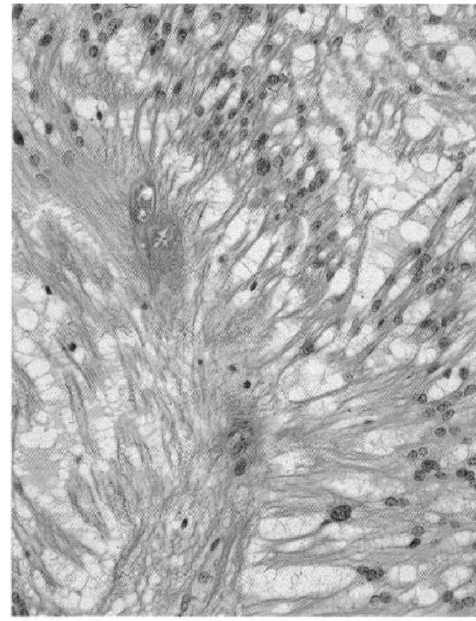

Fig. 3.12 Myxopapillar ependymoma showing radial perivascular arrangement of tumour cell processes.

Electron microscopy

Ultrastructural studies demonstrate few cilia, complex interdigitations and abundant basement membrane structures. A distinctive feature of some examples is the aggregation of microtubules within rough endoplasmic reticulum complexes {2506}.

Cytogenetics and molecular genetics

This entity has not yet been subjected to systematic molecular studies. A rearranged chromosome 1p has been noted in a single case {2205}. Another report revealed dicentric chromosomes and deletions of chromosome 11q in a subcutaneous sacrococcygeal myxopapillary ependymoma {2204}. A recent molecular genetic analysis of 6 myxopapillary ependymomas for allelic deletions on chromosomes 10q and 22q and for point mutations of the *NF2* and *PTEN* tumour suppressor genes did not reveal any changes at these loci {2152}.

Predictive factors

This entity shows good outcome with more than 10 years survival after total or partial resection {1439}. Late recurrence and distant metastases are very uncommon {1028}. Subarachnoid dissemination has occasionally been observed {2207}. The subcutaneous sacrococcygeal myxopapillary ependymoma appears to be associated with a significant rate of regrowth and occasional formation of distant metastases {2202}.

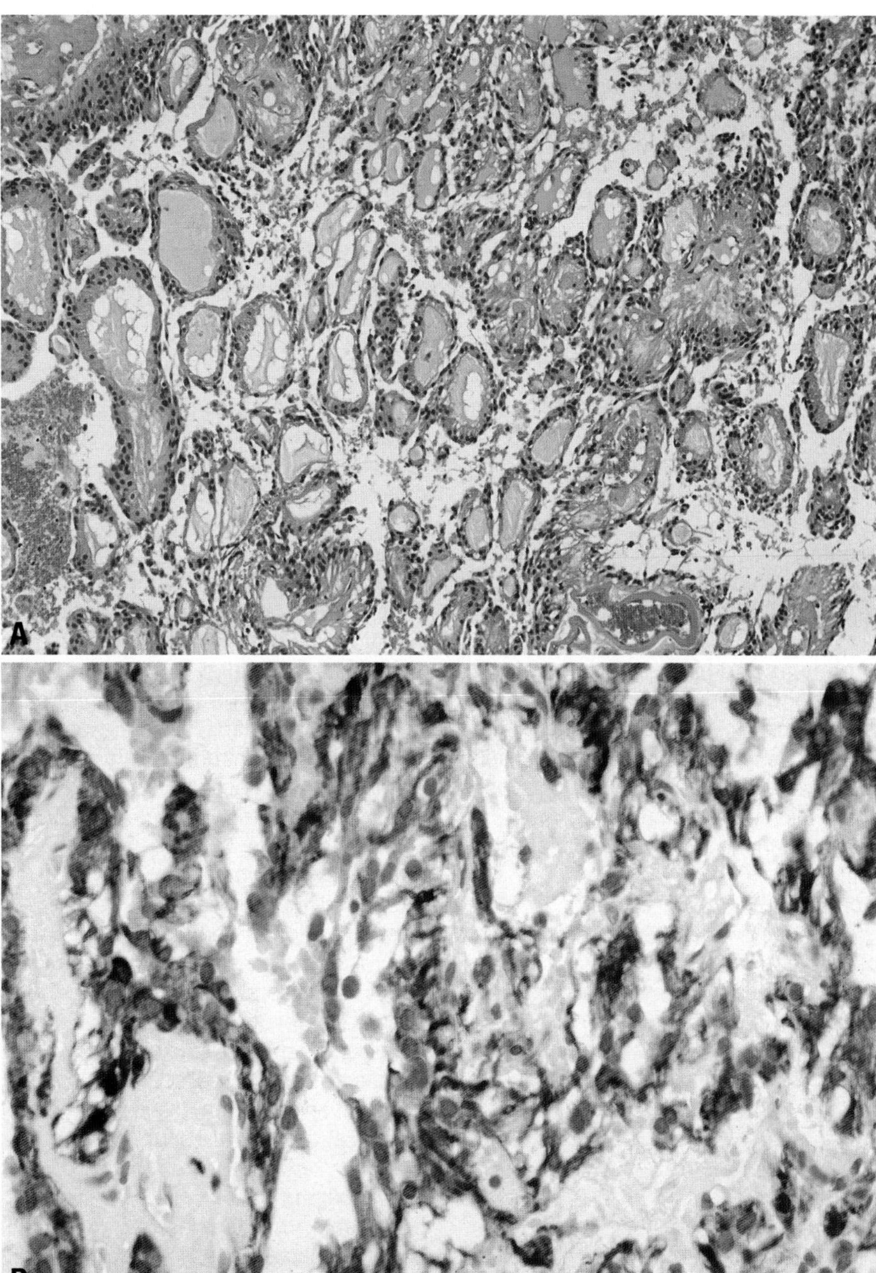

Fig. 3.13 Myxopapillary ependymoma of the cauda equina. **A** Layers of tumour cells around vessels with mucoid degeneration. **B** Perivascular tumour cells consistently express GFAP.

Subependymoma

O.D. Wiestler
D. Schiffer

Definition
A slowly growing, benign neoplasm, typically attached to a ventricular wall, composed of glial tumour cell clusters embedded in an abundant fibrillary matrix with frequent microcystic change.

ICD-O code: 9383/1

Grading
Subependymoma corresponds histologically to WHO grade I.

Synonyms and historical annotation
Subependymoma was originally described by Scheinker in 1945 {2154}. Alternative designations include subependymal astrocytoma and subependymal glomerate astrocytoma {434} but the use of these terms is discouraged.

Incidence
The true incidence of subependymomas is difficult to determine, because these tumours frequently remain asymptomatic and are often found incidentally at autopsy. In a series of 298 cases, they accounted for 8.3% of ependymal tumours {1354}.

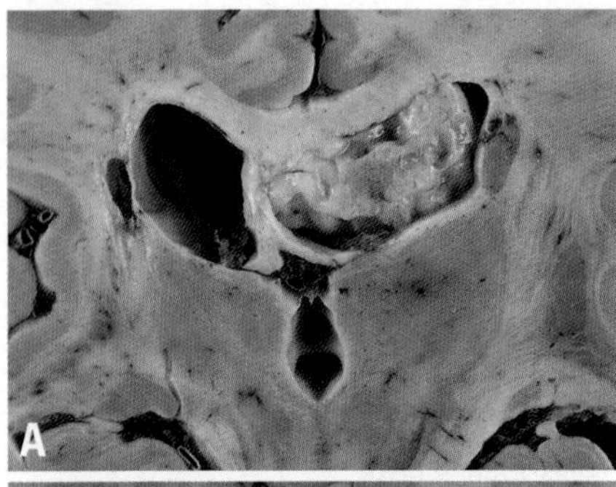

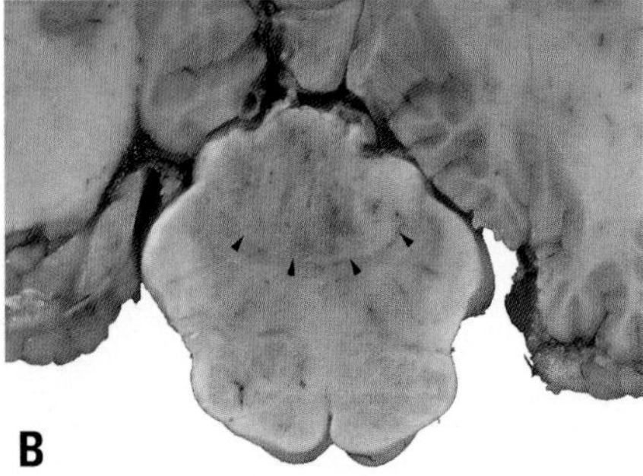

Fig. 3.14 Subependymoma (**A**) originating from the roof of the lateral ventricle, (**B**) attached to the floor of the fourth ventricle (arrow heads).

Age and sex distribution
Subependymomas develop in both sexes and in all age groups, but occur most frequently in middle-aged and elderly males.

Localization
The most frequent site is the fourth ventricle (50–60% of cases), followed by the lateral ventricles (30–40%). Less common sites include the third ventricle and septum pellucidum. In the spinal cord, subependymomas manifest as cervical and cervico-thoracic intramedullary or, rarely, extramedullary mass lesions {673}.

Clinical features
Symptoms and signs
Subependymomas may become clinically apparent through ventricular obstruction and raised intracranial pressure. Spontaneous intratumoral haemorrhage has been observed. Spinal tumours manifest with motor and sensory deficits according to the affected anatomical segment. Incidental detection of asymptomatic subependymomas at autopsy is not uncommon.

Neuroimaging
Subependymomas are sharply demarcated, nodular masses that are usually non-enhancing. Calcification and foci of haemorrhage may be apparent. Intramedullary examples are typically eccentric in location rather than centrally positioned in the manner of intraspinal ependymomas.

Macroscopy
These tumours present as firm nodules of variable size, bulging into the ventricular lumen. In most instances, the diameter does not exceed 1–2 cm. Intraventricular as well as spinal subependymomas are generally well demarcated. Large subependymomas of the fourth ventricle may cause brain stem compression.

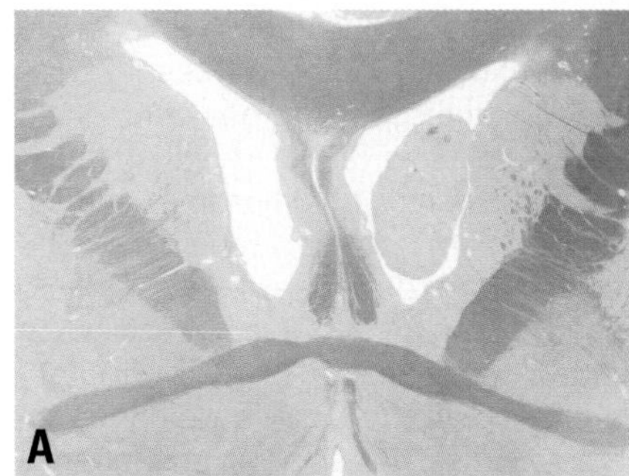

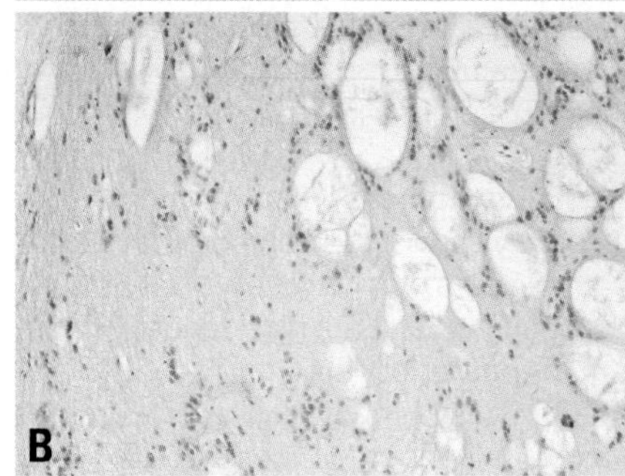

Fig. 3.15 Subependymoma of the lateral ventricle. Higher magnification shows microcystic degeneration and nests of tumour cell nuclei in a fibrillary matrix.

Histopathology
Subependymomas are characterized by clusters of isomorphic nuclei embedded in a dense fibrillary matrix of glial cell processes with frequent occurrence of small cysts. Mitoses are very rare or absent.
Tumour cell nuclei appear isomorphic and resemble those of subependymal glia. Occasional pleomorphic nuclei may be encountered. Some subependymomas exhibit low-level mitotic activity, but this is exceptional. A typical feature are small, sometimes confluent cysts, particularly in lesions originating in the lateral ventricles. Calcifications and haemorrhage can occur. The prominent tumour vasculature may show microvascular proliferations. Occasionally, cell processes arrange around vessels, thus forming ependymal pseudorosettes. In some cases, an additional ependymoma component can be distinguished. Such combined tumours are classified as mixed ependymoma/ subependymoma WHO grade II, assum-

ing that the ependymoma element will determine the outcome. On record are examples of subependymoma with melanin formation {2501}, rhabdomyosarcomatous differentiation {2508}, and sarcomatous transformation of vascular stromal elements {2509}. Immunoreactivity for GFAP is usually present, although to a variable extent.

Electron microscopy

At the ultrastructural level, subependymomas display ependymal as well as astrocytic properties including cilia formation, microvilli and intermediate filament bundles {52, 1347}.

Proliferation

Mitotic activity is usually low or absent. The finding of scattered mitoses and cellular pleomorphism is of no clinical significance {2507}. MIB-1 studies revealed labelling indices below 1%, compatible with the benign nature of this entity.

Genetic susceptibility

Rare familial cases have been described {1309}. One study reports on the simultaneous clinical manifestation of infratentorial subependymomas in identical twins {255}. In the vast majority of cases, subependymomas develop sporadically.

Genetics

Consistent cytogenetic aberrations have not yet been uncovered {2133}. A recent molecular genetic analysis of 2 subependymomas for allelic deletions on chromosomes 10q and 22q and for point mutations of the *NF2* and *PTEN* tumour suppressor genes did not reveal any changes at these loci {2152}.

Histogenesis

Proposed cells of origin include subependymal glia {52, 1042}, astrocytes of the subependymal plate, ependymal cells {1306} and a mixture of astrocytes and ependymal cells {434, 1334}. Development from subependymal glia appears most likely. Due to the small tumour size, low proliferation rate and frequent incidental detection at autopsy, a hamartomatous rather than neoplastic nature has been proposed {1306}.

Prognosis

Subependymomas carry a good prognosis. Surgical removal is usually curative in cerebral as well as spinal subependymomas. Neoplasms with a mixed ependymoma and subependymoma morphology appear to follow a clinical course corresponding to ependymoma WHO grade II.

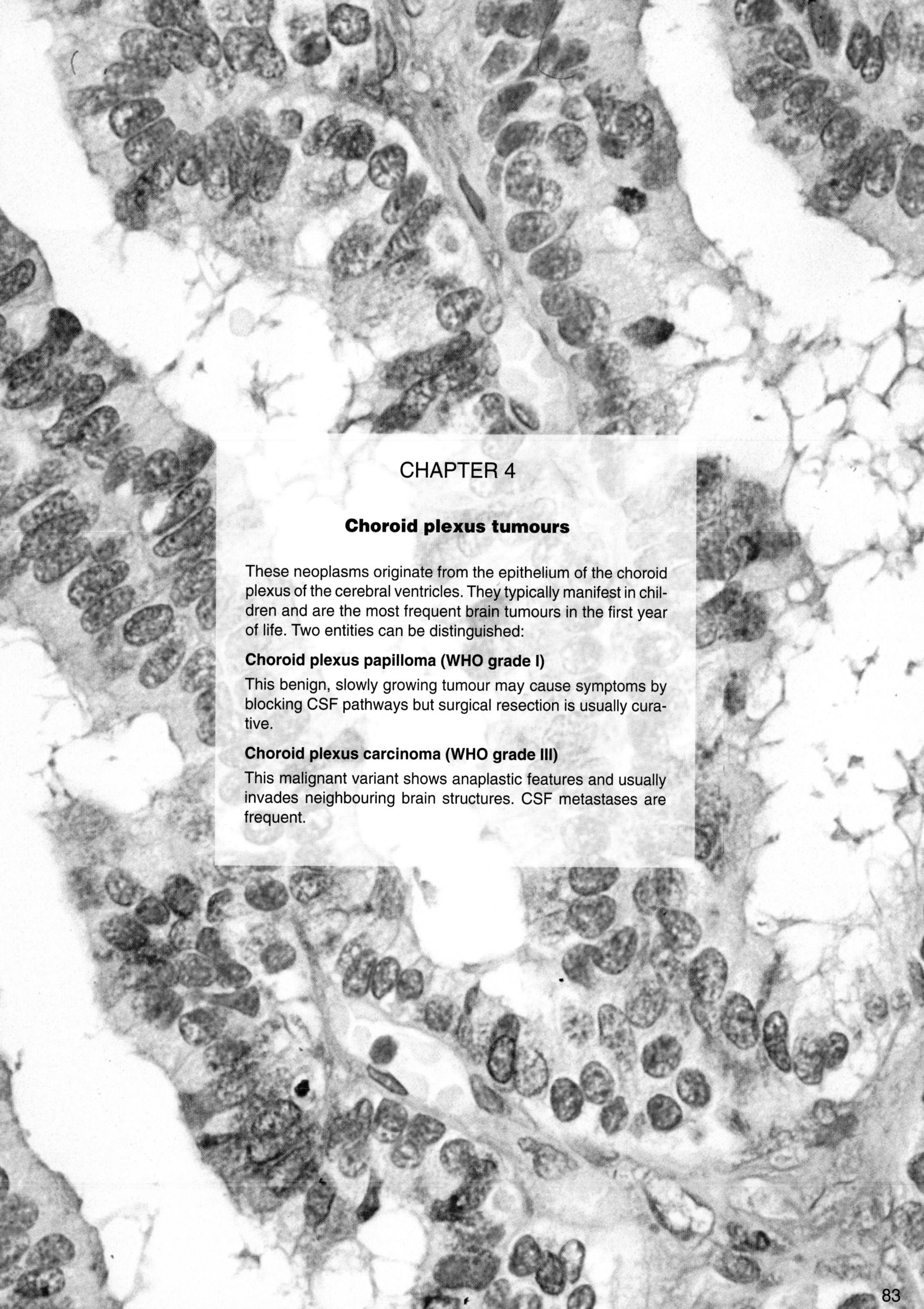

CHAPTER 4

Choroid plexus tumours

These neoplasms originate from the epithelium of the choroid plexus of the cerebral ventricles. They typically manifest in children and are the most frequent brain tumours in the first year of life. Two entities can be distinguished:

Choroid plexus papilloma (WHO grade I)

This benign, slowly growing tumour may cause symptoms by blocking CSF pathways but surgical resection is usually curative.

Choroid plexus carcinoma (WHO grade III)

This malignant variant shows anaplastic features and usually invades neighbouring brain structures. CSF metastases are frequent.

Choroid plexus tumours

A. Aguzzi
S. Brandner
W. Paulus

Definition

Intraventricular, papillary neoplasms derived from choroid plexus epithelium.

ICD-O code

Choroid plexus papilloma: 9390/0
Choroid plexus carcinoma: 9390/3

Grading

Choroid plexus papilloma corresponds histologically to WHO grade I. Choroid plexus carcinoma corresponds to WHO grade III.

Incidence

Although choroid plexus tumours account for 0.4-0.6% of all brain tumours, they represent 2-4% of those that occur in children, and 10-20% of those manifesting in the first year of life. Choroid plexus papillomas outnumber choroid plexus carcinomas by a ratio of at least 5:1. Around 80% of choroid plexus carcinomas arise in children, where they constitute 20-40% of choroid plexus tumours. The average annual incidence is approximately 0.3 per 1.000.000 population {679}.

Age and sex distribution

Around 80% of lateral ventricle tumours present in patients younger than 20 years, whereas fourth ventricle tumours are evenly distributed in all age groups (see Fig. 4.1). Congenital tumours have been described and even foetal tumours have been observed *in utero* by using ultrasound techniques {2511}. The male: female ratio for lateral ventricle tumours is 1:1; for fourth ventricle tumours, this ratio is 3:2.

Localization

Choroid plexus papilloma and choroid plexus carcinoma are confined to areas where choroid plexus is normally found, *i.e.* the lateral (50%), third (5%) and fourth (40%) cerebral ventricles, with two or three ventricles being involved in 5% of cases. Primary manifestation in the cerebellopontine angle near the openings of the fourth ventricle is rare. Exceptional cases of ectopic, *i.e.* intraparenchymal or suprasellar choroid plexus papilloma are on record {773}.

Clinical features

Symptoms and signs

Choroid plexus tumours tend to block CSF pathways. Accordingly, patients present with signs of hydrocephalus (in infants increased circumference of the head) and raised intracranial pressure, *e.g.* vomiting, strabism and headache.

Neuroimaging

CT and MRI show hyperdense, contrast-enhancing masses within the ventricles, generally associated with hydrocephalus {2512}.

Macroscopy

Choroid plexus papillomas are circumscribed cauliflower-like masses that may adhere to the ventricular wall, but are usually well-delineated from brain tissue. Cysts and haemorrhages may occur. Choroid plexus carcinomas are invasive tumours that may appear solid, haemorrhagic and necrotic.

Histopathology

Choroid plexus papilloma

This benign, papillary tumour is composed of delicate fibrovascular connective tissue fronds covered by a single layer of uniform cuboidal to columnar epithelial cells with round or oval, basally situated monomorphic nuclei. Conspicuous mitotic activity, brain invasion and necrosis are absent.

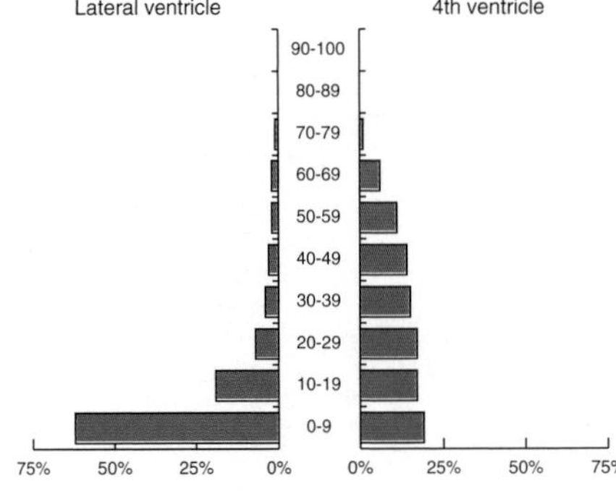

Fig. 4.1 Age vs. localization of choroid plexus tumours, based on a compilation of published cases.

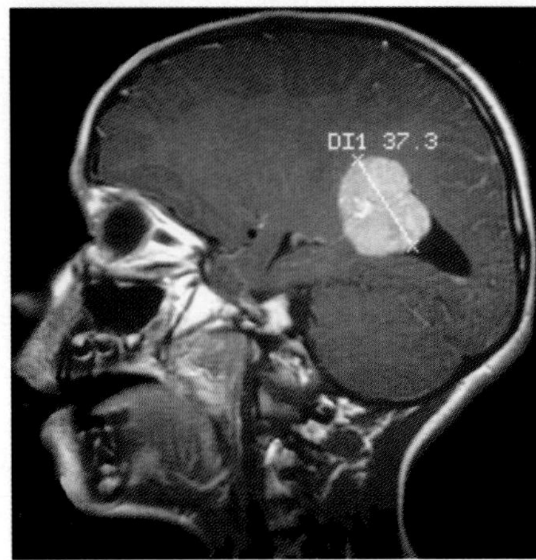

Fig. 4.2 MRI of an anaplastic choroid plexus tumour in the lateral ventricle of a 5 year-old child with a *TP53* germline mutation.

Choroid plexus papilloma closely resembles non-neoplastic choroid plexus, but cells tend to be more crowded and elongated. Rarely, choroid plexus papillomas may acquire unusual histological features, including oncocytic change, mucinous degeneration, melanization and tubular glandular architecture of tumour cells, as well as degeneration of connective tissue, such as xanthomatous change, angioma-like increase of blood vessels, and bone and cartilage formation {336, 345, 1547, 1583}. Immunohistochemically, cytokeratins and vimentin are expressed by virtually all choroid plexus papillomas. S-100 protein is present in about 90% of cases. Prominent staining for epithelial membrane antigen is typically not found. GFAP is absent from normal choroid plexus, but is present focally in 25-55% of choroid plexus papillomas. Electron microscopy shows interdigitating cell membranes, tight junctions, microvilli, occasional apical cilia and a basement membrane at the abluminal pole.

Choroid plexus carcinoma

This solid tumour shows frank signs of malignancy, including nuclear pleomorphism, frequent mitoses, high nucleus: cytoplasm ratios, increased cellular density, blurring of the papillary pattern with poorly structured sheets of tumour cells, necrotic areas and often diffuse brain invasion.

Immunohistochemically, choroid plexus carcinomas express cytokeratins, while positivity for S100 protein and transthyretin is less frequent than in choroid plexus papillomas. About 20% of choroid plexus carcinomas are GFAP-positive. Epithelial membrane antigen is usually not expressed. In rare instances, choroid plexus carcinoma is made of atypical clear cells arranged in a solid pattern; this renders diagnosis very difficult. In such cases, electron microscopy may be required.

Atypical choroid plexus papilloma

The distinction between choroid plexus papilloma and choroid plexus carcinoma is not always clear-cut, as some tumours show only one or a few histological features of malignancy, *e.g.* increased mitotic activity. These tumours have been termed 'atypical choroid plexus papilloma', but clear diagnostic criteria have not been established.

Differential diagnosis

A wide variety of lesions are relevant in the differential diagnosis of choroid plexus tumours. Villous hypertrophy is a diffuse enlargement of the choroid plexus in both lateral ventricles with normal histological appearance, often associated with hypersecretory hydrocephalus {157}. Distinction between choroid plexus carcinoma and the more common metastatic carcinoma is essential. Co-expression of vimentin, cytokeratins and S-100 protein is a helpful feature in distinguishing epithelial choroid plexus tumours from metastatic carcinomas. In addition, a variety of other immunostains have been recommended. The antibodies HEA125 and BerEP4 may be useful, because they label more than 95% of cerebral metastatic carcinomas, but only 10% of choroid plexus papillomas or choroid plexus carcinomas {495}. Transthyretin (pre-albumin), involved in the transport of thyroxin and retinol, is a marker for normal and neoplastic choroid plexus epithelia. However, up to 20% of choroid plexus papillomas are negative, and other brain tumours as well as metastatic carcinomas may be positive {19, 261, 1148}. Staining for synaptophysin has recently been reported to be strongly positive in normal choroid plexus, plexus papilloma and plexus carcinoma {2025}, but this finding has not been confirmed by others (S. Brandner, W. Paulus, unpublished). In one study, expression of insulin-like growth factor II (IGF II) has been described in choroid plexus papillomas, but not in other brain tumours {2026}. Because previous studies detected IGF-II in various tumours such as astrocytoma, meningioma and carcinoma, it remains to be determined whether staining for IGF-II is diagnostically useful. Expression of carcinoembryonic antigen (CEA) suggests metastatic carcinoma, although occasional choroid plexus carcinomas are also positive {261, 1148}. A variety of non-epithelial, mesenchymal tumours may originate in the choroid plexus stroma, including meningioma.

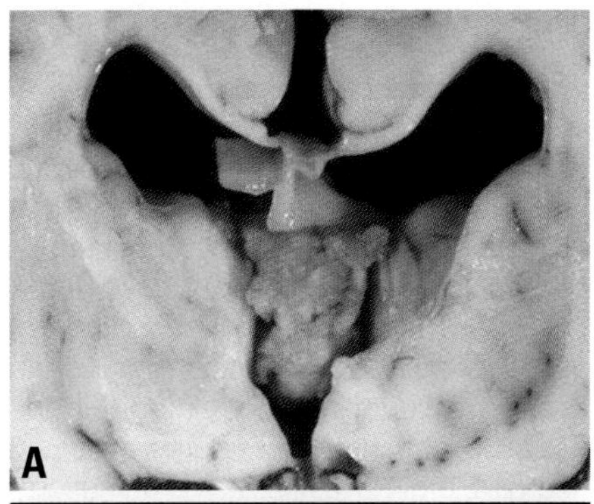

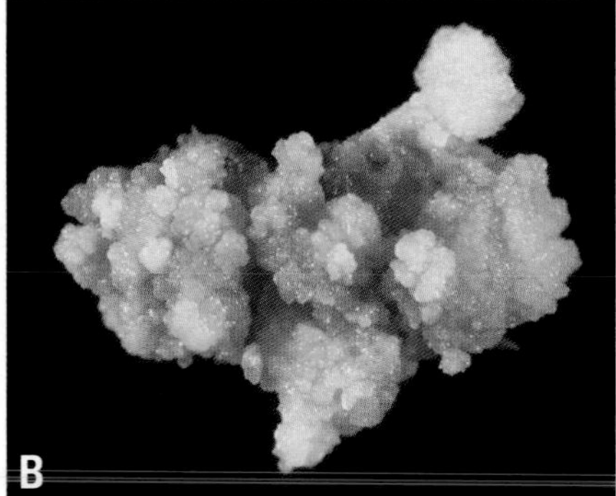

Fig. 4.3 A Choroid plexus papilloma arising in the posterior third ventricle producing partial obstruction with ventricle dilatation. **B** Villous architecture.

Seeding and metastasis

Even benign choroid plexus papillomas may seed cells into the CSF space. Usually, these accumulations are detectable only at the microscopical level and are clinically asymptomatic. In rare instances, extension into epidural fat tissue may occur. In contrast, choroid plexus carcinoma may produce frank metastases along CSF pathways.

Proliferation

Mean Ki67/MIB1 labelling indices for choroid plexus tumours were reported as 1.9% (range, 0.2-6%) for choroid plexus papilloma, and 13.8% (range, 7.3-60%) for choroid plexus carcinoma {1532}.

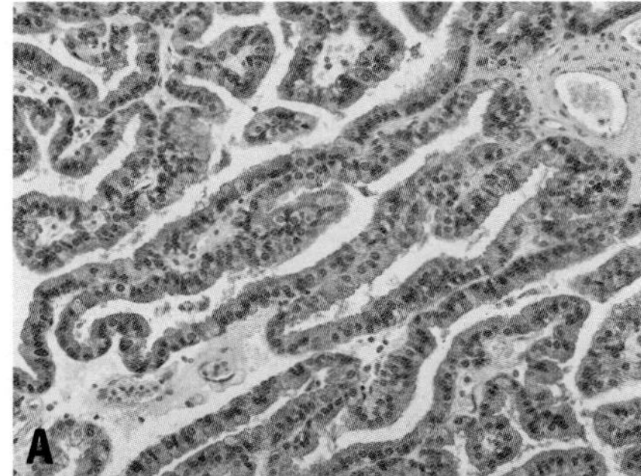

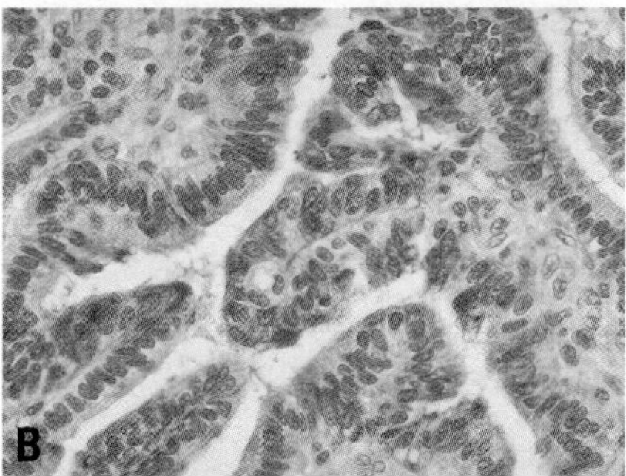

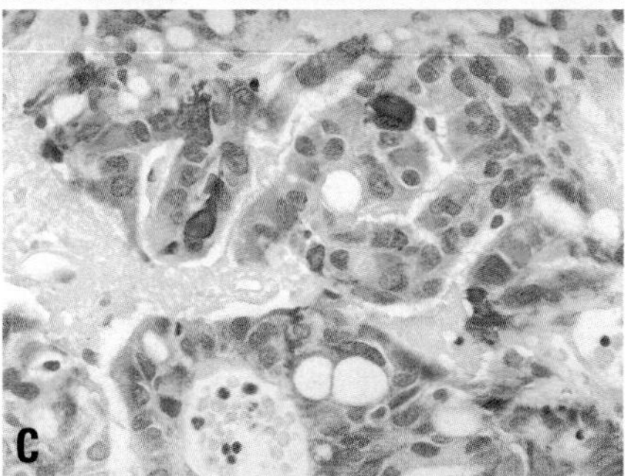

Fig. 4.4 Histological features of choroid plexus tumours. **A** S-100 immunostaining of a plexus papilloma. **B** Atypical papilloma, immunoreactive transthyretin (TTR). **C** Expression of GFAP in a plexus papilloma.

Aetiology

The detection of DNA sequences of the simian virus 40 (SV40), a small primate DNA virus (papova virus) in choroid plexus papillomas, plexus carcinomas and ependymomas suggested a possible role in the evolution of these tumours {1392}. About 40 years ago, the contamination of live polio vaccine with the SV40 virus led to the inadvertent infection of millions of people. SV40 is oncogenic in rodents. Transgenic mice expressing the SV40 large T antigen develop plexus papillomas {156}, and inoculation of newborn rodents induce plexus papillomas and ependymomas {2024, 2028}. However, follow-up studies of persons, who were exposed to

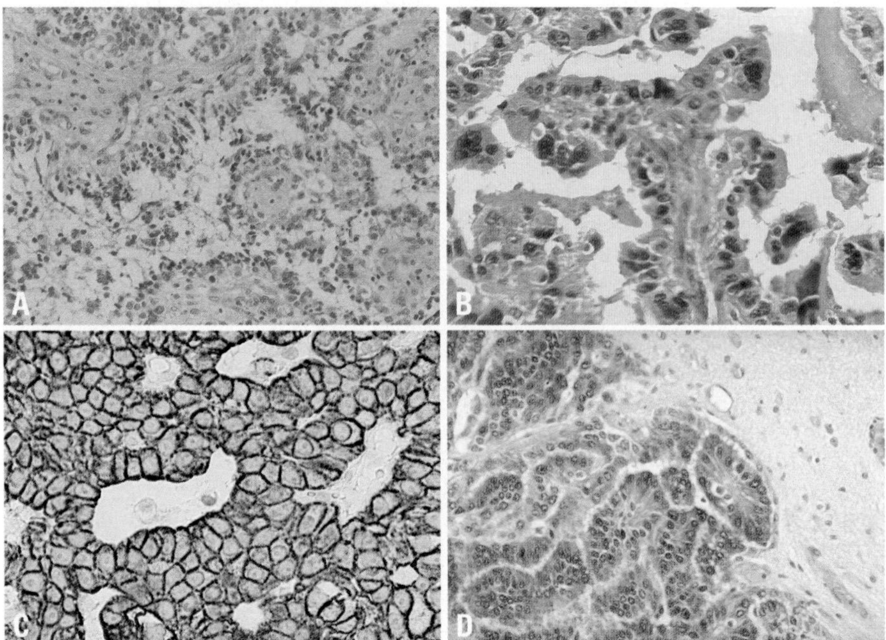

Fig. 4.5 Anaplastic choroid plexus papilloma with **(A)** blurring of the papillary pattern and **(B)** marked nuclear pleomorphism. **C** Choroid plexus carcinoma with striking expression of keratin. **D** Strong immunoreactivity to carbonic anhydrase C of a malignant papilloma invading the brain parenchyma.

the contaminated polio vaccine failed to detect any increase in incidence of cancer {1041}. Several early reports had indicated the presence of SV40-related viral DNA in human brain tumours {984}. An SV40-like virus was isolated from a human glioblastoma {1342}, and was independently cloned from human brain tumours {812}. Nevertheless, in many reports claiming isolation of SV40, contamination with SV40-harbouring cell lines cannot be excluded {812, 984, 1342}. A reinvestigation of the suspected association of SV40 with human tumours {92, 193, 194, 1633, 2231} with PCR revealed SV40-like DNA sequences in about 50% of human choroid plexus tumours and in the majority of ependymomas. More recent studies detected authentic sequences in a variety tumours, among them also tumours outside the CNS (mesothelioma, sarcomas) and, to a lesser extent, in normal tissues, such as sperm fluids, B-, and T-lymphocytes {2027}. It was assumed from these findings, that these cells may be vectors spreading SV40 infection in the human population. The presence of a virus in a tumour does not necessarily indicate that it has a role in its aetiology.

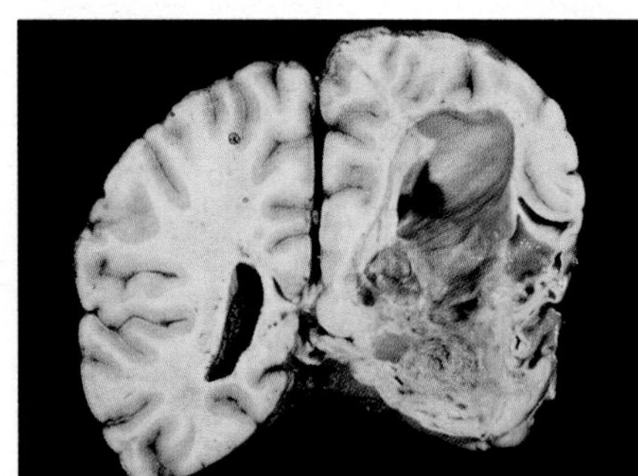

Fig. 4.6 Large choroid plexus carcinoma in the atrium of the right lateral ventricle with extensive invasion of the adjacent brain.

Genetic susceptibility

Choroid plexus papilloma and carcinoma occasionally occur in the setting of Li-Fraumeni syndrome. Of a total of four cases reported, three carried a *TP53* germline mutation in codon 248 {784, 2030}. No *TP53* mutations have been detected in sporadic choroid plexus tumours {1096}.

Cytogenetics and molecular genetics

Classical cytogenetics and FISH of choroid plexus papilloma typically shows hyperdiploidy with gains particularly on chromosomes 7, 9, 12, 15, 17 and 18 {2513}. The occasional association of choroid plexus papilloma or hyperplasia with constitutional duplication of the short arm of chromosome 9 suggests a relationship between 9p abnormality and abnormal growth of the choroid plexus {2514}. It has been suggested that hyperhaploidy may characterize choroid plexus carcinoma {2515}.

Predictive factors

Choroid plexus papilloma can be cured by surgery, with a 5-year survival rate of up to 100% {2512}. Choroid plexus carcinomas grow more rapidly and have a less favourable outcome, with a 5-year survival rate of 40% {2512}; meningeal dissemination and systemic metastasis may occur. Gross total resection, but not adjuvant therapy, appears to be the treatment of choice for choroid plexus carcinoma {1115}. In a clinicopathological study of 52 patients, poor prognosis (recurrence and/or fatal outcome) correlated with the following pathological features: mitoses, necrosis, brain invasion, lack of immunoreactivity for transthyretin, and decreased expression of S100 protein {1148}.

CHAPTER 5

Neuroepithelial Tumours of Uncertain Origin

This chapter deals with three rare lesions that have distinct histological features or growth patterns. Although their neuroepithelial nature is undisputed, their precise histogenesis remains enigmatic. At this time, no genetic data which could aid in defining their aetiopathogenesis are available.

Astroblastoma

Despite its designation, the astroblastoma is not considered to be an embryonal neoplasm. It is characterized by a radial arrangement around vessels of tumour cells with phenotypic characteristics, suggesting that it may have an astrocytic lineage.

Chordoid glioma of the third ventricle

This rare but very typical lesion has now been included in the WHO classification. It is slowly growing, and exhibits epithelial features but strongly expresses the astrocytic protein GFAP.

Gliomatosis cerebri

This neoplasm is defined by an unusually diffuse infiltration of several cerebral lobes, predominantly along myelinated pathways. It is considered likely to have an astrocytic origin, although GFAP expression may be scant or absent. The diagnosis of gliomatosis requires diffuse infiltration of at least two lobes and is usually made on the basis of both histology and neuroimaging.

Polar spongioblastoma

This lesion has been deleted from the WHO classification since it is considered a growth pattern rather than a clinico-pathological entity.

Astroblastoma

P. L. Lantos
M.K. Rosenblum

Definition

A rare glial neoplasm with preferential manifestation in young adults, histologically characterized by a typical perivascular pattern of GFAP-positive astrocytic cells with broad, non-tapering processes radiating towards a central blood vessel.

ICD-O code: 9430/3

Grading

The biological behaviour of astroblastomas is variable. In the absence of sufficient clinico-pathological data, it has been decided not to establish a WHO grade at this stage.

Historical annotation

Astroblastomas were originally described in 1930 by Bailey and Bucy, who considered them to be a clinico-pathological entity with a prognosis intermediate between astrocytomas and glioblastomas {56}. Subsequent studies have, however, revealed that both the nosological definition and the histogenesis of astroblastomas are controversial. Their previous grouping with astroglial neoplasms was revised. Since publication of the 1993 WHO classification, they are listed in the category of neuroepithelial tumours of unknown origin {779}.

Incidence, age and sex distribution

Since these are rare tumours and uniform criteria have not been applied to their definition, reliable epidemiological data are not readily available. Astroblastomas occur most frequently in young adults, occasionally in children and rarely in infants {1306}. A case of congenital astroblastoma has also been reported {1181}. There is apparently no predominance of either sex {1306}.

Localization, neuroimaging and macroscopy

The cerebral hemispheres are most often affected, but tumours may also develop in the corpus callosum, cerebellum, optic nerves, brain stem and cauda equina {1306, 639}. On CT scans and on MRI, they are often enhancing, well defined lesions. Macroscopically, they are usually well circumscribed and solid masses with a homogeneous cut surface, although larger examples may show both cyst formation and necrosis.

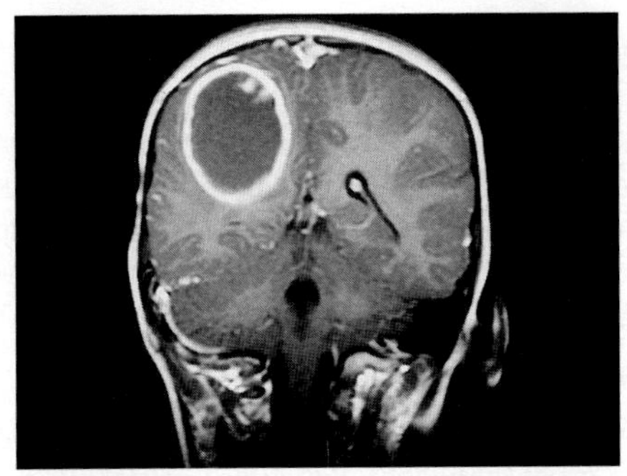

Fig. 5.1 MRI of a well circumscribed cystic astroblastoma without oedema and mass effect. The mural tumour component exhibits contrast enhancement.

Histopathology

Astroblastoma is a structurally homogeneous glial neoplasm characterized by a typical perivascular pseudorosette pattern of GFAP-positive cells with broad, non-tapering processes radiating towards a central blood vessel. As a similar histological pattern may occur in low- and high-grade astrocytomas, as well as in glioblastomas, the designation astroblastoma should be reserved for those rare tumours in which the pattern prevails throughout a well demarcated lesion that does not contain foci of conventional, infiltrative, fibrillary or gemistocytic astrocytoma or ependymoma.

The histology is far from bland: the hallmark lesions are the perivascular pseudorosettes formed by stout, usually non-tapering cell processes which radiate towards a central blood vessel. These pseudo-rosettes resemble ependymal structures, but the cell processes of astroblastomas are usually thicker, shorter and less variable in diameter than those of ependymal cells. The cell bodies from which these processes emanate are moderately pleomorphic and often angulated or club-shaped. The oval, round or indented nucleus is often eccentric, with moderately coarse chromatin. These neoplastic cells may fill all the available space amongst the perivascular pseudorosettes, but more often the extracellular space is ample, giving way to loose areas. The blood vessels frequently have thickened hyalinized walls and this, presumably progressive sclerosis, may result in large, hyalinized stromal areas.

In two published series totalling 30 cases, it was possible to distinguish two histological groups: low-grade and high-grade {144, 1831}. The low-grade tumours had a uniform architecture of perivascular pseudo-rosettes, low-to-moderate mitotic activity, little cellular atypia, minimal or no proliferation of vascular endothelium and prominent sclerosis of the vascular walls. In contrast, the high-grade neoplasms showed increased cellularity with multiple cell layers piled upon the vascular walls, high mitotic rate, cellular atypia, and hypertrophy and hyperplasia of the vascular endothelium without significant hyalinization of the vascular walls. Necrosis was encountered in both of these broad histological groups.

Immunohistochemistry

Immunohistochemistry with antibodies to GFAP, vimentin and S100 protein shows positive immunostaining {1306, 1181, 187}. Positivity was also noted for epithelial membrane antigen {187, 685} and Leu-7 {1306}. Whereas immunostaining for CAM 5.2 was negative {1181, 187}, one example displayed focal labelling for low molecular weight cytokeratins {685}. Reaction with an antibody to neuron-specific enolase was positive in some {1181, 187}, but not in other studies {639}. The tumour cells expressed adhesion molecules, including CD44 and neural cell adhesion molecule, but failed to express Thy-1, epidermal growth factor receptor or epithelial membrane antigen {1181} and synaptophysin {685}.

Electron microscopy

Electron microscopy shows abnormal blood vessels with abundant basal lamina and collagen formation. The neoplastic

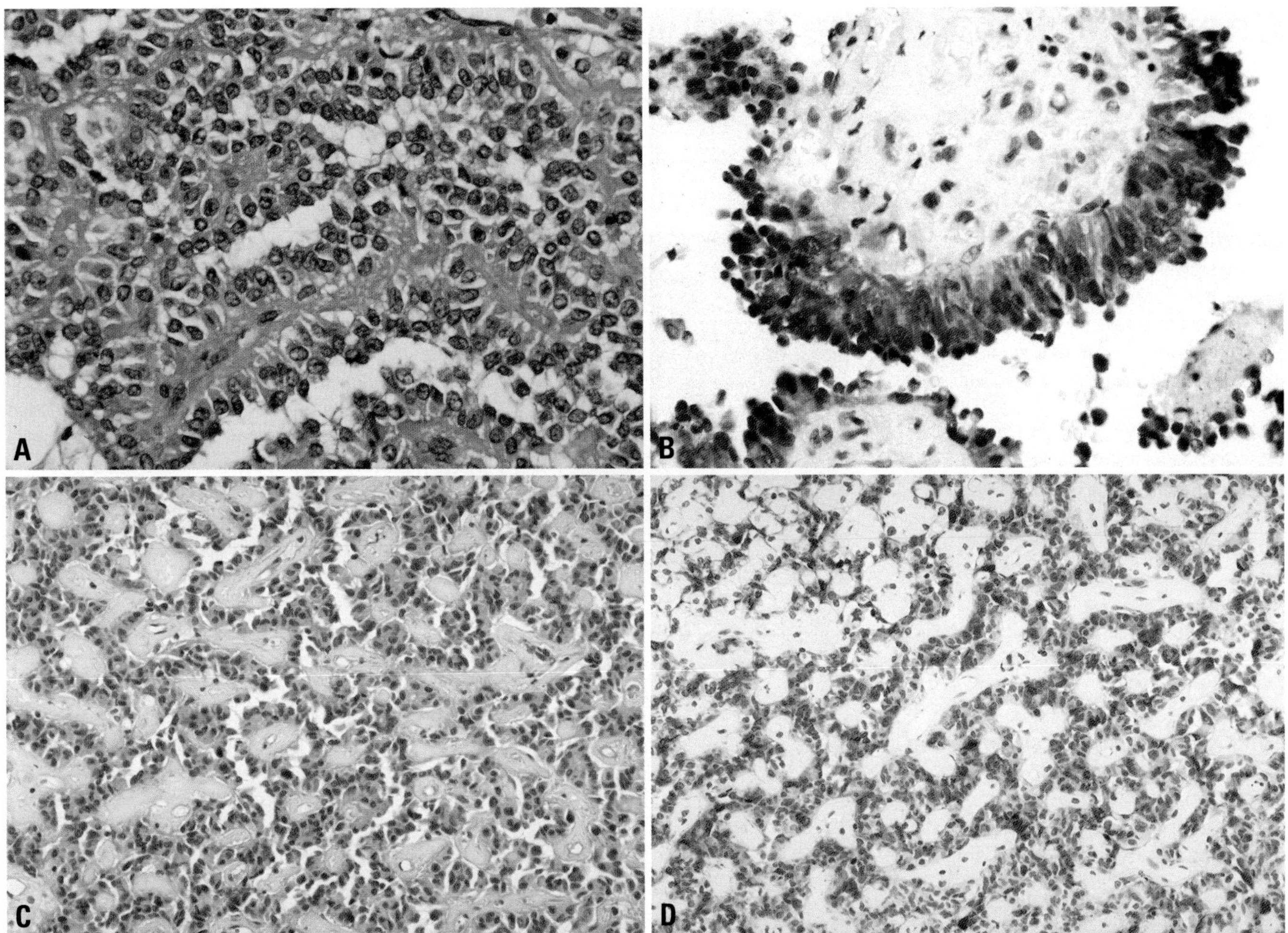

Fig. 5.2 Patterns recognized in astroblastoma. **A** Anchoring of tumour cells to blood vessels by short, stout cytoplasmic processes. **B** Tumour cell processes radiating towards fibrovascular cores show strong immunoreactivity to GFAP. **C** Astroblastoma with extensive vascular sclerosis (trichrome stain) and (**D**) variable GFAP immunoreactivity.

cells, often radially oriented towards the blood vessels, contain intermediate filaments of 10 nm in addition to the usual cell organelles. Importantly, no convincing evidence of neuronal differentiation has been found {1181, 639}. Two studied cases exhibited "purse string" constrictions at cytoplasmic apices and at the bases of budding microvilli, lamellar cytoplasmic interdigitations ("pleatings"), intercellular junctions and microrosette formation with rare cilia {1295}. These features suggested an origin of the tumours from tanycytes (see Histogenesis).

Proliferation

Reported Ki-67/MIB-1 labelling indices vary between 1 and 18% {685, 2595}, while flow cytometry revealed 96% of cells being in the G_0G_1 phase and 4% of cells in the G_2M phase {685}. Cytogenetic analysis revealed an abnormal hypodiploid karyotype with 45 chromosomes and monosomies of chromosomes 10, 21 and 22, and two marker chromosomes in all cells examined {685}. One case showed alterations of chromosomes 17p and 22q {2595}.

Histogenesis

The histogenesis of astroblastomas is controversial and the entity is not universally accepted. The original concept of Bailey and Cushing who considered them to arise from an embryonic cell programmed to become the astrocyte, has subsequently gained some support. The presence of intermediate filaments of 10 nm and the lack of neuronal or ependymal specialization, together with positive immunostaining for GFAP, vimentin and S-100 protein provide evidence of a putative astrocytic derivation. On the basis of immunohistochemical, ultrastructural, as well as tissue- and organ culture studies, the tanycyte, a cell with intermediary features between astrocytes and ependymal cells, was considered to be the cell of origin of at least some astroblastomas {1295}.

Predictive factors

The so-called low-grade astroblastomas are thought to have better prognosis than those with high-grade histological features {144, 1831}. Gross total resection of these sharply circumscribed lesions may result in long-term survival, and account for the unexpectedly favourable course of some patients with frankly malignant-appearing examples {144}. Anaplastic histology has been associated with recurrence and progression, suggesting that more aggressive treatment is necessary for high grade lesions {144, 1831}. None of 13 totally resected astroblastomas (10 with radiotherapy) did recur within 24 months {2595}.

Chordoid glioma of the third ventricle

D.J. Brat
B.W. Scheithauer
S.C. Cortez
G. Reifenberger
P.C. Burger

Definition

A rare, slowly growing, glial tumour located in the third ventricle of adults, histologically characterized by clusters and cords of epithelioid, GFAP expressing tumour cells within a variably mucinous stroma typically containing a lymphoplasmacytic infiltrate.

ICD-O code:

The provisional code proposed for the third edition of ICD-O is 9444/1.

Grading

On the basis of limited clinico-pathological data this neoplasm has been provisionally assigned WHO grade II.

Synonyms and historical annotation

In 1987, Wanschitz, *et al.* {1740} described a solid, third ventricular tumour occurring in a 24-year-old woman and having histologic and immunohistochemical features of a chordoid glioma. The authors concluded the tumour was a meningioma with 'peculiar expression of GFAP'. Subsequent immunohistochemical and ultrastructural studies of similar cases have not supported a meningothelial derivation; rather, evidence indicates that they are glial in nature. Based on a series of eight cases of a third ventricular mass with identical histologic features, chordoid glioma was described as a distinct entity in 1998 {1739}.

Incidence

The tumours are rare, but must enter into the limited differential diagnosis of a solid, contrast-enhancing third ventricular mass.

Age and sex distribution

Chordoid gliomas occur in adults {1739}, their ages distributed rather evenly between 30 and 70-years (mean, 46-years). In cases reported to date, there is a 3:1 female predominance.

Localization

Chordoid gliomas occupy the anterior portion of the third ventricle and displace normal structures in all planes. Their site of origin has not been well defined. In at least some instances, radiographic analysis of anterior third ventricular structures have demonstrated an intraparenchymal hypothalamic component.

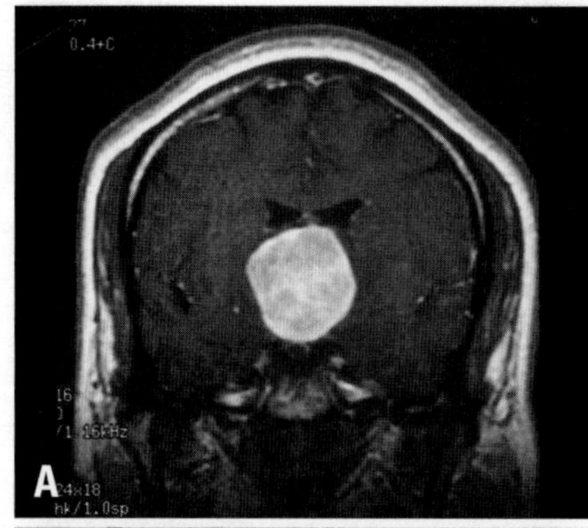

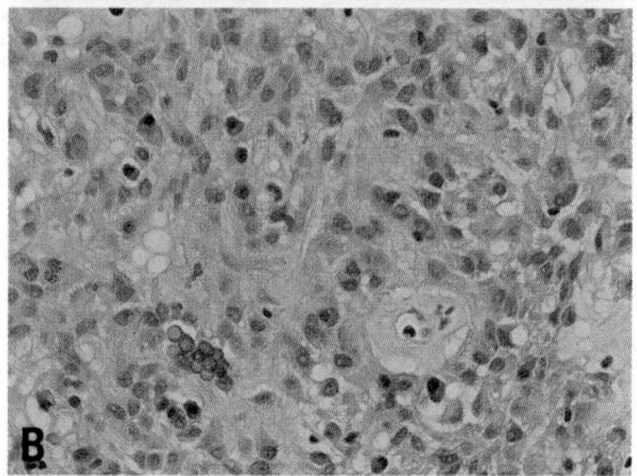

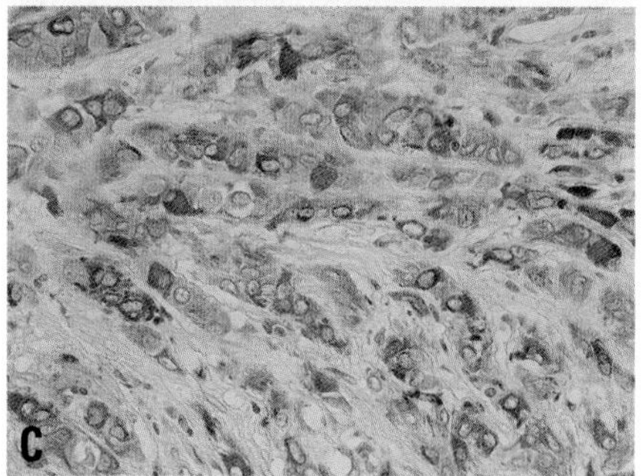

Fig. 5.3 A MRI of a chordoid glioma of the 3rd ventricle presenting as solid, sharply delineated, gadolinium enhanced mass. **B** Histological features include lymphoplasmacytic infiltrates, Russell bodies and a mucinous stroma. **C** Cords of epithelioid cells with marked GFAP expression.

Clinical features

Symptoms and signs

Chordoid gliomas occur in adults, and to date have arisen only in the third ventricular region. Most present with signs and symptoms of obstructive hydrocephalus, including headache, nausea, and ataxia. Others cause hypothyroidism and/or visual disturbances due to inferior displacement of hypothalamus and/or chiasm. Psychiatric and memory abnormalities have also been noted, presumably due to compression of the medial temporal lobes.

Neuroimaging

Magnetic resonance imaging typically demonstrates a bulky, well-circumscribed 2 to 4 cm, third ventricular mass (Fig. 5.3 A). Cystic components have been noted but are uncommon. Aside from cystic elements, the tumours are uniformly contrast-enhancing and appear contiguous with hypothalamic or suprasellar structures.

Histopathology

Chordoid gliomas are solid neoplasms composed of clusters and cords of epithelioid tumour cells within a variably mucinous stroma typically containing a lymphoplasmacytic infiltrate. Immunohistochemical and ultrastructural features indicate glial derivation.

The oval-to-polygonal epithelioid cells with abundant eosinophilic cytoplasm are embedded in a mucinous, often vacuolated stroma (Fig. 5.3 B). In many instances, obvious but limited glial differentiation in the form of coarsely fibrillar processes can also be seen {1739}. Neoplastic nuclei are moderate in size, and relatively uniform. The majority of tumours lack mitoses; in the remainder, they are rare (<1 per 10 high power fields, HPF). A stromal lymphoplasmacytic infiltrate, often with numerous Russell bodies, is a consistent finding. Conforming to radiographic impressions, tumours are architecturally solid, and show little tendency to microscopic infiltration of surrounding brain structures. Reactive astrocytes, Rosenthal fibers, and chronic inflammatory cells are seen in adjacent non-neoplastic tissue.

Immunohistochemistry

The most distinctive immunohistochemical feature of chordoid gliomas is their strong, diffuse reactivity for GFAP (Figure 5.3 C). Staining for vimentin is also strong, while S-100 protein immunoreactivity is variable. EMA staining can be seen focally, but it is usually more prominent in stromal plasma cells. Further, tumors show immunoreactivity for the epidermal growth factor receptor and schwannomin/merlin but no nuclear accumulation of the TP53, p21 (Waf-1) or MDM2 proteins {2544}.

Proliferation

The proliferative potential of chordoid gliomas corresponds to that a low-grade glioma. Mitoses are either exceedingly rare or absent, and the MIB-1 labeling index index is very low, with values of 0 to 1.5% in one study {1739} and <5% in another {2544}.

Differential diagnosis

The strikingly 'chordoid' appearance of these neoplasms, with their eosinophilic clustered tumour cells in a blue mucinous matrix is distinctive among other regional lesions, including pituitary adenoma, craniopharyngioma, pilocytic astrocytoma, and meningioma. The presence of GFAP reactivity and the absence of synaptophysin staining is inconsistent with pituitary adenoma. Pilocytic astrocytoma and craniopharyngioma bear even less of a morphologic resemblance to chordoid glioma. While there are histologic similarities between chordoid gliomas and so-called "chordoid" meningioma, the latter are GFAP-negative {755}. Similarities include the clustering of epithelioid cells and the presence of a lymphoplasmacytic infiltrate, but in contrast to chordoid gliomas, these meningiomas are typically dura-based, and have a more prominent lymphoplasmacytic component often featuring germinal centers.

Genetics

Analysis of 4 chordoid gliomas by comparative genomic hybridization (CGH) did not reveal chromosomal imbalances. None of the neoplasms contained genetic aberrations of the *TP53* and *CDKN2A* tumor suppressor genes. Amplification of the *EGFR, CDK4*, and *MDM2* proto-oncogenes was also absent {2544}.

Histogenesis

Although ultrastructural study of chordoid gliomas lends support for their glial derivation, further subclassification as astrocytic or ependymal has not been possible. The presence of focal basal lamina formation and of microvilli in most cases suggests the possibility of ependymal derivation. More definitive ultrastructural features of ependymoma, such as cilia and desmosomal junctions in series have not been noted.

Prognosis

The location of chordoid gliomas within the third ventricle and their attachment to hypothalamic and suprasellar structures often precludes their complete resection. Postoperative tumour enlargement has been noted in half of the patients undergoing subtotal resections. In addition, deaths due to tumour regrowth have been recorded. The role of adjuvant therapy following incomplete resection remains unsettled; indeed, some residual tumours have regrown despite radiotherapy.

Gliomatosis cerebri

P.L. Lantos
J.M. Bruner

Definition

Gliomatosis cerebri is a diffuse glial tumour infiltrating the brain extensively, involving more than two lobes, frequently bilaterally and often extending to infratentorial structures and even to the spinal cord.

Grading

Gliomatosis cerebri is a malignant lesion usually corresponding to WHO grade III.

ICD-O code: 9381/3

Historical annotation

The nosological definition and histogenesis of gliomatosis cerebri have remained disputed. The term gliomatosis cerebri was originally coined by Nevin in 1938 {1069} to describe diffuse infiltration by glial cells of extensive areas of the brain without formation of an obvious tumour mass. While today this name is generally accepted, there have been more than a dozen synonyms in the literature, ranging from the incorrect (*e.g.*, central diffuse schwannosis) to the meaningless (*e.g.*, diffuse systematic overgrowth of the glial apparatus). The uncertainty concerning histogenesis is reflected by the fact that gliomatosis cerebri has been removed from the category of undifferentiated and embryonic tumours of the 1979 WHO classification {1685} and is since the 1993 WHO classification {780, 779} in the category of neuroepithelial neoplasms of unknown origin.

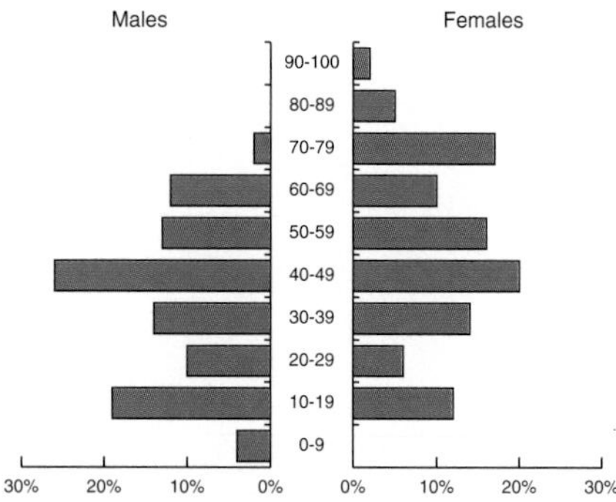

Fig. 5.4 Age distribution of 151 patients with gliomatosis cerebri. Modified, from Jennings *et al.* {698}.

Incidence, age and sex distribution

The rarity of gliomatosis cerebri and the uncertainty of its nosology have prevented large-scale and meaningful epidemiological studies. However, in a recent review of 160 cases, age at diagnosis was available for 151 patients, and the peak incidence was between 40 and 50 years, with males presenting somewhat earlier than females {698}. The age ranged from neonates to 83 years. Both sexes were equally affected.

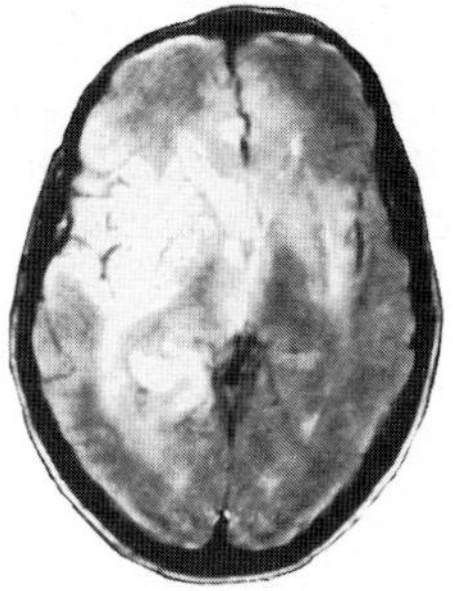

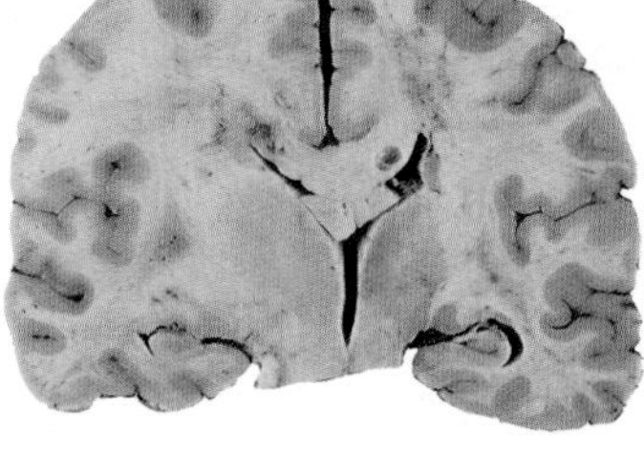

Fig. 5.5 A T2-weighted MRI of a patient with gliomatosis cerebri showing extensive infiltration of white and grey matter of both hemispheres. **B** Gliomatosis cerebri infiltrating the left hemisphere with enlargement of anatomic structures, in particular the thalamus.

Localization

The chief morphological characteristic of gliomatosis cerebri is its diffuse growth pattern. The most commonly involved areas, based on postmortem studies {698} rather than on neuroimaging, are the cerebrum (76%), the mesencephalon (52%), the pons (52%), the thalamus (43%), the basal ganglia (34%),the cerebellum (29%), the medulla oblongata (13%), the hypothalamus, the optic nerve and chiasm, and the spinal cord (each at 9%). When the lesion involves the cerebral hemispheres, the centrum semiovale is always affected, whereas the cerebral cortex is infiltrated only in 19% of such cases, with spread to the leptomeninges in 17%.

Clinical features

Symptoms and signs

On the bases of an evaluation of 139 patients {698}, the most frequent clinical features are: corticospinal tract deficits (58%), dementia (44%), headache (39%), seizures (38%), cranial nerve signs (37%), increased intracranial pressure and papilloedema (34%), spinocerebellar deficit (33%), alterations of mental status, *e.g.* lethargy (20%), behavioural changes including psychosis (19%), sensory deficits and paraesthesia (18%), visual disturbances (17%), pain (3%) and myelopathy (1.4%).

Neuroimaging

Both by CT scan and MRI, the pattern is infiltrative, with enlargement of the involved cerebral structures, usually without their destruction {1213, 328, 1409}. However, MRI gives superior results: on CT scan the lesions may appear as poorly defined areas of subtle low density or isodensity and are usually smaller when compared to T2-weighted MR images {328, 1409}. T1-weighted images are also iso- or hypointense compared to the normal brain, whereas proton density- and T2-weighted images reveal the full extent of the tumour with hyperintensity; overall these images correlate best with postmortem investigations {328, 1409}. Nevertheless, the antemortem diagnosis of gliomatosis cerebri remains difficult even with MRI and brain biopsy. A thorough postmortem examination is necessary to establish the definitive diagnosis {1084, 1622}.

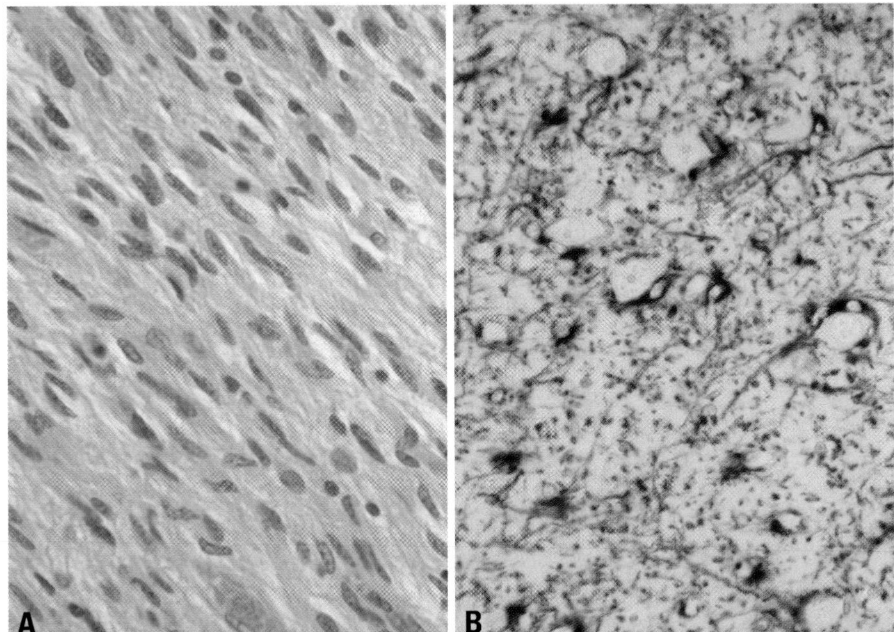

Fig. 5.6 Gliomatosis cerebri. **A** Diffuse infiltration by tumour cells arranged in a parallel fashion. **B** Expression of GFAP in small tumour cells around neurons and in neuropil.

Macroscopy

Two types of gliomatosis cerebri have been distinguished {1213}. Type I is the classical lesion in which there is a diffuse neoplastic growth and enlargement of the involved existing structures, without the formation of a circumscribed tumour mass. Type II gliomatosis, which may develop from Type I, is associated with the presence, in addition to the diffuse lesion, of an obvious neoplastic mass, usually showing features of a malignant glioma.

Histopathology

Gliomatosis cerebri is histologically composed of elongated glial cells that typically resemble astrocytes. The nuclei are oval or fusiform, and often hyperchromatic. When infiltrating myelinated tracts, the cells often form parallel rows among nerve fibres, reflecting local histoarchitecture. Mitotic activity is variable; microvascular proliferation is usually absent.

Histological variation exists not only between different lesions, but also within the same neoplasm. In some areas, the tumour cells are more obviously astrocytic, and gemistocytic forms may also be seen {1084}. Cases of gliomatosis cerebri consisting predominantly of oligodendroglia have also been described {60}. When infiltrating white matter, myelin sheaths may be destroyed, but neurons and axons appear to survive {46}. A morphometric analysis has shown that most cellular parameters of cerebral gliomatosis is comparable with those in the periphery of low grade astrocytomas {449}. However, in type II lesions, the neoplastic mass may have the features of a high-grade glioma.

Immunohistochemistry

The results of immunostaining with antibodies to GFAP and S-100 protein are somewhat variable: while some of the cells are positively stained, many remain unstained {449}; indeed reactive astrocytes dispersed throughout some lesions give a more convincingly positive reaction {1622}. Thus, lack of labelling with GFAP, particularly in a biopsy specimen, does not exclude the diagnosis of gliomatosis cerebri.

Proliferation

In two cases, the mean number of AgNOR-positive cells was only marginally higher than for low-grade diffuse astrocytomas, and was significantly lower than in high-grade astrocytomas {538}. In a single case in which both biopsy and autopsy were performed, the MIB-1 labeling indices were 6.3% and 7.6%, respectively {1084}.

Cytogenetics

Chromosomal analysis revealed the most frequent karyotype being 44,XY, del(6)(q25), del(14)(q21), der(15;21)(q10;q10), add(18)(q22), del(19)(p12), add(20)(p13) ,-21. A smaller proportion of tumour cells had 88 chromosomes with a doubling of this abnormal karyotype. These findings are important for two reasons. First, they are consistent with a clonal neoplasm originating from a single cell. Second, the chromosomal changes, with the possible exception of the chromosome 6 deletion, are not similar to those seen in astrocytomas, thus suggesting that gliomatosis cerebri may belong to a separate category of brain tumours {561}. A single case of gliomatosis cerebri showed microsatellite instability: the opposite skewing patterns in distant areas were consistent with oligoclonal derivation {1833}.

Histogenesis

The cell of origin of gliomatosis cerebri is controversial. While some phenotypic features are similar to those of astrocytomas, other manifestations do not support the view that the lesion is merely a diffuse variety of astrocytoma. The occasional case in which the predominant cell type is oligodendroglial, further undermines this concept, as do the limited data from cytogenetic analyses (see above). There are many hypotheses of pathogenesis: blastomatous dysgenesis, diffuse infiltration, multicentric origin, *in situ* proliferation, and so-called field transformation {698}.

Therefore, it seems preferable to regard gliomatosis cerebri as a neoplasm of unknown histogenesis until further molecular genetics data define the cell of origin.

Prognosis

The prognosis is generally poor. A survival analysis of a cohort of 124 patients has shown that 52% died within 12 months after the onset of symptoms, 63% by 24 months and 73% within 36 months {698}. In a review of 16 histologically verified cases, the Ki-67 labelling index significantly correlated with survival time {1832}. In a case involving the entire neuraxis from the frontal lobe to the conus medullaris of the spinal cord, a focal increase of the Ki-67 labeling index of up to 30% was noted {2596}.

CHAPTER 6

Neuronal and Mixed Neuronal–Glial Tumours

The neoplasms described in this chapter occur at a low frequency and usually carry a favourable prognosis. They have in common a variable extent of neuronal and, less consistently, glial differentiation. Knowledge and precise classification of these entities is important so as to avoid unnecessary radio- or chemotherapy.

Gangliocytoma and ganglioglioma

These benign neoplasms are characterized by the presence of mature ganglion cells with or without a gliomatous component. As CNS neurons are considered to be postmitotic, their cell of origin remains enigmatic.

Desmoplastic infantile astrocytoma and ganglioglioma

These two lesions occur almost exclusively in infants and share most clinical and histological features, the only difference being an additional neuronal component in the ganglioglioma. Despite their usually large size at clinical presentation, the prognosis is favourable.

Dysembryoplastic neuroepithelial tumour

This recently identified lesion occupies a border zone between malformation and neoplasm. Two major histological variants are now recognized, although their distinction does not influence the generally benign clinical course.

Central neurocytoma

This intraventricular neuronal neoplasm is now a well-recognized entity, but must be delineated from neoplasms with neurocytic differentiation occurring in other CNS regions. Its histogenesis remains obscure.

Cerebellar liponeurocytoma

Previously termed lipomatous medulloblastoma, this lesion is a new addition to the WHO classification and has been grouped together with other neurocytic neoplasms.

Paraganglioma

Although morphologically indistinguishable from similar lesions at other locations, the paraganglioma of the filum terminale is unique in that it occurs alone, without association with systemic or inherited disease.

Ganglioglioma and gangliocytoma

J.S. Nelson
J.M. Bruner
O.D. Wiestler
S.R. VandenBerg

Definition

Well differentiated, slowly growing neuroepithelial tumours composed of neoplastic, mature ganglion cells, either alone (gangliocytoma), or in combination with neoplastic glial cells (ganglioglioma).

ICD-O codes:

Gangliocytoma: 9492/0
Ganglioglioma: 9505/1
Anaplastic ganglioglioma:
The provisional code proposed for the third edition of ICD-O is 9505/3.

Grading

Histologically, gangliocytomas correspond to WHO grade I, while gangliogliomas may be WHO grade I or II. Some gangliogliomas show anaplastic features in their glial component and are considered to be WHO grade III (anaplastic ganglioglioma). There are rare cases of newly diagnosed gangliogliomas with grade IV (glioblastoma) changes in the glial component {1866}.

Incidence

The available data indicate that gangliocytoma and ganglioglioma together represent 0.4% of all CNS tumours and 1.3% of all brain tumours {722,1686}. There are no population based epidemiological data on gangliogliomas.

Table 6.1
Tumours causing chronic temporal lobe epilepsy

Diagnosis	Percentage
Ganglioglioma WHO grade I-III	40%
Dysembryoplastic neuroepithelial tumour	18%
Pilocytic astrocytoma WHO grade I	17%
Astrocytoma WHO grade II	9%
Oligodendroglioma WHO grade II	6%
Pleomorphic xanthoastrocytoma WHO grade II	4%
Subependymal giant cell astrocytoma WHO grade I	1%
Other glial tumours	4%
Epidermoid	1%

Based on a series of 209 cases from the Neuropathology Department, University of Bonn. Modified, from Blümcke *et al.* {2215}.

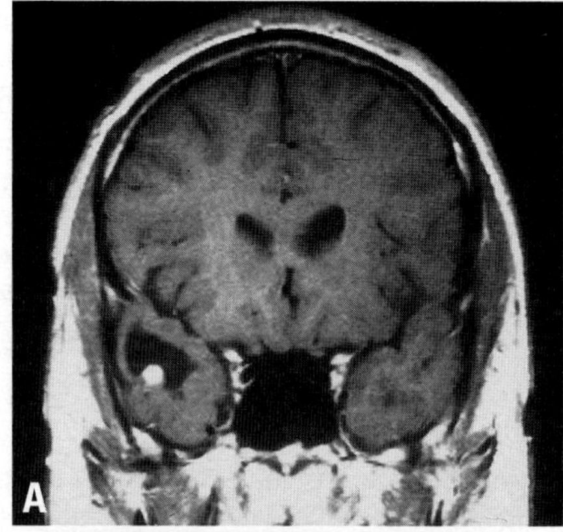

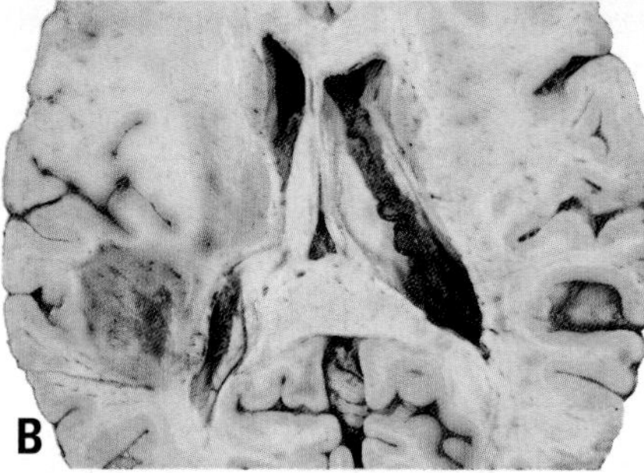

Fig. 6.1 **A** MRI of a cystic ganglioglioma in the left temporal lobe with an intramural nodule. **B** Well-delineated supratentorial ganglioglioma; the central necrosis is due to prior therapeutic irradiation.

Age and sex distribution

The age of patients ranges from 2 months to 80 years {859, 1878}; age-specific incidence rate are not available. Data from four large series with a total of 206 patients indicate a mean or median age at diagnosis ranging from 8.5 to 25 years. The male: female ratio varied from 1.1:1 to 1.9:1 {594, 854, 1205, 1629}. In 99 cases involving only children, the mean age at diagnosis was 9.5 years, with 52% of patients being females {1874}.

Localization

Tumours may occur throughout the CNS, including the cerebrum, brain stem, cerebellum, spinal cord, optic nerves, pituitary gland and pineal gland. The majority are supratentorial and involve the temporal lobe {594, 854, 1205, 1629}.

Clinical features

Symptoms and signs

Symptoms vary according to the site of the tumour. Tumours in the cerebrum are associated with a history of seizures ranging in duration from 1 month to 50 years before diagnosis, with a mean or median interval of 6–25 years {854, 1205, 1629}. For tumours involving the brain stem or spinal cord, the mean duration of symptoms before diagnosis is 1.25 and 1.4 years, respectively {854}. Gangliogliomas have been reported in 15-25% of cerebral cortical resections for control of pharmacoresistant seizures {1877,1632}. They are the most common tumours associated with chronic temporal lobe epilepsy (Table 6.1).

Neuroimaging

CT shows a circumscribed solid mass or cyst with a mural nodule. The tumour is isodense or hypodense and may show calcifications. Some gangliocytomas may be hyperdense. Contrast-enhancement is typical but may be faint or absent. Scalloping of the calvarium may be seen adjacent to superficially located cerebral tumours. MRI shows a T1-weighted hypointense, T2-weighted hyperintense circumscribed mass. Enhancement varies in intensity from none to marked, and may be solid, rim, or nodular {511, 1111}.

Macroscopy

These are solid or cystic tumours that are not usually accompanied by a significant mass effect. Calcification may be present. Haemorrhage and necrosis are rare.

Histopathology

Gangliocytomas are composed of irregular groups of large, multipolar neurons that often show dysplastic features. The stroma consists of non-neoplastic glial elements and a network of reticulin fibres, which may be perivascular. Gangliogliomas show an additional neoplastic glial component, usually astrocytes, surrounded by a reticulin network. Occasional mitoses are compatible with the diagnosis of ganglioglioma. Necrosis is absent, unless the glial component is undergoing malignant change.

Perivascular lymphocytic infiltration is frequent and typical, but not diagnostic. Other features include rounded, eosinophilic granular or hyalin bodies which appear interstitially or within tumour astrocytes, as well as microcysts, calcification, and, occasionally, desmoplastic foci. The astrocytic component frequently has a pilocytic appearance. Neurons can be identified using conventional Nissl and silver impregnation methods or immunohistochemistry (see below). Gangliocytomas and gangliogliomas are generally circumscribed tumours. Gangliogliomas may extend locally into the adjacent leptomeninges and the glial component may give rise to an infiltrative appearance at the border between tumour and parenchyma. Neither of these features appears to correlate with aggressive behaviour. Anaplastic gangliogliomas, however, have been documented. Malignant change almost invariably involves the glial component, which eventually may lead to the histological features of glioblastoma {594, 722, 1205, 1629}.

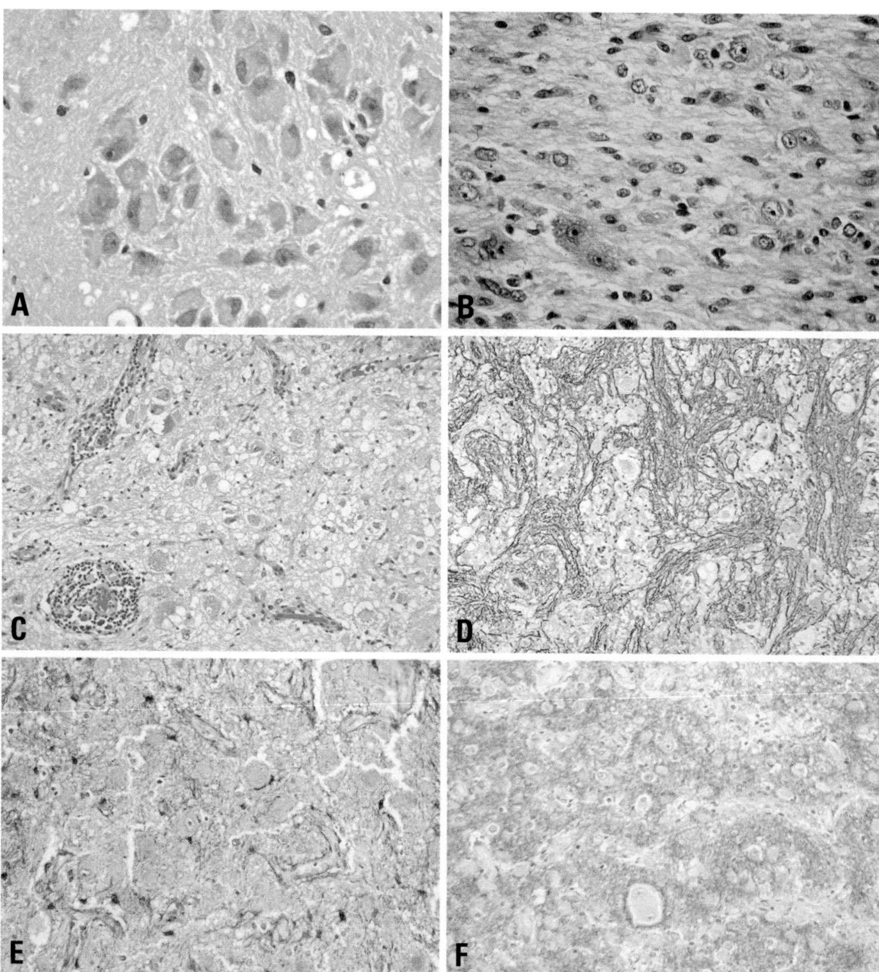

Fig. 6.2 **A** Gangliocytoma with clusters of mature, irregularly shaped ganglion cells. **B** Ganglioglioma with the characteristic combination of dysmorphic, occasionally binucleate neurons and neoplastic glial cells. **C** Ganglioglioma with marked perivascular lymphocytic infiltrations. **D** Lobular pattern with stromal reaction. **E** GFAP expression by neoplastic astrocytes and **(F)** strong immunoreactivity to synaptophysin of ganglion cells and their processes. Note the binucleate neuron with synaptophysin staining of persomatic synapses.

Histopathological variants

A variant of ganglioglioma is the *papillary glioneuronal tumour* {1842, 1841, 1840}. It is characterized by pseudopapillary appearance with a single layer of pseudostratified, small, cuboidal cells around hyalinized blood vessels, associated with sheets or focal collections of neurocytes mingled with ganglion cells and cells with morphology intermediate between neurocytes and ganglion cells. Macroscopically, this tumour arises in deep white matter in paraventricular location and is typically associated with prominent cystic change. Radiographically, this variant is contrast-enhancing. Its histological appearance must be distinguished from pilocytic astrocytoma, ependymoma, and neuroblastoma, because the few cases reported today exhibit a prognosis similar to that of other gangliogliomas.

Neoplasms containing small neurons ('neurocytes') occur occasionally in sites other than the region of the foramen of Monro. Such lesions form a clinically and pathologically heterogeneous group {465, 921, 1008, 1081, 1654}. Children and young adults have been affected. Both supratentorial and infratentorial sites have been described. The lesions are radiologically well-circumscribed, focally contrast-enhancing, often cystic, and sometimes calcified. Histologically, some are similar to the central neurocytoma, with or without focal evolution into ganglion cells. Both well-differentiated and mitotically active types occur. Others are less cellular, and a fibrillary background is more prominent. Some include a glial component and the terms 'gangliocytoma' or 'ganglioglioneurocytoma' have been applied. The glial component is a paucicellular astrocytic proliferation. Many of the lesions mimic oligodendrogliomas. Immunohistochemistry may be necessary to distinguish the lesion, especially when the perinuclear halos are prominent. The fibrillary background in the neurocytic and ganglion cell lesions is immunoreactive for synaptophysin. Ganglion cells stain for synaptophysin and, less predictably, for chromogranin. The astrocytes are GFAP-positive. Clinical follow-up of cases has been limited but, in general, the lesions behave in a benign fashion and lend themselves to surgical resection {465}. Leptomeningeal dissemination has been noted in just one case {1654}.

Immunohistochemistry

Immunostains may be used to demonstrate neuronal features, such as expression of synaptophysin or the presence of neurofilament epitopes in neuronal processes or perikarya. Numerous neuropeptides and biogenic amines have been detected in the neuronal components of CNS ganglion cell tumours. Staining for GFAP demonstrates the astrocytes that usually form the neoplastic glial component of gangliogliomas. A recent study found 74% of gangliogliomas to exhibit CD34 immunoreactivity {2485}.

Electron microscopy

Neurons with dense core granules are a characteristic and diagnostically useful ultrastructural feature of these tumours. Synaptic junctions may be absent, or may be present in only small numbers {594, 859, 1878, 1009}.

Proliferation

Mitotic figures are rare. Ki-67/MIB-1 labelling indices involve only the glial component, mean values ranging from 1.1 to 2.7% {594, 1205, 1629}. Increased growth fraction (MIB-1) and p53 labelling may be associated with tumour recurrence {594}.

Genetic susceptibility

Dysplastic gangliocytoma of the cerebellum (Lhermitte-Duclos) occurs in the setting of Cowden disease, caused by a *PTEN* germline mutation (see Chapter 14). One case of spinal cord ganglioglioma has been reported in a child with neurofibromatosis type 2 {1875}.

Cytogenetics

Abnormal karyotypes were observed in 3/14 gangliogliomas and included a ring chromosome 1, trisomies of chromosomes 5–7, and deletion of chromosome 6 {1067}. A complex abnormal karyotype with three sublines showing inversion, translocations, and gains or losses of long or short chromosome arms and involving chromosomes 6, 7, 11, 13, 15, 16, 18, 19 and Y was observed in a rare case of ganglioglioma with malignant transformation {686}. In addition, a ganglioglioma with an abnormal karyotype involving translocations and deletions of chromosomes 1, 5, 21, 12, 8, 13, 10 and X has been reported {799}. Deletions on chromosome 17p were observed in an anaplastic ganglioglioma with diffuse leptomeningeal spread {1572}. Paracentric inversion of chromosome 7 was noted in a temporal lobe ganglioglioma without anaplastic features that recurred with radiological evidence of intracranial and spinal metastases {1871}.

Molecular genetics

In a study of six gangliogliomas, microsatellite instability was not observed {1677}. A recent study suggests that a splice-site-associated polymorphism in the tuberous sclerosis 2 gene (*TSC2*) may predispose to the development of sporadic ganglioglioma {1188}.

Histogenesis

Gangliocytomas/ gangliogliomas may represent highly differentiated remnants of embryonal neuroblastomas or related primitive neuroectodermal tumours (see Chapter 8, medulloblastoma). A monoclonal origin was shown for 5 of 7 gangliogliomas by both methylation-based and transcription-based clonal analysis. The other 2 cases were polyclonal by the methylation-based technique, but monoclonal with transcription-based analysis {1873}. Neoplastic transformation of subpial granule cells or of glial cells within hamartomas has also been discussed {722, 1629}.

Predictive factors

Anaplastic changes in the glial component and high MIB-1 and TP53 labelling indices may indicate aggressive behaviour and less favourable prognosis {594, 722, 1205}. However, the correlation of histological anaplasia with clinical outcome is inconsistent {722, 854}.

Desmoplastic infantile astrocytoma and ganglioglioma

A.L. Taratuto
S.R. VandenBerg
L.B. Rorke

Definition

Large cystic tumours of infants that involve superficial cerebral cortex and leptomeninges, often attached to dura, with a generally good prognosis following surgical resection. They consist histologically of a prominent desmoplastic stroma with a neuroepithelial population, mainly restricted to neoplastic astrocytes (desmoplastic infantile astrocytoma, DIA) or to astrocytes together with a variable neuronal component (desmoplastic infantile ganglioglioma, DIG), in addition to aggregates of poorly differentiated cells, which are present in both.

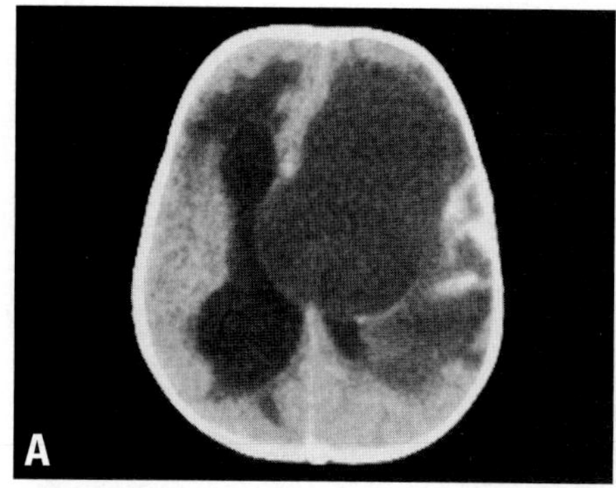

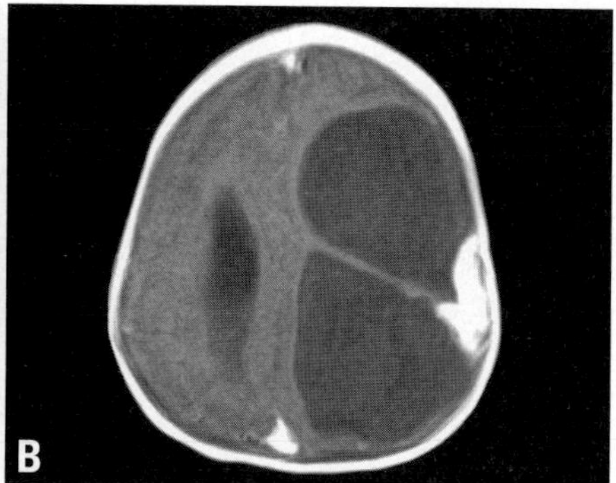

Fig. 6.4 **A** T1 MRI of a desmoplastic astrocytoma in a five-month-old infant presenting as a contrast-enhancing mass on the surface of the parietal lobe overlying a large complex cyst. **B** Desmoplastic infantile ganglioglioma with similar location and large cysts causing mass shifting to the contralateral hemisphere.

ICD-O code:

The provisional code proposed for the third edition of ICD-O is 9493/0.

Grading

Histologically, desmoplastic infantile astrocytoma/ganglioglioma correspond to WHO grade I.

Synonyms and historical annotation

The desmoplastic infantile astrocytoma (DIA) was originally defined in 1982 by Taratuto *et al.* {1487} as meningocerebral astrocytoma attached to dura with desmoplastic reaction. In 1984, the lesion was described as superficial cerebral astrocytoma attached to dura {1488}, thus delineating an entity previously unrecognized or probably regarded as a form of malignant mesenchymal tumour. It was later included in Russell & Rubinstein's classification of astrocytic tumours {1306} and in the first edition of this book {779} under the term 'desmoplastic cerebral astrocytoma of infancy (DCAI).

In 1987, VandenBerg *et al.* described desmoplastic supratentorial neuroepithelial tumours of infancy with divergent differentiation ('desmoplastic infantile ganglioglioma', DIG), occurring in the same clinical setting, but with an additional, variable neuronal component {1543}. They stressed the presence of immature neuroepithelial cell aggregates which initially were suggestive of 'desmoplastic neuroblastomas' in some of their cases. Since both lesions have similar clinical features, including a favourable prognosis, they are, in this edition of the WHO classification, listed together as desmoplastic infantile astrocytoma/ganglioglioma. Surgical pathologists may use the terms desmoplastic infantile astrocytoma (DIA) or desmoplastic infantile ganglioglioma (DIG), depending on the pattern of differentiation of the neuroepithelial component.

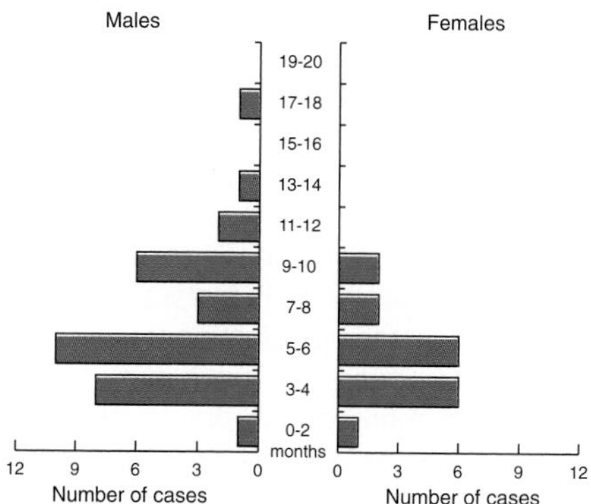

Fig. 6.3 Age and sex distribution (months) of desmoplastic infantile astroctyoma and ganglioglioma, based on 49 published cases.

Incidence

Desmoplastic infantile astrocytoma/ganglioglioma are rare neoplasms. In a series of 6,500 CNS tumours, 22 cases of desmoplastic infantile ganglioglioma were reported {1541}, with at least a further 20 cases being reported from other laboratories diagnosed on the basis of a widely variable number of cells displaying morphological or immunohistochemical ganglion cell features, together with the astrocytic component {11, 355, 450, 966, 1077, 1132, 1154, 1444, 1480, 1495, 2221, 2219}. In a paediatric series of CNS intracranial tumours, 6 desmoplastic infantile astrocytomas were found, representing 1.25% of all {1488}, but 15.8% among cases in infants {1682}. Fourteen additional cases have since been reported {50, 146, 315, 923, 1223,1303, 1387, 1491, 2216, 2217}.

Age and sex distribution

The age range for 60 reported cases of desmoplastic infantile astrocytoma/

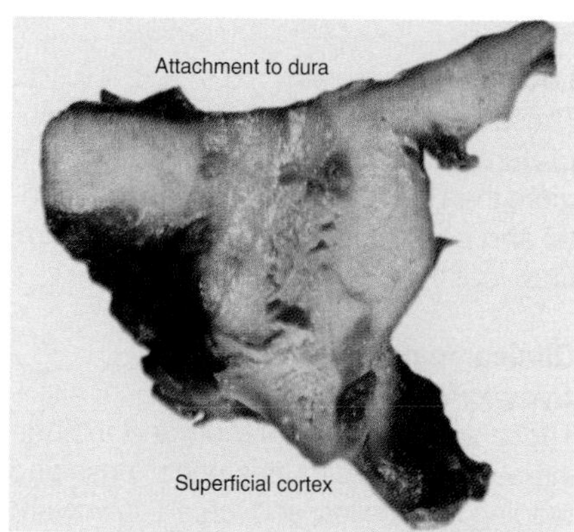

Fig. 6.5 Surgical specimen of a desmoplastic astrocytoma showing a firm ivory-coloured tumour attached to the dura and leptomeninges. There is no clear-cut demarcation between the tumour and the cerebral cortex.

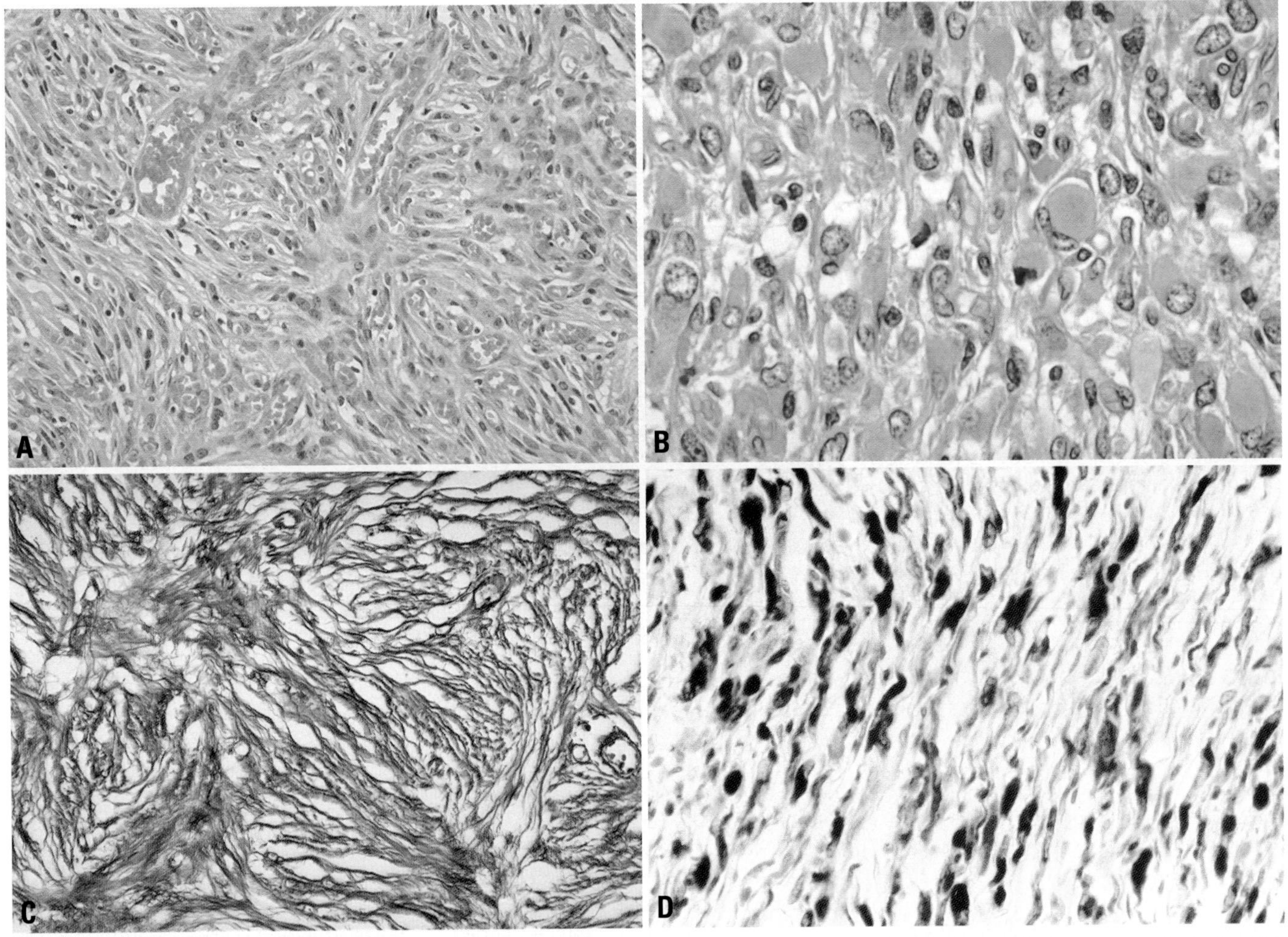

Fig. 6.6 Desmoplastic cerebral astrocytomas of infancy. **A** Neoplastic astrocytes arranged in streams, with a (**C**) marked desmoplastic component (reticulin stain). **B** Field of gemistocytic neoplastic astrocytes. **D** GFAP-expressing neoplastic astrocytes: the desmoplastic component remains unstained.

ganglioglioma is 1–24 months, with a and a male: female ratio of 1.7:1. Several non-infantile cases, with ages ranging from 5 to 17 years, have recently been reported {2222, 2218, 2220, 2219}.

Localization

These tumours invariably arise in the supratentorial region and commonly involve more than one lobe, preferentially the frontal and parietal, followed by the temporal and, least frequently, the occipital.

Clinical features

Symptoms and signs

These are of short duration and include increasing head circumference, tense and bulging fontanelles, and forced downward ocular deviation ('sunset sign'). There may be paresis, seizures, increase in muscle tone with hyperactive reflexes and, rarely, palsy of the sixth and seventh cranial nerves.

Neuroimaging

Plain skull films show sutural diastasis with or without erosion of the inner table adjacent to the tumour. On CT scan, the lesion is a large, hypodense cystic mass with a solid isodense or slightly hyperdense superficial portion which shows contrast enhancement (Fig. 6.4). The T1-weighted image on MRI is characterized by a hypointense cystic mass with an isointense peripheral solid component that enhances with gadolinium. On T2-weighted images, the cystic component is hyperintense and the solid portion is heterogeneous.

Macroscopy

These tumours are large, measuring up to 13 cm in diameter, and have deep uni- or multiloculated cysts filled with clear or xanthochromic fluid. The solid superficial portion is primarily extracerebral, involving leptomeninges and superficial cortex and is commonly attached to the dura, firm or rubbery in consistency, and grey or white in colour. There is no gross evidence of haemorrhage or necrosis.

Histopathology

Diagnostic features are those of a slowly growing superficial glioma mainly composed of neoplastic astrocytes and a prominent reticulin-rich, desmoplastic stroma (desmoplastic infantile astrocytoma, DIA), in some cases together with a variable extent of neuronal differentiation (desmoplastic infantile ganglioglioma, DIG). Aggregates of poorly differentiated cells are present in both lesions.

Astrocytes are the predominant neuroepithelial component, and are particularly present in more desmoplastic regions. These elements, as well as a population of neoplastic ganglion cells, are characteristic of desmoplastic infantile ganglioglioma. The main leptomeningeal portion consists of spindle, elongated astrocytic cells, and of processes arranged in fascicles or in a storiform or whorled pattern, intermixed with collagen and reticulin fibres surrounding tumour cells, mimicking a mesenchymal tumour. The neoplastic astrocytes may include gemistocytic forms. In desmoplastic infantile ganglioglioma, there may be a heterogeneous neuronal component with small polygonal cells and atypical or typical ganglion cells, which are more readily discerned in areas with scanty extracellular matrix {1539, 1543}. Aggregates of poorly differentiated neuroepithelial cells with small, round, deeply basophilic nuclei and minimal surrounding perikarya are present to a variable extent in both DIA and DIG. There is a sharp demarcation between the cortical surface and the desmoplastic tumour, although Virchow-Robin spaces in the underlying cortex are often filled with tumour cells. The parenchymal component may be observed as micro-infiltration or microcysts with reactive cortical gliosis. Mitotic activity and necrosis are uncommon, but when present are mostly restricted to the population of poorly differentiated neuroepithelial cells {1539, 1541}. Some tumours may contain angiomatoid vessels, but microvascular proliferation is not evident {315, 923}.

Immunohistochemistry

Antibodies specific for glial, neuronal and mesenchymal cells are essential in the evaluation of tumour cell phenotypes. Glial cells express both GFAP and vimentin, while neuronal differentiation in desmoplastic infantile ganglioglioma is disclosed by synaptophysin, NF-H and class III beta-tubulin (TUJI) {1541, 1543}, among other markers. Poorly differentiated cells within aggregates sometimes prove reactive for GFAP {1077, 1490, 1541} or vimentin, but immunostaining for synaptophysin, neurofilament protein {1303}, class III beta-tubulin and MAP2 {1154, 1541} has also been reported. Mesenchymal cells express vimentin {923}, whereas antibodies to type IV collagen react in a reticulin-like pattern around tumour cells {50, 923}. Desmin expression has been observed in two tumours {1303}, which might reflect an aberration dating back to early foetal development.

Electron microscopy

Astrocytic cells contain intermediate filaments which may be arranged in bundles together with a few cisternae of rough endoplasmic reticulum and mitochondria, while an extensive basal lamina completely surrounds them {50, 315, 923, 1487, 1488}. Fibroblasts containing granular endoplasmic reticulum and well-developed Golgi complexes may also be disclosed, particularly in collagen-rich areas {50, 315}. Neuronal cells with dense core secretory granules as well as clusters of small processes containing neurofilaments have been described in desmoplastic infantile ganglioglioma, where immuno electron microscopy has shown filamentous reactivity to NF-H in cell bodies and processes lacking a basal lamina. Synapses, myelinated processes and Schwann cell differentiation were not evident {1539, 1541}.

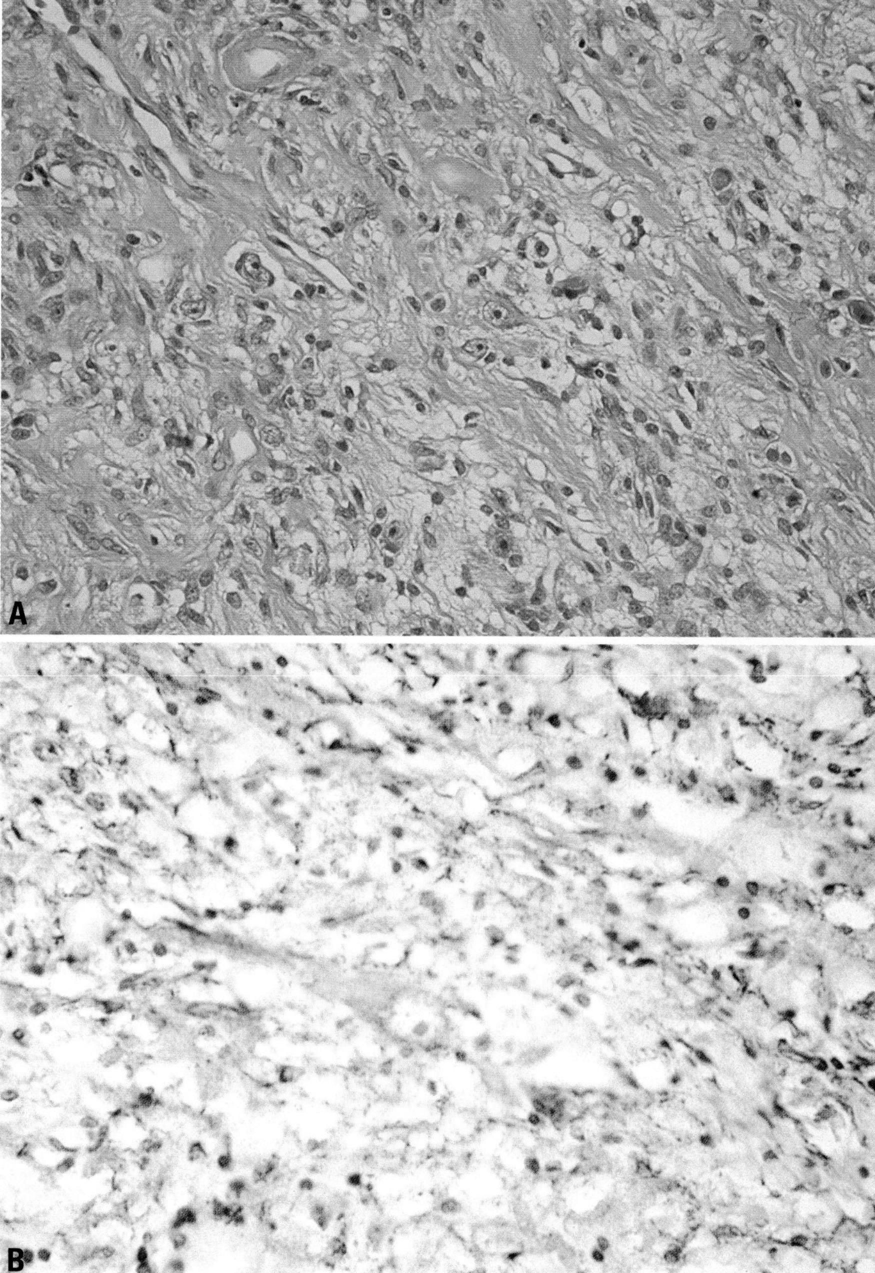

Fig. 6.7 Desmoplastic infantile ganglioglioma with (**A**) scattered ganglion cells and (**B**) marked synaptophysin immunoreactivity of ganglion cells and their processes.

Proliferation

Mitotic activity is rare and is, when present, mostly restricted to the undifferentiated mean age at manifestation of 6.3 months, small cell population {1539, 1541}. Ki-67 labelling indices range from less than 0.5% in one desmoplastic infantile ganglioglioma case {1495}, to 5% (mean, 3.5%) in three desmoplastic cerebral astrocytoma of infancy cases {1491}. DNA analysis of six cases of DIA showed a major, well-differentiated diploid component and a minor, poorly differentiated aneuploid one. In three cases analyzed by flow cytometry of cells from paraffin-embedded material, the S-phase fraction ranged from 3.7% to 12 %, with a mean of 6.6% {1491}. In a single report {50}, mitotic figures were found to correlate with high PCNA labelling index, as well as an elevated S-phase fraction (11%) and a 15% hypertetraploid cell population.

Cytogenetics
No clonal abnormalities were found in short-term cultures of tumours, but several non-clonal aberrations were observed in a desmoplastic infantile astrocytoma case {146}; a second report described a normal karyotype {1387}.

Molecular genetics
In one study of DIA, no loss of heterozygosity was found on chromosomes 10 and 17, including the *TP53* suppressor gene {923}. Another study of four DIA cases also reported the absence of *TP53* mutations {1491}. These findings suggest that the molecular genetics of these tumours is different from that of other supratentorial astrocytomas.

Histogenesis
As in pleomorphic xanthoastrocytoma (Chapter 1), the superficial cortical location and the presence of neoplastic astrocytes surrounded by basal lamina {761} suggests these tumours may originate from subpial astrocytes {842, 1225}, {50, 315, 923, 1488, 1543}. As normal basal lamina matrix proteins have been reported to inhibit growth and promote differentiation of glioma cell lines {1307}, the favourable prognosis of these tumours may be due to growth inhibition mediated by autocrine production of basal lamina components {923} and/or extracellular-matrix-induced maturation of undifferentiated cells {50, 1539, 1541}.
Developmental abnormalities, such as glial and/or neuronal ectopia within the subarachnoid space, arising as the result of a gene mutation, hypoxia, chemical or physical injury to the developing brain have been discussed as possible etiological factors {238}.

Predictive factors
Clinical
Follow-up studies indicate that gross total resection results in long term survival in cases of DIA and DIG despite the presence of primitive-appearing cellular aggregates with (low) mitotic activity and foci of necrosis. In a follow-up study of 8.3–20 years (median 15.1 years), six of eight patients with desmoplastic infantile astrocytoma survived (two died peri-operatively) {1488, 1491}. Fourteen patients with desmoplastic infantile ganglioglioma survived for 8.7 years (range, 1–14.1 years), and no death resulted from a residual or recurrent tumour {1541}.

Histopathological
Two year follow-up of DIG with a high mitotic rate, microvascular proliferation and perinecrotic palisading tumour cells did not show recurrence after macroscopically complete removal {2486, 2487}. Only one death due to tumour progression has been recorded in an unusually deep-seated DIG that could not be completely resected {1132}. CSF metastasis at presentation has been reported in a case described as a DIA, but the appropriate classification of this lesion is open to question as it was basally located, lacked a primitive-appearing small cell component and exhibited relatively inconspicuous basal lamina deposition around neoplastic astrocytes {2223}.

Dysembryoplastic neuroepithelial tumour

C. Daumas-Duport
T. Pietsch
P.L. Lantos

Definition

Benign, usually supratentorial, glial-neuronal neoplasms characterized by a predominantly cortical location and occurrence in children and young adults with a long-standing history of partial seizures. Dysembryoplastic neuroepithelial tumours typically exhibit a multinodular architecture and may be associated with cortical dysplasia.

Grading

These lesions correspond histologically to WHO grade I

ICD-O code:

The provisional code proposed for the third edition of ICD-O is 9413/0.

Synonyms and historical annotations

This tumour entity was originally identified in patients who had undergone epilepsy surgery for the treatment of long-standing drug-resistant partial seizures.

They showed unusual morphological features including cortical topography, multinodular architecture, a 'specific glioneuronal element' with a columnar structure, and foci of cortical dysplasia. Long-term follow-up demonstrated no clinical or radiological evidence of recurrence, even in patients with incomplete surgical removal. Moreover, several factors strongly suggested that these tumours might have a dysembryoplastic origin (see below).

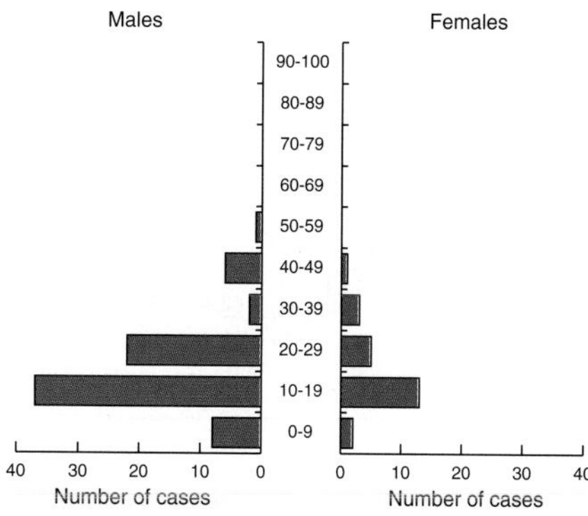

Fig. 6.8 Age distribution of dysembryoplastic neuroepithelial tumours, based on 99 cases from the St Anne Hospital, Paris.

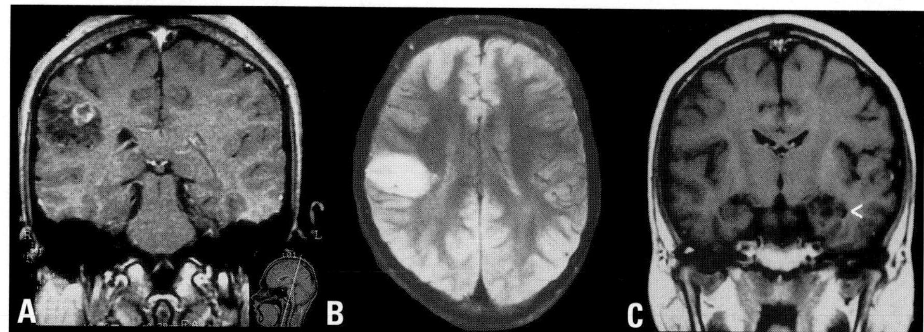

Fig. 6.9 A,B MRI of a complex histological form of DNT. **A** T1 MRI showing a nodule of contrast-enhancement within an area of hypointensity. **B** On T2 MRI, the tumour presents as a well-delineated area of hyperintensity. **C** MRI of a cystic DNT in the medio-basal temporal lobe (arrow).

Therefore the term "dysembryoplastic neuroepithelial tumour" (DNT) was proposed for these distinctive lesions {305}.

In the revised WHO classification of 1993 {779}, DNTs were included in the category of "neuronal and mixed neuronal-glial tumours". These histological criteria were based on the initial description of DNTs and allow only for the diagnosis of a morphological variant now referred as to the "complex form". A "simple form" of DNT with a unique glioneuronal element has later been described {301}.

More recently, it has been suggested that DNTs include a large spectrum of tumours that cannot be distinguished histologically from ordinary gliomas, and that the diagnosis of such "non-specific histological forms" requires that clinical presentation and imaging features be taken into consideration {301, 611, 1836}.

Furthermore, recent studies have demonstrated that DNTs are not exclusively located within the supratentorial cortex, but may also arise in various locations corresponding to the topography of the secondary germinal layers {217, 305, 830, 882}. Thus, the concept of the dysembryoplastic neuroepithelial tumour is evolving further as new investigations are carried out.

Incidence

Large variations are observed in the reported incidence of DNTs according to the surgical protocol and/or to the criteria used for their diagnosis. In epilepsy surgery, the incidence of "typical" DNTs ranged from 0.8% {1632} to 5% {1040}, whereas, in a series that included "non specific" variants, DNTs were identified in 19% of the patients {1836}. In another study, 87% of the lesions associated with drug-resistant seizures were interpreted as DNTs. Among all neuroepithelial tumours diagnosed in a single institution, "typical" DNTs were identified in 1.2% of the patients under age 20 years and in 0.2% of those aged more than 20 years {1835}.

Age and sex distribution

Age at diagnosis are most frequently the second and third decade. Males are more frequently affected.

Localization

A large majority of DNTs that are identified during surgery for epilepsy are located in the temporal lobe and preferentially

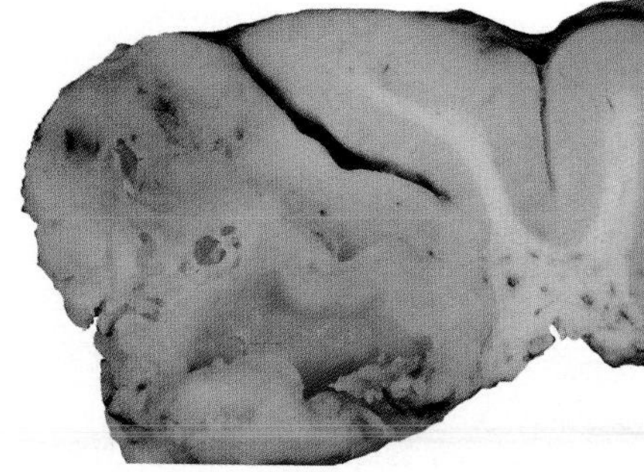

Fig. 6.10 Surgical specimen of the complex form of DNT illustrated in Fig. 6.9 A and B, showing the cortical topography of the lesion and several cysts.

involve the mesial structures {301, 302, 303, 305, 611, 1202, 1836}. However, they may develop in any part of the supratentorial cortex. In series based on general neurosurgical practice, the temporal lobe accounts for less than 50% of the cases {301, 1489}. Recent reports demonstrated that these tumours may also arise in the area of the caudate nucleus {217} and in the cerebellum {305, 830, 1834}. Multifocal examples have been observed and show that these tumours may also be found in the region of the third ventricle and in the pons {882}.

Clinical features

Symptoms and signs

Patients who harbour supratentorial DNTs typically present with long-standing drug-resistant partial seizures, with or without secondary generalisation, that begin before the age of 20 years and are either unassociated with focal neurological deficits or occur in the setting of complex congenital neurological abnormalities {301, 305, 1202, 1236, 1489, 1836}. Late onset of seizures has been reported, with the oldest patient aged 38 years {301, 1236}.

Neuroimaging

Cortical topography of the lesion is an important criterion for differentiating between these tumours and gliomas. Overall, MRI demonstrates the cortical location of the lesion better than the CT scan. On MRI, the tumour may look like macrogyri, but the lesion usually largely encompasses the thickness of the normal cortex. In superficial examples, deformation of the overlying calvarium is often seen on CT scan and this finding further supports the diagnosis of a DNT {301, 303, 792, 840, 1236, 1489, 1836}.

These tumours are hypointense on T1-weighted and hyperintense on T2-weighted MRI. On unenhanced CT scan, their appearance is variable: they may be either hypodense with a pseudocystic appearance, isodense or hypo-isodense; they also often contain calcifications. True cyst formation is seen in a minority of cases. About one-third show contrast enhancement on CT scan or MRI, which often appears as multiple rings. It is noteworthy that neither peritumoural oedema, nor mass effect, is observed {1, 301, 303, 840, 1836}.

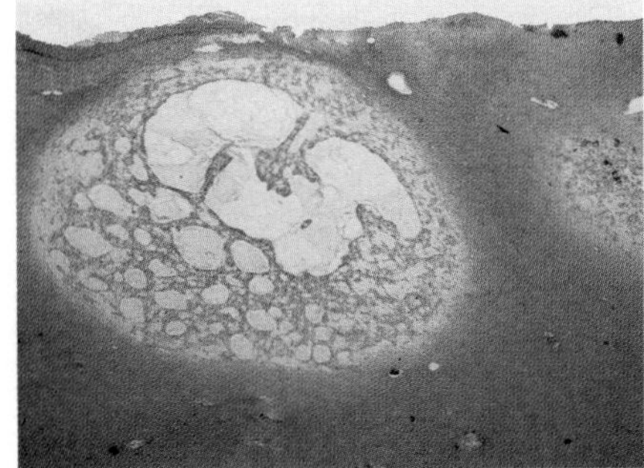

Fig. 6.11 Low-power micrograph of a cortical lesion showing the typical nodular structure of the complex form of DNT.

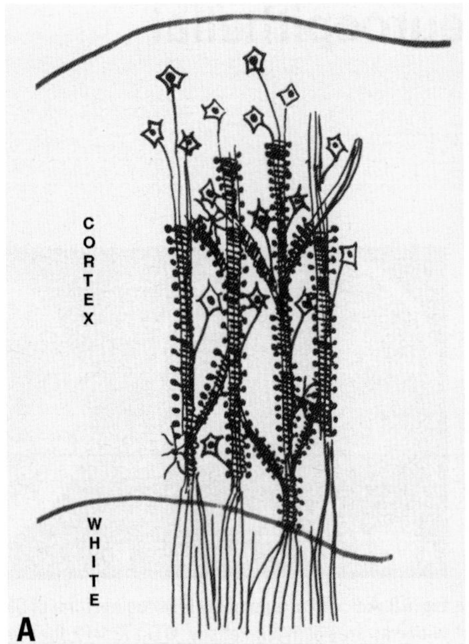

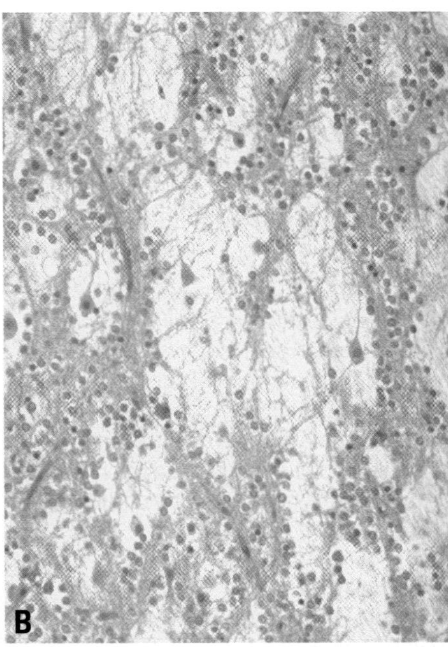

Fig. 6.12 Schematic drawing of the glioneuronal element: bundles of axons (black) are attached to oligodendroglia-like cells while neurons float in the interstitial fluid. Histology shows the glioneuronal elements in a columnar orientation. In this case, the oligodendroglia-like cells exhibit a 'fried egg' appearance. Drawing reproduced from Daumas-Duport *et al.* {301}.

Macroscopy

Appearance on macroscopy may reflect the complex histoarchitecture of the lesion. The most typical feature is the viscous consistency of the glioneuronal component. This may be associated with multiple firmer nodules. The affected cortex is often expanded and although the tumour is predominantly intracortical, the subcortical white matter may also be involved, particularly in temporal examples.

Histopathology

Histological hallmark of the classical DNT is the 'specific glioneuronal element', characterized by columns oriented perpendicularly to the cortical surface. They are formed by bundles of axons lined by small S-100-positive and GFAP-negative oligodendroglia-like cells. Between these columns, neurons with normal cytology appear to float in a pale, eosinophilic matrix. Associated with this element are scattered GFAP-positive stellate astrocytes. The complex form of DNT has a highly characteristic nodular structure.

Depending on the amount of fluid extravasation, subtle variation from a columnar to an alveolar or a more compact structure may be observed {301}. This constituent may easily be recognized when the samples are adequately oriented. As a result of their semi-liquid consistency and of fragmentation during fixation and embedding procedures, the typical architecture may be obscured. Also, microcystic areas in oligodendrogliomas may closely resemble the glioneuronal element.

Several histological forms of DNTs have been described but this subclassification has no clinical or therapeutic implication.

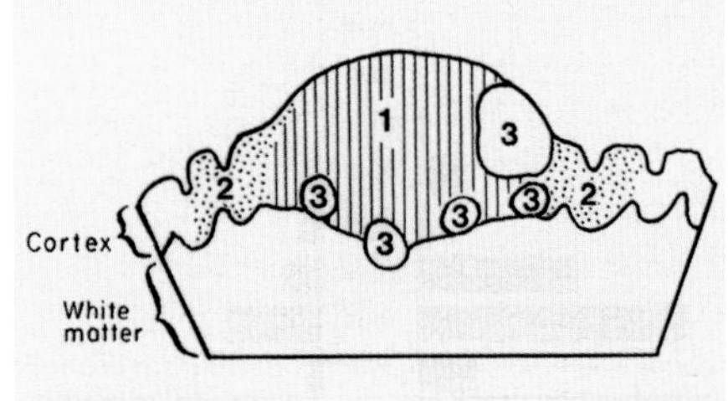

Fig. 6.13 Schematic representation of complex forms of DNTs. 1, Glioneuronal element; 2, cortical dysplasia; 3, glial nodules. Reproduced from Daumas-Duport *et al.* {305}.

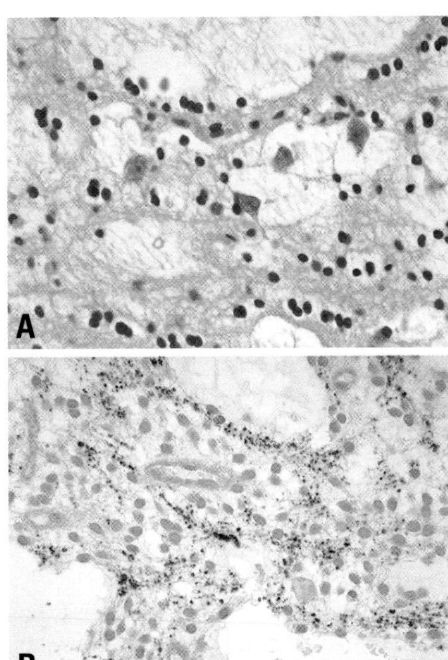

Fig. 6.14 **A** Specific glioneuronal element of DNT with floating neurons and (**B**) synaptophysin immunoreactivity of neuronal cell processes.

Simple form
In this morphological variant, the tumour consists of the unique glioneuronal element. It may show a patchy pattern {301}, owing to the juxtaposition of foci of tumour and of well-recognisable cortex.

Complex form
In this variant, glial nodules, which lend the tumour a characteristic multinodular architecture, are seen in association with the specific glioneuronal element and/or foci of cortical dysplasia. The heterogeneous appearance of these tumours is due to the presence of astrocytic, oligodendrocytic and neuronal components. These constituent cell populations may vary from case to case, and from area to area within the same tumour.
The glial components seen in the complex forms of DNTs have a highly variable appearance: (i) they may form typical nodules, but may also show a rather diffuse pattern; (ii) they may closely resemble conventional categories of gliomas or may show unusual features; (iii) they often mimic low-grade gliomas, but may show nuclear atypia, rare mitosis, necrosis or microvascular proliferation; (iv) their microvascular network may also vary from poor to exuberant, including glomerulus-like formations. In these vessels, the endothelial cells may be hyperplastic and mitotically active. Within the glial components, frankly hamartomatous, usually calcified vessels are not uncommon {301, 1236, 1836}. They may behave as vascular malformations and be responsible for haemorrhages.
On the basis of its similar clinical presentation, neuroradiological profile and failure to show growth on long-term follow-up by CT and MRI, a *'non-specific' variant of DNT* has been proposed. It lacks the glioneuronal component and multinodular architecture. However, since these lesions include tumours histologically indistinguishable from fibrillary or pilocytic astrocytomas, oligodendrogliomas or oligoastrocytomas, the concept of 'non-specific' variants of DNTs remains controversial {302, 303, 1836}.

Cortical dysplasia
Foci of cortical dysplasia are often observed when adequate sampling is available. In association with the tumour, the cortex may show disorganization of the histoarchitecture and loss of normal lamination {301, 303, 305, 1202, 1204, 1236, 1631, 1836}. Note that foci of cortical dysplasia are often difficult to distinguish from secondary changes caused by the growth of gliomas.

Neuronal populations of DNTs
Supratentorial cortical DNTs usually contain mature neurons. Both in the tumour itself and in the area of cortical dysplasia, the neurons may show various degrees of cytological anomalies. However, DNTs do not contain atypical neurons that resemble ganglion cells, such as those found in gangliogliomas. It is also noteworthy that lymphocytic cuffing, a common feature of gangliogliomas, is generally absent in DNTs {301, 303, 305, 1236, 1836}.
As might be expected, intralesional neurons and/or neuropil stain positively with a large panel of neuronal antibodies, including synaptophysin, neuronal nuclear antigen (NeuN), and N-methyl-D-aspartate receptor subunit NR1 {1838}.
Tumour cells with an oligodendrocytic appearance were also found to occasionally express synaptophysin and to exhibit axo-somatic synapses {593, 1837}. Occasionally, "oligodendroglia-like cells" (OLC) were also found to stain positively for NeuN and NR1 {1838}, suggesting that the so-called OLC of DNTs may show an early neuronal differentiation {593, 1838, 1837}. However, recent results with *in situ* hybridisation demonstrated that OLC transcribe myelin genes, indicating oligodendroglial differentiation {1839}. Thus, the origin of OLC remains controversial.
The presence of OLC {1837}, or of NeuN positive OLC {1838}, has been proposed as a diagnostic criterion for the distinction of DNTs from oligodendrogliomas. It is, however, noteworthy that the small granu-

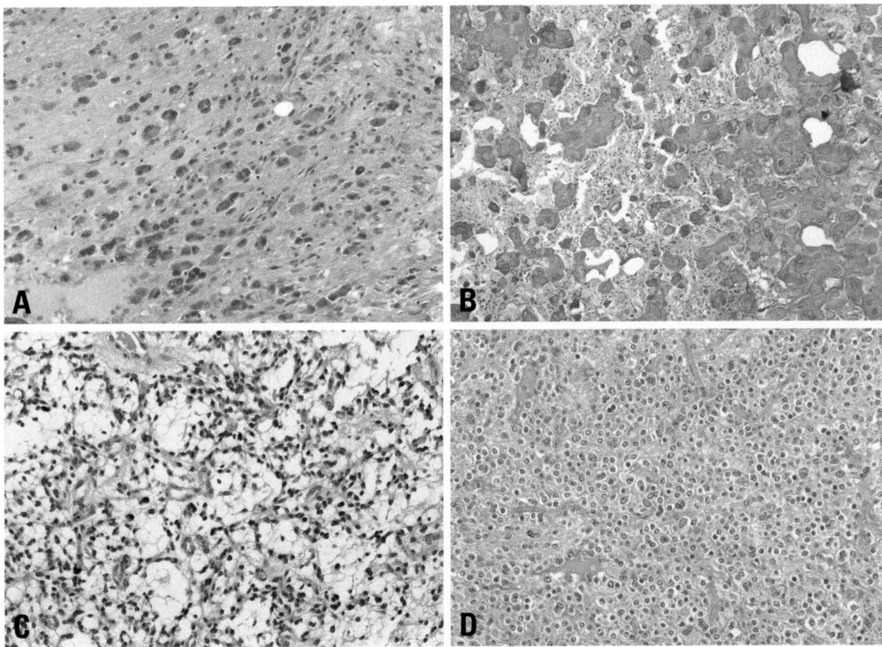

Fig. 6.15 Histological features observed in a complex form of dysembryoplastic neuroepithelial tumour. **A** Marked nuclear atypia, (**B**) calcification of hamartomatous-like vessels, and areas resembling (**C**) astrocytoma and (**D**) oligodendroglioma.

lar neurons of the cortex, or those found in an ectopic location, may easily be misinterpreted as OLC and that both DNTs and infiltrative oligodendrogliomas may contain such small neurons.

Cortical topography

Favourable anatomical orientation of specimens demonstrates that the limits of the lesion most often coincide strikingly with that of the cortex, whereas in other instances, the tumour seems also to involve the adjacent white matter. However, even in the deeper part of the tumour, neurons may usually be identified either within the tumour and/or in the adjacent white matter. In DNTs, neurons may thus be found in an ectopic situation similar to megagyri; it is likely that this reflects disordered neuronal migration {1631, 1836}.

Diagnostic criteria

As a definitive diagnosis may be difficult with limited material, it is important that the diagnosis of DNTs should be taken into consideration whenever all the following criteria are present: (i) partial seizures with or without secondary generalization, usually beginning before the age 20 years; (ii) no progressive neurological deficit; (iii) predominantly cortical topography of a supratentorial lesion, best demonstrated on MRI; and (iv) no mass effect on CT or MRI, except if related to a cyst, and no peritumoural oedema {302, 303, 1836}. The presence of these clinical and radiological features help in distinguishing DNT from other low-grade gliomas, particularly oligodendrogliomas.

Proliferation

These lesions generally have a very low proliferative potential although MIB-1 labeling indices of DNTs have been reported to vary from 0% to 8% {301, 303, 1202, 1489, 1836}.

Genetic susceptibility

It is now recognized that DNTs may occasionally occur in patients with neurofibromatosis type 1 {877}.

Histogenesis

Several factors strongly suggest that DNTs have a dysembryoplastic origin, including the presence of focal cortical dysplasia, the young age at the onset of symptoms, and bone deformity adjacent to the tumours {301, 303, 305, 1836}. The sites in which these tumours have thus far been observed are in accordance with a hypothesis suggesting that DNTs may be derived from the secondary germinal layers {305}. The question remains as to why these tumours behave as stable lesions. On the basis of experimental studies, Pierce {1172} has demonstrated the capacity of embryonic tissue to regulate or to induce maturation of its neoplastic counterpart. According to this theory, DNTs – which arise during embryogenesis – may be regulated by their normal embryonic environment. This hypothesis goes a long way towards explaining the benign biological behaviour of DNTs.

Predictive factors

DNTs are benign lesions. Their stability has been demonstrated in all cases for which successive pre-operative CT or MRI were available, including 52 patients with mean duration of follow-up of 4.5 years {302, 303, 1836}. Long-term clinical follow-up demonstrates neither clinical nor radiological evidence of recurrence, even in patients with partial surgical removal {301, 303, 305, 776, 1236, 1489, 1836}.

Central neurocytoma

D. Figarella-Branger
F. Söylemezoglu
P. Kleihues
J. Hassoun

Definition
A neoplasm composed of uniform round cells with neuronal differentiation, typically located in the lateral ventricles in the region of the foramen of Monro. It affects mostly young adults, and has a favourable prognosis.

ICD-O code:
The provisional code proposed for the third edition of ICD-O is 9606/1.

Grading
Central neurocytoma corresponds histologically to WHO grade II.

Synonyms and historical annotation
The term central neurocytoma was coined by Hassoun *et al.* {550} to describe a neuronal tumour occurring in young adults, located in supratentorial ventricles, and histologically mimicking an oligodendroglioma. These tumours were previously published as ependymomas of the foramen of Monro or intraventricular oligodendrogliomas. Given the benign course of the tumour, it should not be confused with primary cerebral neuroblastoma. Over the past ten years, various tumours mimicking central neurocytomas to some extent, but occurring outside the supratentorial ventricular system have been reported. To avoid any ambiguity, the term "central neurocytoma" should be restricted to neoplasms located within the lateral and third ventricles and the term extraventricular central neurocytoma given to other tumours. Some tumours diagnosed as cerebral neurocytomas {1083, 1215}, may represent dysembryoplastic neuroepithelial tumours (DNTs). Doubt remains concerning the nosology of cases reported as intramedullary and cauda equina neurocytomas {258, 1494, 2254}. In addition, extraventricular neoplasms with neurocytoma features have been reported {465, 1840}. All of these tumours contained "neurocytes", ganglion cells, and hyalinized vessels, occasionally associated with a benign astrocytic component. These tumours, including the cerebellar liponeurocytoma and the recently described 'papillary glioneuronal tumour' {1840} expand the morphological spectrum of neuronal and mixed neuronal/glial neoplasms.

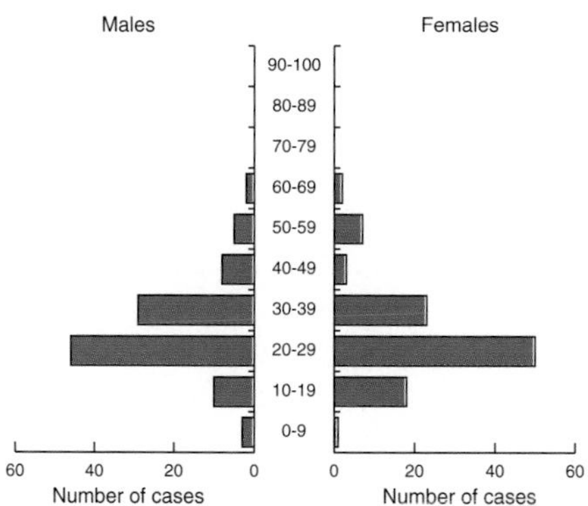

Fig. 6.16 Age and sex distribution of central neurocytoma, based on 207 published cases.

Incidence, age and sex distribution
Population-based incidence rates for central neurocytoma are not available. In large surgical series, incidence ranged from 0.25-0.5% {612, 551} of all intracranial tumours. In the 207 cases published to date (Fig. 6.16), the age at clinical manifestation ranged from 8 days to 67 years, (mean age, 29 years); 46% were diagnosed in the third decade of life, and 72% between the ages of 20 and 40 years. Both sexes are equally affected.

Localization
Central neurocytomas are typically located supratentorially in the lateral ventricle(s) and/or the third ventricle. The most common site is the anterior portion of one of the lateral ventricles (50%), with a preference for the left, followed by combined extension into the lateral and third ventricles (15%), and by a bilateral intraventricular location (13%). In only 3% of cases is the tumour restricted to the third ventricle.

Clinical features
Symptoms and signs
The majority of patients present with symptoms of increased intracranial pressure, rather than with a distinct neurological deficit. The clinical history is short (mean 3.2 months). Occasionally, visual and mental disturbances may be observed. Hormonal dysfunction may be associated with neurocytomas of the septum, third ventricle and hypothalamus {551}.

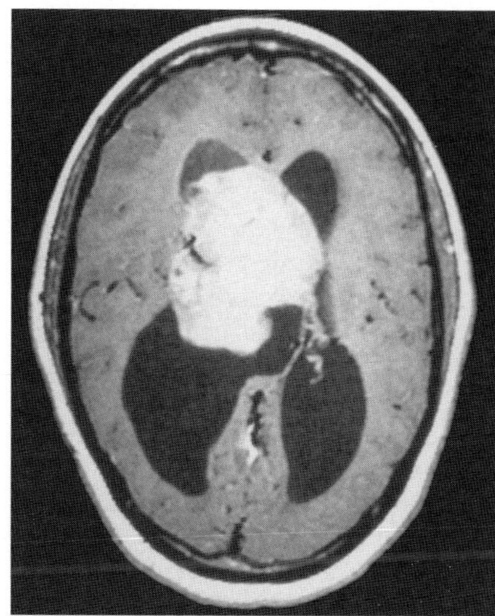

Fig. 6.17 MRI of a large, hyperintense central neurocytoma in the region of the foramen of Monro (gadolinium injection).

Neuroimaging
On CT scan, the mass is usually spontaneously isodense or slightly hyperdense. Enhancement is observed after administration of contrast medium. Calcifications and cystic changes may be seen.
MRI shows normal to high signal intensity on T1- and T2-weighted images and, in all cases, moderate-to-strong enhance-

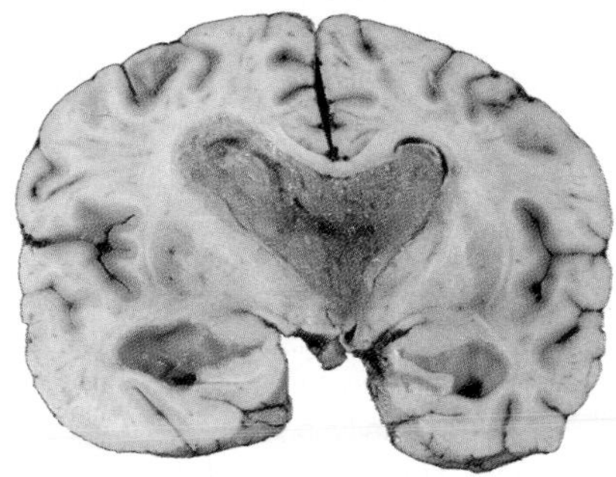

Fig. 6.18 Large central neurocytoma filling both lateral ventricles.

ment after gadolinum injection. Cerebral angiography demonstrates homogeneous vascular staining with a blush persisting into the late venous phase.

Macroscopy

These intraventricular tumours are usually greyish and friable, with varying calcifications and occasional haemorrhage.

Histopathology

A neuroepithelial tumour composed of uniform round cells that show immunohistochemical and ultrastructural features of neuronal differentiation. Additional features include fibrillary areas mimicking neuropil, and a low proliferation rate.

Central neurocytomas have a benign histological appearance. Various architectural patterns may be observed, even in the same specimen. They include an oligodendroglioma-like feature with honeycomb appearance, large fibrillary areas mimicking the irregular "rosettes" in pineocytomas, cells arranged in straight lines, or perivascular pseudorosettes as observed in ependymomas. Cells are isomorphous, having a round or oval nucleus with a finely speckled chromatin and an occasional nucleolus. Capillary-sized blood vessels, usually arranged in a linear arborizing pattern, give the tumours an endocrine appearance. Calcifications are seen in half the cases, usually distributed throughout the tumour. Rarer findings may include Homer-Wright rosettes and ganglioid cells {1264, 1560}. The main differential diagnoses include oligodendroglioma, ependymoma, pineocytoma and DNT.

In rare instances, anaplastic histological features including brisk mitotic activity {551, 1560, 1561} and microvascular proliferation have been observed {829, 1560, 1661}. In some cases, necrosis was associated with anaplastic features {1139, 1560, 1661}. Necrosis may also be observed in rare cases that are otherwise devoid of any malignant features, perhaps as an effect of blood vessel compression {407, 584, 829}.

Immunohistochemistry

Synaptophysin is the most suitable and reliable diagnostic marker. Typically, the immunostaining is diffusely observed in neuropil, especially in fibrillary zones and perivascular cell-free cuffs {407}. The use of antigen retrieval techniques and/or polyclonal anti-synaptophysin antibody may lead to strong intracytoplasmic labelling in central neurocytoma but also to false positive results in other tumours such as oligodendrogliomas. In case of extraventricular neoplasms, intracytoplasmic and paranuclear immunolabeling must be cautiously interpreted whenever other histological, immunohistochemical or ultrastructural evidence of neuronal differentiation is lacking. Moreover, in small biopsies, pre-existent neuropil or neuronal structures can complicate the interpretation of immunoreactivity {2263}. In rare instances, a lack of synaptophysin immunoreactivity is found. Other neuronal markers are expressed, including NSE, synapsin {1561}, neuron-associated class III beta-tubulin, tau, MAP2 and calcineurin {494, 584}. Of particular interest is the anti-Hu antibody because it labels the nuclei of "neurocytes" {2262}. The neuron-specific antigen L1 and the 180 kDa isoform of neural cell adhesion molecule were demonstrated in two cases by Western blot analysis {407}. Chromogranin A and neurofilaments are usually absent {551}, except when ganglion cells are present. With the exception of one series {1264}, HNK1 (Leu7) was invariably present. Although most reports find a lack of GFAP expression, GFAP has been detected by some authors in few cases {1441, 1520, 1560, 1561, 2260}.

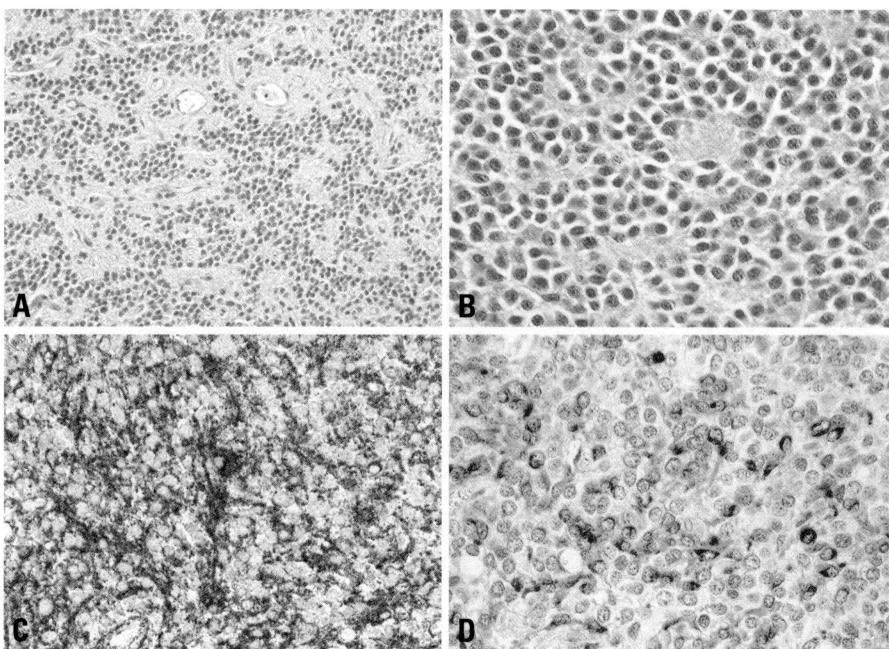

Fig. 6.19 Central neurocytoma. **A** Overview showing nucleus-free areas of neuropil. **B** High-magnification shows isomorphous tumour cells with small neuropil islands. **C** Tumour cells and their processes consistently express synaptophysin. **D** In about 10% of cases, a fraction of tumour cells shows immunoreactivity for GFAP.

Electron microscopy

Electron microscopy is required when

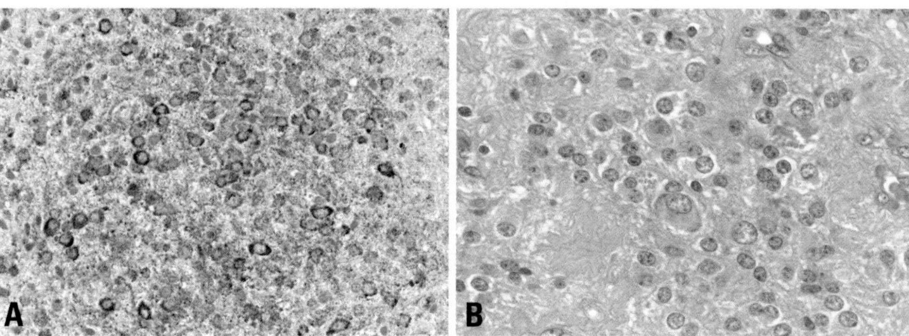

Fig. 6.20 In exceptional cases, neurocytomas display features of advanced neuronal differentiation with neurocytes and small ganglion cells ('ganglioneurocytoma'), associated with strong cytoplasmic expression of chromogranin.

synaptophysin expression is lacking or doubtful and in all extraventricular neoplasms mimicking central neurocytomas. Typically, central neurocytoma cells show regular round nuclei with a finely dispersed chromatin and a small distinct nucleolus in a few cells. The cytoplasm contains mitochondria, a prominent Golgi apparatus and some cisternae of rough endoplasmic reticulum often arranged in concentric lamellae. Numerous thin and intermingled cell processes with features typical of neurites, including microtubules, intermediate filaments and dense core and clear vesicles, are always observed {212, 551}. Furthermore, well-formed synapses may be observed, but are not required for the diagnosis.

Proliferation

Proliferation potential, as measured by Ki67 labelling {1264}, immunostaining for proliferating cell nuclear antigen (PCNA), or silver colloidal staining for nucleolar organizer regions (AgNOR-counts) usually show a low proliferative index {537, 769}. DNA flow cytometry, performed in ten cases revealed diploidy in all {769}. Recent studies using the MIB-1 antibody have revealed that tumours with a labelling index greater that 2% frequently showed vascular proliferation and had a significantly shorter recurrence-free interval {1441, 2255}.

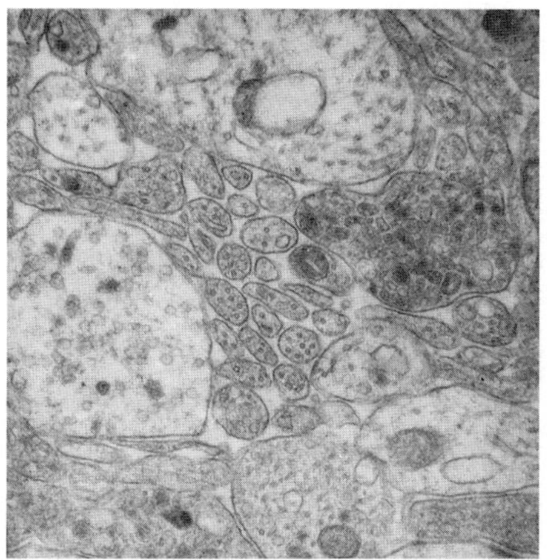

Fig. 6.21 Ultrastructure of a central neurocytoma showing numerous cell processes filled with neurotubules and synaptic bags containing dense core granules and clear vesicles.

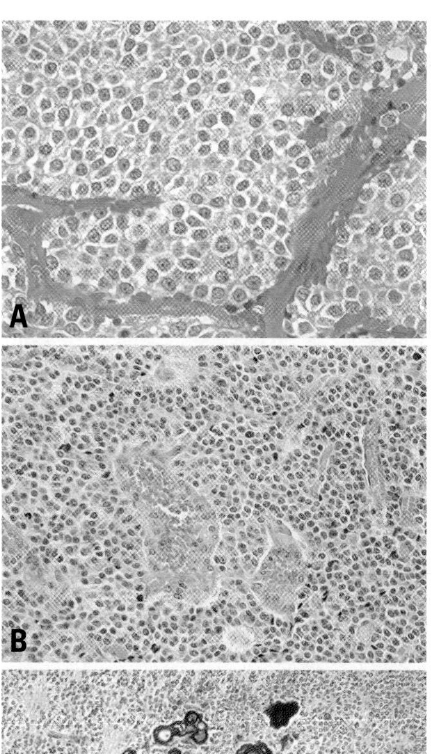

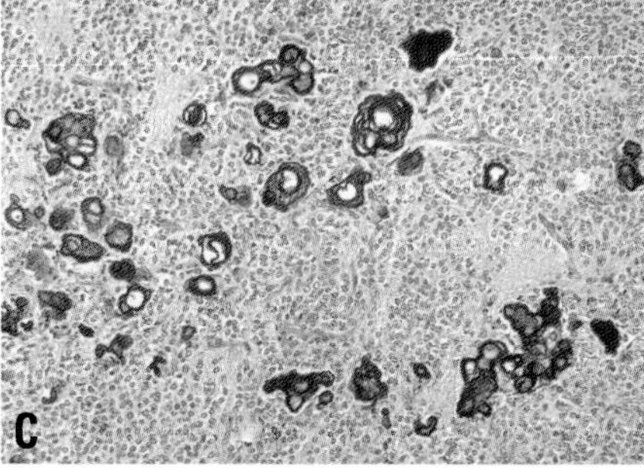

Fig. 6.22 Histopathological features observed in central neurocytoma. **A** Oligodendroglioma-like appearance of tumour cells. **B** Microvascular proliferation associated with mitotic activity. **C** Focal microcalcifications.

Genetic susceptibility

One case of central neurocytoma, although originally reported as intraventricular cerebral neuroblastoma, was associated with von Hippel-Lindau disease {1160}.

Molecular genetics

Gain on chromosome 7 was observed in three of nine neurocytomas {1492}. In two others, an isochromosome 17 and complex karyotype were reported {216, 2256}. *TP53* mutations and *MYCN* amplification were not detectable {1096, 1561, 2256}.

Histogenesis

Although important arguments favour the neuronal nature of the central neurocytoma, including evidence of expression of neuronal markers with immunohistochemistry or Western-blot analysis and the observation of synapses by electron microscopy, some reports demonstrate co-expression of GFAP and synaptophysin {1520, 1561}. In addition, two studies have shown that cultured human neurocytoma cells show characteristics of astroglial differentiation {1613, 2261} although others reveal only neuronal physiological properties and ultrastructural features {1142, 2257}. It remains a matter for debate whether central neurocytomas arise from cells committed to a neuronal phenotype {407}, or from bipotential progenitor cells in the periventricular matrix {1561}.

Clinical course and predictive factors

In accordance with its histopathological features, the clinical course of central neurocytoma is usually benign. Local recurrence may occur but craniospinal dissemination remains exceptional {375, 2258}. Involvement of periventricular parenchyma is associated in some cases with poor outcome {769, 1264}.

The treatment of choice is complete surgical excision. Subtotal excision is associated with shorter local control and shorter survival rate {2260}. The management of patients who underwent subtotal resection has not reached a consensus and three alternatives may be considered: post-operative radiotherapy, radiotherapy at the first sign of progression or re-operation only {2260, 2259}. It is worth of noting that histological findings alone cannot predict adverse outcomes {769, 375}. Moreover central neurocytomas showing aggressive histological features have been described in few patients {1560, 1561, 1661}. These features were not generally associated with poor prognosis. Central neurocytomas with a MIB-1 labelling index (LI) >2% have a significantly shorter recurrence-free interval than others {1441, 2255}. Interestingly, 5 out of 8 central neurocytomas showing GFAP immunostaining in tumour cells had high MIB-1 LI and poor outcome {1441, 375}.

Cerebellar liponeurocytoma

P. Kleihues
L. Chimelli
F. Giangaspero

Definition

A rare cerebellar neoplasm of adults with advanced neuronal / neurocytic and focal lipomatous differentiation, a low proliferative potential, and a favourable clinical prognosis.

Grading

Histological features and the available data on postoperative survival suggest that this tumour corresponds to WHO grade I or WHO grade II.

ICD-O code:

The provisional code proposed for the third edition of ICD-O is 9506/1.

Synonyms and historical annotation

In 1978, Bechtel et al. reported a case of lipomatous medulloblastoma in a 44-year-old man {79}. Subsequently, 15 more cases were reported {169, 232, 309, 372, 467, 1442, 2086, 2087, 2088, 2335, 2404}. Clinical, morphological and immunohistochemical data strongly suggest that the cerebellar liponeurocytoma constitutes a rare but distinct clinico-pathological entity {169, 1442}. The terms neurocytoma / lipoma (neurolipocytoma) {372}, medullocytoma {466, 467}, lipomatous glioneurocytoma {2404}, and lipidized mature neuroectodermal tumour of the cerebellum {2335} have been proposed, so as to emphasize its similarity to central neurocytoma and the prognostic difference from the ordinary medulloblastoma. In accordance with this, the WHO working group proposes the term 'cerebellar liponeurocytoma' since the label medulloblastoma may lead to unnecessary aggressive adjuvant therapy.

Age and gender distribution

Patients typically present during their fifth or sixth decade of life; their age ranged from 36 to 67 years (mean age, 51 years). This is in sharp contrast with the age distribution of medulloblastomas, more than 70% of which occur in children {632}. Medulloblastomas that do occur in adults usually manifest before the age of 40 {202, 632}. Similarly, the age distribution differs from that of central neurocytoma, which occurs in younger age. In the small cohort of 15 patients reported to date there was no significant gender predilection {1442}.

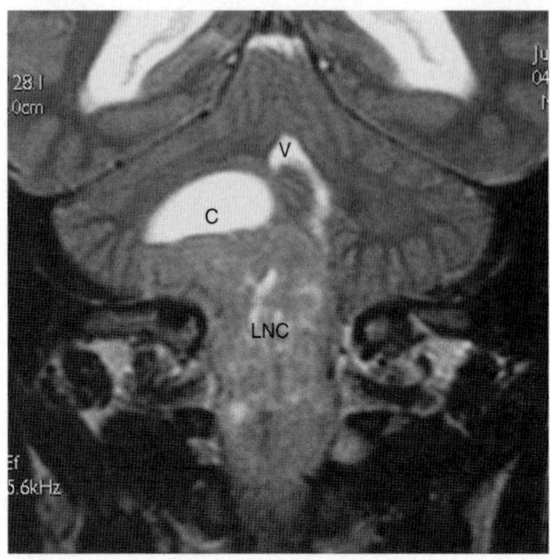

Fig. 6.23 T2 weighted MRI of a cerebellar liponeurocytoma (LNC) with an adjacent cyst (C) and compression of the fourth ventricle (V).

Clinical features

Patients develop typical symptoms of a posterior fossa tumour. The lipomatous component may cause a bright signal in pre-contrast T1-weighted MRI {467, 1207}.

Localization

All 15 tumours reported arose in the cerebellum, 8 from the cerebellar hemispheres, 6 from the vermis; two cases presented as an exophytic mass in the cerebellopontine angle.

Histopathology

An isomorphic round cell neoplasm with consistent neuronal and focal lipomatous differentiation and a low rate of proliferation.

Despite the cellularity of the lesion, tumour cells have a uniform cytological appearance, with few mitotic figures. They contain round or oval nuclei and often show a clear cytoplasm resembling neoplastic oligodendrocytes. Except for the focal accumulation of lipidized tumour cells,

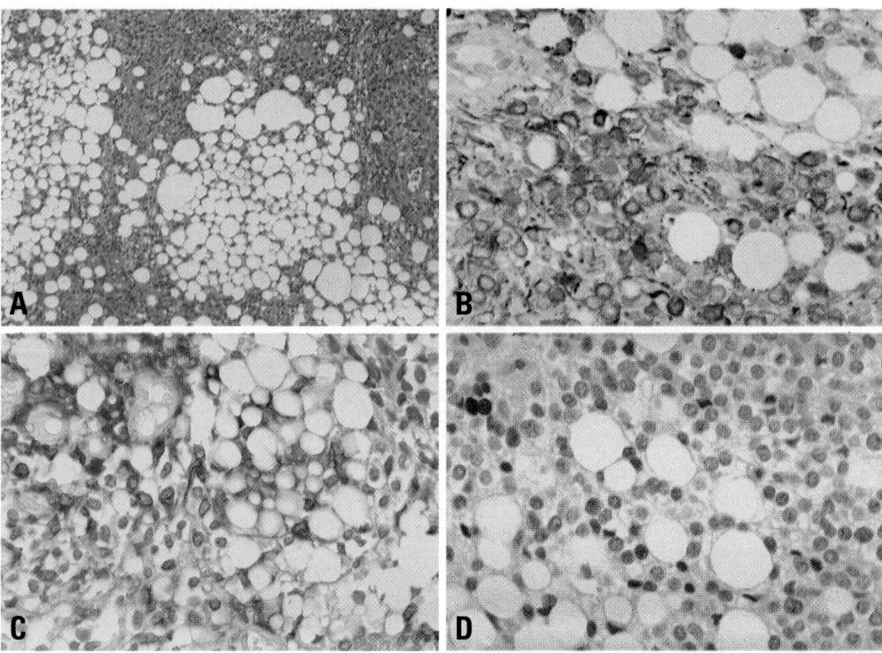

Fig. 6.24 Cerebellar liponeurocytoma. **A** Accumulation of adipocytes on the background of a small round-cell tumour. Small tumour cells and adipocytes focally express the (**B**) neuronal marker MAP-2 and (**C**) GFAP. **D** Low MIB-1 labeling index reflecting the slow growth of liponeurocytomas.

there is no distinctive tissue pattern. Xanthomatous histiocytes, as occasionally observed in ordinary medulloblastomas, are not considered as evidence of lipomatous differentiation. Necrosis and microvascular proliferation are typically absent in primary lesions but may be found in recurrences. Advanced neuronal differentiation is a histopathological hallmark. Accordingly, the majority of reported cases were diagnosed as neurocytoma or neuroblastoma rather than medulloblastoma. Immunohistochemically, there is a consistent expression of NSE, synaptophysin and MAP-2. Electron microscopy shows dense-core and clear vesicles, microtubule-containing neurites and rare synapse-like structures. Focal GFAP expression by tumour cells, indicating astrocytic differentiation, is observed in the majority of cases {1442}. One tumour also showed immunoreactivity to desmin and morphologic features suggesting incipient myogenic differentiation.

Proliferation

The mitotic activity of these tumours is low. The growth fraction, as determined by the Ki-67/MIB-1 labelling index, ranges from <1% to 6%, with a mean value of approximately 2.5 {372, 1442}.

Histogenesis

Immunoreactivity to neuronal antigens and GFAP includes cell bodies embracing fat globules. This suggests that the fat-containing cells result from lipomatous differentiation of tumour cells, rather than being an admixture of non-neoplastic, *e.g.* hamartomatous {168}, adipocytes. It remains to be shown whether this lesion is histogenetically related to the cerebellar medulloblastoma {169, 232, 309}. Lipomatous differentiation has occasionally been observed in neuroectodermal tumours outside the cerebellum {1415, 2497}. Recently, a case of cerebellar neurocytoma/rhabdomyoma (myoneurocytoma) has been reported {2543].

Predictive factors

The low proliferative activity is paralleled by a favourable clinical outcome. Most patients with sufficient follow-up survived more than 5 years, largely irrespective of whether or not adjuvant radiotherapy was applied. The longest known survival is 18 years in a patient whose treatment was confined to surgical excision {467}.

Paraganglioma

D. Soffer
B.W. Scheithauer

Definition

A unique neuroendocrine neoplasm, usually encapsulated and benign, arising in specialized neural crest cells associated with segmental or collateral autonomic ganglia (paraganglia) throughout the body. In the CNS, paragangliomas are almost exclusively located in the cauda equina. They consist of uniform cells with neuronal differentiation forming compact nests (zellballen), surrounded by sustentacular cells and a delicate capillary network.

ICD-O code: 8680/1

Grading

Filum terminale paragangliomas correspond histologically to WHO grade I.

Synonyms and historical annotation

The terminology surrounding paragangliomas is confusing. Early authors divided them into chromaffin and non-chromaffin on the basis of their reaction with chromic acid. However, as the chromaffin reaction does not reliably reflect their functional activity, current terminology is based upon anatomic site, *e.g.*, carotid body paraganglioma (chemodectoma), jugulotympanic paraganglioma (glomus jugulare tumour), etc. Usually, descriptor of functional status is also appended, *i.e.* "functional" or "non-functional" {379}.

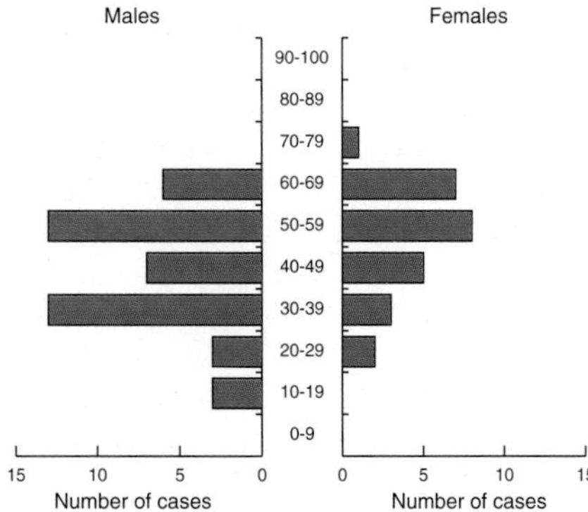

Fig. 6.25 Age and sex distribution of paragangliomas of the cauda equina, based on 71 published cases.

Incidence and location

Paragangliomas of the CNS are uncommon. Most present as spinal intradural tumours in the cauda equina region {179}. The first description of a cauda equina paraganglioma in 1970 {1005} was soon followed by additional case reports {614, 880, 1436}. In 1986, Sonneland *et al.* {1438} reported their study of 56 examples, including 31 Mayo Clinic cases. To date, approximately 120 cases have been reported. Other spinal levels are far less often affected {130, 143, 271, 1847}. Some spinal paragangliomas represent intradural extensions of mediastinal or retroperitoneal tumours {295}.

Intracranial paragangliomas are usually extensions of jugulotympanic paraganglioma. Rare examples of purely intracranial paragangliomas have also been described. These include tumours of the sellar region {1336, 1845, 1843, 1844} which may be associated with von Hippel-Lindau disease {1336}, and of the cerebellopontine angle {677} and pineal region {1433}.

Age and sex distribution

Cauda equina paragangliomas generally occur in adults, the reported age range being 13 to 71 years. In Sonneland's series, the mean age was 47 years, with a predominance in males (M:F 1.4:1) {1438}. Incorporation of an additional 29 non-selected cases from the literature yields similar results (Fig. 6.25). Jugulotympanic paragangliomas show a strong female predilection {379, 849}, their peak incidence being in the fifth decade {379}.

Clinical features

Symptoms and signs

Cauda equina paragangliomas exhibit no distinctive clinical features. They typically present with lower back pain of days or even years duration. Accompanying radicular pain (sciatica) is common. Sensorimotor deficits, include paraplegia and sphincter disturbances, are also frequent. Only two endocrinologically functional tumours have been reported {143, 1511}. Rare thoracic tumours, as well as spinal axis-invasive mediastinal paragangliomas, present with spinal cord compression {143, 271, 295}.

About 40% of glomus jugulare paragangliomas extend into the cranial cavity {379}. These cause not only progressive hearing loss and a sensation of otic fullness or pounding, but multiple cranial nerve palsies (glomus jugulare syndrome) as well. Signs of catecholamine secretion include hypertension, palpitation, and sweating. Intraoperative hypertensive crises may result from tumour manipulation {379}.

Neuroimaging

Radiographically, cauda equina paragangliomas lack specific features {1611}. Most appear as isodense, homogeneously enhancing masses on computed tomography. Magnetic resonance imaging shows them to be hypo- or isointense to spinal cord parenchyma on T1-weighted images, markedly contrast enhancing, and hyperintense on T2-weighted images (Fig. 6.26).

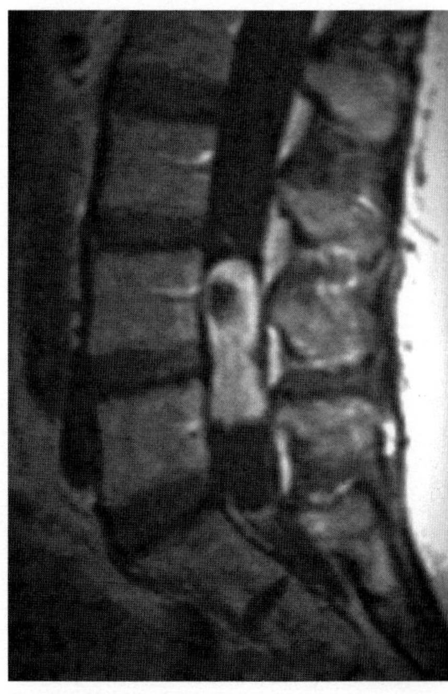

Fig. 6.26 MRI of a paraganglioma of the cauda equina with a cystic component.

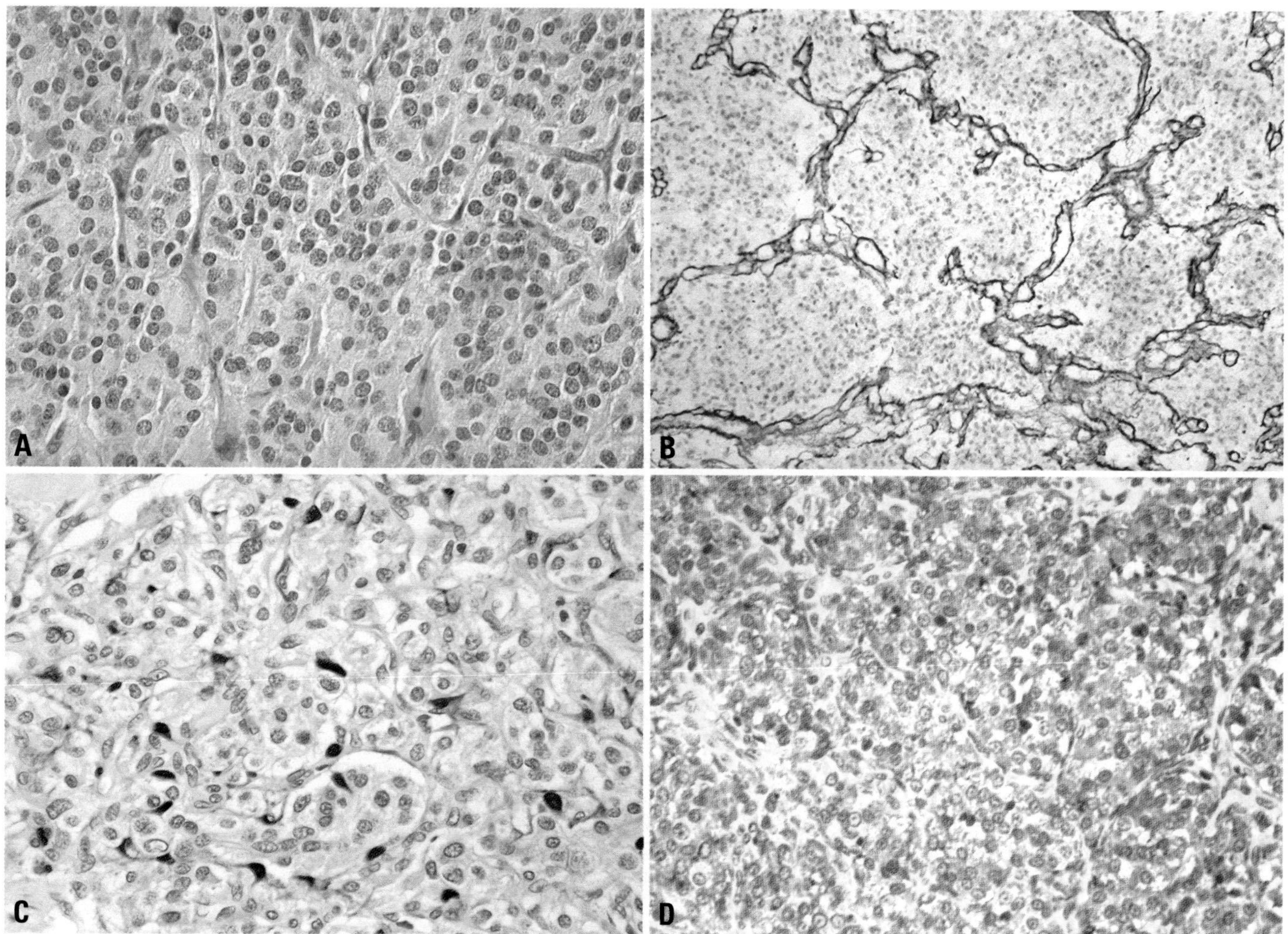

Fig. 6.27 Paraganglioma. **A** Typical zellballen architecture. **B** Reticulin stain showing the septae delineating zellballen. **C** Sustenticular cells identified by immunoreacivity to S-100. **D** Diffuse staining of tumour cells with synaptophysin.

Plain X-rays are usually non-informative, but may show erosion (scalloping) of vertebral laminae due to chronic bone compression.

Macroscopy

Most paragangliomas of the cauda equina are entirely intradural and are attached either to the filum terminale or less often to a caudal nerve root. They are typically oval to sausage-shaped, delicately encapsulated, soft, red-brown tumours measuring from 1.5 to 13 cm. Cystic components may be found within the neoplasm. An occasional tumour penetrates dura to invade bone.

Histopathology

A well differentiated tumour resembling normal paraganglia, composed of chief (type I) cells disposed in nests or lobules (zellballen), surrounded by an inconspicuous, single layer of sustentacular (type II) cells.

The zellballen are surrounded by a delicate capillary network that may undergo sclerosis. The uniform round or polygonal chief cells possess central, round-to-oval nuclei with finely stippled chromatin and inconspicuous nucleoli. Degenerative nuclear pleomorphism ("endocrine anaplasia") is generally mild. Cytoplasm varies somewhat in quantity and is usually eosinophilic and finely granular. In some instances it is amphophilic or even clear. Sustentacular cells are spindle shaped. Encompassing the lobules, their long processes are often so attenuated as to be undetectable by routine light microscopy and visible only on immunostains for S-100 protein (Fig. 6.27). Nearly half of cauda equina paragangliomas contain mature ganglion cells, as well as cells transitional between chief and ganglion cells {179, 379}. Such "gangliocytic paragangliomas" are also found in the duodenum and are analogous to pheochromocytoma with neuronal differentiation.

Some paragangliomas of the cauda equina region show architectural features reminiscent of carcinoid tumours, including angiomatous, adenomatous and pseudorosette patterns {1438}. Tumours composed predominantly of spindle cells {1847}, melanin-containing cells (melanotic paragangliomas) {1847}, and granular eosinophilic cells (oncocytes) {1847, 1846} have also been described. Foci of haemorrhagic necrosis may occur and scattered mitotic figures can be seen. Neither these features nor nuclear pleomorphism are of clinical significance {1438}.

Immunohistochemistry

Markers permit the identification of both chief and sustentacular cells. Neuron-specific enolase (NSE), although a sensitive marker of chief cells lacks specificity, but synaptophysin and chromogranin {787, 1438} are sensitive and reliable. Chromogranin A reactivity parallels the Grimelius (argyrophil) reaction {179}. Neurofilament proteins are also useful markers of chief cells. Expression of serotonin (5H-T) and of various neuropeptides (somatostatin, leu- and metenkephalin) has been demonstrated in paraganglioma of the cauda equina region {1438, 1847}. Paranuclear cytokeratin immunoreactivity is particularly prominent in cauda equina examples {1850}. Sustentacular cells are uniformly reactive for S-100 protein and usually show staining for glial fibrillary acidic protein (GFAP) as well. It is of note that chief cells may also show variable S-100 protein labelling.

Electron microscopy

The distinctive ultrastructural feature of chief cells is the presence of dense core (neurosecretory) granules measuring 100 to 400 nm (mean, 140 nm) {381} (Fig. 6.28). Depending on their cytoplasmic electron density, "light" and "dark" chief cells are recognized. Both feature interdigitation of cell processes and rudimentary junctions. A layer of basal lamina is present at the interface of zellballen and surrounding stroma. In addition to well-developed Golgi, extensive smooth endoplasmic reticulum and lysosomes, chief cells may contain numerous atypical mitochondria as well as paranuclear whorls of intermediate filaments {381, 1438}. Sustentacular cells are characterized by an elongated nucleus with marginal chromatin, increased cytoplasmic electron density, relative abundance of intermediate filaments, and lack of dense core granules {381, 1438}.

Genetic susceptibility

Systemic paragangliomas may be multifocal but to date there has been no reported association of cauda equina or other spinal examples with paraganglioma at other sites. The concurrence of spinal paraganglioma with brain tumours {189, 271}, spinal epidural haemangioma {1611}, syringomyelia {1848} and intramedullary cysts {1849} is of note, but these associations may be coincidental. There are no reports of familial cauda equina paragangliomas and virtually nothing is known of their cyto- or molecular genetics.

Tumours of the carotid body may show familial clustering. The observed inheritance pattern is autosomal dominant with genomic imprinting; tumours arise only after paternal transmission {1851}. Analysis has established genetic linkage to two distinct chromosomal loci, thus suggesting heterogeneity. One locus, perhaps the most common, is in the region of 11q22.3-q23; the other is in the 11q13.1 region {1851, 1853}. Recently, the putative PGL1 gene on chromosome band 11q23 has been localized to an approximately 1.5 Mb region between D11S1986 and D11S1347 {1852}. Complete loss of heterozygosity (LOH) at the 11q11-q23 region was found in microdissected chief cells of two carotid body paragangliomas with unknown family history, thus lending support to the view that the chief cells are a major if not the sole neoplastic component of paragangliomas {1851}. Also using microdissection techniques, another study of sporadic extra-adrenal paragangliomas revealed LOH at chromosomal region 3p21 in 2 of 4 informative tumours {1854}. LOH at this locus had been reported in 40% of pheochromocytomas, thus suggesting that this particular locus contains a gene common to both pheochromocytoma and extra-adrenal paraganglioma {1854}. Although both extra-adrenal paragangliomas and pheochromocytomas are paraganglionic tumours, the findings of Vargas et al {1854} suggest that different molecular mechanisms are involved. LOH at chromosome 1p was found in 45% of informative pheochromocytomas and on chromosome 3p25, the von Hippel-Lindau (VHL) gene locus, but no such losses were detected in paragangliomas.

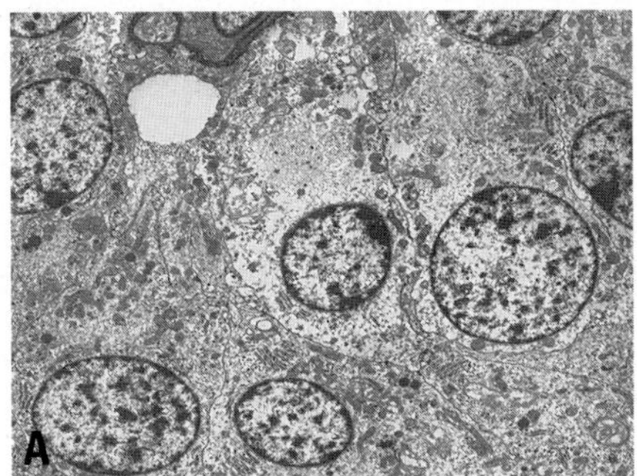

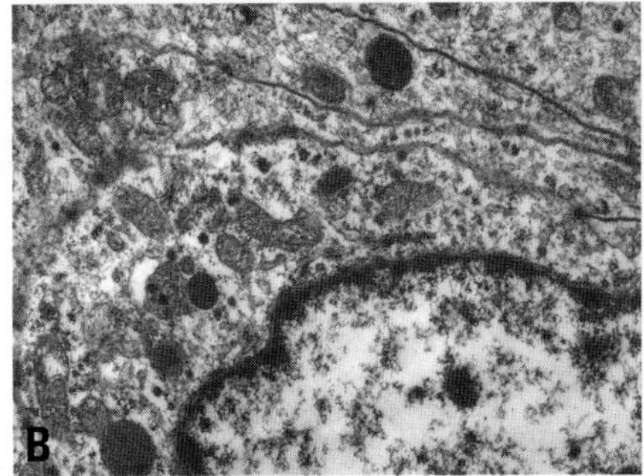

Fig. 6.28 A Electron microscopy of a paraganglioma. The cell in the upper center shows paranuclear filamentous whorls. **B** Detail of a paragangioloma cell showing perinuclear dense core vesicles.

Other familial settings in which paragangliomas occur include multiple endocrine neoplasia (MEN) types 2A and 2B {849}, as well as von Hippel-Lindau syndrome {1336}.

Histogenesis

The histogenesis of cauda equina paraganglioma is a matter of debate. Some authors favour an origin from paraganglion cells associated with regional autonomic nerves and blood vessels {901}, despite the fact that such cells have not been identified at this site {1306}. Others have suggested that peripheral neuroblasts normally present in the adult filum terminale undergo paraganglionic differentiation {189, 1306}. Jugulotympanic paragangliomas presumably arise from microscopic paraganglia within temporal bone {849}.

Prognostic factors

Tumour location is often more relevant than histology in assessing the prognosis of paraganglioma patients {788}. For example, the metastatic rate of para-aortic paraganglioma is high (28 to 42%), whereas that of carotid body tumours is only 2 to 9% {788}. Nearly half of the glomus jugulare tumours recur locally {850} and 5% metastasize {849}.

The vast majority of cauda equina paragangliomas are slow-growing tumours potentially cured by total excision. Nonetheless, based on long-term follow-up, it is estimated that 4% will recur after a gross total removal {1465}. CSF seeding has been documented in occasional spinal paragangliomas {130, 271, 1267, 1465}. Metastasis outside the CNS (bone) has been reported only once {1847}.

Although it is not possible to predict the biological behaviour of cauda equina paraganglioma on the basis of histologic criteria alone, it has been shown that truly anaplastic and metastasizing extraneural paragangliomas are either devoid or markedly depleted of sustentacular cells {787, 788}. It remains to be seen whether these observations are applicable to paragangliomas affecting the central nervous system.

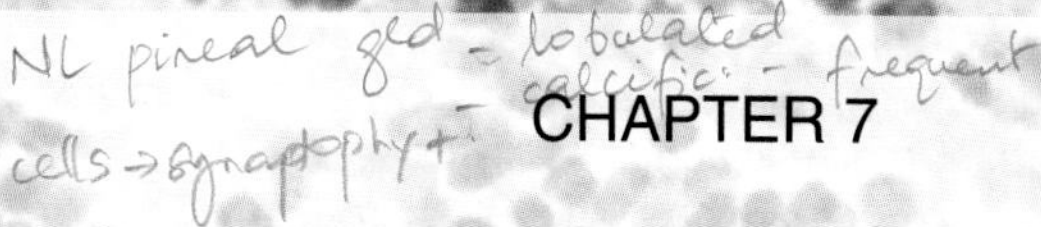

CHAPTER 7

Pineal Parenchymal Tumours

The histogenesis of pineal parenchymal tumours is linked to the pineocyte, a cell with photosensory and neuroendocrine functions. Neoplasms derived from pineocytes or their embryonal precursors span a wide spectrum ranging from tumours composed of mature elements to ones consisting of primitive, immature cells. Between these extremes are tumours demonstrating an intermediate degree of differentiation or, rarely, tumours that are histologically biphasic with fully differentiated as well as poorly differentiated cells. The extent of differentiation is paralleled by differences in biological behaviour and clinical outcome. The following entities are distinguished:

Pineoblastoma

This malignant, embryonal neoplasm is poorly differentiated and has many features in common with the medulloblastoma and related primitive neuroectodermal tumours. Metastasis via cerebrospinal fluid pathways constitutes a frequent complication and is often associated with fatal outcome.

Pineocytoma

This slowly growing tumour may show a wide range of divergent phenotypes, including neuronal, glial, melanocytic, photoreceptor and mesenchymal differentiation. It carries, in most cases, a relatively favourable prognosis.

Pineal parenchymal tumour of intermediate differentiation

This group of neoplasms comprises pineal parenchymal tumours with intermediate differentiation and usually unpredictable growth rate and clinical behaviour.

Other neoplasms located in the pineal gland region but not originating from pineocytes or their precursors include astrocytomas, in particular pilocytic astrocytomas (see Chapter 1), and germ cell tumours (see Chapter 13).

Pineoblastoma

H. Mena
Y. Nakazato
A. Jouvet
B.W. Scheithauer

Definition

A highly malignant, primitive embryonal tumour of the pineal gland with preferential manifestation in children, composed of patternless sheets of densely packed small cells with round-to-irregular nuclei and scant cytoplasm.

ICD-O code: 9362/3

Grading

Pineoblastomas correspond histologically to WHO grade IV.

Incidence, age and sex distribution

Pineoblastomas are rare intracranial tumors that constitute approximately 45% of all pineal parenchymal tumours. They can arise at any age, but usually occur in the first two decades of life with a predilection for children {223, 582, 604, 992, 1361}. There is a slight male preponderance (Fig. 7.1).

Clinical features

Symptoms and signs

The clinical presentation of pineoblastoma is similar to that of other tumours of the pineal region (see pineocytoma). The interval between initial symptoms and surgery may be as short as one month or less {148, 223, 671}. Median post-surgical survivals vary from 24 to 30 months {223, 582, 992}.

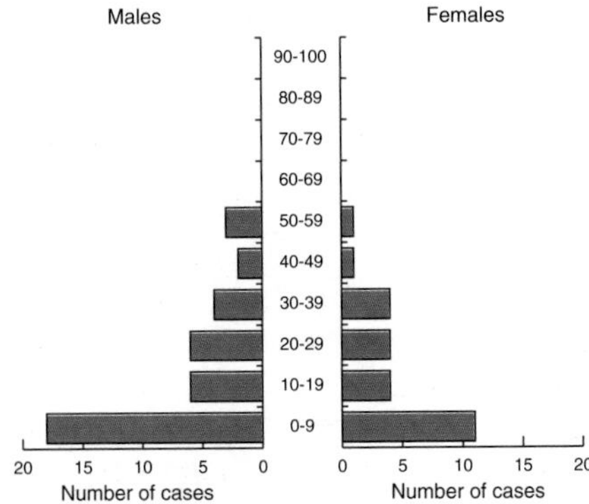

Fig. 7.1 Age and sex distribution of pineoblastoma, based on 64 published cases.

Neuroimaging

In contrast to pineocytoma, the CT appearance of pineoblastoma is that of a large, lobulated or poorly demarcated, homogeneous mass, which is hyperdense after contrast enhancement. Calcification is infrequent. On T1-weighted MRI scan, pineoblastomas are hypo-to-isointense, but are heterogeneous upon contrast administration {231, 356}.

Macroscopy

Pineoblastomas are soft, friable and poorly demarcated {148}. Haemorrhage and/or necrosis may be present, but calcification is rare. Infiltration of surrounding structures, including the meninges is common. The same is true of craniospinal dissemination {148, 223, 326, 356, 582, 604, 671, 992, 1546}.

Histopathology

Constituting the most primitive of pineal parenchymal tumours, pineoblastomas are composed of patternless sheets of densely packed small cells with round-to-irregular nuclei and scant cytoplasm. Pineocytomatous rosettes are lacking, but Homer-Wright and Flexner-Wintersteiner rosettes may be seen.

Pineoblastomas are highly cellular neoplasms resembling other small cell, embryonal and primitive neuroectodermal tumours of the CNS. Primitive in appearance, the cells have a high nuclear cytoplasmic ratio, round-to-irregular, hyperchromatic nuclei with occasional, small, single nucleoli, scant cytoplasm, and indistinct cell borders. The cells are arranged in a diffuse pattern, interrupted only by the occasional formation of Homer-Wright or Flexner-Wintersteiner rosettes. The latter indicating retinoblastic differentiation as do fleurettes. Rarely a papillary pattern may be seen. Necrosis is common, but mitotic activity varies considerably, and may be accompanied by microcalcifications. Silver stains for pineal parenchymal cells demonstrate scant cytoplasm and few cellular processes {1881}. Melanin production, cartilaginous and rhabdomyoblastic differentiation may be present in rare pineoblastomas, such tumors are referred as pineal anlage tumors {582, 1089, 976}. Occasionally, pineoblastomas

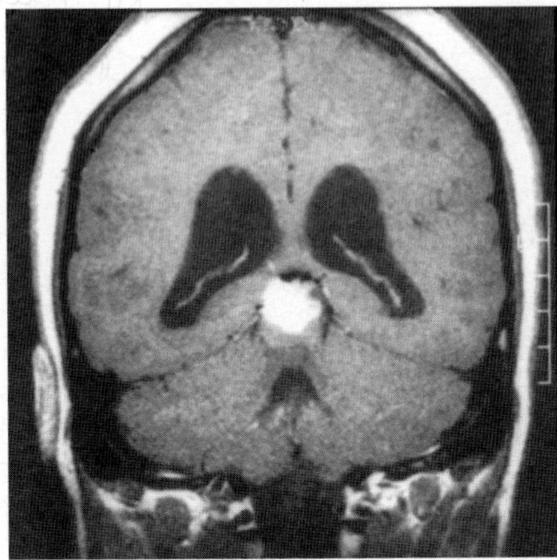

Fig. 7.2 On T1-weighted MRI, pineoblastoma shows homogeneous contrast enhancement.

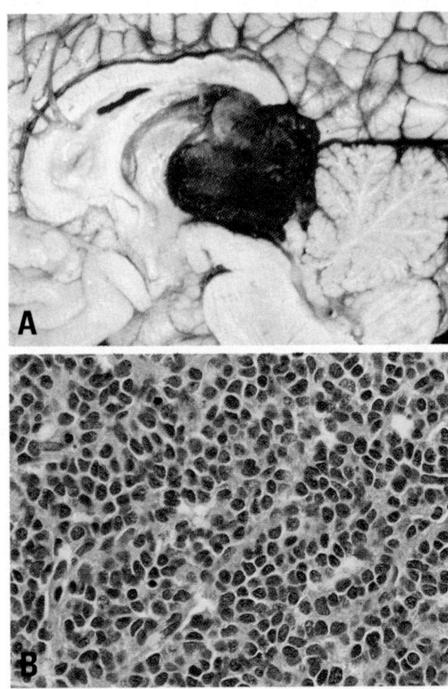

Fig. 7.3 A Large, haemorrhagic pineoblastoma **B** Highly cellular pineoblastoma showing undifferentiated small cell histology.

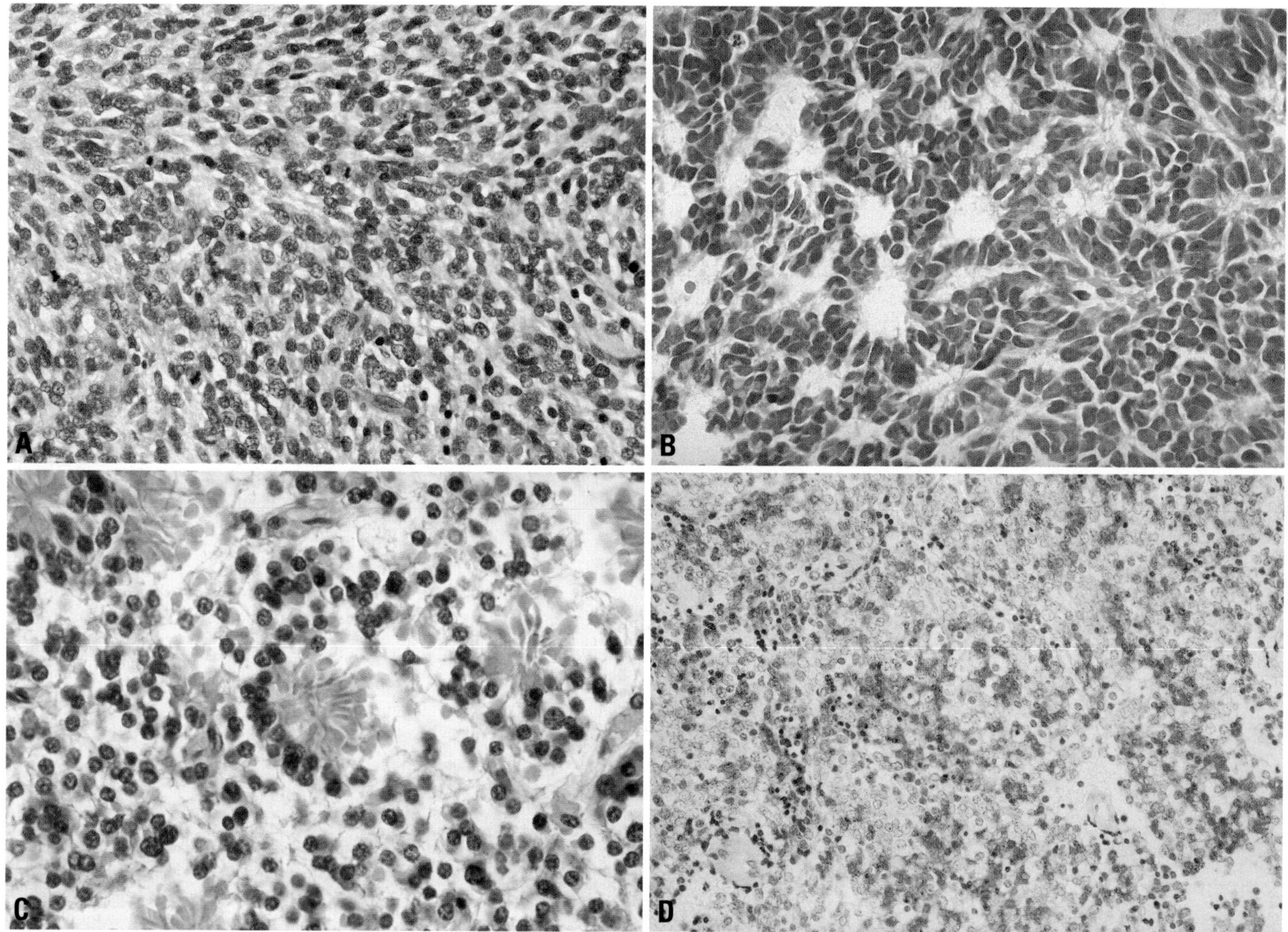

Fig. 7.4 Histopathological features of pineoblastoma. **A** High cellularity with numerous mitotic figures. **B** Homer-Wright and Flexner-Wintersteiner rosettes. **C** Fleurettes. **D** Focal expression of retinal S-antigen.

may exhibit a biphasic pattern, with alternating areas resembling pineocytoma and pineoblastoma.

Immunohistochemistry

The immunophenotype of pineoblastomas in terms of neuronal, glial and photoreceptor markers is similar to that of pineocytomas. Reactivity is variable, but include positivity for synaptophysin, NSE, NFP, class III beta-tubulin, chromogranin A, and retinal S- antigen {992, 1089, 1167}. Reactivity for beta-crystallin, GFAP and desmin has been reported on rare occasions; in such instances, every effort should be made to exclude the presence of entrapped reactive astrocytes.

Electron microscopy

Characterized by a relative lack of significant differentiation, the fine structure of pineoblastoma is similar to that of any poorly differentiated neuroectodermal neoplasm. Cells have round-to-oval, or slightly irregular nuclei and abundant euchromatin as well as heterochromatin. Cytoplasm is scant and contains polyribosomes, few profiles of rough endoplasmic reticulum, small mitochondria, as well as occasional microtubules, intermediate filaments, and lysosomes {965, 1013, 1089}. Dense core granules are rarely seen in the cell body {965, 1013}. Cell processes, poorly formed and short, may contain microtubules as well as scant dense core granules {965}. Bulbous endings are not identified {1013}. Junctional complexes of zonula adherens and zonula occludens type may be present between cells and processes {717, 965, 1013, 1089}. Synapses are absent {1089}. Cilia with a 9+0 microtubular pattern are occasionally seen {965}. Rarely, cells radially arranged around a small central lumen may be encountered {1089}.

Genetic susceptibility

Primitive neuroepithelial tumours of the pineal region having a pineoblastomatous appearance may be seen in patients with familial (bilateral) retinoblastoma, an occurrence termed "trilateral retinoblastoma syndrome" {319, 928} and have also been reported in a patient with familial adenomatous polyposis {1884}.

Genetics

Few studies deal with the cytogenetic aberrations of pineoblastoma. Chromosomal analysis of cultured cells from a pineoblastoma showed an interstitial deletion of the long arm of chromosome 11, del(11)(q13.1q13.5) {1888}. In vitro, the pineoblastoma cell line PER-480 showed evidence of neuronal differentiation and two karyotype abnormalities, a der XXX (10)t (10;17) and a der XXX (16) t (1;16), as well as enhanced expression but not amplification of a member of the MYC family of proto-oncogenes. {1885}. In one study of four pineoblastomas and pineocytomas, no *TP53* gene mutations were found {1522}.

Histogenesis

Pineal parenchymal tumours share morphologic and immunohistochemical features with cells of the developing human pineal gland and retina (see histogenesis of pineocytoma). Evidence for this ontogenic concept include the finding of interphotoreceptor retinoid-binding protein and its mRNA in a mixed pineocytoma/pineoblastoma, and the occasional development of bilateral retinoblastoma and pineoblastoma (trilateral retinoblastoma) {319, 911, 928, 1879}.

Prognosis and predictive factors

With the exception of pineocytomas, pineal parenchymal tumours are potentially aggressive, as is demonstrated by the occurrence of craniospinal seeding and, rarely, of extracranial metastases {582, 1119, 1170, 1361}. Extent of disease at the time of diagnosis, as determined by CSF examination and MRI of the spine, directly affects the survival of patients with pineoblastoma {223}. The prognosis for patients with sporadic and familial trilateral retinoblastoma is dismal, with less than one year survival after diagnosis {319, 1886}. Metastasis of the pineal tumour to the CNS and vertebral column is the most common cause of death {1886}. Occasionally, the pineal tumour remains asymptomatic and is discovered on routine imaging studies; in such instances, the outcome is better {1886, 319}. Projected 1-, 3-, and 5-year survival rates of pineoblastoma patients treated by various modalities are 88%, 78% and 58%, respectively {1361}.

Pineocytoma

H. Mena
Y. Nakazato
A. Jouvet
B.W. Scheithauer

Definition

A slow-growing pineal parenchymal neoplasm with predominant manifestation in young adults, composed of small, uniform, mature cells resembling pineocytes with occasional large pineocytomatous rosettes.

ICD-O code: 9361/1

Grading

Pineocytomas correspond histologically to WHO grade II.

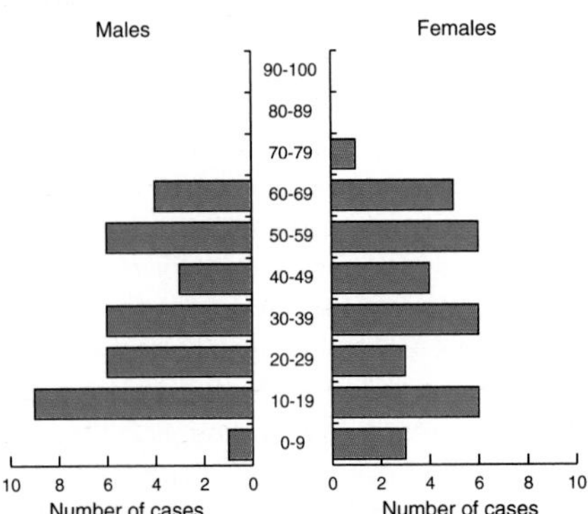

Fig. 7.5 Age and sex distribution of pineocytoma, based on 69 published cases.

Incidence, age and sex distribution

Pineal region tumours account for less than 1% of all intracranial neoplasms. Approximately 14–30% are of pineal parenchymal origin {1546}. Of these, pineocytomas represent approximately 45%. Pineocytomas occur throughout life, but most frequently affect adults 25-35 years of age {582, 992, 1237, 1361}. There is no sex predilection (Fig. 7.5).

Localization

Pineocytomas typically remain localized to the pineal area and they compress adjacent structures, including the cerebral aqueduct, brain stem and cerebellum. Extended growth into the third ventricle may be seen.

Clinical features

Symptoms and signs

Clinically, it is not possible to differentiate pineocytoma from other pineal region lesions. The clinical signs and symptoms vary, and relate to increased intracranial pressure, neuro-ophthalmologic dysfunction, changes in mental status, dysfunction of the brain stem, and/or cerebellum, and hypothalamic-based endocrine abnormalities {148, 340, 344, 604, 1361, 1880}. The majority of patients exhibit neuro-ophthalmologic findings, particularly Parinaud syndrome {344, 604, 1883}. In rare cases, a patient may present with intramural haemorrhage ("pineal apoplexy") {604, 1456}.

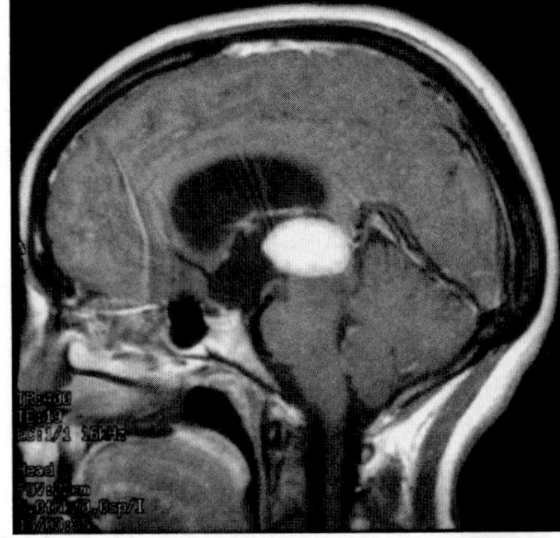

Fig. 7.6 Pineocytoma showing rounded contours and homogeneous enhancement on a T1-weighted MRI.

Neuroimaging

On CT scans, pineocytomas are usually round, demarcated masses, measuring less than 3 cm in diameter. They appear hypodense and homogeneous, but some feature peripheral calcification or occasional cystic changes {231, 1361}. Most tumours show heterogeneous contrast enhancement. Accompanying hydrocephalus is a common feature. On magnetic resonance imaging (MRI), the tumours tend to be hypointense on T1 and hyperintense on T2-weighted images {231}.

Macroscopy

Pineocytomas are well-circumscribed lesions with a grey-tan, homogeneous or granular cut surface {148, 582}. Degenerative changes, including cysts and small areas of haemorrhage, may be present {992, 1026, 1545}. Necrosis has been reported, but in most reported instances, this is a reflection of misdiagnosis. If necrosis does occur in pineocytoma, it is likely to be due to large tumour size and vascular compromise.

Histopathology

A well-differentiated neoplasm composed of small, uniform, mature cells resembling pineocytes. It grows primarily in sheets, but also features large pineocytomatous rosettes composed of abundant, delicate tumour cell processes.

Pineocytomas are tumours of moderate cell density exhibiting a sheet-like or an ill-defined lobular growth pattern. The latter differs from the defined lobules that characterise normal pineal parenchyma. The cells are uniform and rather small in size, with round-to-oval nuclei, inconspicuous nucleoli, finely dispersed chromatin, and moderate quantities of homogeneous eosinophilic cytoplasm. The short cytoplasmic processes of pineocytoma cells often end in club-shaped expansions that are optimally demonstrated on histochemical and silver impregnation stains, including the Bielschowsky or Bodian methods and the Achucarro or DeGirolami and Swalezne methods for pineal parenchymal cells.

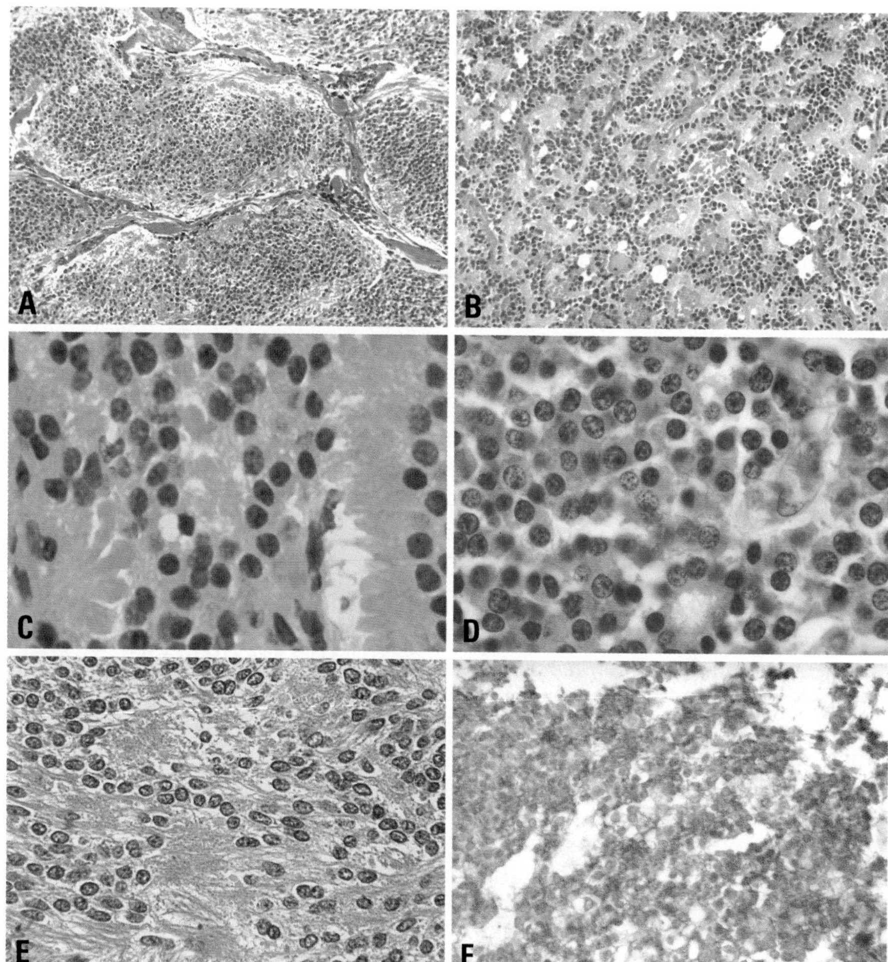

Fig. 7.8 Histopathological features typical of pineocytoma. **A** Lobular pattern with groups of tumour cells separated by mesenchymal septae. **B** Large, partly confluent rosettes. **C** High magnification shows tumour cells with irregular hyperchromatic nuclei and prominent processes with bulbous extensions. **D** Tumour cells with finely granular chromatin. Note the small rosette with clearing of the central area. **E** Pineocytomatous rosettes with nucleus-free spaces filled with a fine meshwork of cell processes. **F** Diffuse staining with synaptophysin.

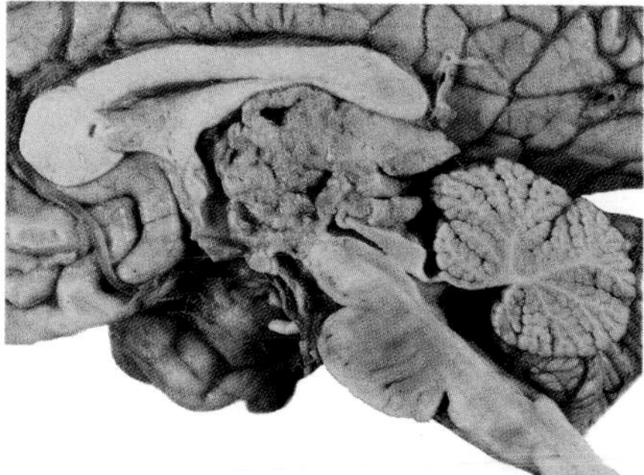

Fig. 7.7 Large pineocytoma extending into the third ventricle.

Pineocytomatous rosettes, a characteristic feature of this variant of pineal parenchymal tumour, vary in number and size, their centres being composed of delicate, enmeshed cytoplasmic processes {148}. Nuclei surrounding the periphery of the rosette are not regimented. The tumour stroma consists of a delicate network of vascular channels lined by a single layer of endothelial cells and supported by scant reticulin fibres. Other features include virtual lack of mitoses, occasional multinucleated tumour giant cells with bizarre nuclei, and layered microcalcifications. Necrosis is only occasionally seen; when present, it usually accompanies other degenerative changes and lacks peripheral nuclear palisading.

Morphologically recognizable neuronal or ganglionic differentiation occurs rarely {148, 582, 992, 1361}; such cells may be bi- or multinucleated. Identification of glial or photoreceptor elements requires the use of immunohistochemistry and/or electron microscopy; reactive astrocytes must be excluded. A *papillary variant* of pineal parenchymal tumour with aggressive clinical behaviour has been reported but is still poorly characterized{1515, 1545}.

Immunohistochemistry

Pineocytoma cells usually show strong immunoreactivity for synaptophysin and NSE. Also reported is variable staining for other neuronal markers, including NFP, class III beta-tubulin, tau protein, PGP 9.5 as well as for chromogranin and the neuropeptide serotonin {259, 647, 717, 831,

1089}. Photosensory differentiation is associated with immunoreactivity for retinal S-antigen and rhodopsin {647, 992, 1089, 1167}. In culture, pineocytoma cells are capable of synthesizing serotonin and melatonin {1882}. Astrocytic differentiation, suggested by immunoreactivity of tumour cells for GFAP, is not generally agreed upon {259, 582, 992}.

Electron microscopy

Pineocytoma cells are characterized by moderate size, oval nuclei with smooth nuclear envelopes, and moderate amounts of heterochromatin. Their cytoplasm is abundant and contains well-developed organelles, including smooth and rough endoplasmic reticulum, Golgi zones, mitochondria and lysosomes {1013}. Membrane-bound, electron-dense granules and clear vesicles are present in both cytoplasm and cellular processes {717}. Small junctional complexes join plasma membranes. Nuclear-free areas are occupied by abundant cytoplasmic processes containing microtubules and ending in club-like expansions rich in clear vesicles {582, 1013}. Such processes may show synapse-like junctions and synaptic ribbons. When present, ganglion cells contain abundant rough endoplasmic reticulum and numerous neurosecretory granules {1013}. Retinoblastic differentiation may be indicated by the presence of cytoplasmic annulate lamellae, intercellular lumen formation, cilia with a 9+0 microtubule configuration, and synaptic ribbons {582, 717, 1013}. The occasional finding of cells with processes containing intermediate filaments suggests astrocytic differentiation, but this is difficult to confirm at the ultrastructural level.

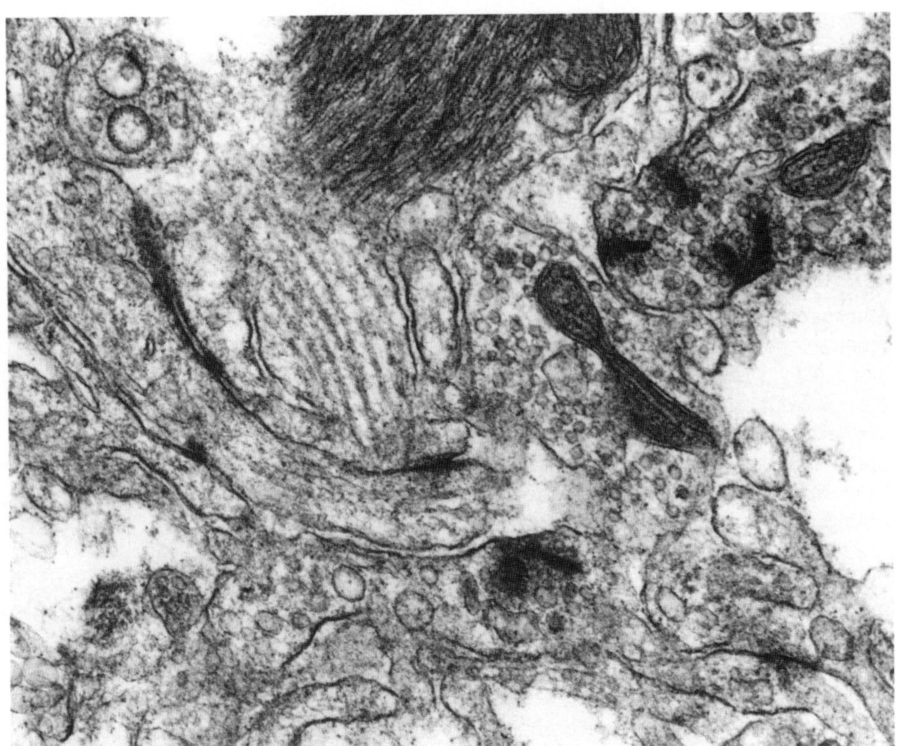

Fig. 7.9 Electron micrograph of pineocytoma. Terminal cell processes show synaptic vessicles and rods.

Genetics

Cytogenetic studies of two pineocytomas have been reported. In one tumour, numerical alterations were present in chromosomes X, 5, 8, 11,14 and 22, together with structural changes in chromosomes 1, 3, 12 and 22. In the other case, numerical alterations were noted on chromosomes Y, 10, 18, 21 and 22 and structural alterations in chromosomes 2, 6, 11 and 12. It is possible that monosomy or loss of chromosome 22, deletions in the distal 12q region, and partial deletion or loss of chromosome 11 are related to tumour progression {84, 1221}.

Histogenesis

The histogenesis of pineal parenchymal tumours is linked to the pineocyte, a cell with photosensory and neuroendocrine functions. The ontogeny of the human pineal gland recapitulates the phylogeny of the retina and the pineal organ {1014}. During late stages of intrauterine life and the early post-natal period, the human pineal gland consists primarily of cells arranged in rosettes similar to those of the developing retina. These feature abundant melanin pigment as well as cilia with a 9+0 microtubular pattern. By the age of three months, the number of pigmented cells gradually decreases, so that pigment becomes undetectable by histochemical methods {1014}. As differentiation progresses, cells strongly immunoreactive for NSE accumulate. By age one year, pineocytes predominate. To a variable extent, pineal parenchymal tumours mimic the developmental stages of the human pineal gland.

Prognosis and predictive factors

The clinical course of pineocytomas is characterised by an interval of four years between the onset of symptoms and surgery {148}. Cases with cerebrospinal seeding or remote metastases have been reported but probably represent examples of inadequately sampled or misclassified tumours {298, 582, 652}. In a recently reported series of strictly defined tumour, no pineocytomas metastasized, the 5 year patient survival rate was 86% {1887}. The prognosis of patients with pineocytomas with divergent differentiation including glial, neuronal and retinoblastic elements appears to be similar to that of pineocytomas without such elements {992, 1293}.

Pineal parenchymal tumour of intermediate differentiation

Pineal parenchymal tumours with intermediate differentiation (provisional ICD-O code 9362/3) are monomorphous tumours characterized by moderately high cellularity, mild nuclear atypia, occasional mitosis, and the absence of large pineocytomatous rosettes {1361}. Such neoplasms constitute approximately 10% of all pineal parenchymal tumours. They occur at all ages, from young children to adults, with a peak incidence in adulthood {717, 992, 1361}. The clinical behaviour of these tumours is variable, as reflected in a review of 28 published cases {165, 340, 363, 604, 717, 992, 1089, 1237, 1361}. Survival for longer than four years has been observed in a group of 7 patients with pineal parenchymal tumours with intermediate differentiation who underwent gross total excision at the same institution {717}. Only occasional pineal parenchymal tumours with intermediate differentiation are associated with central nervous system or extraneural metastases {1361}. In one example, photosensory differentiation has been demonstrated by the detection of interphotoreceptor retinoid-binding protein and its mRNA {911}.

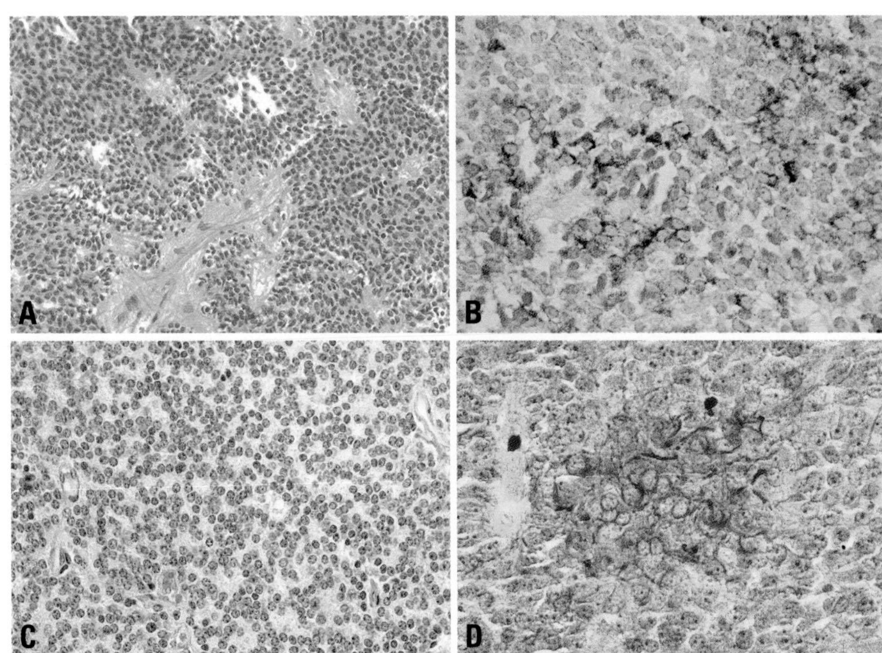

Fig. 7.10 A Highly cellular pineal parenchymal tumour of intermediate differentiation. Note the absence of rosettes and the tendency to form nucleus-free perivascular spaces. **B** Moderate cellularity, nuclear pleomorphism, and formation of small rosettes. **C** Focal chromogranin staining of a pineal parenchymal tumour of intermediate differentiation. **D** Fine tumour cell processes visualised by pineal silver carbonate staining.

CHAPTER 8

Embryonal Tumours

Embryonal tumours constitute a large and important fraction of paediatric brain tumours. Considerable progress has been made in their diagnosis and treatment but their origin and histopathological classification remain, to some extent, controversial. The following histologically identifiable entities all develop on the backgound of an undifferentiated round-cell tumour but show a variety of divergent patterns of differentiation. It has been proposed that they be merged under the term primitive neuroectodermal tumours:

Ependymoblastoma

Medulloblastoma

Supratentorial PNETs

Two other entities should be kept separate as they have a distinctly different histology and also appear to evolve by different genetic pathways:

Medulloepithelioma

Atypical teratoid/rhabdoid tumour

Medulloepithelioma

L.E. Becker
M.C. Sharma
L.B. Rorke

Definition

A rare, malignant embryonal brain tumour affecting young children, histologically characterized by papillary, tubular or trabecular arrangements of neoplastic neuroepithelium mimicking the embryonic neural tube.

ICD-O code: 9501/3

Grading

Medulloepitheliomas are highly malignant and correspond histologically to WHO grade IV.

Age and sex distribution

Medulloepitheliomas are rare tumours that typically affect children between 6 months and 5 years. Congenital tumours have been described. No gender preference is apparent.

Localization

Medulloepitheliomas develop in both the supra- and infratentorial compartments {1024}. The most common site is periventricular, within the cerebral hemispheres, involved in order of frequency are temporal, parietal, occipital and frontal lobes. They have been described in the cauda equina, presacral area {2496}, outside the central nervous system along nerve trunks (sciatic) {1056, 2495}, and in the eye. The medulloepitheliomas of the eye characteristically occur intraorbitally but may also involve the optic nerve {1929}.

Clinical features

The tumour is often large at the time of clinical presentation with symptoms of increased intracranial pressure such as headaches, nausea and vomiting. All patients have had abnormal neurological examination at clinical presentation. CT and MR imaging characteristics have been variable. At initial presentation, these tumours have been described as well circumscribed and isodense to minimally hypodense on CT and non-enhancing with intravenous contrast {1024}. On T_1 weighted MR imaging, medulloepitheliomas have been either hypointense or isointense. Gadolinium enhancement appears with tumour progression. Cysts and calcifications have been reported.

Macroscopy

Medulloepitheliomas are often massive and well circumscribed with areas of haemorrhage and necrosis. Occasionally, there is infiltration of the subarachnoid space at the initial presentation while diffuse dissemination is frequent at the time of death.

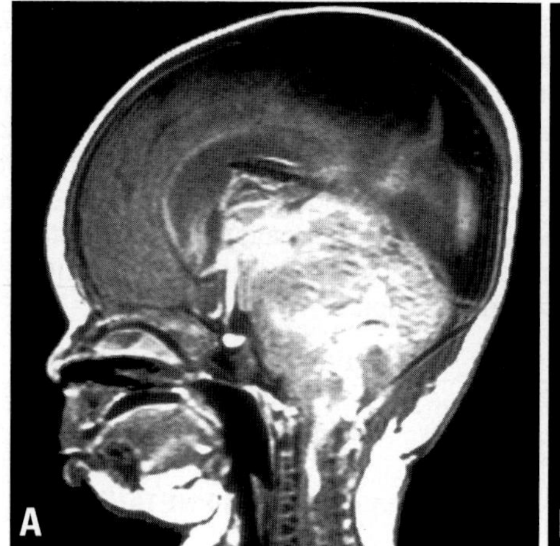

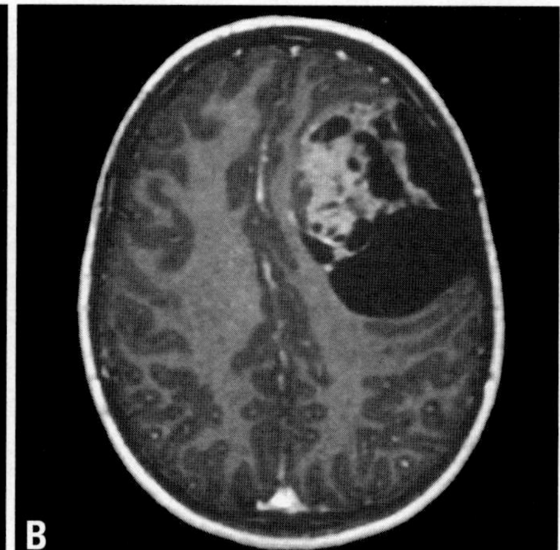

Fig. 8.1 **A** MRI of a large medulloepithelioma occupying the posterior fossa. **B** T1 weighted gadolinium enhanced MRI of a cystic medulloepithelioma in the frontal lobe.

Histopathology

A malignant neoplasm that mimics the embryonic neural tube, characterized by papillary, tubular or trabecular arrangements of neoplastic neuroepithelium with an external limiting membrane. Medulloepitheliomas often display multiple lines of differentiation, including neural, glial and mesenchymal elements.

The diagnostic feature of medulloepithelioma is the distinctive pseudostratified epithelium arranged in papillary and tubular patterns that resembles the structure of the primitive neural tube {729}. On the luminal (inner) marginal surface of the tubules there are no cilia or blepharoblasts but there may be discrete protruding blebs. On the outer surface of the epithelium is an external limiting membrane which stains with PAS and is immunopositive with antiserum to collagen type IV. This basement membrane rests on a delicate network of reticulin. The cells have a columnar to cuboidal shape. The nuclei are oval to piloid and are perpendicular to the inner and outer surfaces and are characterized by coarse chromatin and multiple nucleoli. Mitotic figures are abundant and tend to be located near the luminal surface similar to the early stages of neural tube development.

In areas distinct from the neuroepithelium there are sheets of tumour cells with hyperchromatic nuclei and a high nuclear to cytoplasmic ratio. These cells may show a range of differentiation; neuronal, astrocytic, ependymoblastic or oligodendroglial {48, 323}. There is also a spectrum in the degree of differentiation from embryonic early differentiated cells to mature neurons and astrocytes. In medulloepitheliomas, ependymoblastomatous rosettes are more common than ependymal rosettes, but both may occur. Areas of oligodendroglial differentiation are suggested by round regular nuclei and white halos and negative immunocytochemistry with antiserum to synaptophysin. A primitive neuroectodermal tumour with tubules containing melanin pigment has been described as a pigmented medulloepithelioma {1930}. Rare tumours may manifest development along mesenchymal lines that range from a prominent vascular and fibrous connective tissue stroma to areas of cartilage, bone and striated muscle {48, 188}.

Immunohistochemistry

The medulloepitheliomatous components show extensive nestin immunoreactivity which appears confined to the basal area of the epithelium leaving the luminal surface non-reactive or slightly immunoreactive {1932, 1504}. These cells also display an ·immunoreactivity to vimentin and to microtubule associated protein type 5, similar to the immunoreactivity of cells of the primitive neural tube. Neurofilament, cytokeratin and epithelial membrane antigen have been focally described in isolated cases {188, 1932, 1517}. These neuroepitheliomatous areas do not exhibit GFAP, neuron specific enolase or S-100 protein immunoreactivity. Antisera to basic fibroblast growth factor and insulin-like growth factor I (IGF-I) have been shown to be immunoreactive in medulloepithelioma {1411}.

In areas away from the neuroepithelium, the immunoreactivity reflects the cell lineage. Antisera to neuron specific enolase (NSE), synaptophysin, neurofilament and microtubule associated proteins reveal an increasing degree of positivity commensurate with the degree of differentiation {188}. Astrocytic differentiation spans the spectrum, from densely cellular areas and high mitotic activity with variable *GFAP* expression to areas of mature differentiation, of low to moderate cellularity with consistently strong immunoreactivity to GFAP.

Proliferation

Medulloepitheliomas have a high rate of proliferation. The epithelium is also mitotically active, with mitotic figures tending to be located near the luminal surface.

Electron microscopy

Ultrastructural examination of the neuroepitheliomatous areas reveals extensive primitive lateral cell junctions (zonulae adherentes) and a basal lamina on the outer surface of the epithelial cells, consisting of a distinct, continuous, often folded, basement membrane {1194, 1517}. On the luminal side, there is an amorphous surface coating but no true membrane. Cells appear poorly differentiated with sparse cytoplasmic organelles and absence of cilia or microvilli.

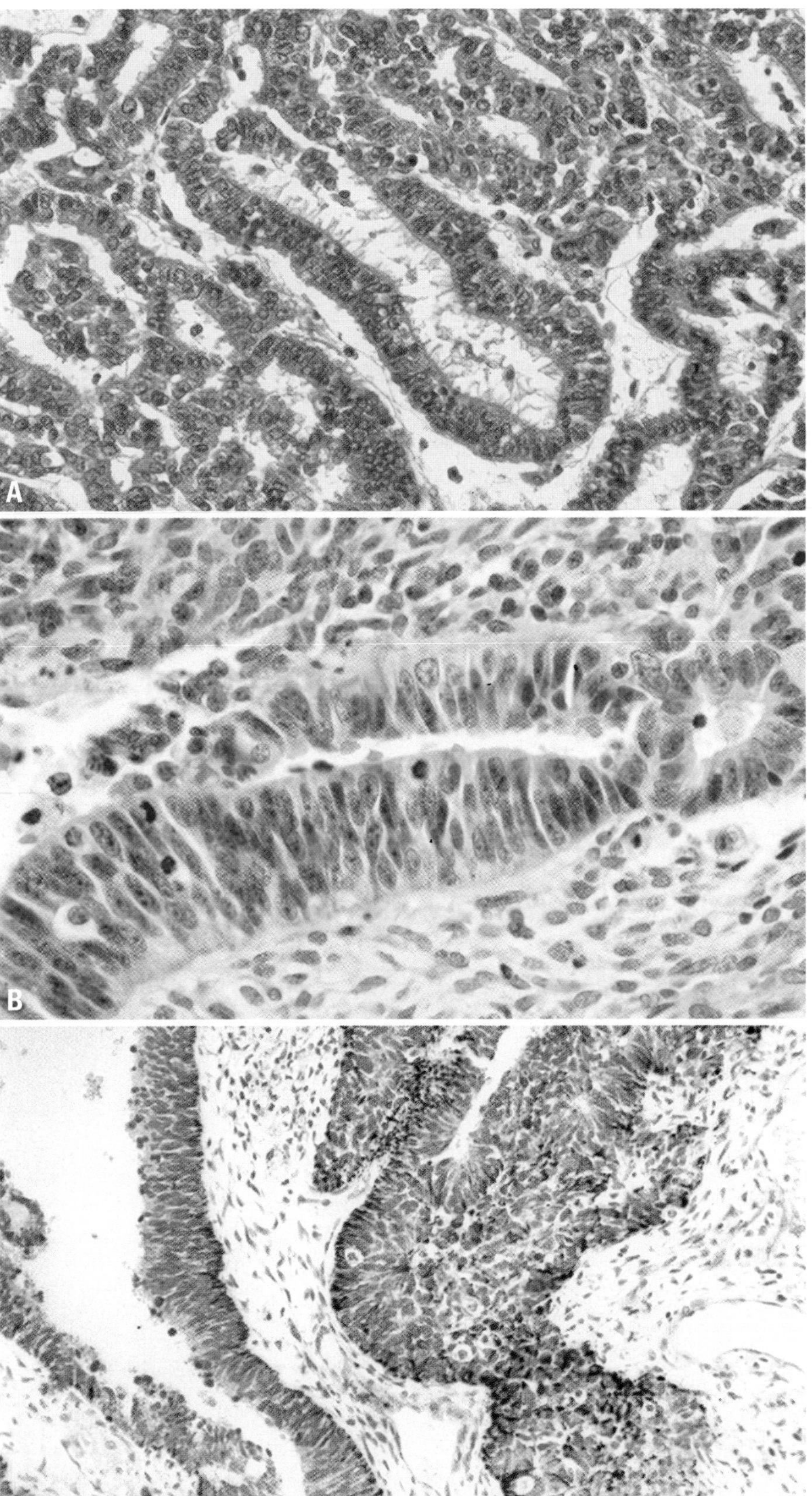

Fig. 8.2 **A** Typical glandular pattern of medulloepithelioma. **B** Immature neuroepithelial cells resting on a basement membrane. Mitotic cells tend to be located towards the luminal surface. **C** Nestin expression predominates on the apical side of neoplastic neuroepithelial cells.

Histogenesis

Microscopy, immunohistochemistry and electron microscopy of the medulloepithelioma reveal features that resemble the primitive neural tube {1291, 1932, 1504}. Developmentally, the transformation of the neuroepithelium into ependyma occurs only after all neuroblasts and glioblasts have migrated from the epithelium.

Medulloepithelioma is probably derived from a type of primitive cell in this subependymal location either as the result of neoplastic transformation at some stage of fetal or early postnatal development or as a result of abnormal re-expression of genes for early neural tube determinants. Because both teratomas and medulloepitheliomas are embryonal and multipotential tumours, there is a conceptual relationship accentuated by the occasional presence of mesenchymal elements in medulloepitheliomas. The mesenchymal elements in medulloepitheliomas have been explained on the basis of a teratoid element, stromal metaplasia or neuroectodermal origin {48, 188}.

Differential diagnosis

Although the characteristic neuroepithelium of medulloepithelioma is usually apparent, the frequent predominance of undifferentiated neuroectodermal cells includes the differential diagnosis of primitive neuroectodermal tumours such as medulloblastoma. Because of the frequent presence of ependymoblastomatous rosettes in medulloepitheliomas, the distinction between these tumours can be difficult. Choroid plexus carcinomas are papillary and lack the spectrum of neuroectodermal differentiation frequently seen in medulloepitheliomas. Immature teratomas are included in the differential diagnosis because they frequently contain primitive medullary epithelium, together with neuroectodermal differentiation. The distinction from medulloepithelioma is that immature teratomas contain tissue of foetal appearance from other germ layers.

Prognosis and prognostic factors

Medulloepitheliomas are rapidly growing tumours that arise at a young age and their optimal management is unknown. Treatment with gross total resection is a feature of long-term survivors {1024}. Radiation may also provide some benefit. However, most children with medulloepithelioma die within a year of diagnosis, often with cerebrospinal fluid dissemination but rarely with systemic metastases.

Ependymoblastoma

L.E. Becker
F.F. Cruz-Sanchez

Definition
A rare, malignant, embryonal brain tumour manifesting in neonates and young children, histologically characterized by distinctive multilayered rosettes.

ICD-O code: 9392/3

Grading
Ependymoblastomas are highly malignant and correspond histologically to WHO grade IV.

Age and sex distribution
Consistent with the primitive neuroepithelial nature of the tumour, the ependymoblastoma occurs in young children including neonates {342, 955}. Males and females appear to be equally affected.

Localization
These neoplasms are often large and supratentorial and generally relate to the ventricles although they do occur at other sites {905, 1038}. A sacrococcygeal congenital ependymoblastoma with elevated serum alpha-fetoprotein {1936} and a primary leptomeningeal ependymoblastoma have been documented {1940}.

Clinical features
In the first and second year of life, the most common clinical manifestation is increased intracranial pressure and hydrocephalus. Focal neurological signs are more common in older children. Neuroimaging criteria do not allow a distinction from other primitive neuroectodermal tumours {1934}. CT and MR usually show a contrast enhancing, large tumour mass, surrounded by an extensive area of oedema.

Macroscopy
The ependymoblastoma tends to be well circumscribed, with a distinct tumour margin, although focal microscopic extension and leptomeningeal invasion are common. Widespread leptomeningeal invasion and extraneural metastases have been described {48, 191}. The unusual extension of a supratentorial ependymoblastoma through the tentorium into the cerebellum has been documented {1935}

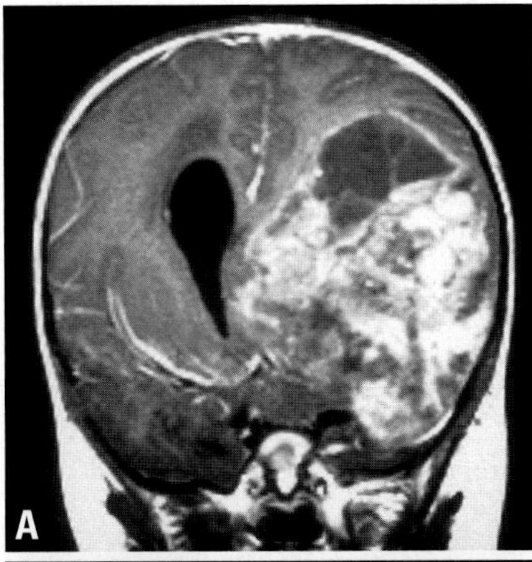

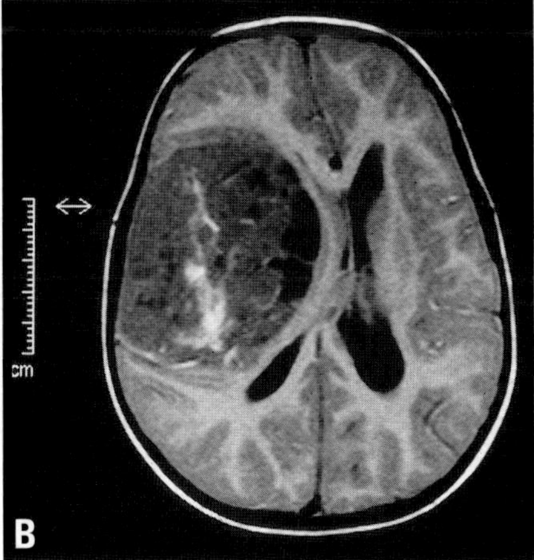

Fig. 8.3 A MRI of a large hemispheric ependymoblastoma with a cystic component. **B** MRI of an ependymoblastoma bordering the lateral ventricle.

Histopathology
Diagnostic features are those of a central primitive neuroectodermal tumour with distinctive multilayered rosettes, with cells in the outer rim of the rosette merging with the surrounding undifferentiated neuroectodermal cells.

The chief histological characteristic of ependymoblastoma is the dense cellularity with distinctive and numerous rosettes. These rosettes are multi-layered and form concentric cellular rings around small round lumina. The nuclei of these cells tend to be pushed away from the lumen towards the outer cell border and the chromatin is coarse and nuclei distinct. The cells have a high mitotic activity. The cells facing the lumen have a defined apical surface beneath which is a faint stippling which corresponds to blepharoplasts. These apical surfaces may form a prominent internal limiting membrane. The outer layer of cells merges with the background of undifferentiated cells with small round-to-oval nuclei and wispy cytoplasmic processes.

Immunohistochemistry
Expression of S100, vimentin, cytokeratin, GFAP and carbonic anhydrase isoenzyme II has been demonstrated {364, 955, 289, 1937}. One report describes immunoreactivity to NF 68, 160 and 200 kDa neurofilaments {364}.

Electron microscopy
Tumour cells are compactly arranged and poorly differentiated with large nuclei and a high nuclear to cytoplasmic ratio. Cytoplasm is scanty with few organelles. In rosettes the cells are united by long or short junctional complexes featuring thickened and electron dense membranes. Frequent "abortive" cilia {289} and a few basal bodies oriented toward the lumen of the rosette {857} have been observed, as have short bands of glial-like filaments.

Aetiology
Of interest is a single case report of an ependymoblastoma occurring in an HIV-positive haemophilic girl {954}.

Differential diagnosis
The histological differential diagnosis includes *anaplastic ependymomas*, characterized by prominent perivascular pseudorosettes in which radially-oriented cell processes form nuclei-free zones around blood vessels and ependymal rosettes with a limited, often single, circumferential layering of cells. *Medulloepitheliomas* may contain ependymoblastoma type rosettes but also have distinctive diagnostic neuroepithelium characterized by an outer basement membrane arranged in

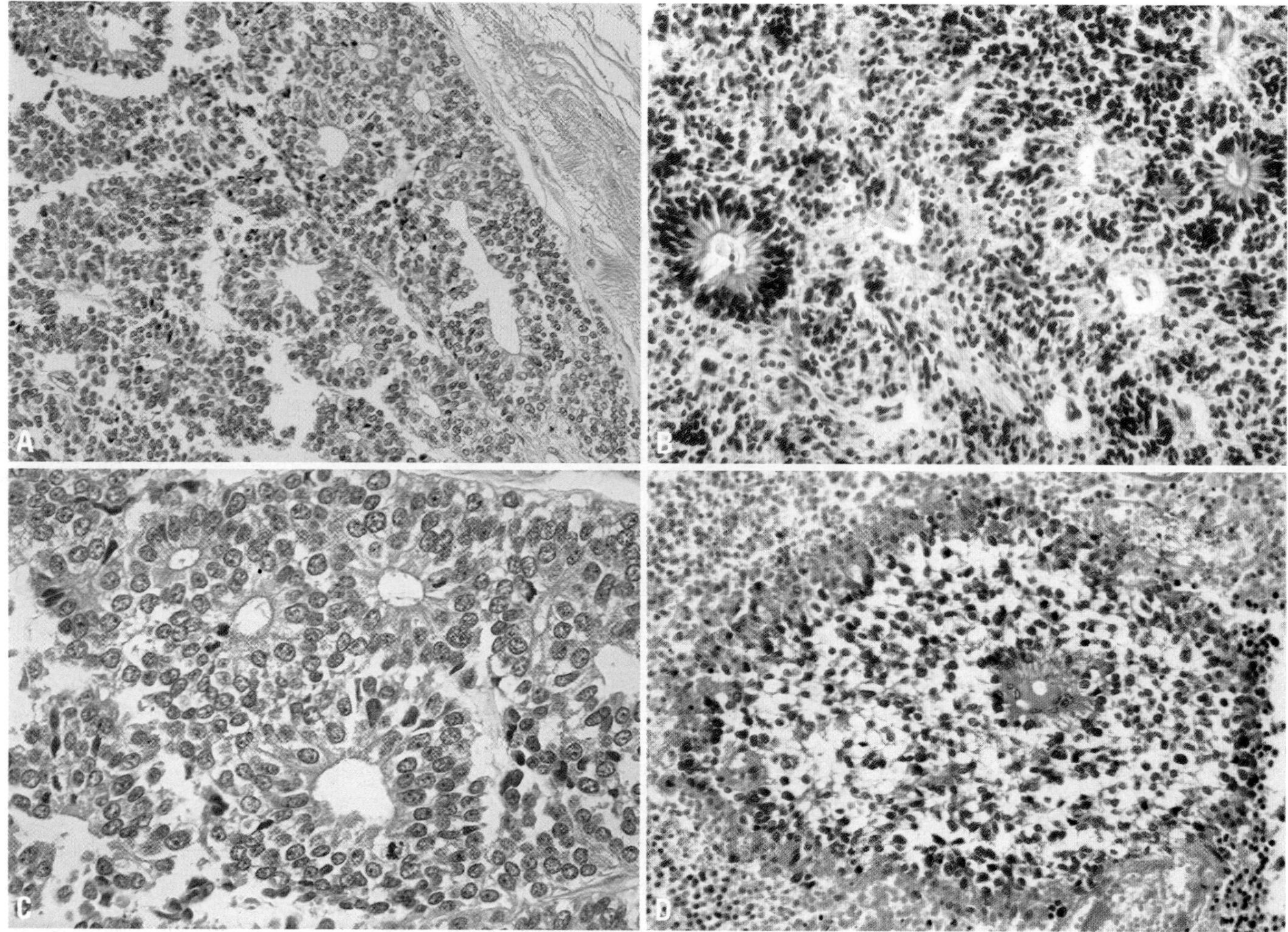

Fig. 8.4 Histopathological features encountered in ependymoblastoma. **A** Low-power micrograph showing the ependymoblastoma rosettes as predominant histological feature. **B** Moderately cellular ependymoblastoma with ependymal rosettes. **C** Highly differentiated area with ependymal rosettes. Note the numerous, sometimes atypical, mitoses. **D** Well-delineated circular tumour area with a central rosette within a geographic necrosis.

tubular, canalicular and papillary patterns. These tumours often display a spectrum of neuroectodermal differentiation including ependymal, glial, neuronal and oligodendroglial features. *Medulloblastomas* are distinct by their cerebellar location and characterized by Homer-Wright rosettes which lack a central lumen {1933, 1939}.

Histogenesis

It is presumed that these tumours arise from periventricular neuroepithelial precursor cells. The term 'ependymoblast' implies an incompletely differentiated ependymal cell showing some phenotypic features of ependyma together with immature characteristics, such as a high nucleus to cytoplasmic ratio, dense chromatin and mitotic activity {289, 1291}.

Prognosis and prognostic factors

Biological characteristics are similar to other embryonal neuroepithelial tumours {1933}. Ependymoblastomas grow rapidly, with craniospinal dissemination and fatal outcome within 6 months to one year of diagnosis. Development of effective treatment protocols for ependymoblastomas is limited by rarity of occurrence, young age of onset and aggressive tumour behaviour. Some studies suggest that gross total resection of ependymoblastoma is a predictor of outcome {1938}. Consistent with the response of other embryonal neuroepithelial tumours, post-operative irradiation may prolong survival.

Medulloblastoma

F. Giangaspero
S.H. Bigner
P. Kleihues
T. Pietsch
J.Q. Trojanowski

Definition

A malignant, invasive embryonal tumour of the cerebellum with preferential manifestation in children, predominantly neuronal differentiation, and an inherent tendency to metastasize via CSF pathways.

ICD-O code: 9470/3

Grading

Medulloblastomas correspond histologically to WHO grade IV.

Incidence

The annual incidence has been estimated at 0.5 per 100'000 children less than 15 years {1919, 214}.

Age and sex distribution

The peak of occurrence is 7 years of age (Fig. 8.5). Seventy percent of medulloblastomas occur in individuals younger than 16 {45, 1265}. In adulthood, 80% of medulloblastomas arise in the 21–40 years age group {632, 1897}. This tumour rarely occurs beyond the fifth decade of life. Approximately 65% of patients are male.

Localization

At least 75% of childhood medulloblastomas arise in the vermis, and project into the fourth ventricle. Involvement of cerebellar hemispheres increases with the age of the patient.

Clinical features

The presenting clinical manifestations include truncal ataxia, disturbed gait, intracranial hypertension secondary to obstruction of CSF-flow and lethargy, headache, and morning vomiting. On computerized tomography (CT) or magnetic resonance imaging (MRI), medulloblastomas appear as solid, intensely and homogeneously contrast-enhancing masses. CSF-borne metastases are seen as foci of nodular or diffuse contrast enhancement in the leptomeninges or on the ventricular surface. They are present in one-third of patients at presentation.

Macroscopy

Medulloblastomas vary considerably in their texture and degree of circumscription. Some are firm and discrete; others are soft and less well defined. Massive haemorrhage occurs in some examples.

Histopathology

Classic medulloblastoma is composed of densely packed cells with round-to-oval or carrot-shaped highly hyperchromatic nuclei surrounded by scanty cytoplasm. Neuroblastic rosettes are a typical but not constant feature.

Round cells with less-condensed chromatin are frequently intermingled, and occasionally form the main population. Neuroblastic rosettes, which consist of tumour cell nuclei disposed in a circular fashion around tangled cytoplasmic processes, are observed in less than 40% of cases. Occasional ganglion cells are seen. Neuroblastic rosettes are frequently associated with marked nuclear polymorphism and high mitotic activity. Although usually numerous, mitoses are infrequent in about 25% of the cases {174, 180}. Apoptosis is frequent, whereas geographic areas of necrosis are less common; pseudopalisading may be observed. Occasionally, nuclear gigantism, multinucleated giant cells and atypical mitoses are seen. Vascular proliferation, calcification and massive haemorrhages are observed in a minority of cases.

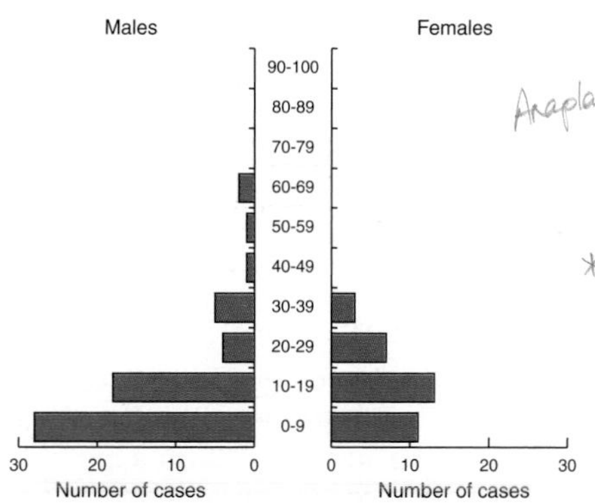

Fig. 8.5 Age and sex distribution of medulloblastoma, based on 89 cases treated at the University Hospital, Zurich.

Desmoplastic medulloblastoma. This lesion shows nodular, reticulin-free zones ('pale islands') surrounded by densely packed, highly proliferative cells that produce a dense intercellular reticulin fiber network {180, 468, 738}. The nodules have reduced cellularity, a rarified fibrillar matrix and marked nuclear uniformity. Nuclei of cells between nodules are usually more irregular and hyperchromatic. Medulloblastomas showing only an increased amount of collagenous and reticulin fibers without the nodular pattern are not classified as desmoplastic variant.

Medulloblastomas with extensive nodularity and advanced neuronal differentiation show intranodular nuclear uniformity and cell streaming in a fine fibrillary background and have also been termed 'cerebellar neuroblastoma' {180, 1159, 1900}. The intranodular round cells resemble the neurocytes of central neurocytoma. Mature ganglion cells may be observed. These neoplasms occur predominantly in children less than 3 years of age. The extreme lobularity is appreciable by neuroimaging as a "grape-like" appearance (Fig. 8.13). Neoplasms of this type occasionally undergo maturation to more-differentiated ganglion cell tumours {314}. It has been suggested that they constitute a pathogenetically separate group {1372}.

Large cell medulloblastoma is a variant representing approximately four percent of cases {470, 1899}. Tumour cells have large, round and/or pleomorphic nuclei with prominent nucleoli and a more abundant cytoplasm than that found in the classic medulloblastoma. Nuclear molding is also frequently present. Large areas of necrosis, high mitotic activity and high apoptotic rate are common findings. This variant resembles the rhabdoid/atypical teratoid tumours of the cerebellar region but it differs on the basis of immunophenotype and cytogenetic findings {1899}.

Immunohistochemistry

Synaptophysin

Synaptophysin expression has been demonstrated in a subset of CNS tumours of presumed neuronal lineage, including medulloblastomas, but not in glial or mesenchymal brain tumours {1023}. Immunoreactivity to synaptophysin is a characteristic feature of medulloblastomas and most prominent in nodules and in the centers of neuroblastic rosettes {180, 260, 742}.

Intermediate filament proteins

The expression patterns of intermediate filament (IF) proteins have been exploited as molecular markers of developing CNS cells {1516}. They have also been used to identify cell lineages in medulloblastomas. *Nestin* is a class VI IF protein with a molecular weight of 210–240 kDa. It is expressed in neuroepithelial progenitor cells of the developing human CNS, but is almost completely eliminated toward the end of gestation {1504, 1533}. Thus, nestin is a marker of CNS precursor cells; however, it is also widely expressed by many types of embryonic cells outside the CNS {1504}. Nestin expression has been demonstrated in several types of brain tumours including medulloblastomas, astrocytomas, glioblastomas, ependymomas, gangliogliomas and meningiomas {1504}. *Vimentin and glial fibrillary acidic protein (GFAP)* are class III IF proteins with a molecular weight of 57 and 52 KD, respectively {1023}. During CNS development, the expression of vimentin closely parallels that of nestin {1504}. Classic medulloblastoma may be strongly immunoreactive for vimentin {180}. The expression of GFAP is restricted almost exclusively to developing and mature astrocytes in the CNS. The majority of medulloblastomas contain stellate GFAP-positive cells. These could be trapped astrocytes, but could also be terminally differentiated neoplastic astrocytes, because they have been found in medulloblastoma metastases {180}. However, unquestionably GFAP-positive neoplastic cells have been noted in classic and desmoplastic medulloblastomas {174, 180}.

There are three different groups of *neuron-specific IF proteins*, including the triplet of neurofilament (NF) proteins, alpha-internexin and peripherin. The triplet of NF subunits are class IV IF proteins and the expression of NF proteins in embryonic CNS cells is a specific indicator of commitment to the neuronal lineage. Neurofilaments are composed of the low (NF-L, 68 kDa), middle (NF-M, 150 kDa) and high (NF-H, 200 kDa) molecular weight NF subunits. In the developing CNS, the more heavily phosphorylated isoforms of NF-M and NF-H are expressed in more advanced stages of neuronal development than their less phosphorylated counterparts. The expression of NF proteins has therefore been used to identify neoplastic cells of the neuronal lineage in medulloblastomas {439, 496, 957, 1504}.

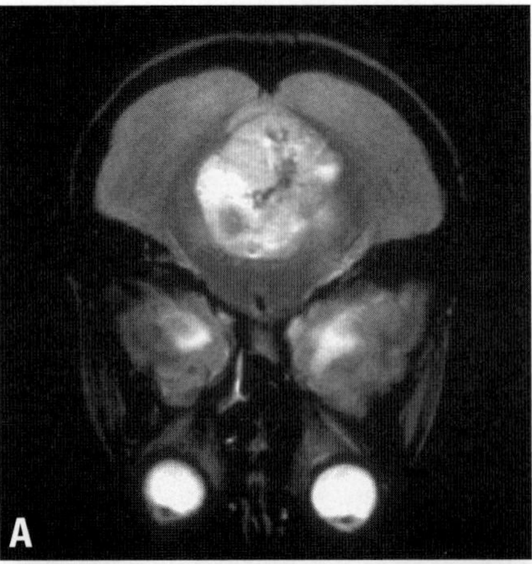

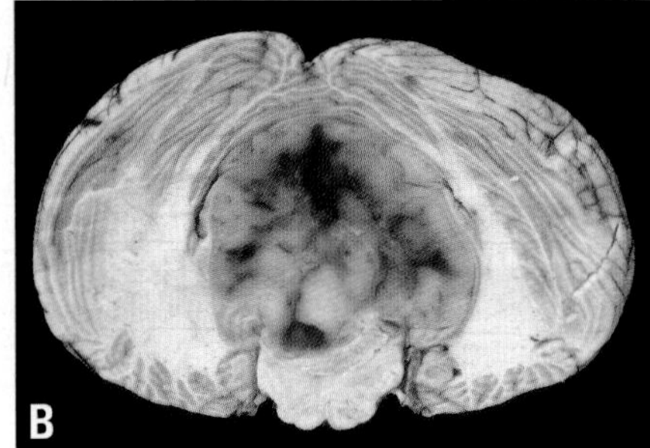

Fig. 8.6 MRI and gross macroscopic images of medulloblastomas of the cerebellar vermis compressing the brainstem.

Photoreceptor cell proteins

Retinal S-antigen, rhodopsin and interphotoreceptor retinoid-binding protein (IRBP) are photoreceptor proteins that have been demonstrated in a variety of brain tumours. Focal expression of rhodopsin and retinal S-antigen is a typical though not a regular feature of medulloblastomas {297, 957}.

Neural cell adhesion molecules

Neural cell adhesion molecules (N-CAMs) belong to the immunoglobulin superfamily and appear to play an important role in cell migration in the developing nervous system. Expression of N-CAMs has been described in medulloblastomas as well as in gliomas and a variety of other intracranial neoplasms {406, 433, 1021}, suggesting that N-CAMs are not lineage-specific markers, but may reflect the level of differentiation in a tumour.

Growth factors and their receptors

Nerve growth factor (NGF) was the first growth factor identified, and has been the most extensively studied member of the neurotrophin family. NGF receptors exist in high- and low-affinity forms. The low-affinity NGF receptor is a protein with a molecular weight of 75 kDa (p75-NGFR), while the high-affinity receptors are a family of proteins with a molecular weight of 140 kDa, known as Trk A, B, and C, expression of which has been demonstrated in medulloblastomas {1382, 1582}. The p75-NGFR is expressed in a small proportion of medulloblastomas {59}. Follow up immunohistochemical studies of biopsy samples of medulloblastomas using antibodies to NGF, BDNF and NT3, as well as to their cognate receptors, *i.e.* TrkA, TrkB and TrkC, respectively, suggest that neurotrophins might modulate the behaviour of these tumours in a paracrine or autocrine manner {1921}. Although NGF and TrkA did not co-distribute in the same medulloblastoma samples, BDNF co-distributed with TrkB and NT3 co-distributed with TrkC in some tumours, several of which showed evidence of neuronal differentiation {1921}.

Electron microscopy

In areas of neuroblastic differentiation, such as rosettes, and 'pale islands', the cells elaborate neurite-like cytoplasmic processes joined by specialized adhesion plaques and are laden with microtubules in parallel array. Dense-core vesicles and synapses may also be observed, *i.e.* features seen in embryonal neurons {742}. Abundant intermediate filaments may be noted in areas of glial differentiation. Tissue from histologically and immunohistochemically undifferentiated areas may reveal few, if any, specific ultrastructural features.

Apoptosis

Apoptosis is a major contributor to cell loss in medulloblastomas. Apoptotic nuclei can be recognized in H&E slides as compact, round masses, or as crescentic caps at the nuclear periphery, or as small spherules corresponding to apoptotic bodies. By electron microscopy, the chromatin appears compact, split into blocks or con-

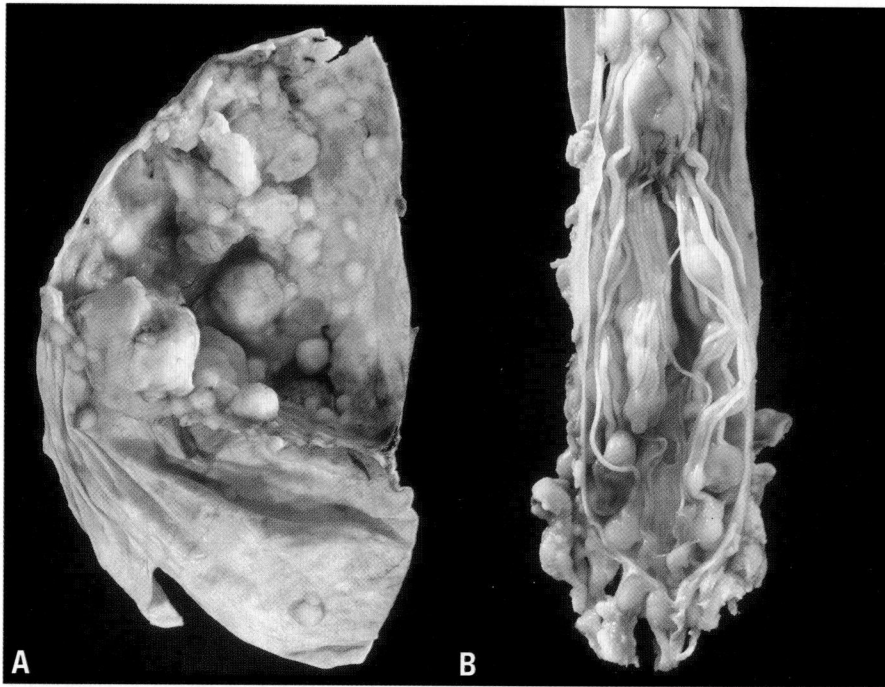

Fig. 8.7 Numerous CSF metastases of cerebellar medulloblastoma (**A**) at the inner surface of the dura mater and (**B**) in the cauda equina.

densed on the nuclear membrane; apoptotic bodies or phagocytosed chromatin masses are also identifiable. By *in situ* end labelling (ISEL), apoptotic nuclei are present in classic and desmoplastic medulloblastoma, comprising 1.3 ± 0.5% of nuclei {1348}. The distribution of apoptotic nuclei is uneven; they are generally more frequent in areas with higher mitotic index and higher numbers of Ki67-positive cells {1349}. The Bcl-2 proto-oncogene prevents apoptosis under many conditions, and is expressed in 30% of medulloblastomas {1350}. This relationship is consistent with the high number of apoptotic cells in medulloblastoma. A positive correlation between apoptosis and expression of cell-cycle inhibitor p27/Kip-1 has been observed {1916}. Tumours expressing Bcl-2 have been found to show features of neuronal differentiation {1350}. Recent data suggest that NGF, acting through TrkA {1048}, may induce apoptosis in medulloblastomas. However the absence of co-distributed NGF and TrkA in the same biopsy samples may signify that NGF induces apoptosis through TrkA signalling pathways thereby eliminating neoplastic cells that express NGF and/or TrkA in proximity to each other.

Proliferation

The growth kinetics of medulloblastomas have been studied by *in vivo* uptake of tritiated thymidine (^{3}H-thymidine), bromodeoxyuridine and iododeoxyuridine. The labelling index (LI) of ^{3}H-thymidine ranges from 8 to 14.4%, appreciably higher than that found in malignant gliomas {619}. Iododeoxyuridine LI ranged from 3.9 to 38.2% (mean 11.7 ± 1.3%, SE) {650}. Younger patients have a higher LI than older patients. In addition, the LI of medulloblastomas in the cerebellar vermis tends to be higher than that of hemispheric medulloblastomas {650}.

The S-phase duration (Ts) and potential doubling time (Tp), calculated on the basis of the double-staining with bromodeoxyuridine and iododeoxyuridine, are 8.0 ± 0.8 hours, and 25–82 hours (mean 51 ± 7 hours, SE), respectively {650}. The actual doubling time as estimated from serial CT scans {1656} and from serial MR images {650} was considerably longer (19–24 days), suggesting that extensive cell loss affects the rate at which cells are added to the population by mitosis. A cell-loss factor of 0.89–0.96 has been calculated {650}.

The growth fraction, as revealed by the fraction of medulloblastoma cells expressing Ki-67, is often >20% {1348}. In the most active areas, the MIB-1 proliferating cell index was found to range from 15 to >50%, with considerable regional variability {2549}. Nuclei positive for Ki-67 are more regularly distributed in classic medulloblastomas and infrequent in the pale islands of desmoplastic medulloblastomas {1348}.

Some cases of medulloblastoma have a diploid DNA status, others are hyperdiploid, and yet others are aneuploid

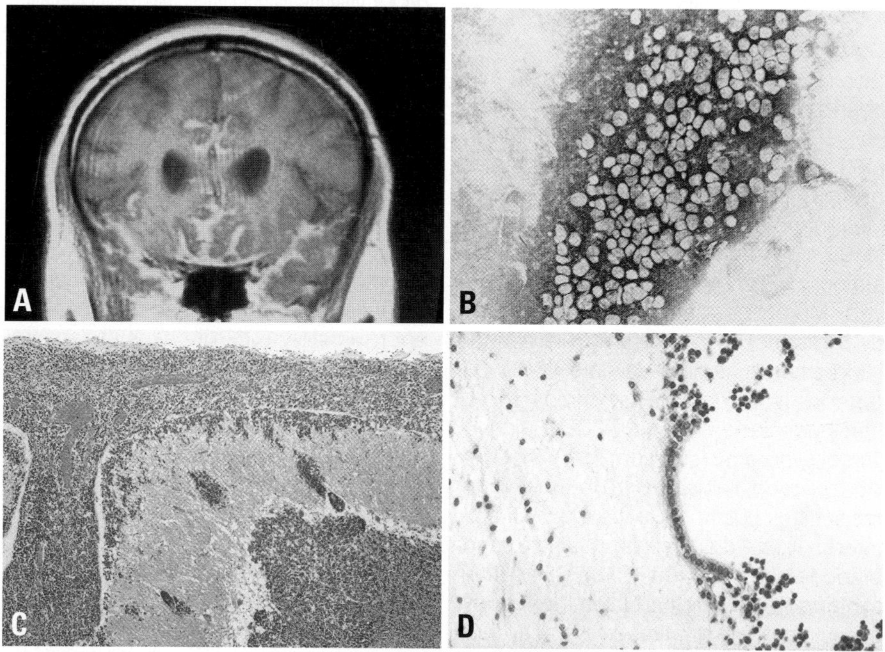

Fig. 8.8 A MRI of a medulloblastoma with extensive meningeal spread. **B** CSF cytology showing a cluster of medulloblastoma cells strongly expressing N-CAM. **C** Infiltration by a cerebellar medulloblastoma of the subarachnoidal space. Note clusters of tumour cells in the molecular layer, particularly in the subpial region. **D** CSF metastases in the ependymal lining of a lateral ventricle.

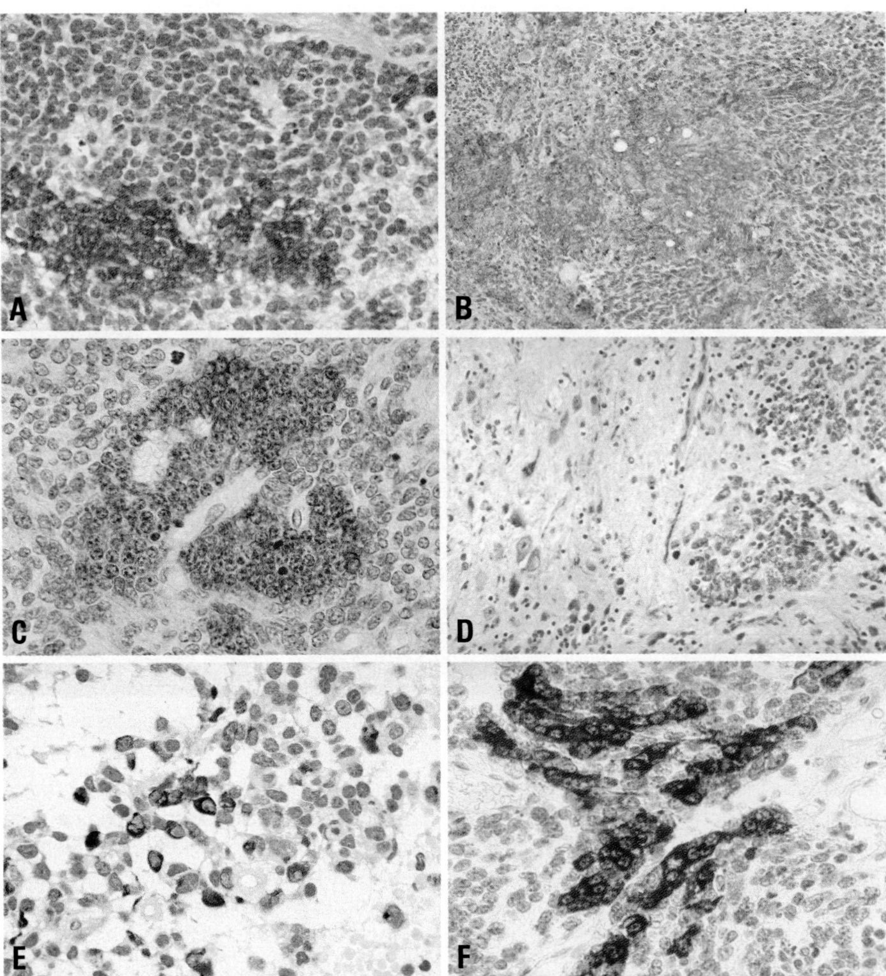

Fig. 8.9 Immunohistochemical features of medulloblastoma. Focal expression of (**A**) neuron-specific enolase (NSE), (**B**) synaptophysin, (**C**) neurofilament protein (NF). **D** Area with advanced neuronal differentiation showing NF labelling of a mature ganglion cell and of neurites. **E** Focal GFAP staining of tumour cells. **F** Clusters of medulloblastoma cells expressing retinal S-antigen.

in varying proportion {447, 1506, 1662, 1675}. More diploid tumours were found among patients of very young age {1506, 1662, 1675} and among desmoplastic medulloblastomas {468}.

Aetiology

No environmental factors have been implicated in the aetiology of human medulloblastomas. In experimental animals, cerebellar neoplasms with a phenotype similar to that of medulloblastoma have been induced in hamsters by perinatal intracerebral injection with JC virus {970, 1681}, and in rats by retrovirus-mediated transfection of fetal rat brain cells with the large T antigen of SV40 {365}. Other models of medulloblastoma-like PNETs have been produced using transgenic mice that express SV40 large T antigen under the influence of different promoters {439}. A recent study has demonstrated a high frequency of detection of JC virus DNA sequences and the viral oncoprotein, T-antigen, by immunohistochemistry in human medulloblastoma, suggesting that JC virus may play a role in tumorigenesis of this neoplasm {1903, 2550}. However, these findings have not been confirmed by others {2231}. SV40 sequences have also been identified but their possible role in the evolution of medulloblastomas and other brain neoplasms remains to be elucidated {2231}.

Genetic susceptibility

Several cases of medulloblastoma have been reported in monozygotic twins {1895} as well as in dizygotic twins and siblings {103, 637, 1657}. Associations with other brain tumours {392} and extraneural malignancies, including Wilms' tumour {1105, 1222} and renal malignant rhabdoid tumour {145, 424}, have also been observed. Moreover, medulloblastomas have been diagnosed in several familial cancer syndromes, including patients with *TP53* germline mutations, the naevoid basal cell carcinoma syndrome (NBCCS) {851}, and Turcot syndrome (see Chapter 14). Occasionally, medulloblastomas develop within the setting of complex malformations, *e.g.* intestinal malrotation, omphalocele, and bladder extrophy {1095}, and Coffin-Siris syndrome (mental retardation, deficiency of postnatal growth, joint laxity, brachydactyly of the fifth digit with absence of the nail bed) {1274}. Some studies suggest that relatives of patients with medulloblastomas have an increased risk of developing other childhood tumours, particularly leukaemia and lymphoma {391, 834}.

Cytogenetics

Isochromosome 17q

The most common specific abnormality in medulloblastomas, which is present in approximately 50% of cases, is isochromosome 17q [i(17q)] {120, 507}. In the majority of cases, the breakpoint is in the proximal portion of the p-arm, so that the resultant structure is dicentric; this is also the case in the i(17q) that occurs in leukaemia. This observation has been confirmed by restriction-fragment length polymorphism (RFLP) and microsatellite analyses, and it has been demonstrated that most medulloblastomas with 17p loss have breakpoints between D17S689 and D17S95 at 17p11.2 {1345}. This chromosomal region is deleted or duplicated in the Smith-Magenis syndrome, and instability in this region is a plausible explanation for the tendency for 17p loss to occur through isochromosome formation. Isochromosome 17q has been demonstrated in interphase nuclei using fluorescence *in situ* hybridisation (FISH) {109, 1531}. Although i(17q) is the most common mechanism for 17p loss in medulloblastomas, in a small number of cases, partial or complete loss of 17p occurs through interstitial deletion, unbalanced translocation or monosomy 17 {105}.

Chromosome 1

This chromosome is also frequently involved in medulloblastoma, but the types of abnormalities are variable, including unbalanced translocations, deletions and duplications {120, 507}. In contrast to the chromosome 17 defects, rearrangements of chromosome 1 often result in trisomy 1q without loss of the p-arm.

Other chromosomes
Studies using comparative genomic hybridisation (CGH) have demonstrated a greater degree of genomic imbalance in medulloblastoma than previously recognized. They have confirmed loss of 17p with gain of 17q as the most frequent finding {1376, 1911, 1891}. Among other non-random changes, the most frequently observed were losses on chromosomes 10q (41%), 11(41%), and gain of chromosome 7 (44%) {1911}. Although isolated examples of 6q, 9q, 10q and 16q deletions were observed, gains of chromosomal regions were, overall, more prevalent than were losses. Recurrent imbalances included gain of distal regions on 4p, 5p, 5q, 7q, 8q and 9p. Approximately two-thirds of medulloblastoma cell lines and xenografts contain double minutes. In contrast, these structures are seen only occasionally in biopsy material (<5% of samples) {118, 120}.

Molecular genetics

Gene amplification
In most samples of medulloblastoma with double minutes, amplification of *MYC* {53, 74, 118} or less often of the *MYCN* {1507} has been found. The reported frequency of *MYC* gene amplification varies, largely according to the method of analysis. A recent CGH analysis suggested that it may be as high as 20% {1914}. It appears that the large cell variant carries a high incidence of *MYC* amplification {1899}.

Deletion of genetic material on chromosome arm 17p
Studies of loss of heterozygosity (LOH) by both RFLP and microsatellite analysis have shown loss of genetic material of chromosome arm 17p in 30-45% of cases as the most frequent molecular genetic alteration in medulloblastomas {264}. This indicates a medulloblastoma-related tumour suppressor gene located on 17p which has not been identified yet. In the majority of the cases, most of the p-arm is missing with breakpoints in the 17p11 region {1345}. In occasional cases, partial 17p deletions were identified, mapping the smallest overlapping region of deletion to 17p13.3 {105, 974, 1905}.
As *TP53* is located on 17p13 and is mutated in a variety of human tumours, this gene was initially considered as a candidate gene. *TP53* mutations have been identified in a small subset of 5-10% of medulloblastomas {6, 23, 1096}. Because of the low incidence of mutations and the localization of the smallest region of deletion to 17p13.3 (distal to *TP53* at 17p13.1), *TP53* is not considered a major target of chromosome 17p loss.
Three putative tumour suppressor genes *ROX/MNT* {1922}, *HIC1* {1575}, and the active *BCR*-related (*ABR*) {264} have been mapped to the region 17p13.3, but so far no data implicate these genes in medulloblastoma pathogenesis.

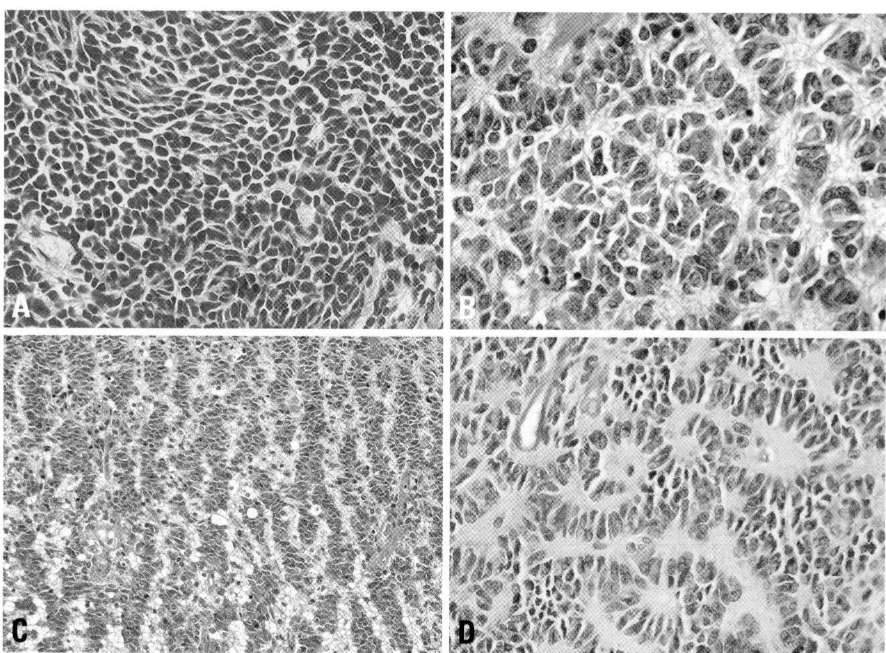

Fig. 8.10 Histopathological features of medulloblastoma. **A** Typical arrangment of sheets of undifferentiated tumour cells. **B** Area with Homer-Wright (neuroblastic) rosettes. **C** Arrangement of tumour cells in parallel rows. **D** Palisading tumour cells creating a pseudoglandular appearance.

Candidate genes on chromosome arms 1q and 10q
Losses of genetic material was also found in approximately 20-40% on chromosome 1q and 10q {1906, 131, 1914, 1911}. The frequency of these alterations varies be-

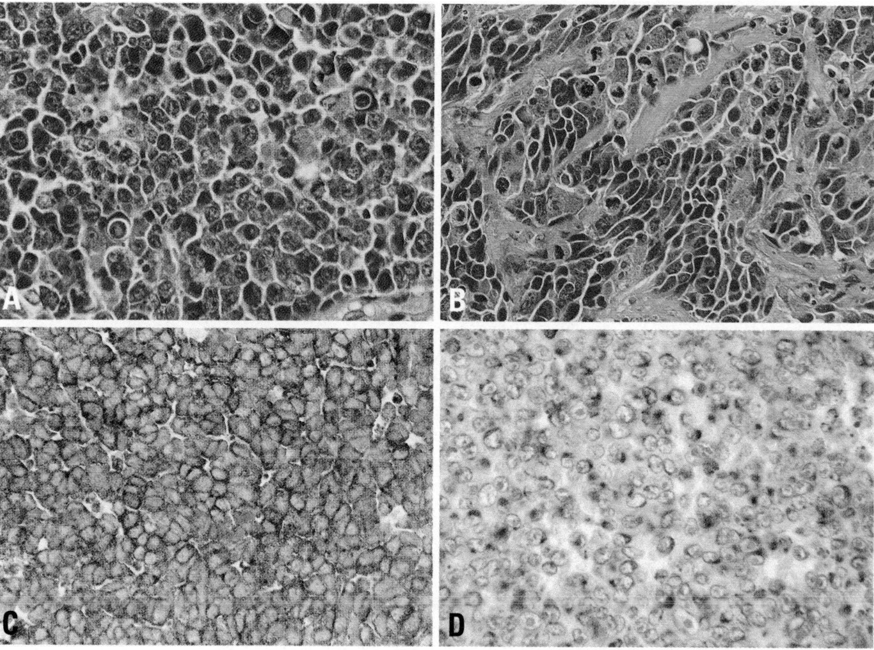

Fig. 8.11 Large cell medulloblastoma displaying **(A)** pleomorphic, large nuclei with prominent nucleoli and **(B)** atypical mitoses. **C** Strong immunoreactivity for synaptophysin and **(D)** neurofilament.

tween different studies, and the target genes are not identified with certainty. The region affected on chromosome 1q has been narrowed to 1q31-32 and corresponds to a locus deleted in breast cancer {1893}. On chromosome arm 10q, two candidate genes have been studied in detail. The tumour suppressor gene *PTEN* located on 10q23 encoding a dual specific phosphatase was found to be frequently affected in glioblastomas but only in a single medulloblastoma case {1910}. Using representational difference analysis, a homozygous deletion at 10q25.3-26.1 was identified in a medulloblastoma cell line and a novel gene, *DMBT1*, spanning this deletion was cloned {1775}. *DMBT1* shows homology to the scavenger receptor cystein-rich (SRCR) superfamily. Intragenic homozygous deletions have been detected in 2/20 medulloblastomas {1775}. Therefore, *DMBT1* represents a putative tumour-suppressor gene implicated in the pathogenesis of a small subset of medulloblastoma.

The hedgehog / patched signalling pathway

Another putative tumour suppressor locus is located on the long arm of chromosome 9 where allelic losses have been described in 10-18% of the cases {20, 1372, 1914}. In this region, the locus of NBCCS has been mapped and the gene responsible for this syndrome has been cloned in 1996 {524}. Patients with NBCCS are predisposed to develop basal cell carcinoma and medulloblastomas mainly of the desmoplastic variant {1372}. They have inactivating germline mutations in the human homologue of the *Drosophila* segment polarity gene *patched, PTCH. Patched* encodes a cell surface receptor which is regulated by binding of its ligands, members of the hedgehog morphogen family and plays an important role during the development of various tissues including the central nervous system {1898}. Sonic hedgehog is a mayor mitogen for cerebellar granule cell progenitors which carry its receptor Patched {1924}. Patched is believed to be a negative growth regulator that complexes and inhibits a second transmembrane, signal transducing component, Smoothened. Activation of this pathway occurs by binding of a Hedgehog ligand which inhibits Patched and results in increased transcription of specific target genes including *GLI1*, *WNT*s and *TGFß*-related genes as well as *PTCH* itself {1896}. The signal transducing cascade is well known from *Drosophila*, but some of the human homologues have still not been identified. Whereas *PTCH* is believed to have tumour suppressor activity both the ligand encoding gene *SHH* and *SMOH* are candidates for putative oncogenes.

Inactivating mutations of the *PTCH* gene have been identified in approximately 8% of sporadic medulloblastomas {1174, 1634, 1218, 1923, 2551}. One study suggests that *PTCH* mutations occur preferentially in desmoplastic medulloblastomas {1174}. Most mutations resulted in truncated proteins. Sonic hedgehog (Shh), produced by Purkinje neurons, regulates the proliferation of granule cell precursors {1924}. Mutational inactivation of *PTCH* may result in inappropriate or sustained proliferation of these progenitor cells in the external granular layer of the cerebellum {1924}, suggesting that developmental control genes play an important role in the pathogenesis of medulloblastoma.

In the Sonic Hedgehog (*SHH*) gene, a point mutation in exon 2 resulting in an amino acid change (His133Tyr) has been identified in 1/14 medulloblastomas {1109}. However, this *SHH* mutation which was claimed to be activating, was not identified in larger studies {1925, 2551}. Mutation analysis of the *SMOH* gene in medulloblastomas uncovered two cases with missense mutations {1912, 1907}, one being an activating mutation at position 1604 in exon 9, recently described in basal cell carcinomas {1926}. However, *SMOH* mutations, too, appear to be very rare {2551}. An inactivating mutation of *PTCH2*, a human homologue of *PTCH* located on chromosome 1p32-34, has been reported in a single case of medulloblastoma {1918}. These data indicate that different genetic alterations may lead to an activation of the hedgehog/patched signalling pathway.

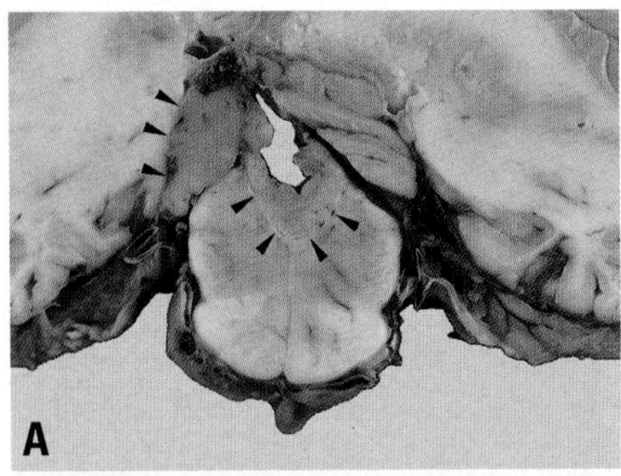

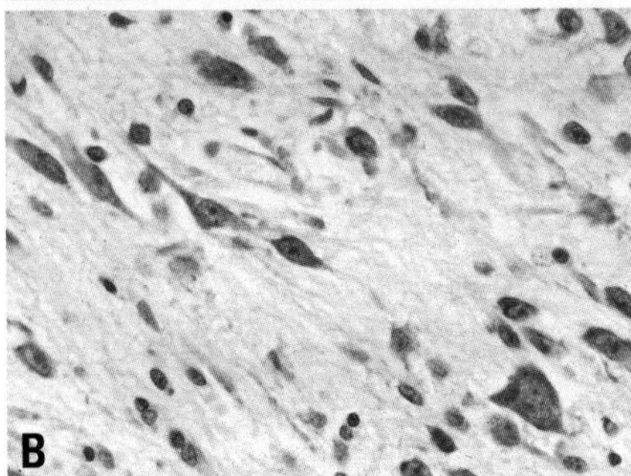

Fig. 8.12 Maturation of a medulloblastoma. Fifteen years after operation and radiotherapy, the patient died from other causes. At the site of surgical intervention a remaining tumour mass (arrowheads) showed the characteristics of a gangliocytoma.

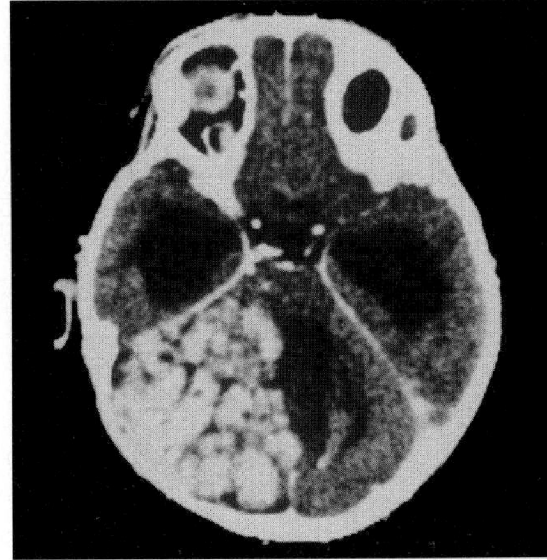

Fig. 8.13 Medulloblastoma with extensive nodularity and grape-like appearance on MRI.

APC and the Wnt signalling pathway

The adenomatous polyposis coli *(APC)* gene was originally identified as the target of germline mutations causing familial adenomatous polyposis (FAP), a syndrome of inherited predisposition to colon cancer {2553}. The APC protein forms a complex with glycogen synthase kinase 3b (GSK-3b), thereby regulating the level of this protein, which functions as a downstream transcriptional activator of the Wnt signaling pathway {2554, 2555} and is also the submembrane component of a cell-cell adhesion system {2554, 2556}. Somatic *APC* mutations are frequently found in sporadic colon cancer {2558, 2559} and typically lead to a truncated protein that lacks regulatory activity, causing β-catenin accumulation {1033}. Colorectal carcinomas without *APC* mutation frequently contain a *β-catenin* mutation, which also activates the Wnt pathway {2559}.

Involvement of the Wnt pathway in the evolution of sporadic medulloblastomas was first indicated by the presence of *β-catenin* mutations in 3/67 (4.5%) of cases {1928}. This raised the question whether sporadic medulloblastomas also contain *APC* mutations. Attempts to identify *APC* mutations by an RNAse protection assay failed {1033} and LOH on chromosome 5q, on which the *APC* gene is located, was not detected in 23 sporadic medulloblastomas {2560}. However, in a recent study using SSCP and direct DNA sequencing, three miscoding *APC* point mutations were found in 2/46 (4.3%) medulloblastomas {2552}. One case contained a GCA->GTA mutation at codon 1296 (Ala->Val) and another case had double point mutations at codons 1472 (GTA->ATA, Val->Ile) and 1495 (AGT->GGT, Ser->Gly). In addition, miscoding *β-catenin* mutations were detected in 4/46 tumors (8.7%). Three of these were located at codon 33 (TCT ->TTT, Ser-> Phe). *APC* and *β-catenin* mutations were mutually exclusive and occurred in a total of 6 of 46 cases, suggesting involvement of the Wnt pathway in approximately 13% of sporadic medulloblastomas {2552}.

Neural transcription factors

The *PAX* (paired-box containing) gene family has nine members, all of which are transcription factors active in neural development. Expression of PAX6 protein was demonstrated in 16/28 (57%) of medulloblastomas by immunohistochemistry, and expression of *PAX5* and *PAX6* mRNA was shown in 70% and 78% of medulloblastomas by *in situ* hybridisation {803, 1552}. Expression of both genes was seen mainly in the most undifferentiated tumour cells. The lack of expression of the *PAX5* gene in normal neonatal cerebellum and its upregulation in medulloblastoma indicate that it may play a role in development of medulloblastoma .

Other neural transcription factors have been found to be expressed in medulloblastomas including the granule cell marker *ZIC*, and transcription factors of the *NEUROD* family {1927, 1913}. Their expression may reflect the phenotype of the cellular origin of medulloblastomas. However, a contribution of these transcription factors in the pathogenesis of medulloblastomas has not been ruled out.

Histogenesis

Bailey and Cushing recognized the medulloblastoma as a distinct clinicopathological entity in 1925 {57}. They assumed a derivation from medulloblasts, *i.e.* undifferentiated, proliferating embryonal cells with the capacity to differentiate into spongioblasts and neuroblasts. The existence of such precursor cells was postulated, but not unequivocally identified, in subsequent neuro-anatomical studies of the developing nervous system {1542}. The histogenesis of medulloblastoma has been a controversial issue for over 75 years. There are three hypotheses. One view suggests that it originates from the external granular layer of the cerebellum, which forms during embryogenesis by migration of undifferentiated cells from the roof of the fourth ventricle to the surface of the fetal cerebellar cortex, where they give rise to cells which later form the internal granular layer neurons {1542}. This view is strongly supported by the recent observation that the proliferation of precursor neurons in the external granular layer of the cerebellum is controlled by sonic hedgehog {1924} whose receptor *PTCH* is mutated in a subset of sporadic medulloblastomas (see above). If medulloblastomas arise from the external granular layer, neuronal differentiation might be expected in these neoplasms; this is indeed observed in the majority of medulloblastomas. However, there is no evidence that the external granular cells have the capacity to differentiate along glial or other lines {1474}.

The second hypothesis is the basis of the PNET concept and assumes that medulloblastomas are derived from subependymal matrix cells, which reside throughout the embryonal CNS, including the fourth ventricle, and which give rise to neuronal and glial cells. The PNET concept implies that medulloblastomas and

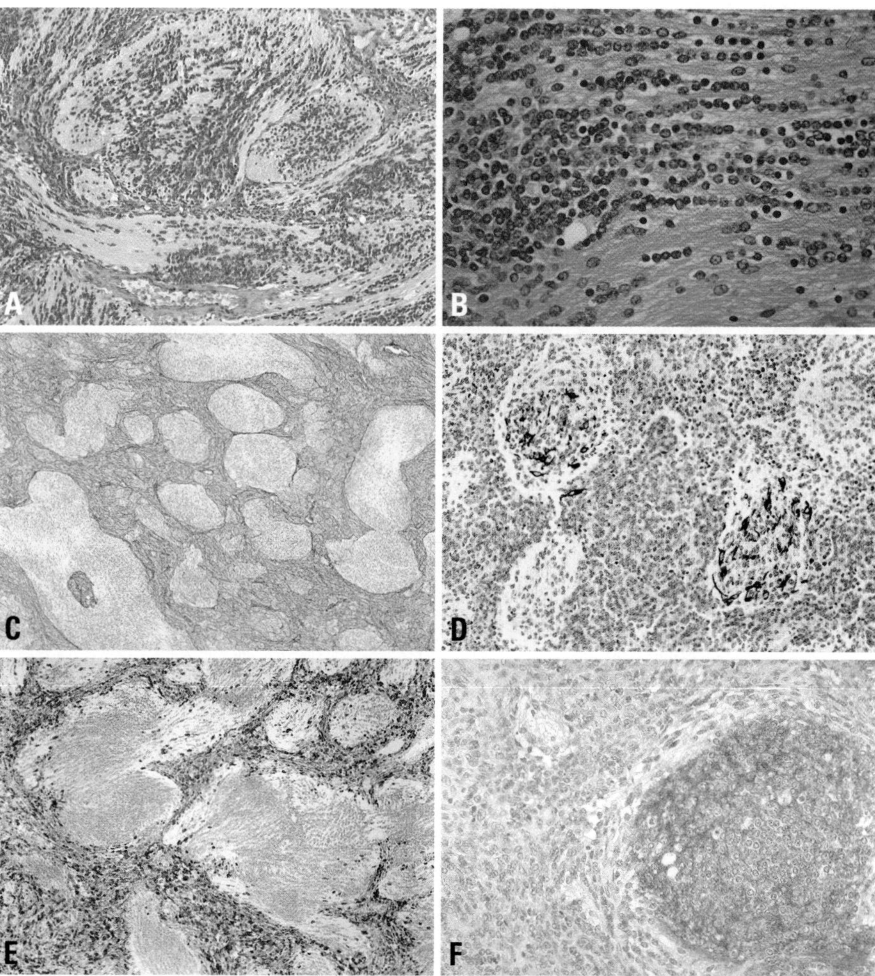

Fig. 8.14 Features of desmoplastic medulloblastomas. **A** Nodular medulloblastoma with advanced neuroblastic differentiation. **B** Streaming of tumour cells on a fibrillary background. **C** Reticulin stain showing the typical biphasic pattern with highly cellular, desmoplastic areas and reticulin-free islands. **D** GFAP immunohistochemistry showing that astrocytic differentiation is restricted to reticulin-free islands. **E** MIB-1 staining shows that the proliferative activity predominates in the highly cellular, desmoplastic areas, whereas **(F)** neuronal differentiation, shown by immunoreactivity to synaptophysin, occurs in the islands.

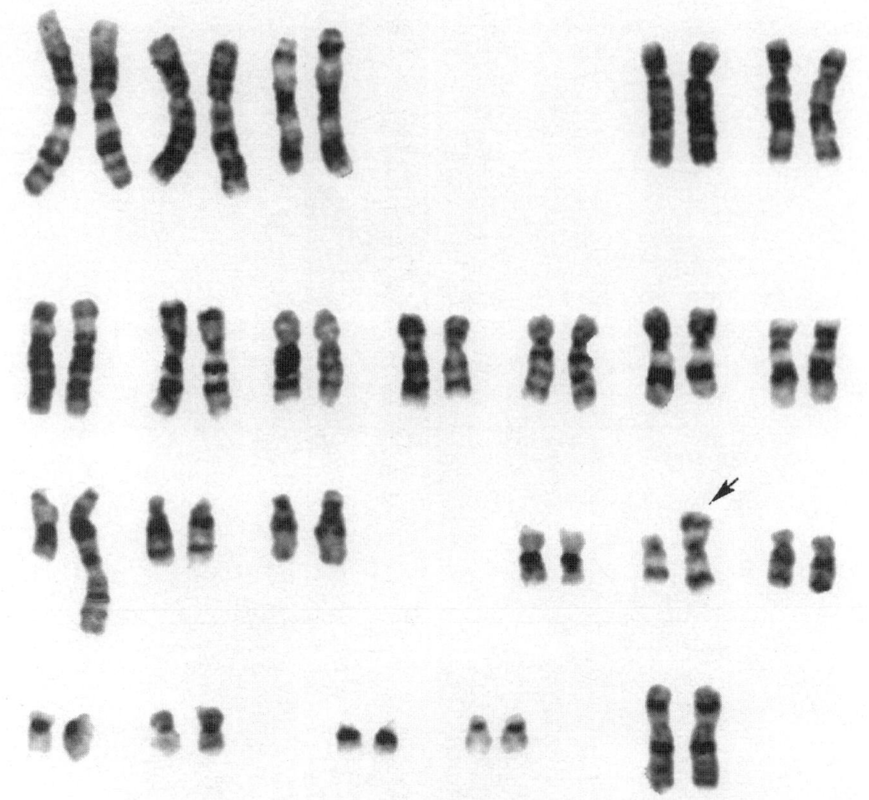

Fig. 8.15 Karyotype of medulloblastoma cell line D-556 MB. The arrow indicates isochromosome i(17q), which is a characteristic finding in these tumours.

supratentorial PNETs originate from a common precursor cell. However, there is emerging evidence that infratentorial PNETs (medulloblastomas) and supratentorial PNETs show different genetic alterations. Recently, Burnett *et al.* described the lack of allelic loss of chromosome arm 17p in supratentorial PNETs {1889}. Similarly, inactivating mutations of the *PTCH* locus seem not to occur in this entity {1634}. Supratentorial PNETs express the human ACHAETE SCUTE homologue (HASH1) which is absent in medulloblastomas {1913}. These findings argue against the hypothesis that PNETs of different locations may derive from closely related progenitor cells by similar genetic mechanisms.

A third hypothesis proposes that medulloblastomas may have more than one cell of origin. This is based on studies showing differential immunoreactivity to calbindin-D28k, a ventricular matrix-associated neuronal calcium-binding protein neither expressed in the external granular layer nor in its progeny, and to the class III beta-tubulin isotype (beta III), which is expressed in the neuronal descendants of both ventricular matrix cells and external granular cells {736, 737, 739}. These studies suggest that classic medulloblastomas arise from the ventricular matrix/velum medullare, whereas the desmoplastic variant originates from the external granular layer {736}.

Predictive factors

Significant advances have been made in the treatment of medulloblastoma: the 5-year survival of 30% in the 1960s has now risen to 50–70%. This improved survival rate has been attributed to improvement in perioperative care, imaging, surgical techniques, chemo- and radiotherapy {308, 474, 1116, 1265, 1909}. A similar increase in survival has been achieved in adult patients {1894}.

Clinical criteria

The prognostic significance of age and extent of surgical resection and tumour location (midline versus lateral) are complicated and controversial issues. In general, "poor risk" medulloblastomas are associated with those patients having one of these features: less than three years of age, metastases at presentation and partial surgical resection {1909}.

Histological criteria

There is increasing evidence that clinical outcome may, to some extent, depend on the histological type of medulloblastoma. *Desmoplastic medulloblastomas* were associated with a somewhat better outcome in some series {946}, but with poorer prognosis in others {474, 632}. Such discrepancy may be explained by the fact that in some of these studies tumours were classified as desmoplastic on the basis of an increased amount of collagen and reticulin fibers but without the typical nodular pattern of this variant. In a single institution study, in which the desmoplastic lesions were defined on the basis of nodularity, the prognosis was significantly better than for patients with classic medulloblastoma {1920}. A more recent study on a series of *medulloblastomas with extensive nodularity* showed a very favourable outcome despite the fact that most of the patients were considered "poor risk" and were treated with chemotherapy only {1900}.

Large cell variant medulloblastomas appear to be biologically aggressive, with frequent CSF dissemination and extra CNS metastases {470,1899}. The survival of children bearing this variant was significantly shorter {1899}.

Cellular differentiation

The prognostic significance of cellular differentiation, whether neuronal or glial, is still controversial {180, 1117}. GFAP expression appears to signify a poor prognosis in medulloblastoma {485, 681}. Expression of retinal S-antigen and rhodopsin {297, 957} have been found to be associated with a better prognosis. Recent *in situ* hybridisation studies of biopsy samples extend earlier reports that TrkC receptor expression correlates with a favourable prognosis {1901}, and *in vitro* studies suggest that NT3 mediated activation of TrkC receptors might induce apoptosis thereby retarding tumour progression and resulting in a more favourable prognosis {1904}.

Proliferation

The prognostic value of tumour cell proliferation is limited. In univariate analyses it appears that the BrdU labelling index (LI) has some bearing on survival; tumours with a LI of more than 20% appeared to have a worse prognosis {650}. The percentage of cells in S-phase, as evaluated by flow cytometry, ranges from 4 to 17%

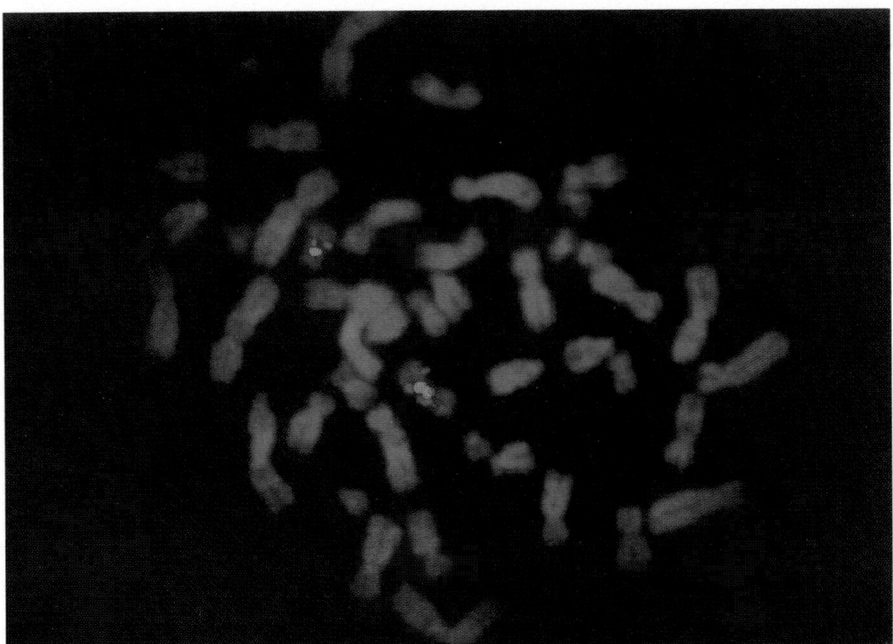

Fig. 8.16 Karyotype of medulloblastoma cell line D-556, containing an isocentric chromosome 17q, as demonstrated by fluorescence *in situ* hybridization (FISH), which shows two copies of the RARA region (red) around the centromere (green). A normal chromosome 17 only contains one copy of the RARA region.

and is unrelated to prognosis {1506, 1662}. A more favourable prognosis has been associated with aneuploidy in medulloblastoma {1506, 1662}.

In a multivariate analysis of postoperative survival of adult medulloblastoma patients, PCNA and Ki-67 LI had no prognostic value {474, 1349}. A comparison of PCNA and Ki67 LI between children and adults showed that the proliferation potential of childhood medulloblastomas may be lower than of those in adults {475}. Although BCL-2 prevents programmed cell death induced by irradiation, BCL-2-positive medulloblastomas do not recur earlier than those lacking BCL-2 expression {1057}.

Apoptosis

The degree of tumour cell apoptosis at diagnosis seems to predict treatment outcome in children with medulloblastoma as demonstrated by a recent study in which patients with a high apoptotic index had substantially improved outcome compared to all other patients, independently from the assignment to a high risk or low risk group at the time of diagnosis {1828}.

Genetic factors

Several investigators have evaluated LOH on 17p as a prognostic indicator {106}. Some studies showed a correlation between LOH on 17p and poor response to therapy {262, 263, 264}, and shortened survival time {73} while another study in 21 patients failed to demonstrate a relationship between 17p loss and survival {373}. In a recent study by Scheurlen *et al.* {1914}, all tumours with amplification of *MYC* were resistant to therapy and had a fatal outcome. Moreover, tumours that displayed LOH on 17p were associated with metastatic disease, but the prognosis of these tumours was worse only when associated with amplification of *MYC*.

Medullomyoblastoma

M.T. Giordana
O.D. Wiestler

Definition
A rare embryonal cerebellar neoplasm with both a primitive neuroectodermal and striated muscle component.

ICD-O code: 9472/3

Grading
Medullomyoblastomas are malignant and correspond histologically to WHO grade IV.

Synonyms and historical annotation
Common histogenesis, age distribution and clinical outcome suggest that the medullomyoblastoma constitutes a variant of medulloblastoma.

Incidence
Originally reported in 1933 {962}, 33 cases have been described to date.

Age and sex distribution
From a clinical viewpoint, the cases are rather homogeneous. All but two cases {448, 1231} were observed in children aged 2.5–10.5 years (mean age, 7.4); the two adults were 26 and 40 years old. There is a predominance of male patients (male: female ratio, 3.8:1).

Localization
In all but two cases, the tumour was in the vermis, with some tumours projecting into, and invading the fourth ventricle, cerebellar hemisphere and brain stem; in the remaining cases, the tumour developed in the cerebellar hemisphere.

Clinical features
The preoperative duration of symptoms and neuroimaging findings are similar to those seen in medulloblastoma {241, 608, 1231, 1358, 1432}.

Macroscopy
The tumour is soft, moderately vascular and may be partially necrotic.

Histopathology
The microscopic aspect is largely that of a medulloblastoma with focal myogenic differentiation.

The additional muscle component consists of striated muscle fibers collected in bundles or around vessels; the spindle cells are occasionally accompanied by round or oval cells with abundant eosinophilic cytoplasm {1432}. Round cells may be numerous. Occasionally, strap-like cells with cross-striation are observed {1231}. An additional smooth muscle component was found in two cases {448, 1683}; however, this was not confirmed immunohistochemically. The muscle cells are either intimately admixed with primitive neuroectodermal cells, or collected in distinct areas. Melanin-containing cells have also been reported {720}.

Immunohistochemical and ultrastructural studies
The immunohistochemical expression of neuronal and/or glial antigen by the small-cell component documents the neuroectodermal nature of this portion of the tumour, and is helpful in the differential diagnosis towards a primitive cerebellar rhabdomyosarcoma. Evidence of advanced neuronal differentiation has frequently been reported, in some cases with features of a hamartomatous component, which contains clusters of neuronal elements and immature oligodendroglia-like cells {608}. The ultrastructural observation of dense-core vesicles, synapse-like structures, rows of microtubules and bundles of intermediate filaments of glial type confirms the neuroectodermal origin. Muscle cells are reactive for myoglobin {335, 608, 1432}, desmin {608, 1358} and fast myosin {720}, and negative for smooth-muscle actin {608, 1358}. Electron microscopy shows thick and thin filaments arranged in sarcomeres and Z-band material {608, 720, 1358, 1432}. The primitive myoblastic cells have rudimentary Z-line-like densities {1432}.

Proliferation
Studies using antibodies to the proliferation-associated Ki-67 antigen usually show significant proliferative activity in the medulloblastoma component. Labelling indices of the muscle element are generally lower but vary considerably.

Histogenesis
Several hypotheses on the nature and origin of medullomyoblastoma have been put forward {1231}. Undifferentiated neuroectodermal cells in medulloblastoma can undergo not only neuronal and/or glial differentiation, but also myoblastic differentiation. Desmin is expressed in primitive

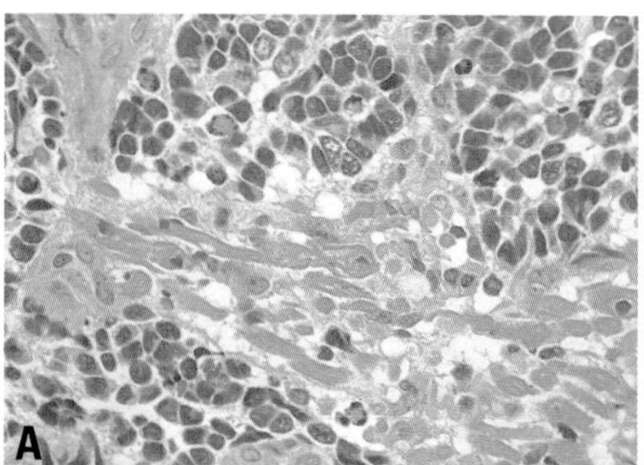

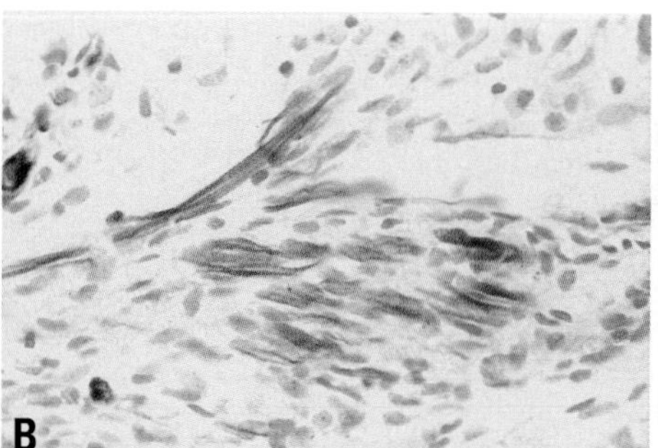

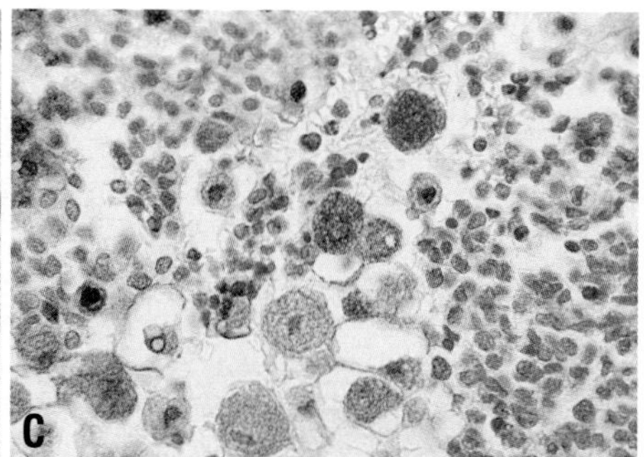

Fig. 8.17 Medullomyoblastoma showing **(A)** striated muscle fibers on the background of a medulloblastoma with brisk mitotic activity, **(B)** anti-fast-myosin immunostaining of highly differentiated, striated myogenic cells, **(C)** biphasic pattern of small undifferentiated medulloblastoma cells and large rhabdomyoblasts immunostaining for myoglobin.

neuroectodermal tumour cells that are devoid of advanced myoblastic differentiation; features of transition from immature tumour cells to frank myocytes can be found in medullomyoblastoma {608}. In addition, there is evidence from neurobiological studies that nestin-positive cerebellar precursor cells may undergo both neuroglial and myogenic differentiation {1533}. These observations point to a neuroectodermal origin for the myogenic tumour component.

The coexistence of areas of well-differentiated teratoma {241} has been viewed as evidence that medullomyoblastoma may constitute a variant of malignant teratoma {1306}. However, the usual absence of other tissue elements argues strongly against this hypothesis.

It has also been proposed that the muscle component may originate from neural-crest-derived ectomesenchyme. Ectomesenchyme gives rise to the leptomeninges; the occasional finding of striated muscle fibers {608} and of primary rhabdomyosarcomas in the leptomeninges lend support to the pluripotential nature of ectomesenchyme.

Predictive factors

The biological and clinical behaviour of medullomyoblastoma is similar to that of the medulloblastoma. A postoperative survival of longer than one year was reported in only four patients, all of whom underwent postoperative radiotherapy.

Melanotic medulloblastoma

H. Kalimo
H. Haapasalo

Definition
A rare tumour of childhood with a predominant element of small round cells closely resembling classic medulloblastoma and a minor component of melanin-forming neuroepithelial cells.

ICD-O code:
The provisional code proposed for the third edition of ICD-O is 9470/3.

Grading
Melanotic medulloblastoma corresponds histologically to WHO grade IV.

Synonyms and historical annotation
Common histogenesis, age distribution and clinical outcome suggest that this tumour constitutes a variant of medulloblastoma.

Incidence
The first melanotic medulloblastoma was described by Fowler and Simpson in 1962 {426}. Since then, only approximately 10 similar tumours have been reported.

Age and sex distribution
All patients reported with these lesions have been children (aged 1–9 years), except for one equivocal case of a 21-year-old male {525}. Only one female patient has been reported {1296}.

Localization
Most often, the primary tumour resides in these cerebellar vermis, though in one case it may have originated in the pineal gland {101}.

Clinical features
The clinical signs and symptoms are those of an expanding process in the posterior fossa and largely correspond to those of the ordinary medulloblastoma.

Histopathology and immunohistochemical findings
This variant of medulloblastoma contains focal accumulations of melanotic tumour cells. As the name indicates, the predominant component closely resembles medulloblastoma. Small cells show immunoreactivity for vimentin, synaptophysin, neurofilament, neuron-specific enolase, or S100 {343, 2336}. Homer-Wright rosettes, vesicular nuclei with prominent nucleoli and/or triangular cell bodies indicate neuronal differentiation. In some neoplastic cells, immunoreactivity to GFAP has also been observed {454, 702}.
The pattern of the melanotic cells and type of melanin vary to such an extent that it has been questioned whether melanotic medulloblastomas represent a single entity. Most often, melanotic cells appear epithelial and form tubules, papillae {101, 343, 426, 454, 1471, 2336}, or clusters {136, 525, 702}. Ultrastructural analysis of some tumours has verified that the pigment is oculocutaneous melanin with distinct melanosomes {136, 343, 454, 702}. This indicates a formation of melanin by enzymatic oxidation of tyrosine into dopa, with further conversion into polymerized 5,6-indolequinone, to be deposited upon the lattice of premelanosomes. In cells with high catecholamine content, neuromelanin is formed by auto-oxidation of catecholamines into quinones to be polymerized within lysosomal residual bodies; thus, ultrastructurally, neuromelanin looks like compact lipofuscin {1046}. It is possible that in some melanotic medulloblastomas, the pigment is neuromelanin. Melanotic cells may, expectedly, immunostain for S100 {454, 2336}, but they may also be negative, as described for cells of the ocular pigment layer at very early stages of development {343}. In one case melanotic cells were vimentin positive, but HMB-45, EMA and cytokeratin negative {2336}.
Melanotic medulloblastomas tend to disseminate via the CSF. Disseminated pigmented cells may appear as black speckling in the subarachnoid space. In a single case, the extracranial metastases did not show pigmentation {343}.

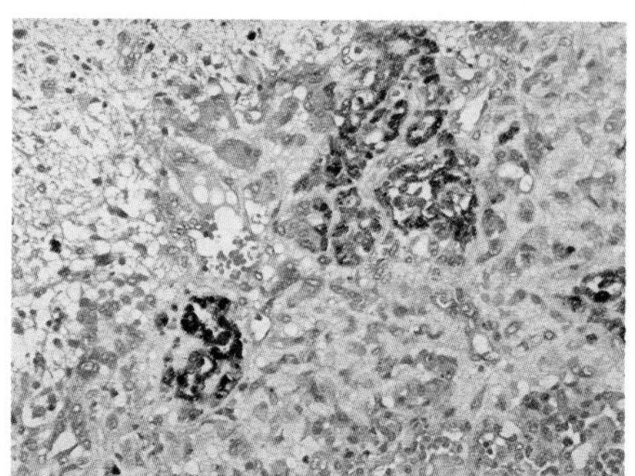

Fig. 8.18 Melanotic cells commonly appear as tubular epithelial structures.

Histogenesis
An origin of melanotic medulloblastomas from neural crest tissue has been proposed. On the other hand, tight junctions and basal lamina like those found in melanotic medulloblastoma have also been described between pigmented cells of the ocular pigment epithelium, which is of neural tube origin {343}.
As pigmented cells may also occur in medullomyoblastoma {720}, myogenic cells should be looked for in cases of melanotic medulloblastomas. This raises the issue of whether melanotic medulloblastomas and medullomyoblastomas simply represent subtypes of medulloblastoma. No molecular genetic data are currently available that could prove or disprove this assumption.
Melanotic medulloblastoma has been related to, or even equated with, the more common melanotic neuroectodermal tumour of infancy (MNTI; melanotic progonoma), which has similar cellular components. MNTI is, however, almost always benign, located extracranially and can be distinguished from melanotic medulloblastoma by immunoreactivity for HMB-45, EMA and cytokeratin {2336}. Thus, there is no compelling evidence to suggest that the two tumour types are closely related.

Predictive factors
The clinical outcome is poor, with postoperative survival ranging from 2 months to 2.5 years. In a single case, the tumour was considered cured by radical surgery and radiation therapy, since it had not recurred 10 years later, when the patient died of a cerebellar glioblastoma regarded as a separate, secondary tumour, possibly related to the radiation and/or growth hormone therapy given {2336}.

Supratentorial primitive neuroectodermal tumour (PNET)

L.B. Rorke
M.N. Hart
R.E. McLendon

Definition

An embryonal tumour in the cerebrum or suprasellar region composed of undifferentiated or poorly differentiated neuroepithelial cells which have the capacity for or display divergent differentiation along neuronal, astrocytic, ependymal, muscular or melanocytic lines. Tumours with a distinct neuronal differentiation are termed *cerebral neuroblastoma* or, if ganglion cells are also present, ganglioneuroblastoma.

ICD-O codes:

Supratentorial PNET	9473/3
Cerebral neuroblastoma	9500/3
Cerebral ganglioneuroblastoma	9490/3

Grading

As other primitive neuroectodermal tumours, supratentorial PNETs correspond histologically to WHO grade IV.

Synonyms

Tumours with these histological features have been called by a number of different names, including cerebral medulloblastoma {57, 292}, cerebral neuroblastoma {615}, cerebral ganglioneuroblastoma {615}, 'blue tumour' {870}, and primitive neuroectodermal tumour {544}. It is suggested to use the term 'supratententorial PNET'; ICD-O codes for lesions with neuroblastic (cerebral neuroblastoma) or advanced neuronal differentiation (cerebral ganglioneuroblastoma) have been retained.

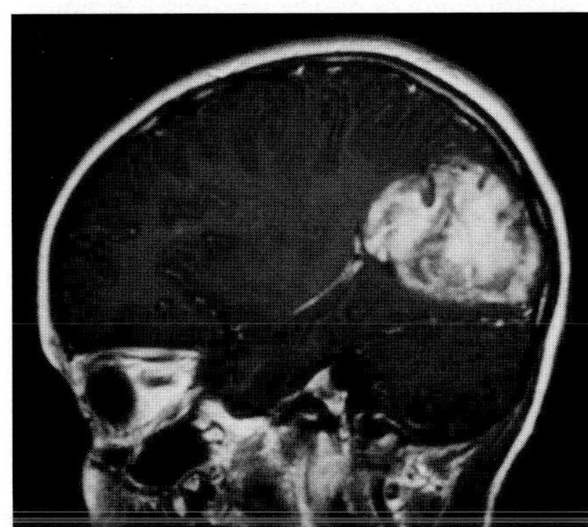

Fig. 8.19 Sagittal, gadolinium enhanced MRI of an occipital PNET that extends to the posterior horn of the lateral ventricle.

Incidence

PNETs in the supratentorial compartment are uncommon. Precise statistics of incidence are difficult to determine because of differing viewpoints regarding classification. One percent of 933 primary paediatric CNS neuroepithelial tumours were found to be located in the cerebrum or suprasellar region; among CNS PNETs, 10 out of 178 (5.6%) were located in these regions [Rorke, unpublished observation].

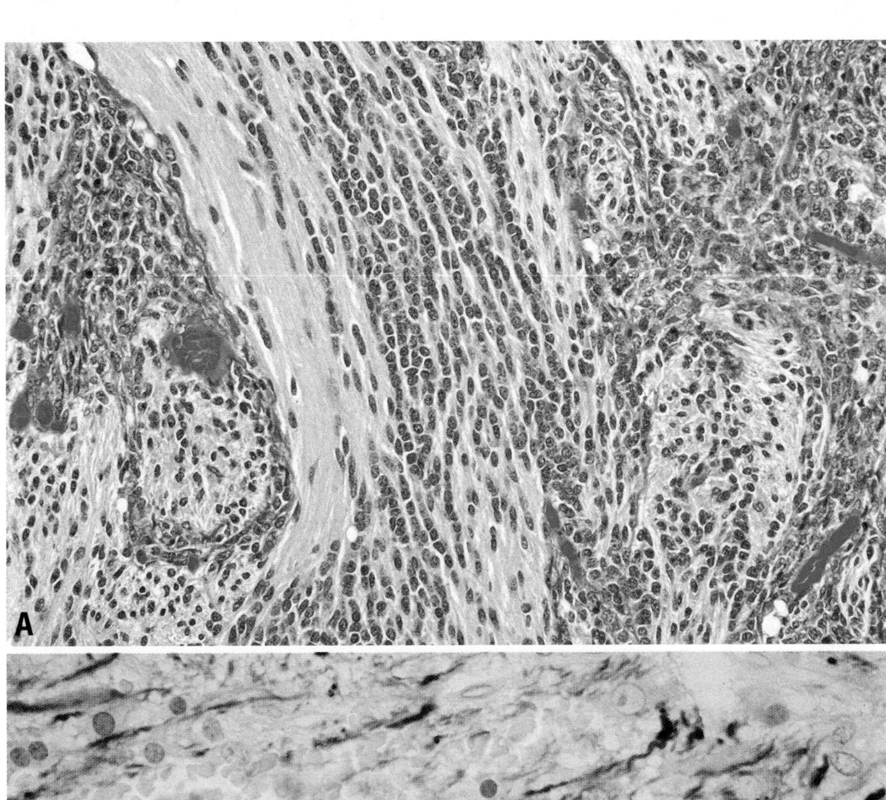

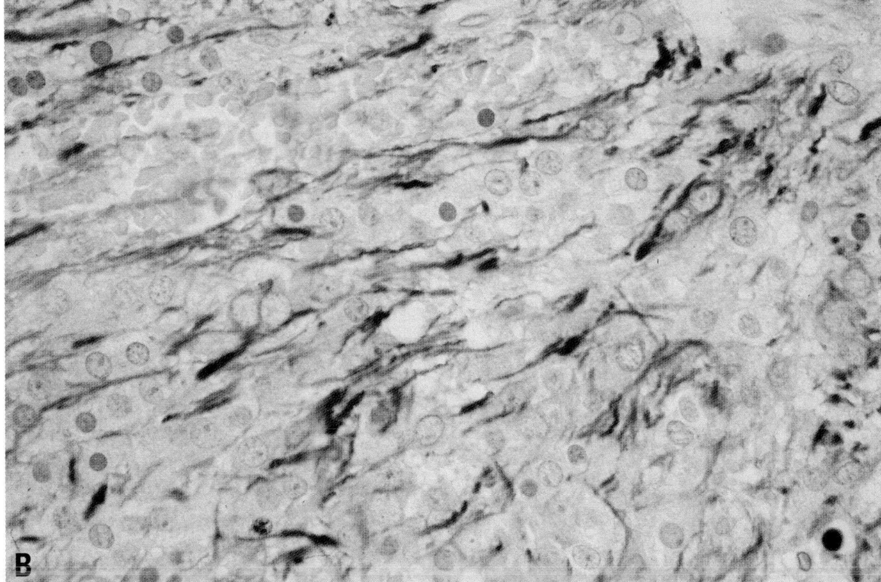

Fig. 8.20 A Supratentorial PNET with advanced neuronal differentiation (cerebral neuroblastoma) exhibiting a nodular architecture with typical streaming of tumour cells. **B** Neurofilament staining predominantly of tumour cell processes.

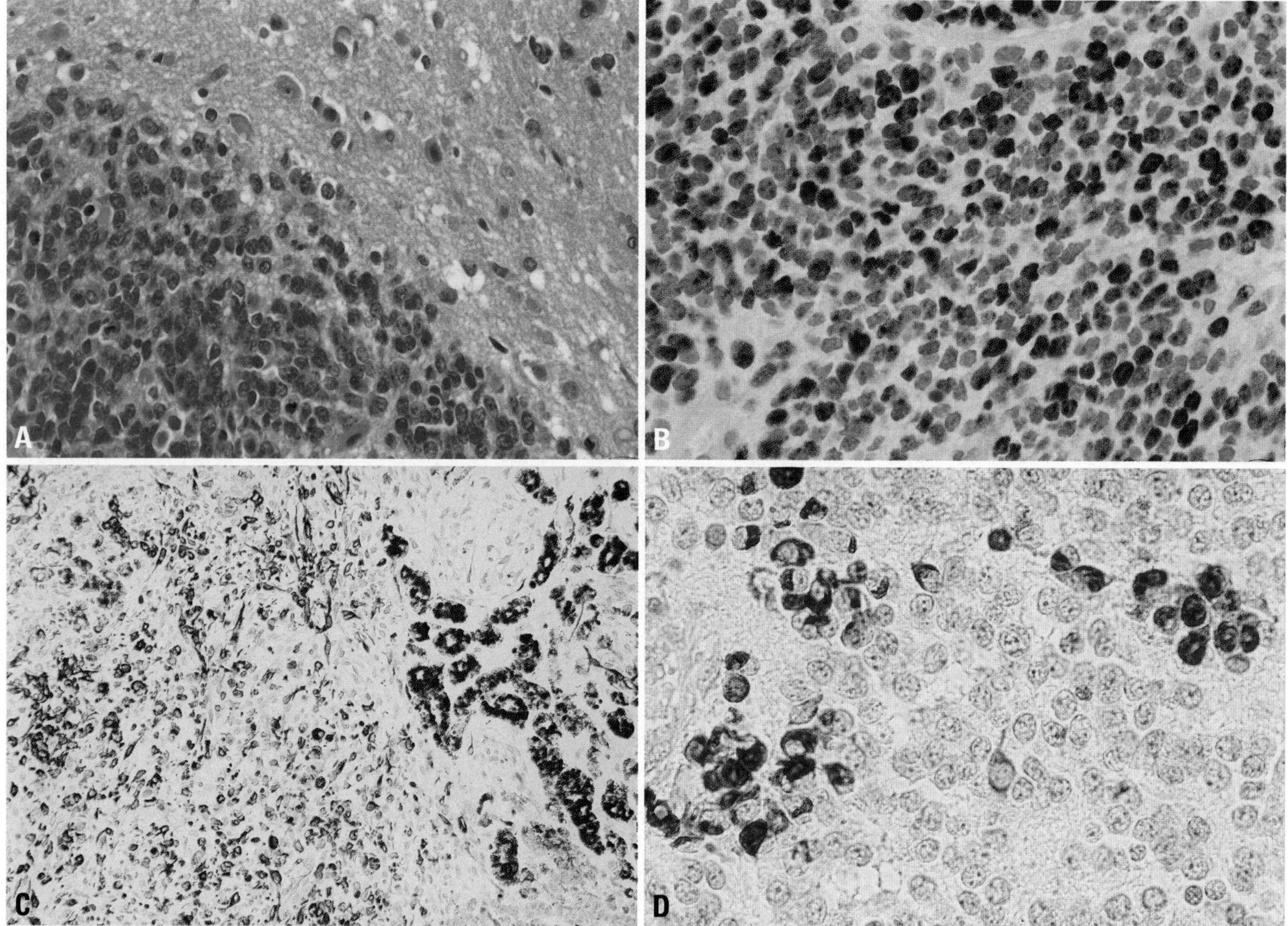

Fig. 8.21 Histological features of supratentorial PNET. **A** Highly cellular tumour, well demarcated from the adjacent brain, with brisk mitotic activity. **B** Very high MIB-1 labeling index. **C** Pineal pigmented PNET with strong neurofilament protein (NFP) expression. **D** Clusters of GFAP-expressing tumour cells suggestive of clonal evolution.

Age and sex distribution

The age range for cerebral-suprasellar PNETs is 4 weeks to 10 years, with a mean of 5.5 years. The male: female ratio is 2:1.

Localization

As indicated by the terminology, these tumours are found in the supratentorial space occupied by the cerebrum or suprasellar region. Pineal region PNETs (pineoblastoma) are considered elsewhere (see Chapter 7).

Clinical features

Signs and symptoms are related to the site of origin of the tumour. Those arising in the cerebrum often present with seizures, disturbances of consciousness, increased intracranial pressure or motor deficit. The suprasellar lesions produce visual and/or endocrine problems. If the patient is an infant, the head circumference may increase more rapidly than normal.

Neuroimaging

Computed tomographic findings in PNETs are similar, regardless of the site of origin of the tumour. They are iso-to-hyperdense, but density increases following injection of contrast material. They may appear as solid masses or may contain cystic or necrotic areas. Between 50 and 70% of all supratentorial PNETs contain calcium. Oedema surrounding parenchymal masses is not usually extensive {1678}.

Appearance of PNETs on magnetic resonance imaging may vary with the site of origin. On T1-weighted MRI, the tumours are hypointense relative to cortical grey matter. They look similar on T2-weighted imaging, but cystic or necrotic areas are hyperintense. There is contrast enhancement with gadolinium or T1-weighted imaging. If the tumour has bled, the region of haemorrhage is hypointense on T2-weighted imaging {1679}.

Macroscopy

The tumours are of variable size at the time of clinical presentation. Those in the suprasellar region tend to be smaller than those in the cerebrum. The parenchymal tumours may be massive growths, with or without cysts or haemorrhages. Demarcation between tumour and brain may range from indistinct to clear-cut. They have a pink-red colour. They are soft unless they contain a prominent desmoplastic component, in which case they are more firm and have a tan colour.

Histopathology

Light microscopic features of cerebral-suprasellar PNETs are basically similar to medulloblastoma. The tumours are composed of undifferentiated or poorly-differentiated neuroepithelial cells, which may vary somewhat in their morphological features.

Most commonly, the component cell has

a small, round, deeply basophilic nucleus, rich in chromatin, and little or no surrounding perikaryon. Cells in some tumours have larger, more pleomorphic nuclei with oval or even angular configurations. Nucleoli are not common but may be seen, and mitotic activity is variable. Cells with the pleomorphic nuclei often have recognizable surrounding cytoplasm. These densely cellular tumours have a relatively inconspicuous background granulo-fibrillar matrix. Individual cell necrosis is common and presents features of karyorrhexis or apoptosis. Field necrosis and/ or haemorrhages may also be present. Homer-Wright rosettes, ependymal canals or Flexner-Wintersteiner rosettes may be found. Rarely, melanin-bearing cells are observed. As in cerebellar medulloblastomas, tumour cells may be distributed in a linear fashion along delicate fibers, or stream within a neuropil-type background. Poorly-defined or discrete fields of more recognizable neuronal or glial cells are sometimes identified.

In rare examples, there is a combination of primitive-appearing and terminally differentiated cells (ganglioneuroblastoma). Cerebral PNETs have a variable desmoplastic component, most typically fibrocollagenous in nature, but in rare examples may consist of mature smooth or striated muscle. Alternatively, the primitive-appearing cells may express muscle antigens.

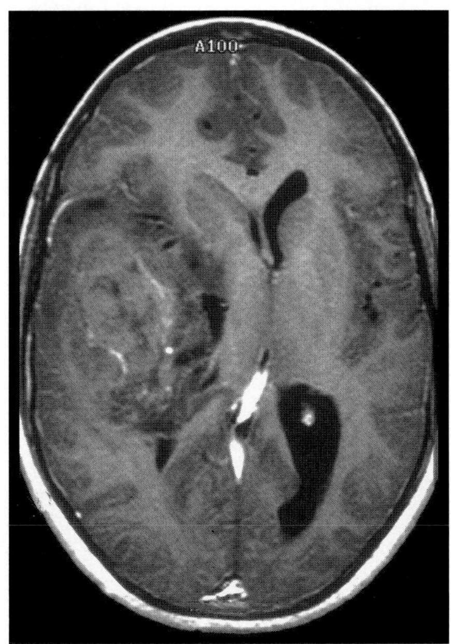

Fig. 8.22 T1-weighted MRI of a large, hemispheric PNET with advanced neuronal differentiation (neuroblastoma).

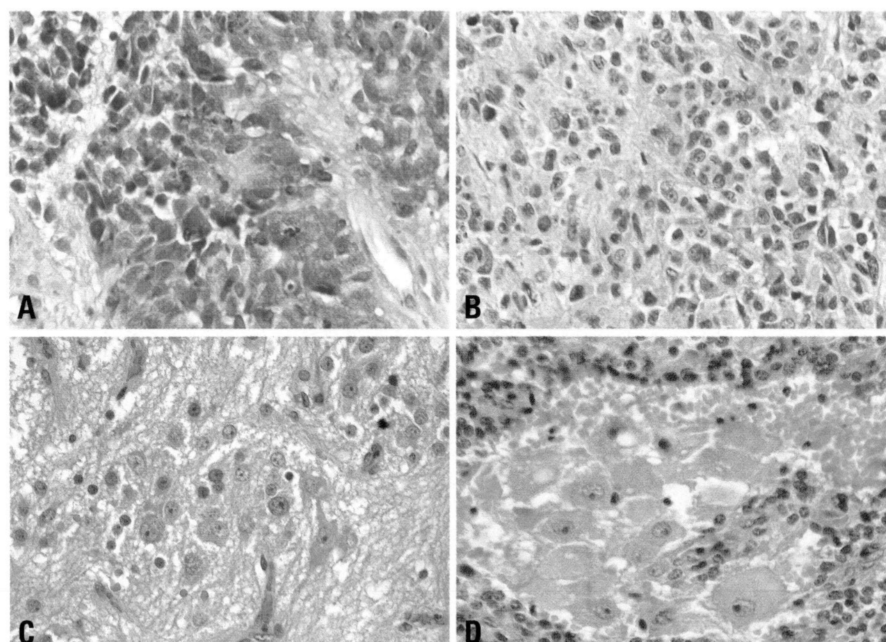

Fig. 8.23 **A** Cerebral neuroblastoma with poorly differentiated, irregularly shaped cells. **B** Tumour cells in different stages of neuronal differentiation. **C** Region of low cellularity in a ganglioneuroblastoma showing some tumour cells with neuronal phenotype. **D** Cluster of mature ganglion cells next to an area of poorly differentiated elements.

Immunohistochemistry

Evidence of divergent differentiation in cells, which with routine staining methods appear to be primitive, is most reliably identified by use of various antibodies. Most useful, because of their general availability, are GFAP, NFP and desmin. Many others, such as synaptophysin, vimentin and keratin could be used, but do not add significant diagnostic information. In fact, synaptophysin and other neuroendocrine markers are consistently identified {497}. If feasible, expression of retinal S-antigen and/or rhodopsin can be investigated {801}. Elaborate studies of neuronal differentiation can also be done provided that appropriate antibodies are available, *i.e.* NFP low-, medium- and high-molecular weight, MAP II, beta tubulin, etc. {1022}. Antigen expression is unique for each tumour, making prediction of patterns of expression for one or a group of tumours unreliable.

Electron microscopy

The typical tumour is very poorly differentiated, revealing only a sparse population of cytoplasmic organelles. While microtubules may be found, dense core vesicles, although not always present, are diagnostic of neuroblastoma. With ganglionic differentiation, some processes may terminate as growth cones containing arrays of microtubules. Demonstration of synapses is exceptional {1256}. Compact arrays of cytoplasmic glial filaments supports glial differentiation, although intervening reactive astrocytes must be ruled out.

Ultrastructural features may also reflect the sample examined and hence present a variable picture, depending upon whether the tumour is differentiating along neuronal, glial (including ependymal) or muscular lines {1306}.

Proliferation

PNETs at any site show a variable amount of mitotic activity that is most accurately measured by use of the proliferation marker Ki-67. The percentage of cells undergoing proliferation is generally high but may vary from 0-85% in any given high power field.

Cytogenetics

Only a limited number of cytogenetic studies of supratentorial PNETs (S-PNET) have been done. The i(17)q abnormality found in 30 to 50% of medulloblastomas has been found in only one S-PNET {1209}. Studies of Burnett *et al.* {2190} of 8 S-PNETs and Feuerstein {2193} of 10 such tumours disclosed a variety of non-random cytogenetic gains and losses, but no i(17)q {121}. Bigner *et al.* {121} noted two cases of neuroblastoma with normal karyotypes.

Scattered reports of other genetic abnormalities in these tumours include identification of *MYCN* expression {2194}, germline mutation of *TP53* {2129}, expression of the Neuro D family of basic helix-loop-helix transcription factors, and achaete scute, another neurogenic transcription factor with homology to *Neuro D* genes {2195}. This latter gene was actually expressed in 3 of 5 S-PNETs but not in medulloblastoma PNETs (MB). Thus, although the number of cytogenetic studies of S-PNETs is small, it appears that genetic events associated with development of PNETs in the supratentorial compartment are different from those that arise in the cerebellum. This view is supported by a recent CGH study comparing S-PNETS with medulloblastomas {2578}.

Histogenesis

The histogenesis of PNETs as a group has been a controversial issue for many years (see Histogenesis of medulloblastoma, this chapter), and the only issue upon which consensus has been achieved is that these embryonal tumours arise from primitive neuroepithelial cells where ever they happen to be located in the CNS {780, 1279}.

Predictive factors

Infants who are less than two years old at the time of diagnosis of a supratentorial PNET have a bleaker prognosis than older children {462}. Children with S-PNET have an overall 5-year survival rate of 34%, in contrast to 85% for children with a PNET arising in the posterior fossa {21,1281}. Many studies have addressed the relationship between survival and various histological features of cerebellar PNETs. However, the rarity of S-PNETs has precluded similar analyses for tumours in cerebral-suprasellar sites.

Atypical teratoid / rhabdoid tumour

L.B. Rorke
J.A. Biegel

Definition

A malignant embryonal CNS tumour manifesting in children and composed of rhabdoid cells, with or without fields resembling a classical primitive neuroectodermal tumour (PNET), epithelial tissue and neoplastic mesenchyme.

ICDO-code: 9508/3

Grading

Histological features and the poor clinical outcome indicate that these tumours correspond to WHO grade IV.

Synonyms and historical annotation

The unique clinical, biological and histological features of this tumour have been defined over the past 14 years {1280}. Its biological characteristics and some of the histological features are similar to those of the malignant rhabdoid tumour of the kidney (MRTK) of infancy {1592}. The first example affecting the CNS was reported in 1985 {7} and simply called 'rhabdoid tumour'. Others, giving attention to the small cell embryonal component, placed these tumours in that category, and ignored the other features. Rorke *et al.* {1280} named them 'atypical teratoid/rhabdoid tumours' (AT/RT) to call attention to the disparate combination of rhabdoid, primitive neuroepithelial, epithelial and mesenchymal components. This suggested a teratomatous tumour, but one which looked different from the more familiar teratomas and, furthermore, was consistently negative for routine germ-cell markers. Complicating the picture was the observation that some infants with MRTK also had a CNS embryonal tumour {145}.

Incidence

Accurate data relative to incidence are difficult to obtain since this tumour has been generally misdiagnosed until the past few years. Although a total of 97 cases had been reported by early 1997 {2191}; 91 additional cases have been documented to date {2174, 2180, 2183, 2175, 2176, 412, 613, 2181, 2184, 2182, 2185, 2192, 2178, 2179, 2177} [Rorke, unpublished observation]. In total, 2.1% of a group of 930 primary CNS tumours in children 18 years or less, diagnosed at The Children's Hospital of Philadelphia between July 1979 and June 1999, were AT/RT [Rorke, unpublished observation].

Age and sex distribution

Of the 188 cases observed to date, 184 have been infants or children, 94% of whom were five years of age or less at diagnosis. The average age of the four adults was 32 years (21-41 years). The male: female ratio in paediatric cases is 1.4:1; males were also predominant among the small group of adults, 3:1 {2174, 613, 2188} [Rorke, unpublished observation].

Localization

Distribution of the 184 primary childhood AT/RTs is as follows: posterior fossa, 52% (cerebellum, cerebello-pontine angle, and/or brainstem); supratentorial, 39% (cerebral or suprasellar); pineal, 5%; multifocal, 2%; spinal, 2%. Tumours in the adults were all located in the cerebrum. The tendency to arise in the cerebello-pontine angle with invasion of surrounding structures is a distinct feature of this tumour. One-third of patients already has metastases throughout the cerebrospinal pathways at presentation.

Clinical features

Symptoms and signs

Clinical presentation is variable, depending upon the age of the patient, location, and size of the tumour. Infants, in particular, present with non-specific signs of lethargy, vomiting, and/or failure to thrive. More specific problems include head tilt and cranial nerve palsy (most commonly sixth and seventh nerve paresis). Headache and hemiplegia are more common in children older than three years.

Neuroimaging

Findings on both computerized tomography (CT) and magnetic resonance imaging (MRI) are similar to those seen in patients with medulloblastoma. Specifically, there is increased density on unenhanced CT images and inhomogeneous contrast enhancement. Cysts and haemorrhage are common. On MRI, there is decreased density on T1-weighted images, iso- or decreased density on T2, isointensity on proton density, and enhancement with gadolinium {1280}.

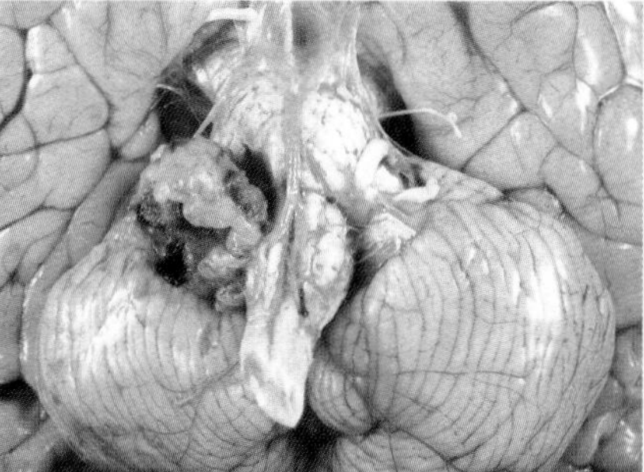

Fig. 8.24 Atypical teratoid/rhabdoid tumour with multiple haemorrhages, arising in the right cerebellopontine angle.

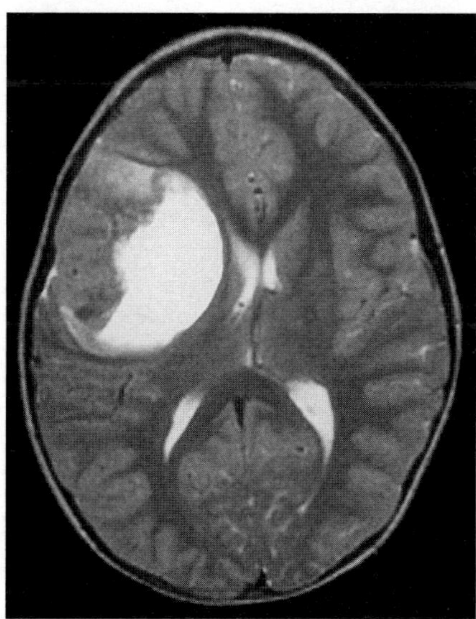

Fig. 8.25 Gadolinium enhanced, T1 weighted MRI of a large, cystic supratentorial atypical teratoid/rhabdoid tumour.

Macroscopy

These tumours have the same basic gross appearance as more classical medulloblastomas. They tend to be soft, pinkish-red, often bulky neoplasms that, in places,

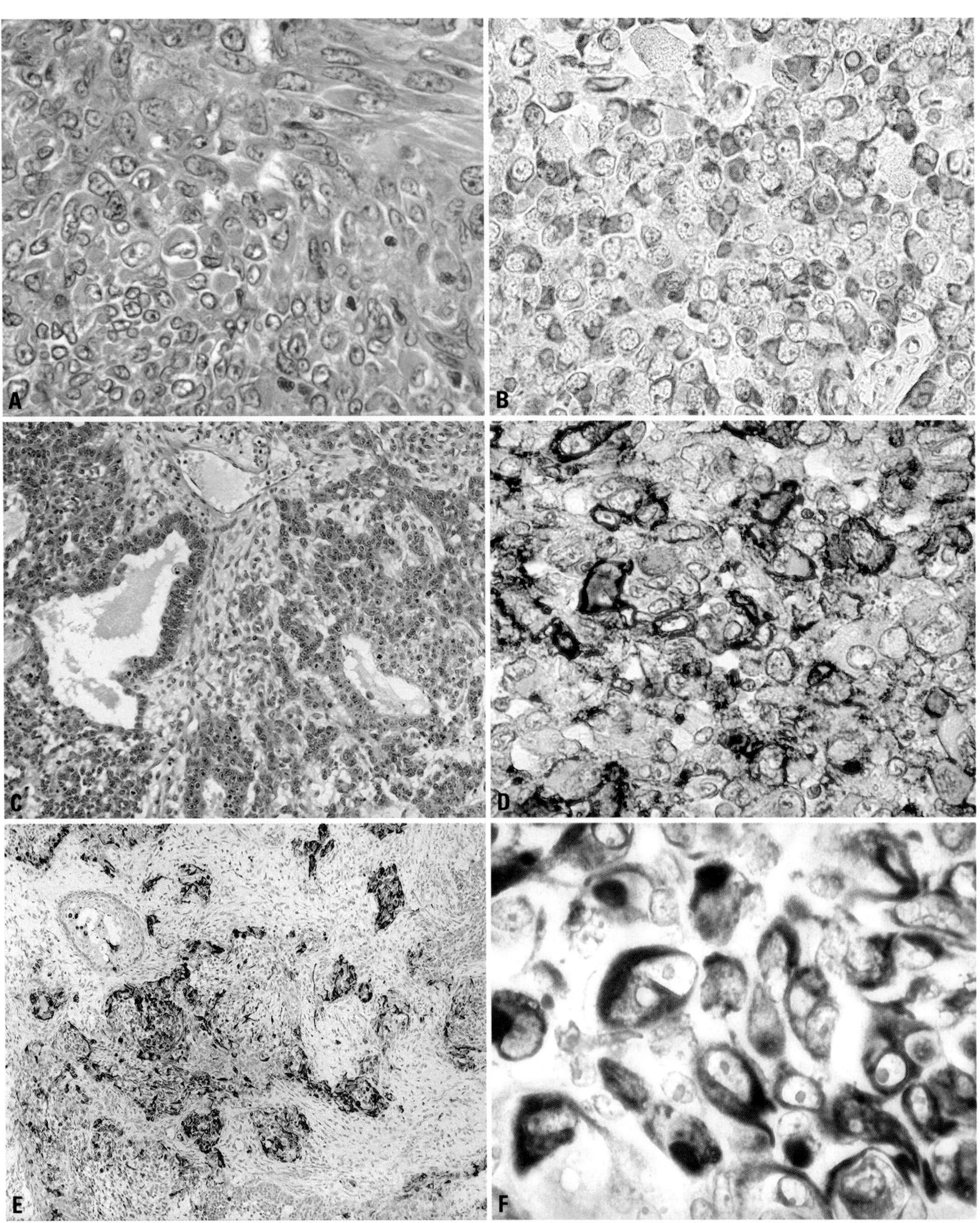

Fig. 8.26 Features of atypical teratoid/rhabdoid tumours. **A** Rhabdoid cells with pink cytoplasm and prominent nucleoli. **B** Expression of smooth muscle actin (SMA) by numerous cells. **C** Glandular component with a central mesenchymal area. **D** Expression of epithelial membrane antigen. **E** Patchy expression of GFAP, accentuated at the interface with mesenchymal tissue. **F** Expression of neurofilament (NF) by rhabdoid cells.

appear to be demarcated from adjacent parenchyma. They typically contain necrotic foci and may be haemorrhagic. Those with significant amounts of mesenchymal tissue are firm and tan-white in some regions. Tumours arising in the cerebellopontine angle wrap themselves around cranial nerves and vessels and invade brainstem and cerebellum to a variable extent. Deposits along cerebrospinal pathways are similar to medulloblastomas and other PNETs.

Histopathology

A tumour containing rhabdoid cells, usually with additional, variable components of primitive neuroectodermal, mesenchymal and epithelial cells.

Histological features are straightforward or complex, depending upon the number of different tissue types that are present {2176, 1280}. Obviously, all tumours contain a population of rhabdoid cells; in some instances, the tumour consists of only such cells. Specific details relative to histological features are not provided in all case reports, hence the frequency of specific component tissue types cannot be gauged against those reported earlier. Evaluation of 52 AT/RTs in children disclosed that 15% consisted only of rhabdoid cells. However, two-thirds have a major small cell embryonal component, one-third a mesenchymal component, in combination with rhabdoid fields with or without small cell embryonal areas, and one-quarter contain neoplastic epithelium, which may be adenomatous, squamous or simply arranged in nests {1280}.

The typical rhabdoid cell is medium-sized, round to oval, with an eccentric nucleus that commonly has a prominent nucleolus. Cytoplasm has a fine granular homogeneous character or may contain a poorly defined denser pink 'body' resembling an inclusion. Cell borders are typically distinct. Mitotic figures are usually abundant. Small rhabdoid cells may have a tapering cytoplasmic tail, whereas others may be huge, bizarre forms with more than one nucleus. Electron microscopically, rhabdoid cells typically contain whorled bundles of intermediate filaments which fill much of the perikaryon {114, 1695}.

The small cell embryonal component may consist only of sheets of primitive neuroepithelial cells or may display Homer-Wright or Flexner-Wintersteiner rosettes. Ependymal canals or neural-tube-like structures are rarely present.

Mesenchymal fields appear either as loose arrangements of small spindle cells or are more tightly arranged in a fascicular pattern resembling frank sarcoma {490}. The epithelial tissue may form an adenomatous pattern suggestive of adenocarcinoma, or may be confused with choroid plexus carcinoma. Rarely, squamous epithelium or nests of cells expressing keratin with no particular distinguishing features are scattered about. Field necrosis is common. The vasculature displays no unique features, but haemorrhages are common.

Immunohistochemistry

Application of a panel of monoclonal antibodies with the immunoperoxidase method yields a unique pattern of expression. This is complex, primarily because of the disparate tissue components forming these tumours. The rhabdoid cells almost always express EMA and vimentin, but not so consistently smooth-muscle actin (SMA). They may also express GFAP, NFP and keratin, but do not express desmin or any of the markers for germ cell tumours. Small cell embryonal portions

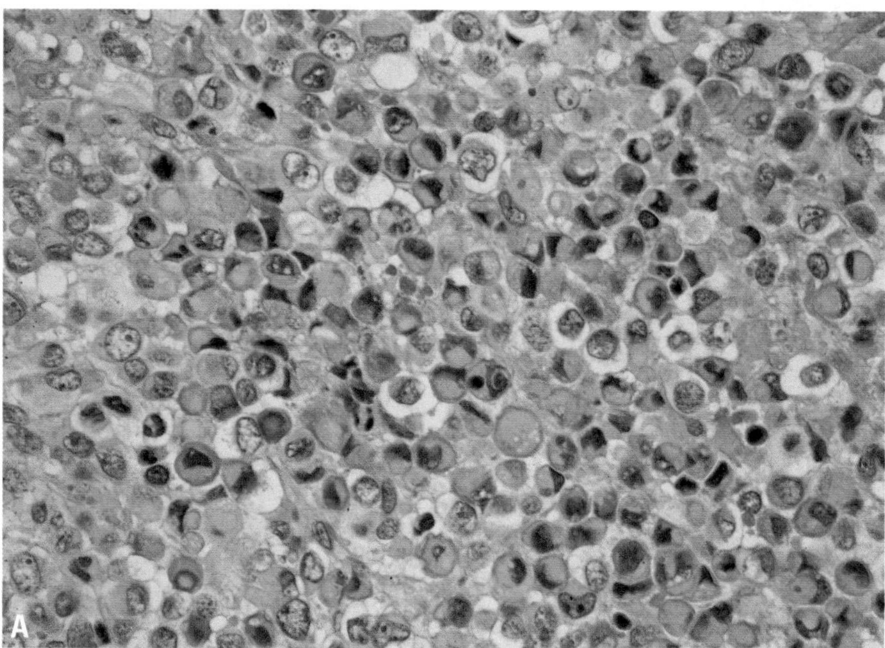

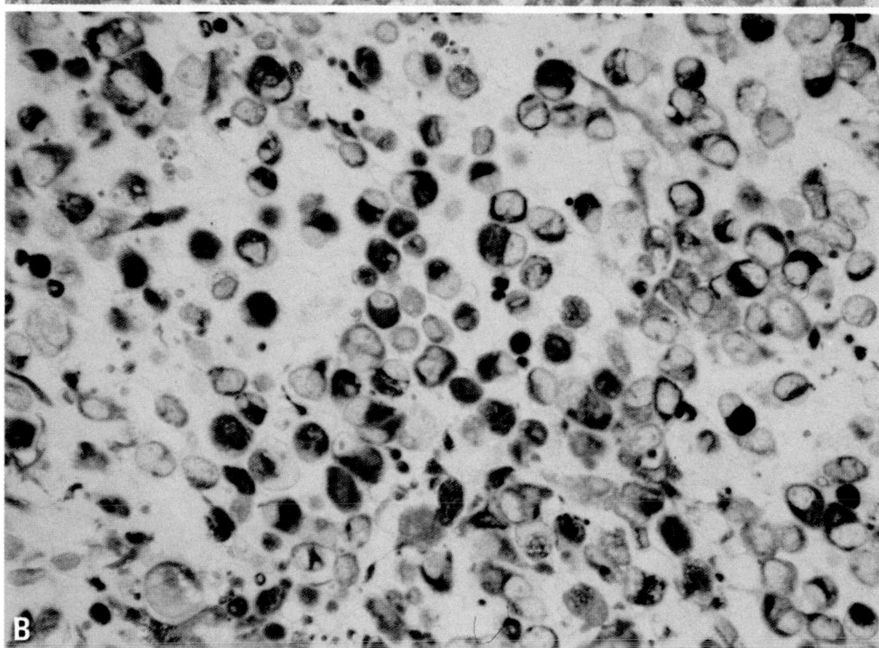

Fig. 8.27 Typical rhabdoid cells with (**A**) eccentric nuclei and prominent nucleoli, most of which show strong cytoplasmic vimentin immunoreactivity (**B**).

variably express vimentin, GFAP, NFP, and/ or desmin, mesenchymal tissue expresses vimentin and occasionally SMA and/or desmin, and epithelial portions express keratin, and less commonly, vimentin and/ or EMA.

Proliferation

These tumours have marked proliferative activity, and labelling indices with Ki67/ MIB-1 indicate a growth fraction of focally up to 80%.

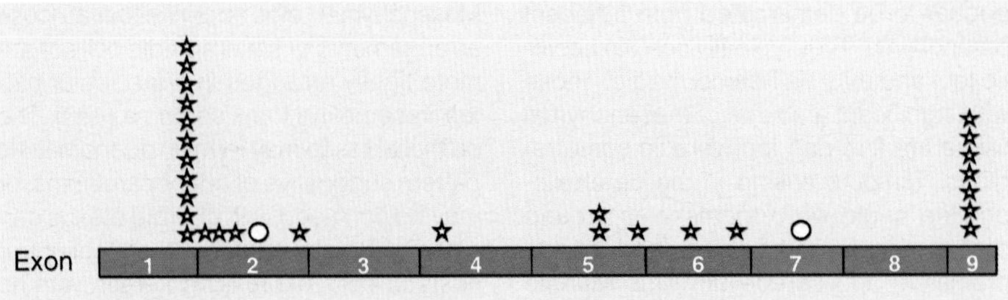

Fig. 8.28 Distribution of germline (circles) and somatic (stars) mutations in exons 1-9 of the *INI1* gene. Results are representative of 29 patients with CNS AT/RT.

Histogenesis

The precise nature of the rhabdoid cell is unknown. Opinions regarding this issue suggest that it is histiocytic {1112}, mesenchymal {114}, neuroectomesenchymal {1112}, meningeal {239} or of germ cell-cell lineage {1280}.

Genetics

Ninety percent of CNS AT/RTs demonstrate monosomy or a deletion of chromosome 22 by fluorescence *in situ* hybridization or loss of heterozygosity studies {2175}. The gene involved in AT/RTs, *hSNF5/INI1*, maps to chromosome band 22q11.2 {2175, 2189}.

The *INI1* gene contains 9 exons and has a coding sequence of approximately 1.2 kb {2187}. This gene is ubiquitously expressed {2187}. A cryptic splice donor site in exon 2 results in an alternate transcript expressed in all tissues. The INI1 protein is a component of the mammalian SWI/ SNF complex, which functions in an ATP-dependent manner to alter chromatin structure {2188}. The specific function of INI1, and its role in malignant transformation is unknown.

Somatic mutations or intragenic deletions have been documented in 22 AT/RTs, most of which create a novel stop codon. Although mutations have been observed throughout the coding sequence (Fig. 14.28), there appear to be two potential hot spots, including a deletion/mutation of exon 1, and a single base pair deletion in exon 9. Germline *INI1* mutations have been detected in two patients with AT/RTs and 4 patients with renal rhabdoid tumours {2175}. One child had a CNS and a renal rhabdoid tumour. The specificity of *INI1* abnormalities for rhabdoid tumours has yet to be determined.

Predictive factors

Experience to date indicates that the majority of patients with AT/RT die within a year of diagnosis {2176, 1280}. There does not appear to be any clear difference in survival as a function of age. Maximum periods of survival have been reported for three patients: one of four years (a five-year old who was still alive at the time of the case report {2181}, another child who survived for 5 years {1280}, and an adult who lived for six years following diagnosis {613}.

CHAPTER 9

Peripheral Neuroblastic Tumours

Neuroblastic tumours outside the central nervous system are clinically important neoplasms constituting a significant diagnostic and research challenge. Like other embryonal tumours of the nervous system, they display a wide range of neuronal differentiation, from highly cellular, immature round cell tumours to lesions with advanced differentiation and formation of mature ganglion cells.

Olfactory neuroblastomas

These rare neuroectodermal tumours are assumed to originate from olfactory receptor cells in the nasal cavity and, unless resected at an early stage, carry a poor prognosis. In addition to the typical neuroblastic pattern with occasional formation of rosettes, some lesions show neuroendocrine differentiation which may dominate the histology and lead to the diagnosis of neuro-endocrine carcinoma.

Neuroblastic tumours of the sympathetic nervous system and the adrenal gland

These neoplasms are among the most frequent paediatric tumours of the nervous system. Considerable progress has been made in their histological classification and grading as well as in regard to the underlying genetic alterations. *MYCN* amplification has remained the most significant predictive marker. Depending on the degree and type of differentiation, three major types are recognized:

Neuroblastoma (NB)

Ganglioneuroblastoma (GNB)

Ganglioneuroma (GN)

Current research concentrates on the identification of a putative tumour suppressor gene on chromosome 1p36, which is deleted in a significant fraction of neuroblastic tumours.

Olfactory neuroblastoma

S.D. Finkelstein
T. Hirose
S.R. VandenBerg

Definition
A malignant neuroectodermal tumour assumed to originate from olfactory receptor cells high in the nasal cavity.

ICD-O code: 9522/3

Synonyms
Aesthesioneuroblastoma, olfactory aesthesioneuroma.

Incidence, age and sex distribution
Olfactory neuroblastoma is a relatively uncommon neoplasm. The age of those affected ranges from 2 to 90 years {133, 1391}, the youngest reported case being in a two-year-old male child presenting with locally advanced disease {1961}. A bimodal age distribution has been noted, with cases tending to cluster around ages 20 and 50 years. The age of onset is to some extent correlated with the morphological pattern of olfactory neuroblastoma; tumours showing the more classical neuroblastic Homer-Wright rosettes tend to arise at an earlier age. The tumour affects both sexes with an approximately equal frequency.

Localization, growth and metastasis
Olfactory neuroblastoma typically involves the cribriform plate which is destroyed, through a process of slow growth and local invasion. Over time, infiltration of adjacent structures takes place in the direction of the paranasal sinuses, oro-nasopharynx, the base of skull, and even the cerebral frontal lobes. Eventually, the malignant nature of the tumour manifests by metastatic spread locally to cervical lymph nodes, distally to lungs and bone, and through leptomeningeal spread into the brain.

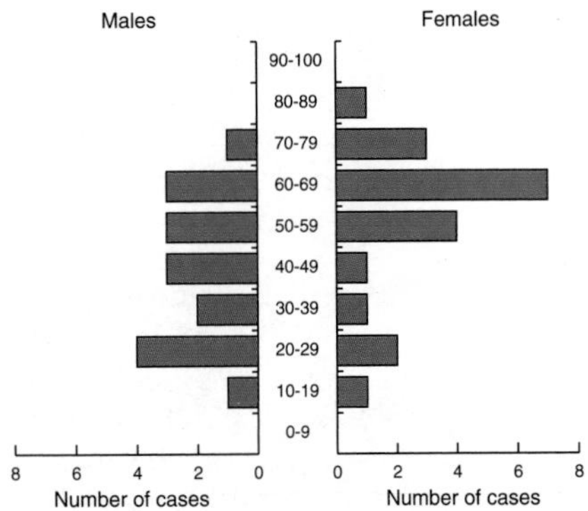

Fig. 9.1 Age and sex distribution of olfactory neuroblastoma, based on 37 patients treated at the University of Pittsburgh Medical Center.

Clinical features and staging
Olfactory neuroblastoma is a slowly growing neoplasm, and is typically associated with long-standing symptoms. Symptoms often experienced at initial presentation include nasal obstruction, anosmia and epistaxis. However, local extension may be asymptomatic, and clinical presentation not uncommonly may be due to extradural compression of the frontal lobes. Unusual presentations include ectopic release of hormones such as ACTH leading to Cushing syndrome {43}, and inappropriate water retention caused by production of antidiuretic hormone {12, 1050}. Ultimately, if left untreated, olfactory neuroblastoma produces life-threatening sequelae in the form of either meningitis secondary to breach of brain coverings, or of tumour metastasis. Early detection is therefore highly desirable, as it may permit tumour resection *en bloc* with negative margins, the single best predictive marker of favourable outcome {133}.
A clinicopathological staging system proposed by Kadish has proven useful in categorising the extent of tumour spread {421, 719}. Four stages are recognised: (A) tumour is confined to the nasal cavity; (B) tumour is limited to the nasal and paranasal sinuses; (C) direct regional spread into adjacent structures; and (D) metastasis, most frequently to the cervical lymph nodes and lung. To enhance the delineation of tumour extent, combined use of computerised tomography and magnetic resonance imaging has been increasing utilised. In addition, the presence of somatostatin receptors on olfactory neuroblastoma tumour cells has led to the use of octreotide imaging with ^{111}In-octreotide as a sensitive means to delineate tumour extent radiologically {1965}.

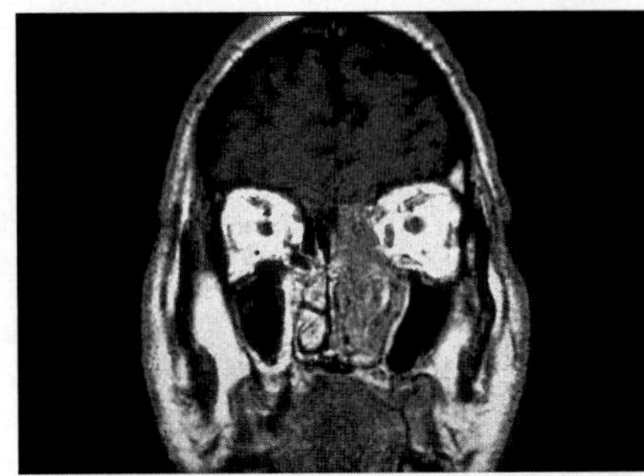

Fig. 9.2 Coronal MRI of an olfactory neuroblastoma that destroys the nasal turbinates and extends through the cribriform plate, reaching the base of the frontal lobe.

Macroscopy
The gross appearance of olfactory neuroblastoma is usually that of a soft, polypoid, richly vascularized tumour {133,1391}. Intratumoural haemorrhage, either intrinsic or induced during surgical exploration, is frequently encountered. Varying degrees of stromal desmoplasia and collagen deposition may render the tumour difficult to demarcate clearly for diagnostic and therapeutic purposes.

Histopathology
The histological appearance of olfactory neuroblastoma is diverse, encompassing a spectrum of morphological subtypes that are often intermingled within an individual case {69, 727}. In the past, two broad growth patterns have been recognised, which have been designated as the 'neuroblastoma-like' and 'neuroendocrine carcinoma-like' patterns. Within this general grouping, several subtypes may be distinguished. This morphological diversity has resulted in a variety of synonyms. More recently, there has been greater acceptance for separating 'neuroblastoma-like' forms of olfactory neuroblastoma from tumours that arise in the same location and manifest morphological and immunohistochemical characteristics of neuroendocrine carcinoma. Previously, these two tumour types were regarded as lying within a spectrum of histological types encompassed by the term olfactory neuroblastoma. Clinical and histopathological evi-

dence supports the separation of the 'neuroendocrine carcinoma' forms as distinct from olfactory neuroblastoma. The following discussion highlights this distinction.

The typical microscopic appearance of olfactory neuroblastoma is that of a cellular tumour composed of uniform small cells with scant fibrillar cytoplasm and round dark nuclei. Tumour cells are arranged in lobules, containing scattered rosettes of the Homer-Wright type.

This morphological pattern is often referred to as aesthesioneuroblastoma, a term that is virtually synonymous with olfactory neuroblastoma. Much less commonly, the tumour may show Flexner rosettes and other characteristics more typical of classic neuroblastoma. Rarely, differentiation to ganglion cells or the presence of teratomatous components may also be seen. Combined presence of olfactory neuroblastoma and craniopharyngioma has recently been reported {1960}.

In contrast to this neuroblastic growth pattern, olfactory neuroblastoma may be composed of larger cells with distinct cytoplasm that have a solid growth pattern and impart a distinct epithelial quality. This basic pattern may be further modified by the presence of intersecting bands of collagen leading to lobulation and a zellballen type of cellular organization, reminiscent of that of paraganglioma.

In the *neuroendocrine carcinoma variant*, tumour cells can take on nuclear and architectural features that are strongly suggestive of neuroendocrine differentiation, as seen in carcinoid tumour or small cell carcinoma of the lung. These histologic differences relate to variations in tumour cell growth pattern for diagnostic purposes only and are not predictive with respect to biological aggressiveness or treatment responsiveness.

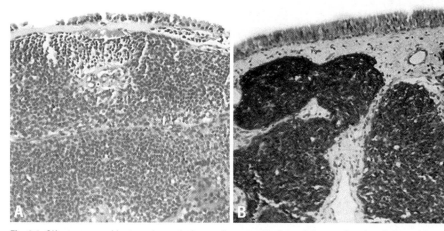

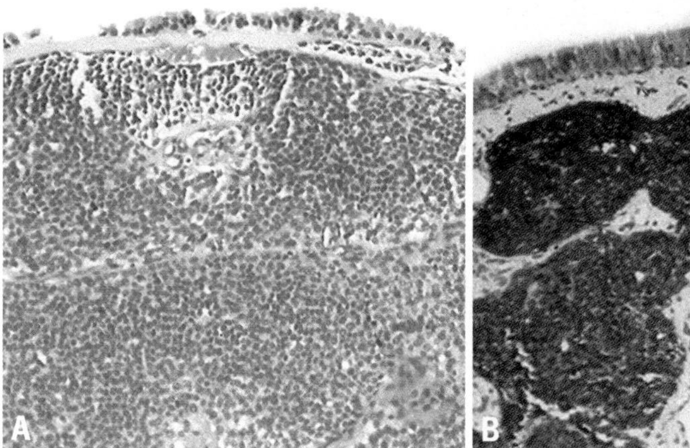

Fig. 9.4 Olfactory neuroblastoma beneath the respiratory epithelium of the nasal cavity. **A** Nests of small tumour cells in neuropil. **B** Tumour cell nodules expressing synaptophysin.

A histologic grading system based on degree of differentiation, cellular anaplasia and mitotic rate has been proposed by Hyams {1966, 1967} and found to correlate with disease outcome {1963}. This four level system has been simplified into low grade (Hyams grades I and II) and high grade (Hyams grades III and IV) with equivalent effectiveness. It should be noted that histologic grading may not be predictive in individual cases due to sampling effects in biopsy or minimal resection specimens.

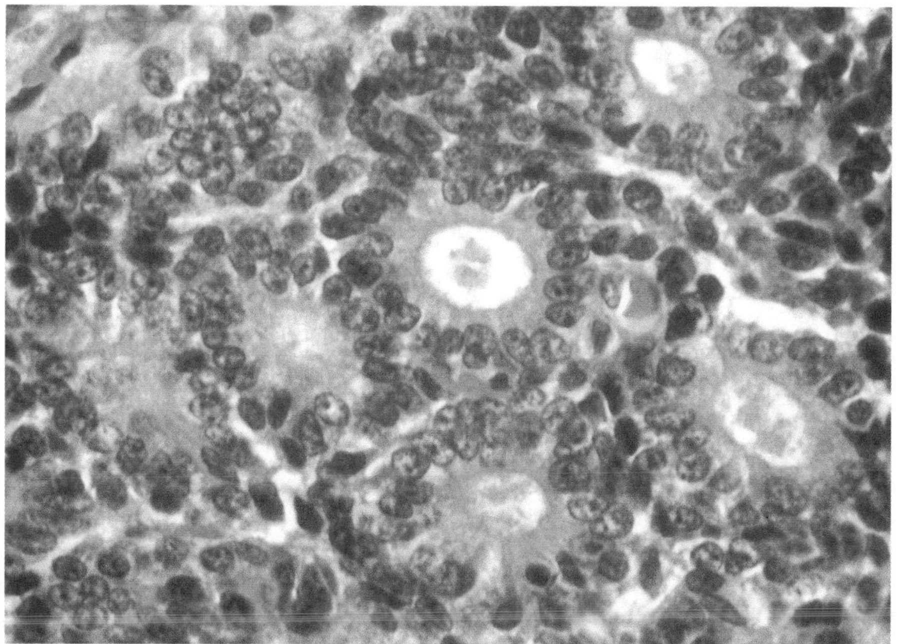

Fig. 9.3 Olfactory neuroblastoma with focal accumulation of rosettes.

Immunohistochemistry

This technique is especially valuable in the evaluation of olfactory neuroblastoma {591}. All forms consistently stain for neural crest markers, including neuron-specific enolase, chromogranin, synaptophysin, neurofilament, microtubule-associated protein, and beta-tubulin. S-100 staining decorates the peripherally oriented sustentacular cells in the paraganglioma variant of olfactory neuroblastoma. Epithelial markers such as cytokeratin and epithelial membrane antigen are absent from the neuroblastoma forms of olfactory neuroblastoma. In contrast, epithelial markers tend to be present in the various neuroendocrine carcinoma-like tumours. Ultrastructural analysis can provide additional support for neuroectodermal histogenesis by demonstrating neuritic processes, neurofilaments, microtubules, and dense core membrane-bound secretory granules {591, 1006, 1548}. At low magnification, olfactory neuroblastoma presents an appearance that is often described as a small round cell tumour, raising the differential diagnosis of lymphoma, undifferentiated sinonasal carcinoma, embryonal rhabdomyosarcoma, Ewing's sarcoma, primitive neuroectodermal tumour, melanoma, pituitary adenoma, and metastatic neuroendocrine carcinoma {133, 331, 1010}. Judicious use of immunohistochemical stains is sufficient to resolve most diag-

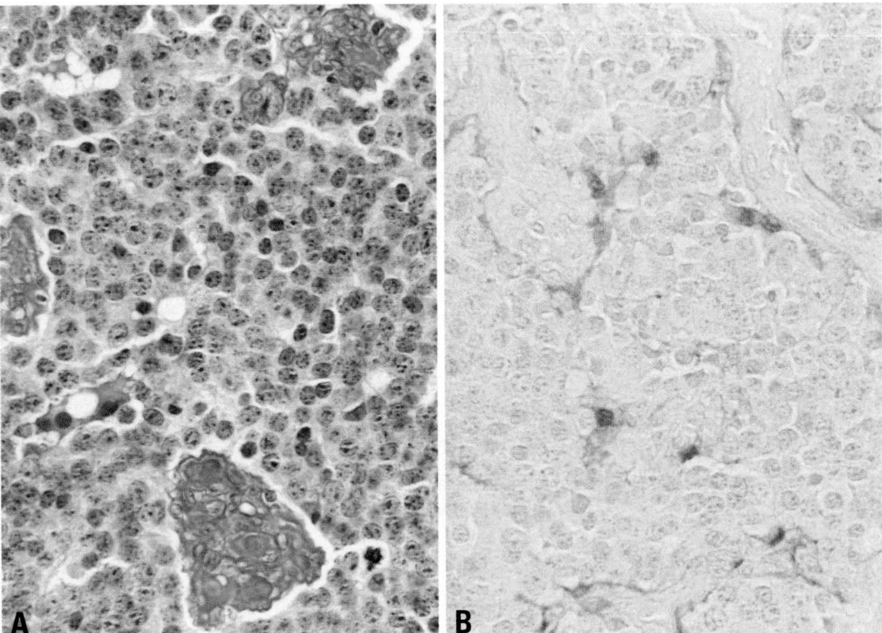

Fig. 9.5 Olfactory neuroblastoma with (**A**) marked PAS staining and (**B**) S-100 immunoreactivity of sustentacular cells.

nostic dilemmas. Ancillary techniques such as electron microscopy or analysis of molecular markers are valuable in difficult diagnostic cases.

Proliferation

Several studies of the neuroblastic form of olfactory neuroblastoma have reported a high proliferative index of 10–50%, as demonstrated by Ki-67 and MIB-1 immunostaining {1493, 1548}. Flow cytometric analyses have consistently confirmed a high rate of polyploidy/aneuploidy present in 66–78% of these neuroblastic tumours {1493, 1548}. Furthermore, both these indices have been shown to correlate with tumour recurrence, metastatic spread, and decreased survival.

Molecular genetics

There is agreement that, despite morphological similarities, olfactory neuroblastoma is genetically distinct from classic neuroblastoma. Studies of the neuroblastic form of the olfactory neuroblastoma have found that it lacks several characteristics typical of classic neuroblastoma including chromosome 1p deletion, *MYCN* amplification, and expression of tyrosine hydroxylase and neurotrophin receptor TrkA. Several reports, based on the analysis of selected cell lines, have proposed that olfactory neuroblastoma has a shared histogenesis with peripheral neuroectodermal tumour {207, 703, 1440}. Three studies have independently demonstrated the common finding of t(11:22) (q24:q12) or t(21:22) (q22:q12) translocations involving a fusion of the *EWS* gene with either *FLI1* or *ERG*. Others have questioned this relationship, using immunohistochemistry to demonstrate the absence in olfactory neuroblastoma of MIC-2 expression, a marker that is strongly associated with peripheral neuroectodermal tumours {1066}. The cytogenetic abnormalities found in peripheral neuroectodermal tumours are detected only inconsistently in olfactory neuroblastoma specimens {1066}. The relationship of olfactory neuroblastoma to primitive neuroectodermal tumours has recently been challenged in a more comprehensive analysis of twenty cases {1959}. A variety of markers for primitive neuroectodermal tumours was studied including immunohistochemistry for O13 antigen, sensitive RT/PCR for chromosomal translocation and Southern blot analysis failed to reveal evidence for such a relationship {1959}.

Combined immunohistochemical/microdissection genotyping showed that subsets of olfactory neuroblastoma demonstrate varying degrees of overexpression of wild-type TP53 protein {1128}.

Histogenesis

Given the diverse morphologic appearance of the tumour, the cellular origin of olfactory neuroblastoma has been the subject of controversy. Histological precursor lesions are still unidentified {199}. The neuroblastic appearance of the tumour cells suggests that they may be derived from the neuroepithelium. The developing olfactory placode of early embryogenesis covers a large portion of the nasal mucosa, from the midpoint of the nasal septum medially, to the roof of the nasal cavity, and over a considerable extent of the superior turbinate. During childhood and adolescence, the neuroepithelium is replaced by respiratory mucosa. However, persistence of neural elements may occur, and may explain the unexpected finding that olfactory neuroblastoma is seen as far afield as the nasopharynx and the maxillary and ethmoid sinuses.

Predictive factors

Subsets of olfactory neuroblastoma that overexpress wild-type TP53 are more likely to recur and to metastasize, suggesting a link between *TP53* overexpression and more aggressive growth {1210, 1391}. The most useful intermediate biomarkers, besides the stage of the tumour and completeness of resection, appear to be histological grade, proliferative index, and *TP53* overexpression.

It has been repeatedly demonstrated that completeness of primary tumour excision is the single best predictive marker and therapeutic measure for treatment effectiveness {1962}. Recent studies have shown the tumour to be sensitive to radiation therapy as well as chemotherapy, especially platinum based regimens {1964}. The most effective strategy for cure that has emerged in recent years has been the use of preoperative chemoradiation followed by a multidisciplinary surgical team approach including neurosurgery, head and neck surgery and neuro-ophthalmology {1963}.

Neuroblastic tumours of adrenal gland and sympathetic nervous system

M. Schwab
H. Shimada
V. Joshi
G.M. Brodeur

Definition
Childhood embryonal tumours of migrating neuroectodermal cells derived from the neural crest and destined for the adrenal medulla and sympathetic nervous system.

ICD-O codes: 9500/3

Synonyms
Neuroblastoma is often used as an omnibus term for all types of neuroblastic tumours. It is recommended that the term be used to designate a specific type of neuroblastic tumour, characterized by the grade of neuroblastic differentiation and the degree of Schwannian stromal development {2327}. The International Neuroblastoma Pathology Committee proposes four types of neuroblastic tumours: they are Neuroblastoma (Schwannian stroma-poor), Ganglioneuroblastoma, intermixed (Schwannian stroma-rich), Ganglioneuroma (Schwannian stroma-dominant), and Ganglioneuroblastoma, nodular (composite, Schwannian stroma-rich/ stroma-dominant and stroma-poor). The WHO working group has retained this nomenclature because it is widely used in clinical practice. The presence or absence of Schwannian stromal development is noted in parentheses after the specific tumour category (see Histopathology).

Incidence
Neuroblastic tumours are the most common solid extracranial malignant tumours during the first two years of life {1285}. In the United States of America, there are 7 new cases per million population per year in black children, and 9.6 per million in white children.

Table 9.1
Age distribution of neuroblastic tumours

Age	Frequency
<1 year	36%
1–4 years	49%
5–10 years	12%
>10 years	~3%

Age and sex distribution
Approximately 96% of cases occur in the first decade of life, and 3.5% in the second decade (Table 9.1) {158}. Neuroblastoma has been detected *in utero* by prenatal ultrasound examination {2287}. There is no sex predilection.

Localization and histogenesis
The primary sites include the adrenals (40% of neuroblastic tumours), followed by the abdominal (25%), thoracic (15%), cervical (5%) and pelvic sympathetic ganglia (5%). These structures are derivatives of migrating neuroectodermal cells originating from the neural crest. It has been suggested that in ganglioneuroblastoma (Schwannian stroma-rich), the diploid Schwann cells are reactive, in contrast to triploid ganglion cells {31}. All ganglioneuromas (Schwannian stroma-dominant), the fully mature form of neuroblastic tumour, were once neuroblastomas (Schwannian stroma-poor).

Clinical features
The common presenting features are a palpable abdominal mass, hepatomegaly and thoracic mass detected on routine chest X-ray. Dumbbell-shaped thoraco-abdominal neuroblastic tumours may cause spinal cord compression. Unusual clinical features include Horner's syndrome, owing to involvement of cervical sympathetic nerves, diarrhoea, caused by secretion of vasoactive intestinal polypeptide (VIP) by neuroblastic tumours, proptosis, owing to an orbital mass, cutaneous nodules and Ondine's curse (impairment of autonomic control of respiration) {747}. Also, opsoclonus syndrome, *i.e.* rapid, irregular non-rhythmic movements of the eye in horizontal and vertical direction, is frequent. Neuroblastic tumours are detected on plain radiographs or other imaging techniques, in which calcification is frequently seen (Fig. 9.6). ^{131}I-meta-iodobenzylguanidine (MIBG), which is taken up by adrenergic secretory vesicles, has been used in recent years to demonstrate both the primary tumour and metastatic disease.

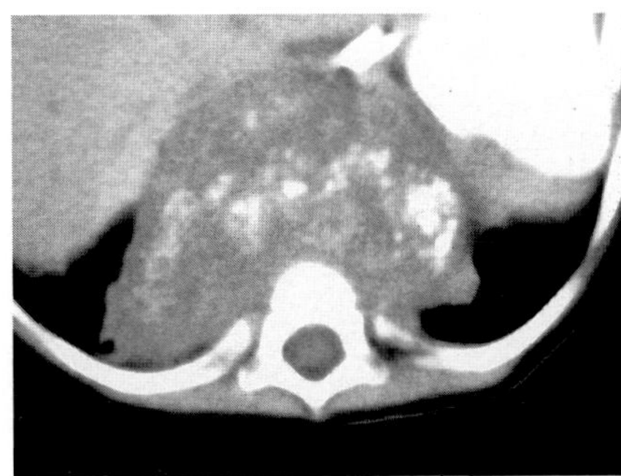

Fig. 9.6 Non-contrast-enhancing CT showing a large paravertebral, retroperitoneal neuroblastoma with focal calcifications.

Macroscopy
Neuroblastomas (Schwannian stroma-poor) can reach 1–10 cm in diameter, and are encapsulated, forming a soft, grey-tan mass, often haemorrhagic with or without foci of calcification. Extra-adrenal neuroblastomas may present as ill-defined infiltrative masses. Cystic change may be seen, particularly in the less differentiated form of neuroblastoma and dural metastasis {700}. Ganglioneuroblastoma (Schwannian stroma-rich) and ganglioneuroma (Schwannian stroma-dominant) have a firmer consistency and a tan-white colour. In the nodular type of ganglioneuroblastoma (composite Schwannian stroma-rich/ stroma-dominant and stroma-poor), one or more grossly visible, usually haemorrhagic nodules of softer consistency (stroma-poor component) and grey-tan colour (stroma-rich/stroma-dominant component) are present.

Histopathological examination
Primary, pre-treatment tumour specimens are optimal material for histologic examination and prognostic evaluation (see below). A diagnosis of neuroblastic tumour may, however, be established by incisional biopsy or fine-needle aspiration biopsy (FNAB) from the primary or metastatic tumour {1420} or by bone marrow biopsy. However, FNAB does not allow for histopathological classification, which is required for proper risk assessment, so it should only be performed if a core needle biopsy or tumour biopsy is impossible for

Table 9.2
Categories and subtypes of neuroblastic tumours (recommendation by the International Neuroblastoma Pathology Committee)

Category	Definition	Subtype	Remarks
Neuroblastoma	Cellular neuroblastic without prominent Schwannian stroma (Schwannian stroma-poor)	undifferentiated	Supplementary techniques required for the diagnosis
		poorly differentiated	The diagnosis can be made by pure morphological criteria due to the presence of characteristic neuropil. Differentiating neuroblasts < 5%
		differentiating	Differentiating neuroblasts > 5%. Usually with abundant neuropil.
Ganglioneuroblastoma	Intermingled microscopic foci of neuroblastic elements in an expanding Schwannian stroma, comprising > 50% of the tumour volume (Schwannian stroma-rich)	intermixed	Neuroblastic foci should be macroscopic without grossly visible nodular formation. Neuroblastic foci composed of a mixture of neuroblastic cells with various stages of differentiation.
Ganglioneuroblastoma	One or more grossly visible neuroblastic nodular component co-existing with ganglioneuroblastoma, intermixed or ganglioneuroma component (Schwannian stroma-rich/ stroma-dominant and stroma-poor)	nodular	Proportion of two components varies. Stroma-poor component usually haemorrhagic.
Ganglioneuroma	Predominantly composed of Schwannian stroma with individually distributed neuronal elements (Schwannian stroma-dominant)	maturing	Presence of differentiating neuroblasts and immature cells along with fully mature ganglion cells.
		mature	Fully mature ganglion cells surrounded by satellite cells, embedded in a Schwannian stroma.

clinical reasons. At the surgical pathology bench, to secure enough sample for histological examination should be the first priority. Then to save snap-frozen material for molecular tests becomes critical for biological characterization of the tumour. It is always recommended to make touch preparation for *MYCN* and chromosome 1p analysis by fluorescence-based *in-situ* hybridization (FISH) test.
Lymph nodes, which may adhere to the capsule, should not be separated from it, but should be included in the histological sections, as metastasis to these contiguous lymph nodes does not indicate stage II disease {158, 159}.

Histopathology

The International Neuroblastoma Pathology Committee has adopted, with some modifications, the classification scheme proposed by Shimada and associates in 1984 {708, 709, 1406, 2326, 2327, 2329}. Neuroblastic tumours are assigned to one of four basic morphologic categories (Table 9.2 and Fig. 9.7):

Neuroblastoma (Schwannian stroma-poor)

A tumour composed of neuroblastic cells forming groups or nests separated by delicate stromal septa with none to limited Schwannian proliferation.

Three subtypes; undifferentiated, poorly differentiated, and differentiating, are recognised in this category. Neuroblastoma, undifferentiated subtype is a tumour that requires supplementary techniques (imunohistochemistry, electron microscopy, and/or cytogenetics) to establish the diagnosis. Neuroblastoma, poorly differentiated subtype is defined as a tumour with a background of readily recognizable neuropil. Most tumour cells in this subtype are undifferentiated and only 5% or less of the cell population has cytomorphologic features of differentiation. Infrequently tumours of the neuroblastoma, undifferentiated and poorly differentiated subtypes show unusual histological features (large, pleomorphic, fusiform, spindle, pseudorhabdoid, *etc.*) focally or diffusely {715, 710}. Neuroblastoma, differentiating subtype is a tumour with usually abundant neuropil and with 5% or more of the tumour cells showing differentiation toward ganglion cells (differentiating neuroblasts). A differentiating neuroblast is characterized by synchronous differentiation of the nucleus (enlarged, eccentrically located with vesicular chromatin pattern and usually a single prominent nucleolus) and of the cytoplasm (eosinophilic/amphophilic with the diameter of twice or more of the nucleus).

Ganglioneuroblastoma, intermixed (Schwannian stroma-rich)

A tumour containing well-defined microscopic nests of neuroblastic cells intermixed or randomly distributed in the ganglioneuromatous stroma.
These nests are composed of a mixture of neuroblastic cells in various stages of differentiation, usually dominated by differentiating neuroblasts and maturing ganglion cells in a background of neuropil.

Ganglioneuroma (Schwannian stroma-dominant)

This variant has two 2 subtypes, maturing and mature.
The *maturing subtype* ("stroma-rich, well differentiated" in the original Shimada Classification) is composed predominantly of ganglioneuromatous stroma with scattered collections of differentiating neuroblasts and/or maturing ganglion cells in addition to fully mature ganglion cells. The *mature subtype* is composed of mature Schwannian stroma and ganglion cells.
Fully mature ganglion cells are usually surrounded by satellite cells. Stromal area

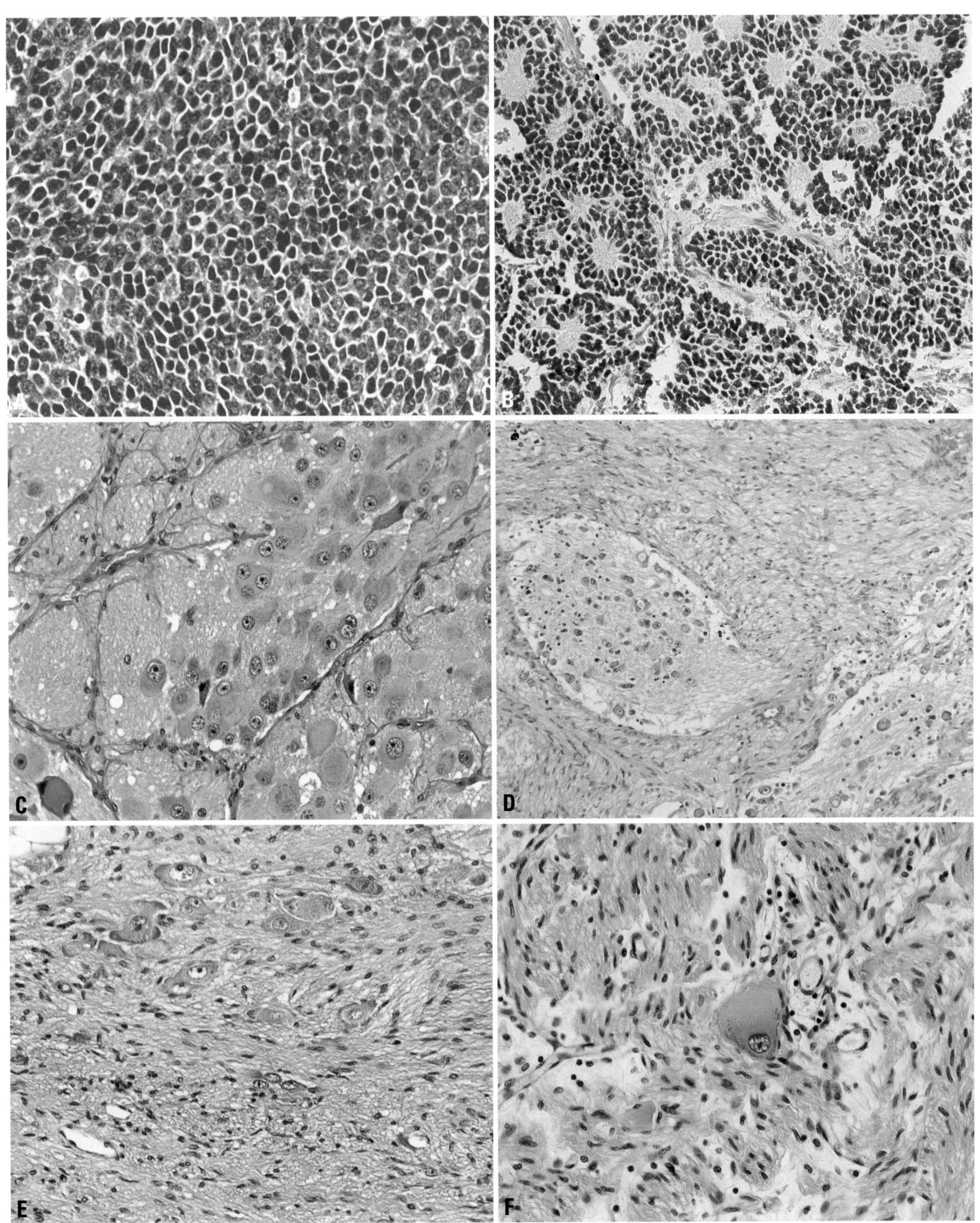

Fig. 9.7 Neuroblastoma (Schwannian stroma-poor). **A** Undifferentiated, (**B**) poorly differentiated, (**C**) differentiating. **D** Ganglioneuroblastoma, intermixed (Schwannian stroma-rich). **E** Ganglioneuroma (Schwannian stroma-dominant) maturing. **F** Ganglioneuroma (Schwannian stroma-dominant), mature.

shows fascicular profile of neuritic processes accompanied by Schwann cells and perineurial cells (Fig. 9.7F).

Ganglioneuroblastoma, nodular (composite Schwannian stroma-rich/ stroma-dominant and stroma-poor)

This lesion is characterized by the presence of grossly visible, usually haemorrhagic neuroblastic nodule(s) (stroma-poor component), co-existing with ganglioneuroblastoma, intermixed (stroma-rich component) or with ganglioneuroma (stroma-dominant component). The term "composite" implies that the tumour is composed of biologically different clones.

Immunohistochemistry

Neuron-specific enolase (NSE) and other neuronal markers (synaptophysin, neurofilament protein, ganglioside GD2, chromogranin A, tyrosine hydroxylase, and protein gene product 9.5) are helpful in diagnosis {747}. While NSE may show positive staining in other small round-cell tumours, for example, in rhabdomyosarcoma, the NSE staining pattern in neuroblastic tumours is diffuse and strongly positive. It is recommended that in the immunohistological diagnosis of neuroblastic tumours, positive staining for neural markers {491}, combined with negative staining for markers of other small round-cell tumours should be considered.

Electron microscopy

The diagnostic ultrastructural features are dense core neurosecretory granules (50–200 nm in diameter), generally of uniform size and located at the periphery of the cytoplasm and in the cell processes containing neurotubules {985}.

Proliferation

Diploid neuroblastomas have higher proliferative activity as indicated by a higher percentage of cells in S/M phase than is seen in aneuploid tumours {633, 909}. Proliferative activity has also been studied by immunohistochemical methods using antigens such as proliferating cell nuclear antigen (PCNA) and Ki-67 {1299}. Overall immunoreactivity to both antibodies as assessed by counting 1000 cells ranged from 0% to 80% (mean, 22.1% for Ki-67; 17% for PCNA).

Central nervous system metastases

While metastases to the CNS are generally rare in children, when it does occur the primary tumour is most commonly neuroblastoma. These metastases typically localize to the dura and display characteristic gross features; namely, multinodular haemorrhagic, papular growth primarily on the epidural surface. These, however, may penetrate the dura and assume a subdural location thereby compressing the underlying neural tissues.

The spinal epidural space is involved most often, and accurate diagnosis requires consideration of other small cell neoplasms, such as Ewing's tumour, lymphoma and rhabdomyosarcoma.

Aetiology

The aetiology of neuroblastoma is unknown, but it appears unlikely that environmental exposure plays a major role. There have been a few reports of neuroblastoma associated with the foetal hydantoin, phenobarbitol or alcohol syndromes, suggesting that prenatal exposure to these substances may increase the risk of neuroblastoma. There have also been studies suggesting a weak association between

Table 9.3
Morphological prognostic markers of neuroblastic tumours

Prognostic feature {Ref.}	Grade[1] /group[2] and criteria	Remarks
Degree of differentiation along gangliocytic line {81}	Grades I, II, III, & IV (>50%, 5–50%, <5% & 0% differentiating cells, respectively)	Lympocytic infiltration also of prognostic value. Statistical analysis not given
Degree of lymphocytic infiltration {2292}	Grades 1, 2, 3, 4, & 5 (no, occasional, moderately dense, dense with and without follicles, respectively)	
Degree of differentiation along gangliocytic line {2294}	Groups 1, 2a, and 2b (no differentiation, some differentiation without ganglion cells and some differentiation with ganglion cells, respectively)	Necrosis, calcification, vascular invasion also of prognostic value
Degree of differentiation along gangliocytic line {2288}	Grades I, II, & III (undifferentiated cells and ganglion cells, undifferentiated cells and differentiating cells, only undifferentiated cells, respectively)	Statistical analysis not given. No relationship between lymphocytic infiltration and survival
Amount of neuropil {2304}	Grades I, II, & III (dominant, moderate, and no neuropil, respectively).	Degree of differentiation but no rosettes found to be of prognostic value
Amount of Schwannian stroma, nuclear morphology (mitosis karyorrhexis index- MKI), degree of differentiation {1405}	Favourable and unfavourable histology	Linkage of age with morphological features is essential for the categorization into favourable and unfavourable histology group
Mitotic rate (MR) and calcification (Ca) {708}	Grades I, II, & III (Low MR & Ca+, low MKI or Ca+, high MKI & Ca-, respectively)	Ganglion cells and tumour giant cells also found to be of prognostic significance. Grades with or with-out linkage to age found to be of prognostic value
Mitosis/karyorrhexis index (MKI) and calcification (Ca) {713}	Grades I, II, & III (Low MKI & Ca+, low MKI or Ca+, high MKI & Ca-, respectively)	Grades with or without linkage to age found to be of prognostic value.

[1] High grades are associated with poor prognosis.
[2] Higher group is associated with better prognosis.

neuroblastoma and paternal occupational exposure to electromagnetic fields, or maternal use of hair colouring products, but none of these associations has been confirmed {805, 2280}. Moreover, no prenatal or postnatal exposure to drugs, chemicals or radiation has been either strongly or consistently associated with an increased incidence of neuroblastoma.

Genetic susceptibility

Constitutional chromosomal abnormalities have been described in patients with neuroblastoma, although there is no apparent pattern {2274}. An interstitial deletion and a reciprocal t(1;17) translocation, both affecting 1p36, have been observed in patients with neuroblastoma {111, 865, 1534}. However, it is unclear if these 1p36 rearrangements contributed to neuroblastoma predisposition.

Although the majority of neuroblastomas are thought to be sporadic, there has been a number of reports of familial neuroblastoma, as well as bilateral or multifocal disease, consistent with hereditary predisposition {99, 843}. The median age at diagnosis of patients with familial neuroblastoma is 9 months, which contrasts with a median age of 22 months for neuroblastoma in the general population. At least 20 percent of patients with familial neuroblastoma have bilateral adrenal or multifocal primary tumours. One report examined the genetic linkage of neuroblastoma predisposition to several candidate loci in families segregating the disease, but linkage was not found {2295}. However, a more recent genome-wide study has identified linkage of familial neuroblastoma to 16p12-13 in 10 families, suggesting that this genomic region may harbour a locus for neuroblastoma predisposition {2325}.

Cytogenetics and molecular genetics

Chromosome arm 1p

Deletion of the short arm of chromosome 1(1p) is a common abnormality that has been identified in 30-40% of cases using DNA polymorphisms {1598, 419, 1380, 2321, 2296}. Distal 1p36 (including 1p36.2-3) appears to be deleted in almost all cases. However, the breakpoints on 1p are quite variable, and there may be more than one site of deletion on distal 1p {1363, 1481, 2281}. There is also controversy about whether distal 1p undergoes genomic imprinting, based on preferential parental allelic loss. The resolution of these controversies must await additional studies, but it appears clear that at least one (and possibly more) tumour suppressor gene resides on distal 1p.

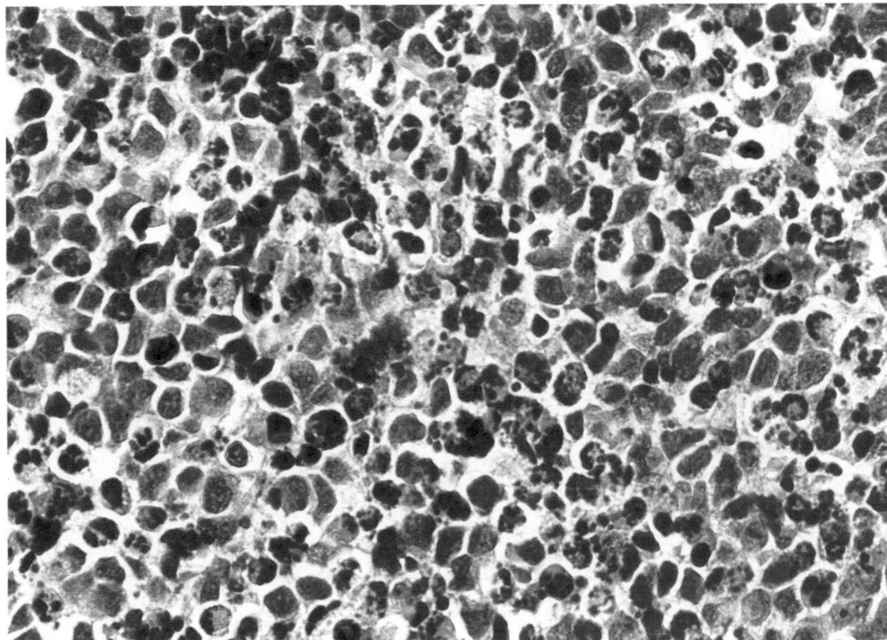

Fig. 9.8 Schwannian stroma-poor neuroblastoma with *MYCN* amplification showing a high mitosis/karyorrhexis index.

Chromosome arm 11q

Allelic loss of 11q has been detected by analysis of DNA polymorphisms and by comparative genomic hybridization (CGH) techniques {2276, 2291, 2301, 2319}. Allelic loss of 11q occurs in 30-50% of cases, making it the most common deletion detected to date in neuroblastomas {2312, 2324}. Loss at 11q23 is the most common site of deletion. Loss of heterozygosity (LOH) on 14q also occurs in ~25% of neuroblastomas {2313, 2315, 2312, 2330}. There was a strong correlation of 11q allelic loss with 14q loss, and an inverse relationship with 1p deletion and *MYCN* amplification, suggesting these genetic changes may characterize two distinct subsets of neuroblastomas. Deletion or allelic loss has been demonstrated at a variety of other sites by genome-wide allelotyping or by CGH, but none of these other sites has been studied in great detail.

Amplification of MYCN and other loci

Gene amplification is the selective increase of gene copy number {2307}. Amplification of different oncogenes has been found sporadically in a large number of tumour types {1377, 1378, 1379}. A novel *MYC*-related oncogene (*MYCN*) was found amplified in a series of neuroblastoma cell lines with double minute chromosomes (DMs) or homogeneously staining regions (HSRs) and in tumour {1377}. *MYCN* is normally located on 2p24, but maps to the DMs or HSRs in tumours with *MYCN* amplification {1381}. Apparently a large region from 2p24 (including the *MYCN* locus) becomes amplified initially as extrachromosomal DMs, but may become linearly integrated into a chromosome as one or more HSR, particularly in established cell lines {2269, 278, 2323}. *MYCN* amplification occurs in about 25 percent of primary neuroblastomas from untreated patients {2278}. Amplified *MYCN* can be detected by Southern blot, fluorescence *in-situ* hybridization, quantitative PCR, CGH or other techniques {2323}. Our studies have also shown a strong correlation between amplified *MYCN* and 1p LOH {1379, 2321}. Both amplified *MYCN* and deleted 1p are strongly correlated with a poor outcome and with each other {419}, and they appear to characterize a genetically distinct subset of aggressive neuroblastomas.

All neuroblastoma cells with double minutes or homogeneously staining regions appear to have amplified *MYCN*. However, there are at least six examples of neuroblastoma cell lines or primary tumours that amplify regions that are remote from the *MYCN* locus at 2p24. These include amplification of genes from 2p22 and 2p13

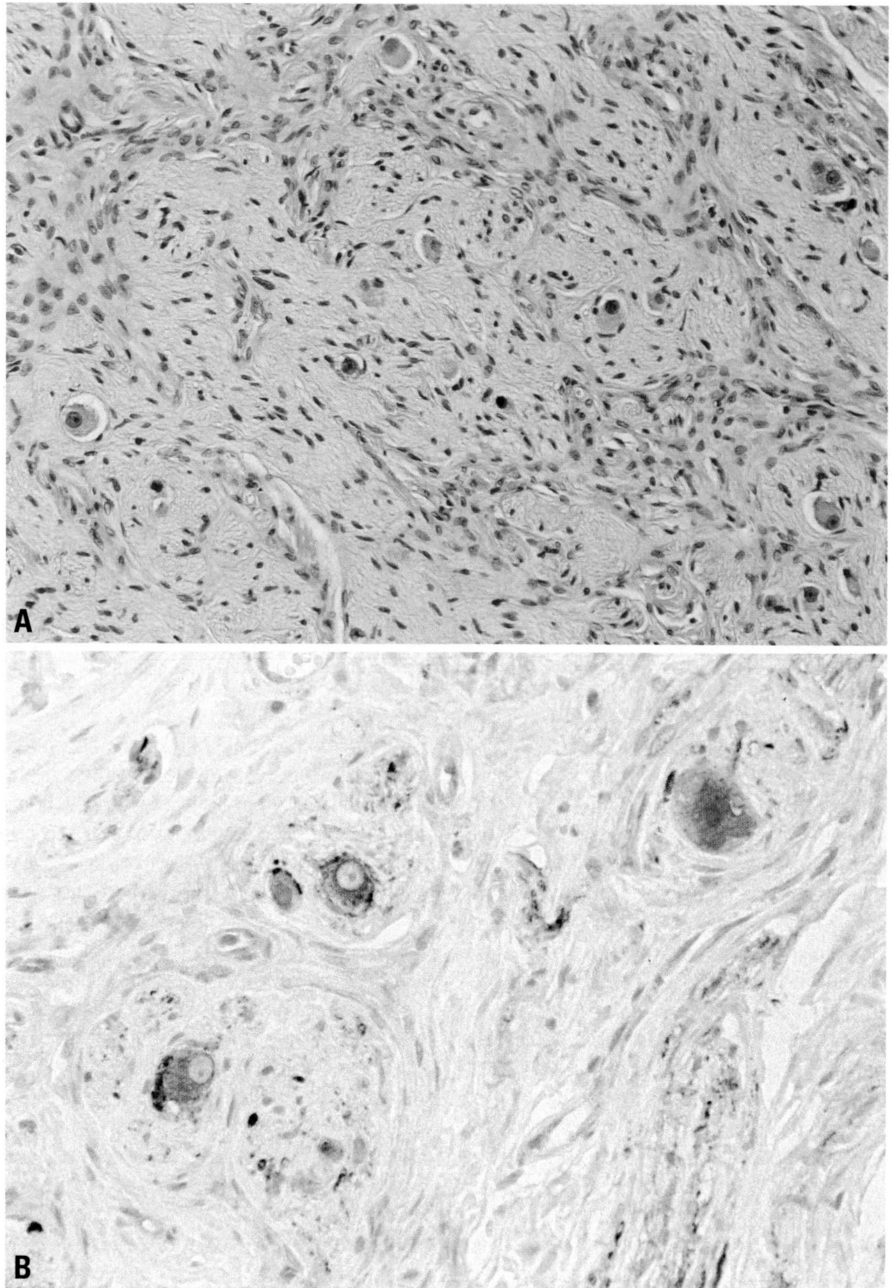

Fig. 9.9 A Neuroblastoma showing variably differentiated neuroblastic cells and mature neurons that strongly express synaptophysin (**B**).

in the IMR-32 cell line, as well as independent amplification of *MYCN* and *MDM2* (from 12q13) in the NGP, TR-14 and LS cell lines {279, 2285, 2310, 2317}. Finally, there is one report of independent amplification of *MYCN* and *MYCL* in a neuroblastoma cell line, and this has been seen in at least one primary tumour as well {2323, 2290}. These findings indicate that more than one locus can be amplified, but no neuroblastoma has been shown to have another amplified gene in the absence of amplified *MYCN*.

Overexpression of MYCN

Consequent to amplification *MYCN* is expressed at high level {2306, 2275}. About 25% of neuroblastomas have amplified *MYCN*, and virtually all of these cases have very high *MYCN* expression at the RNA and protein levels. Indeed, there is heterogeneity in the level of expression of *MYCN* in single-copy tumours, but higher expression in non-amplified tumours does not consistently correlate with a worse outcome {2300, 2311, 2282, 2271}. It is possible that the level of expression in non-amplified tumours seldom if ever exceeds a certain threshold level necessary to confer an unfavourable outcome, whereas almost all tumours with amplified *MYCN* exceed this threshold {2299}. Furthermore, activation of *MYCN* by mechanisms other than amplification or overexpression may play an important role {2283}.

The MYCN protein appears to have an important role during brain development, as indicated by its high expression during foetal stages. This is in contrast to the situation in normal adult brain, where *MYCN* mRNA expression is undetectable {499}. Like the MYC protein, MYCN is a member of a multiprotein complex {2320, 1606}. The only known function of this complex is transcriptional activation. The significance of overexpression in the absence of gene amplification is unclear.

Recent studies suggest a role of the MYCN protein in apoptosis {2293, 2286}. It seems that neuroblastoma cells with high MYCN protein expression have apoptotic dysfunction, which could be related to genomic changes, such as deletions. Defining the mechanisms of apoptosis and apoptotic dysfunction could lead to further understanding of neuroblastoma pathogenesis.

Trisomy for 17q

Trisomy for the long arm of chromosome 17 (17q) is another karyotypic abnormality that has been detected frequently in neuroblastomas. Allelotyping and CGH studies have suggested that gain of the long arm of chromosome 17 may occur in over half of all neuroblastomas {2276, 2291, 2297, 2301, 2316, 2319}. Even accounting for near triploid cases with gain of the entire chromosome, 17q trisomy may be the most prevalent genetic abnormality identified to date in neuroblastomas. Although gain of 17q can occur independently, it frequently occurs as part of an unbalanced translocation between chromosomes 1 and 17 {32, 201, 1329, 2318}. The 17q breakpoints vary, but a region has been defined at 17q22-qter that suggests a dosage effect rather than interruption of a gene. Gain of 17q appears to be associated with a more aggressive subset of neuroblastomas and is of prognostic value for adverse outcome (overall 5-year survival 30.6 % with 17q gain *versus* 86.0% with normal 17q) {2273}.

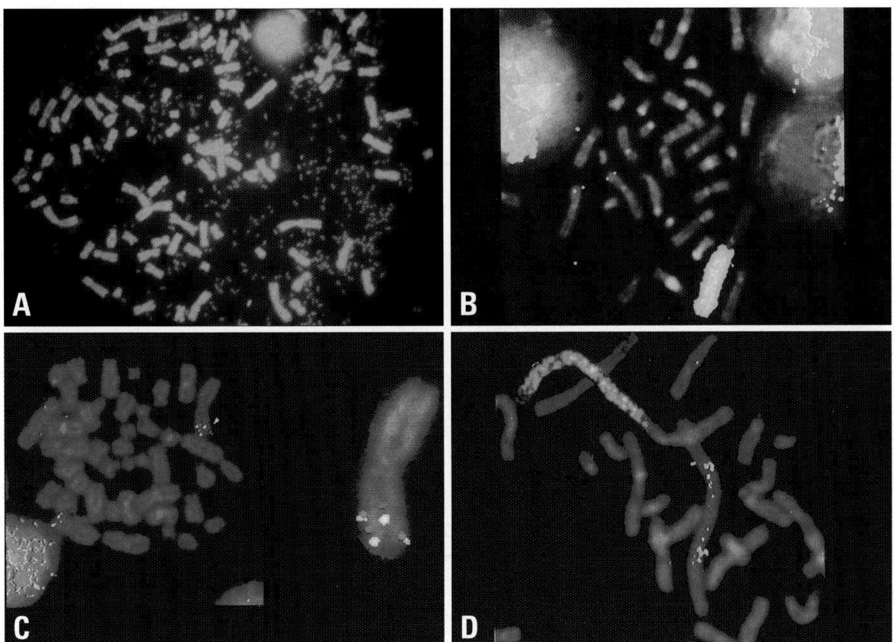

Fig. 9.10 A Cytogenetic evidence of gene amplification in a neuroblastoma. Note the small, extrachromosomal chromatin bodies (double minutes), which contain additional copies of the *MYCN* gene. **B** Metaphase of a neuroblastoma cell showing amplified *MYCN,* integrated as multiple copies in a homogeneously staining chromosomal region (HSR, strong signal), in addition to the single-copy signal on both homologues of chromosome 2. *In situ* hybridization with cosmid pNb-101. **C** Duplicated *MYCN* on chromosome 2 in a human neuroblastoma cell lacking *MYCN* amplification. Fluorescence *in situ* hybridization with cosmid probe pNb-101 (red) and anonymous 2p probe YAC (D2S165). **D** Independent amplification of *MYCN* (red) and *MDM2* (green) in two different HSRs in a neuroblastoma.

Tumour DNA Content: Near-Diploidy versus Hyperdiploidy

Although the majority of tumours that have been karyotyped are in the diploid range, a substantial number of tumours from patients with lower stages of disease are hyperdiploid or near triploid {151, 633, 909, 910}. The modal karyotype number has been shown to have prognostic value. Flow cytometric analysis of DNA content is a simple and semi-automated way of measuring total cell DNA, which correlates well with modal chromosome number. Recent studies by Look and others have demonstrated that the determination of the DNA index (DI) of neuroblastomas from infants provides important information that can be predictive of response to particular chemotherapeutic regimens as well as outcome {909, 910}. Unfortunately, the DNA index looses its prognostic significance for patients over 2 years of age. This is probably because hyperdiploid tumours from infants generally have whole chromosome gains without structural rearrangements, whereas hyperdiploid tumours in older patients usually have a number of structural rearrangements as well.

Expression of neurotrophin receptors

Neuroblastoma cells are derived from sympathetic neuroblasts, and they frequently exhibit features of neuronal differentiation. Indeed, neuroblastomas may show spontaneous or induced differentiation to ganglioneuroblastoma or ganglioneuroma, so the malignant transformation of these cells may result in part from a failure to respond fully to the normal signals to undergo this maturation process. The factors responsible for regulating normal differentiation are not understood well at present, but they probably involve one or several neurotrophin receptor pathways that signal the cell to differentiate. Recently, three tyrosine kinase receptors for a homologous family of neurotrophin factors have been cloned. The main ligand for the TrkA, TrkB and TrkC receptors is nerve growth factor (NGF), brain-derived neurotrophic factor (BDNF) and neurotrophin-3 (NT-3), respectively, and neurotrophin-4/5 (NT-4) appears to function through TrkB. Another transmembrane receptor binds all the neurotrophins with low affinity (P75, LNTR), but its role in mediating responses to the presence or absence of these homologous ligands is controversial.
High level of TrkA expression has been seen in 82% of the neuroblastomas {1055}. All tumours that had low stage and no amplified *MYCN* showed a high level of TrkA expression. However, all but one tumour with amplified *MYCN* had an extremely low or undetectable level of TrkA expression. The expression of TrkA correlated strongly with survival: the 5-year cumulative-survival rate of the group with a high level of TrkA expression was 86 percent, whereas that of the group with a low level of TrkA expression was 14 percent ($p<0.001$). Indeed, the combination of TrkA expression and amplified *MYCN* had a strong influence on overall survival. Similar results have been obtained independently by others, supporting the strong correlation between high TrkA expression and a favourable outcome {2314, 794, 2272}. Thus, the NGF/TrkA pathway may play an important role in the propensity of some neuroblastomas to regress or differentiate in selected patients.

Interestingly, expression of full-length TrkB was strongly associated with *MYCN* amplified tumours {2298}. Because these tumours also express the TrkB ligand (BDNF), this may represent an autocrine or paracrine loop providing some survival or growth advantage. In contrast, the expression of TrkC was found predominantly in lower stage tumours, and, like TrkA, was not detected in *MYCN* amplified tumours {2322, 2303}. This suggests that favourable tumours are characterized by the expression of TrkA, with or without TrkC, but unfavourable tumours express full-length TrkB plus its ligand BDNF.

Predictive factors

Clinical factors

Neuroblastic tumours have favourable prognosis in infants less than one year of age. Adrenal neuroblastic tumours have a worse prognosis than extra-adrenal tumours, particularly thoracic tumours. Children with stage 1 and stage 2 neuroblastic tumours have a longer survival than those with stage 3 and 4 tumours. Spontaneous regression is most apparent in patients with stage 4S tumours, i.e. infants with a local stage 1 or 2 neuroblastoma or unknown primary with involvement of the liver, skin, and/or bone marrow with <10% tumour cells. However, even within stage 4S there is a subset of tumours with poor prognosis, which is characterized by unfavourable histology or amplified *MYCN* {520}.

Regression also occurs in a subset of patients with other stages of neuroblastoma, but predominantly in infants {383}. It is not clear whether spontaneous maturation or an immunological phenomenon {747} is related to regression.

Histopathological criteria

Several investigators have described prognostic classifications of neuroblastic tumours based on their histological features (Table 9.3) {81, 708, 713, 1405, 2292, 2294, 2288, 2304}. Besides these systematized prognostic classifications, the following individual histological features of prognostic value have been described: high mitotic rate of >10 cells per ten high power fields and necrosis and foam cells (poor prognosis); and calcification, S-100-positivity, multinucleation and ganglion cells (good prognosis) {716}. Other notable features include the vascular index which represents total number of blood vessels/mm^2 of the tumour – an index of <4 is associated with good prognosis and on of >4 with poor prognosis {989}.
In 1999 the International Neuroblastoma Pathology Committee proposed the classification by adopting the Shimada system {1405} with minor modifications for prognostic evaluation of the neuroblastic tumours {2329}. This is an age-linked histopathological classification distinguishing 2 prognostic groups; i.e., favourable and unfavourable histology group.

Tumours in the favourable histology group include:
(1) Age < 1.5 years old: neuroblastoma (Schwannian stroma-poor), poorly differentiated subtype with low (<2% or <100/5,000 cells) or intermediate (2-4% or 100-200/5,000 cells) mitosis-karyorrhexis index (MKI) {711};
(2) Age between 1.5 and 5 years old: neuroblastoma (Schwannian stroma-poor), differentiating subtype with low MKI;
(3) Ganglioneuroblastoma, intermixed (Schwannian stroma-rich), usually seen in older children
(4) Ganglioneuroma, maturing and mature subtypes (Schwannian stroma-dominant), usually seen in more older children.
These tumours are within a framework of age-appropriate maturation sequence from neuroblastoma, poorly differentiated and differentiating subtype to ganglioneuroblastoma, intermixed to ganglioneuroma. Cut-off points for MKI also change according to the age of the patients.

Tumours in the unfavourable group include:
(1) Any age: neuroblastoma (Schwannian stroma-poor), undifferentiated subtype;
(2) Age between 1.5 and 5 years old: neuroblastoma (Schwannian stroma-poor), poorly differentiated subtype;
(3) Any age: neuroblastoma (Schwannian stroma-poor) with high (>4% or >200/5,000 cells) MKI;
(4) Age between 1.5 and 5 years old: neuroblastoma (Schwannian stroma-poor) with intermediate MKI;
(5) Age >= 5years old: all neuroblastoma (Schwannian stroma-poor) subtypes
(6) Ganglioneuroblastoma, nodular (composite Schwannian stroma-rich/stroma-dominant and stroma-poor).
Morphologic indicators for the tumours in the unfavourable histology group are inappropriate degree of maturation and/or increased MKI for neuroblastomas, and presence of nodular formation by an aggressive clone for ganglioneuroblastoma, nodular (Table 9.3). It should be noted that prognostic evaluation by this system can only be performed on pre-treatment tumours from either primary or metastatic sites.

Proliferation

Proliferative activity, as assessed by immunoreactivity to Ki-67, defines the growth fraction in tumour tissue {1299}: high Ki-67 scores (>25%) correlate with poor survival after adjusting for stage and Hughes grade defined by degree of differentiation.

Biochemistry

Serum NSE (>100 ng/ml), ferritin (>150 ng/ml), lactate dehydrogenase (>1500 IU/l), and VMA:HVA ratio <1.0 are associated with poor prognosis {716}.

Genetic alterations

Neuroblastoma can have many genetic changes, some have clinical significance {2279, 2277}.
Amplified MYCN. Determination of *MYCN* status is used world-wide by virtually all paediatric group trials, and patients with amplified *MYCN* are usually assigned to more intense therapeutic regimens. Amplified *MYCN* is associated with poor outcome, regardless of clinical stage {70, 151, 269, 910, 2302, 1521, 2309}. In stage IV, amplified *MYCN* has prognostic significance only in children younger than 2 years at the time of diagnosis. Amplified *MYCN* is generally regarded as the reference molecular marker for prognosis of neuroblastoma. The classical technique to determine amplified *MYCN* has been by Southern blotting {1377}. More recent assays use chromosomal fluorescence *in situ* hybridization (FISH) with cosmid probe pNb-101 (Fig. 9.10) {278, 2323}.
Chromosome 1p deletion. Deletion of portions of the short arm of chromosome 1 has been determined by various technical approaches: by inspection of Giemsa-banded metaphase chromosomes; by RFLP analysis of DNA; by PCR of microsatellite loci; and by FISH. The most sensitive and rapid approach appears to be PCR analysis of microsatellites. Only a few nanograms of DNA are required, which should be generally available even from minute tumour samples and from small amounts of blood cells from young children.
Cytogenetics. Early studies indicated a correlation of 1p deletion with poor prognosis {247, 557}. These interpretations should be taken cautiously, however, because the cytogenetic approach introduces sample bias, owing to the fact that only a fraction of tumours will yield karyotypes suitable for evaluation. In an apparent confirmation of cytogenetic approaches {200}, Caron reported that allelic loss of 1p identifies patients at high risk of an unfavourable outcome. It is obvious, though, that roughly one-third of the patients with 1p loss are long-term survivors, thus making 1p loss an unreliable marker and raising the question of how to apply this information to the benefit of the patient. A correlation has not been seen by Gehring *et al.* {460} or Maris *et al.* {963} and was not confirmed in a more recent evaluation by Christiansen *et al.* {248}, suggesting that the value of 1p loss as a marker of prognosis needs to be assessed more rigorously. In a study of 377 patients, a risk estimation of high discriminating power was found only for patients with localized and metastatic neuroblastoma using stage and *MYCN* amplification {248}, but not for 1p. As it now stands, the clinical and biological significance of 1p alterations awaits further clarification {1380}.
TrkA expression. Expression of the nerve growth factor receptor TrkA has been analysed in clinical samples by northern blotting, PCR and by immunological approaches. The immunological technique can be performed most rapidly and provides data on the single-cell level. Lack of

TrkA expression has been identified as indicating poor prognosis in those patients lacking amplified *MYCN* {794, 1055, 1485, 2314, 2272}. Conversely, neuroblastomas expressing TrkA appear to differentiate, regress spontaneously or respond to conventional therapy. An obvious biological interpretation is that loss of functional TrkA/NGF receptor is an important step in the development of undifferentiated progressive neuroblastoma. The clinical significance of TrkA expression for neuroblastoma merits close monitoring in future studies.

CD44 expression. The level of expression is generally assayed at the protein level by an immunological approach at the single-cell level. In general, lack of CD44 expression has been associated with poor outcome {268, 269, 2284, 393}. Independent comparative studies did not find that CD44 added much in prognosis assessment {248, 2270}.

Correlation between morphologic and non-morphologic predictive factors

There is generally a good correlation between morphological and non-morphological markers. A statistically significant association between original and modified grade 3 and DNA index of 1, >1 copy number of *MYCN* per haploid genome and serum LDH of >1500 IU/l has been described {715}. Most importantly, a reproducible correlation between a high MKI (in undifferentiated or poorly differentiated subtype of neuroblastoma) and adverse clinical and biological (*MYCN* amplification) manifestation exists (see below ref. {1406}).

Biological relevance of the International Neuroblastoma Pathology Classification (Shimada system).

There is a significant correlation between morphologic features of the International Neuroblastoma Pathology Classification (Shimada system) and biological properties of the neuroblastic tumours.

Tumour maturation. The classification is based on the concept of tumour maturation according to the morphologic changes of two main cellular populations: *i.e.*, neuroblastic cells and Schwannian cells. It starts with neuroblastoma (poorly differentiated and differentiating neuroblasts in Schwannian stroma-poor background), proceeds to ganglioneuroblastoma, intermixed (differentiating neuroblasts and ganglion cells in Schwannian stroma-rich background), and reaches to the final stage of ganglioneuroma (ganglion cells in Schwannian stroma-dominant background).

Amplified MYCN. There is a significant correlation between *MYCN* amplification and a specific histological appearance in neuroblastic tumours {1406}. Tumours with amplified *MYCN* do not show neuroblastic differentiation (differentiation arrest) and are usually of the undifferentiated or poorly differentiated subtype of neuroblastoma. They also have markedly increased proliferation and apoptosis, i.e. a high MKI (Fig. 9.8). The balance appears to favour cellular proliferation more than cellular death (karyorrhexis) in the *MYCN* amplified tumours, as they usually show an aggressive and rapidly progressive clinical behaviour.

TrkA Expression. Preliminary data {2328} show that neuroblastoma (Schwannian stroma-poor) tumours with favourable histology express significantly higher levels of TrkA than those with unfavourable histology, especially when the *MYCN* oncogene is amplified. Within the favourable histology tumours, there is no significant difference in the expression levels of TrkA between "poorly differentiated" and "differentiating" subtypes. It is noted, however, that tumours of the differentiating subtype are diagnosed in significantly older children (usually over one up to 5 years of age) than those of the poorly differentiated subtype (newborn to 1.5 years of age). These data clearly suggest an *in vivo* latent period required for morphologic evidence of neuroblastic differentiation by the cells expressing higher levels of TrkA in the tumours of the favourable histology group.

Composite Tumour. The term "composite" implies that the tumour is composed of biologically different clones {2305}. The prototype of this composite tumour is designated as the nodular subtype of ganglioneuroblastoma and characterized by grossly visible haemorrhagic nodule(s) of neuroblastoma (stroma-poor component) representing an aggressive clone, and a background of either ganglioneuroblastoma, intermixed (stroma-rich component) or ganglioneuroma (stroma-dominant component) representing a non-aggressive clone. Due to a high potential of the aggressive clone for distant metastasis, this subtype falls into the unfavourable histology group.

Table 9.4
Typing of neuroblastomas according to prognosis.

	Type 1	Type 2	Type 3
MYCN amplification	no	no	yes
1p deletion	no	+/-	yes
Ploidy	hyperdiploidy triploidy	diploidy tetraploidy	diploidy tetraploidy
TRKA expression	A ± C	no	B
Age (years)	0 - 1	> 1	1 - 5
INSS stage	all stages	2, 3, 4	3, 4
Survival	> 90%	50 - 60%	20 - 30%

CHAPTER 10

Tumours of Cranial and Peripheral Nerves

This group of tumours spans a wide range of histopathological features and associated clinical characteristics. More frequently than any other class of nervous system neoplasms, tumours of cranial and peripheral nerves occur in the setting of familial cancer syndromes, in particular the neurofibromatoses. The major clinicopathological entities include:

Schwannoma (WHO grade I)

This benign, slowly growing neoplasm may be located anywhere in the peripheral nervous system but intracranially its most frequent site is the vestibular division of the eighth cranial nerve. Surgical resection is usually curative.

Neurofibroma (WHO grade I)

If solitary, this tumour is usually indolent, with a favourable prognosis. Multiple neurofibromas are the hallmark of neurofibromatosis von Recklinghausen (NF1), which is discussed in Chapter 14.

Perineurioma

This benign tumour consists entirely of perineurial cells and occurs both intraneurally and as soft tissue lesion.

Malignant peripheral nerve sheath tumour (MPNST)
WHO grade III or IV

This malignant neoplasm is morphologically variable, with a distinct tendency towards divergent mesenchymal differentiation. More than half of those affected have inherited mutations of the neurofibromatosis type 1 gene.

Peripheral nerve tumours not discussed in this chapter include nerve sheath myxoma, neurothekeoma, and benign and malignant granular cell tumours. A detailed discussion of these neoplasms can be found in the AFIP Tumour Atlas: Tumours of the Peripheral Nervous System {Ref. 1977}.

Schwannoma

J.M. Woodruff
H.P. Kourea
D.N. Louis
B.W. Scheithauer

Definition
A usually encapsulated benign tumour composed of differentiated neoplastic Schwann cells.

ICD-O code: 9560/0

Grading
Schwannoma corresponds histologically to WHO grade I.

Synonyms
Neurilemoma and neurinoma.

Incidence
Schwannoma is a common tumour of peripheral nerves. It also accounts for an estimated 8% of intracranial {204} and 29% of primary spinal tumours {581}. There is a high incidence of schwannomas in patients with neurofibromatosis 2 (NF2). In the absence of NF2, multiple, often subcutaneous schwannomas are indicative of "schwannomatosis", a rare genetically distinct disorder {933}.

Age and sex distribution
All ages are affected, but there is a peak incidence in the fourth to sixth decades. Generally, there is no sex predilection, the exception being a female:male ratio of 2:1 among patients with intracranial tumours {204}.

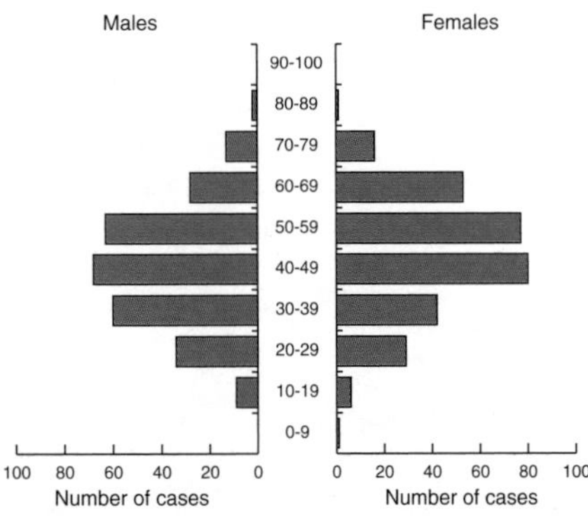

Fig. 10.1 Age and sex distribution of schwannomas, based on 582 patients treated at the University Hospital, Zurich.

Localization
Schwannomas most commonly arise from peripheral nerves in the head and neck region and extensor aspects of the extremities. Cutaneous lesions are well described. The tumours also arise from spinal and cranial nerves, notably the vestibular division of the eighth cranial nerve. Around 40 cases each of intracerebral and intramedullary schwannomas have been reported {204, 581}, as have a few intraventricular tumours {1177, 1595}. Although sensory nerves are the preferred site of development, motor and autonomic nerves may also be affected. Visceral schwannomas are rare {1977}.

Clinical features
Symptoms and signs

Peripherally situated schwannomas commonly present as asymptomatic masses, paravertebral tumours as incidental findings on imaging studies, spinal column tumours with radicular pain and signs of nerve root and spinal cord compression, and eighth cranial nerve examples with symptoms of a cerebellopontine angle lesion (e.g. tinnitus, hearing difficulties and facial paresthesias). Motor symptoms are uncommon since schwannomas favour sensory nerve roots.

Neuroimaging

MRI reveals a well-circumscribed, sometimes cystic and often heterogeneously enhancing mass which in paraspinal sites may be associated with bone erosion that is sometimes evident on plain x-rays {204}.

Macroscopy
The majority of schwannomas are globoid masses measuring from a few centimeters to 10 cm in size. With the exception of examples arising in bone or intraparenchymal CNS sites, viscera and skin, they usually are encapsulated. In peripheral tumours, a nerve of origin is identified in less than half of cases. The cut surface of the tumour reveals a light tan glistening tissue that may be interrupted by bright yellow patches, cysts and hemorrhage. Typically, no necrosis is evident.

Histopathology
A tumour composed of spindle-shaped neoplastic Schwann cells with alternating areas of compact, elongated cells with occasional nuclear palisading (Antoni A pattern) and less cellular, loosely textured, often lipidized tumour areas (Antoni B). The Schwann cells comprising the tumour have relatively abundant, faintly eosinophilic cytoplasm without discernible cell margins, and normochromic spindle nuclei. The latter are approximately the same size as those of smooth muscle, but are tapered instead of blunt-ended. In loose-textured areas, tumour cells often have ovoid, smaller nuclei. Nuclear pleomorphism, including bizarre forms ("ancient

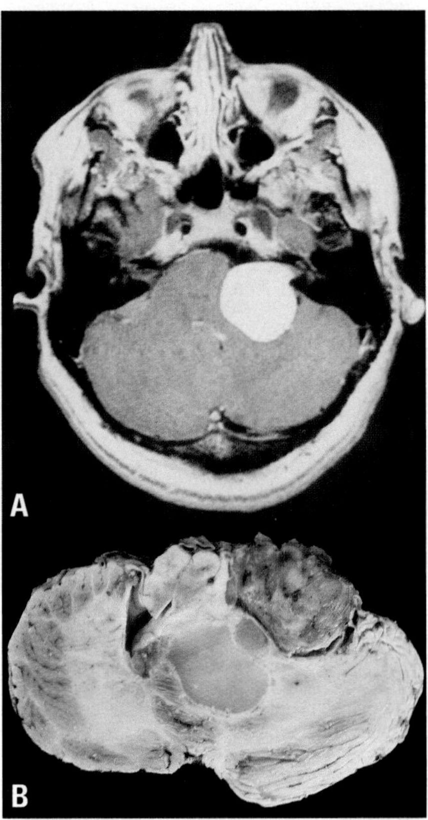

Fig. 10.2 Vestibular schwannoma. **A** MRI showing location in the cerebello-pontine angle. Note the tumour protrusion at the upper margin extending into the internal acoustic canal. **B** Large schwannoma causing compression of and cyst formation in the cerebellum, and displacement of the medulla.

schwannoma"), and occasional mitotic figures may be seen, but should not be mistinterpreted as indicating malignancy. The growth pattern consists of Antoni A areas, represented by closely packed tumour cells, and Antoni B areas, where tu mour cells are loosely arranged. Commonly found in Antoni A areas are nuclear palisades and often Verocay bodies. These bodies are formed by roughly parallel arrays of tumour cell nuclei separated by dense closely aligned cell processes and basement membranes which are hypereosinophilic. Collections of lipid laden cells may be present within either Antoni A or B areas. Schwannoma vasculature is typically thick-walled and hyalinized, and the observation of dilated blood vessels surrounded by or invested by haemorrhage is common. Eighth cranial nerve schwannomas are known for the infrequent presence of Verocay bodies, predominance of Antoni B tissue, and often clusters of lipid-laden cells.

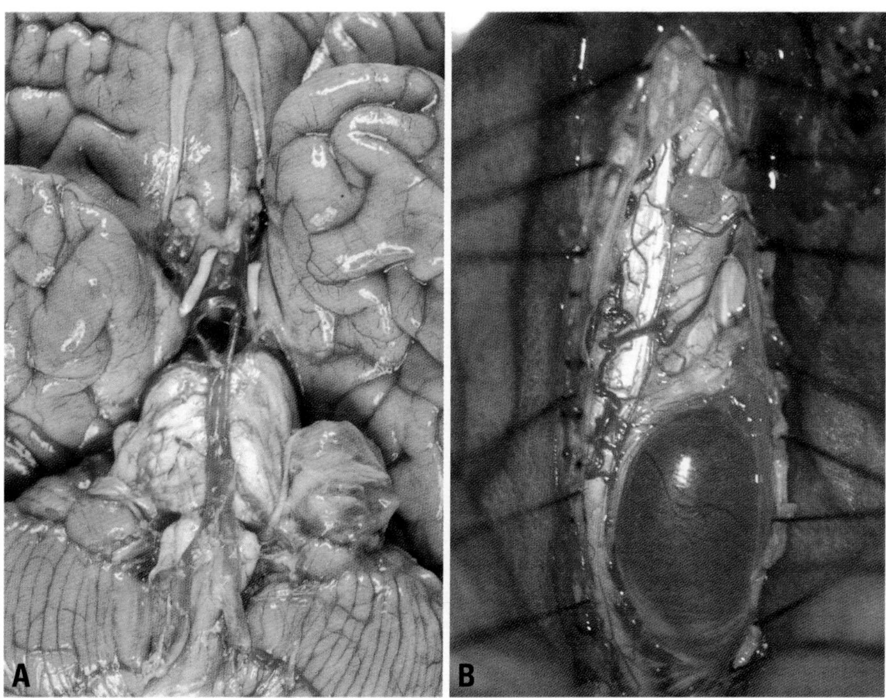

Fig. 10.3 A Macroscopic appearance of a vestibular schwannoma in the left cerebello-pontine angle and (**B**) a spinal schwannoma (intraoperative view).

Cellular schwannoma
This variant is defined as a hypercellular schwannoma composed exclusively or predominantly of Antoni A tissue, and devoid of formed Verocay bodies {1643}. The most common location of cellular schwannoma is at paravertebral sites in the pelvis, retroperitoneum and mediastinum {1616, 1643}. Cranial nerves, especially the fifth and eighth, may be affected {205}. Clinical presentation of cellular schwannoma does not differ from that of conventional schwannoma, but the histological features of hypercellularity, fascicular growth of cells, occasional nuclear hyperchromasia and atypia, as well as hypercellularity and readily identified mitotic activity, may lead to a mistaken diagnosis of malignancy. Reported labeling indices for the proliferation markers PCNA and MIB-1 were 5.6 and 6% in non-recurrent tumours {205}. On flow cytometry, two thirds were diploid, and the rest either tetraploid or aneuploid {205}. p53 immunostaining has been reported in 52% of 71 tumours, but generally with few positive cells {205}. Cellular schwannomas are benign, although recurrences are seen, notably in spinal examples. No cellular schwannoma has metastasized or been reported to follow a clinically malignant course.

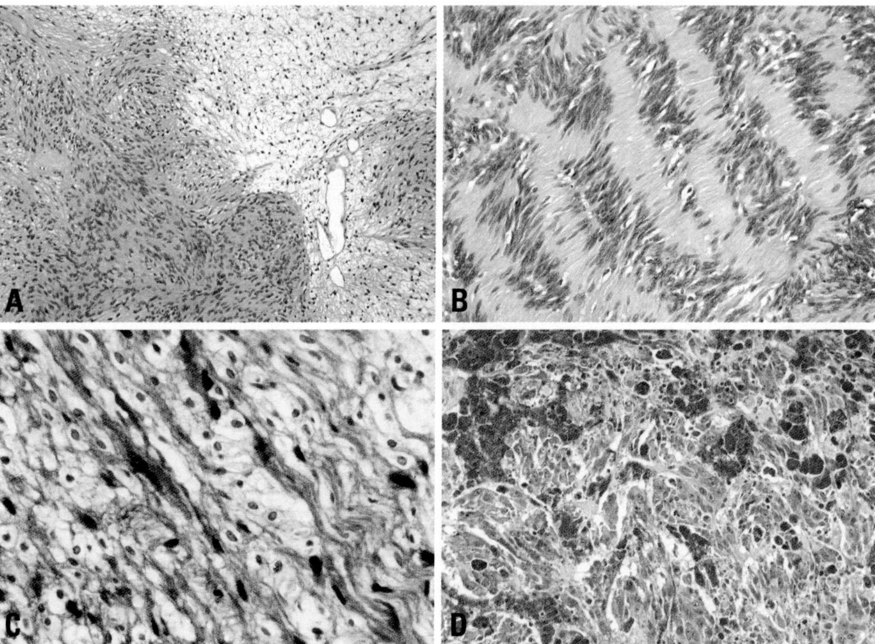

Fig. 10.4 Histological features of schwannoma. **A** Biphasic pattern with cellular Antoni A and hypocellular Antoni B areas. **B** Schwannoma cell nuclei forming palisades. **C** S-100 immunostaining of elongated tumour cells in a predominantly immunonegative Antoni B area. **D** Melanotic schwannoma with clusters of plump, spindled, heavily pigmented tumour cells.

Melanotic schwannoma
This circumscribed, grossly pigmented tumour is composed of cells having the ultrastructure and immunophenotype of Schwann cells but containing melanosomes and being reactive for melanoma markers. Rare in occurrence, their peak incidence is a decade earlier than that of conventional schwannoma. Melanotic schwannomas are divided roughly equally into non-psammomatous {420} and psammomatous {197} varieties. The vast majority of non-psammomatous tumours affect spinal nerves, whereas the psammo-

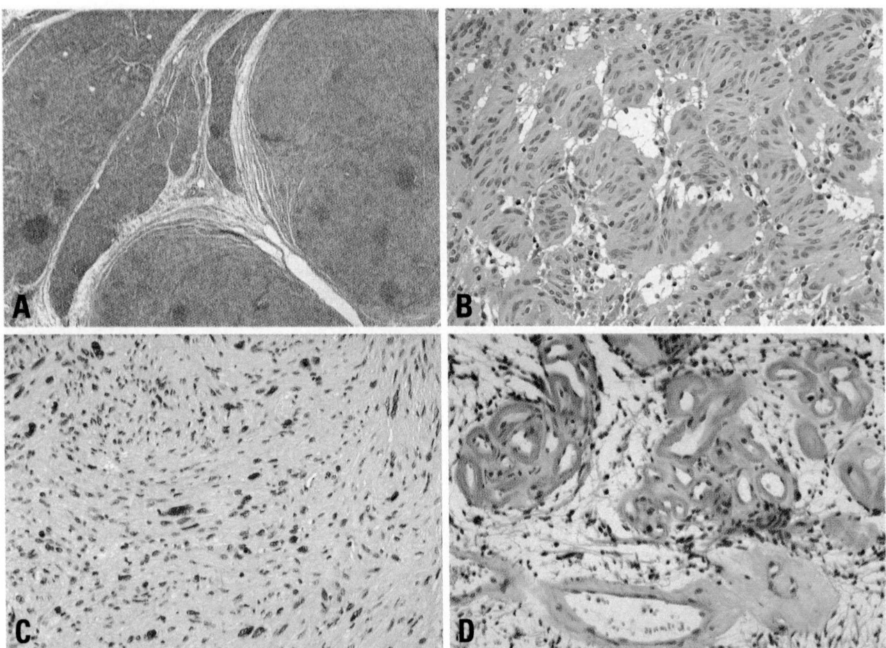

Fig. 10.5 **A** Plexiform schwannoma involving multiple small nerves. **B** Numerous Verocay bodies in a schwannoma. **C** Nuclear polymorphism seen in many cellular schwannomas from any site, not to be interpreted as a sign of malignancy. **D** Hyalinized vessels in a Antoni B area of a conventional schwannoma.

matous lesions also involve nerves of the intestinal tract and heart. Cranial nerves may be affected. Distinction between these two varieties of melanotic schwannoma is important, since about 50% of patients with psammomatous tumours have Carney complex, an autosomal-dominant disorder {198} characterized by lentiginous facial pigmentation, cardiac myxoma and endocrine overactivity. Endocrine manifestations include Cushing syndrome associated with multinodular adrenal hyperplasia or acromegaly due to pituitary adenoma which may be either related or unrelated to a tumour. Slightly over 10% of melanotic schwannomas follow a malignant course.

Plexiform schwannoma

This variant is defined as schwannoma growing in a plexiform or multinodular manner {1644}. Presumably involving a nerve plexus, the vast majority arise in skin or subcutaneous tissue of an extremity, head and neck, or trunk. The tumour is associated with NF2 but not with NF1, and has been noted in non-NF2 patients with multiple schwannomas (schwannomatosis) {414, 658}. Cranial and spinal nerves are usually spared.

Immunohistochemistry

Tumour cells routinely strongly and diffusely express S-100 protein {1597}, often express Leu-7, and may focally express GFAP {1978}.

Electron microscopy

Ultrastructural features are diagnostic and consist of cells with convoluted, moderately thin cytoplasmic processes that are essentially devoid of pinocytotic vesicles, but are lined by a continuous basal lamina {382}. Stromal long-spacing collagen (Luse body) is a common finding.

Genetics

Although most schwannomas are sporadic tumours, multiple schwannomas occur in two inherited tumour syndromes. Bilateral vestibular (eighth cranial nerve) schwannomas are pathognomonic of neurofibromatosis 2 (NF2, see Chapter 14), while multiple peripheral schwannomas in the absence of other NF2 features is characteristic of schwannomatosis, a newly described syndrome {933}. As previously noted, psammomatous melanotic schwannoma is a component of Carney complex. Extensive analyses have implicated the *NF2* gene as a tumour suppressor integral to the formation of sporadic schwannomas {667,1383}. The *NF2* gene and the merlin protein which it encodes (also termed schwannomin) are discussed in detail in the chapter on NF2. Inactivating mutations of the *NF2* gene have been detected in approximately 60% of schwannomas {124, 667, 666, 1289, 1514}. These genetic events are predominantly small frameshift mutations that would be predicted to result in truncated protein products {919}. Mutations occur throughout the coding sequence of the gene and at intronic sites, although they have not been described in exons 16 and 17. In most cases, such mutations are accompanied by loss of the remaining wild-type allele on chromosome 22q. Still other cases demonstrate loss of chromosome 22q in the absence of detectable *NF2* gene mutations. Nonetheless, loss of merlin expression, demonstrated by Western blotting or immunohistochemistry, appears to be a universal finding in schwannomas, regardless of their mutation or allelic status {596, 643, 1311}. This suggests that abrogation of merlin function is an essential step in schwannoma tumourigenesis. Loss of chromosome 22 has also been noted in cellular schwannoma {908}. With the exception of chromosome 1p loss in a small number of cases, consistent genetic alterations have not been documented at other loci in schwannomas {1970}.

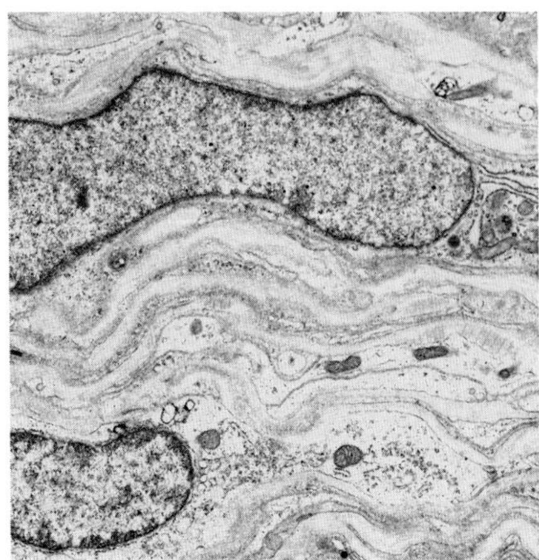

Fig. 10.6 Ultrastructural features of a schwannoma showing a continuous lining of tumour cells by basal lamina.

Prognosis

Schwannomas are slowly growing benign tumours that only rarely undergo malignant change {1646}.

Neurofibroma

J.M. Woodruff
H.P. Kourea
D.N. Louis
B.W. Scheithauer

Definition
A well-demarcated intraneural or diffusely infiltrative extraneural tumour consisting of a mixture of cell types including Schwann cells, perineurial-like cells, and fibroblasts. Multiple neurofibromas are typically associated with neurofibromatosis 1 (NF1).

ICD-O code: 9540/0

Grading
Neurofibroma corresponds histologically to WHO grade I.

Incidence
Neurofibromas are common and occur either as sporadic solitary nodules unrelated to any apparent syndrome, or, far less frequently, as solitary, multiple or numerous lesions in individuals with neurofibromatosis 1 (NF1).

Age and sex distribution
All ages and both sexes are affected.

Localization
Neurofibroma presents most commonly as a cutaneous nodule (localized cutaneous neurofibroma), less often as a circumscribed mass in a peripheral nerve (localized intraneural neurofibroma), or as a plexiform enlargement of a major nerve trunk. Least frequent are diffuse but localized involvement of skin and subcutaneous tissue (diffuse cutaneous neurofibroma), or extensive to massive involvement of soft tissue of a body area (localized gigantism and "elephantiasis neuromatosa"). Neurofibromas occasionally involve spinal roots {1386} but are almost unknown on cranial nerves.

Clinical features
Symptoms and signs

Rarely painful, the tumours present as a mass. The presence of multiple neurofibromas is the hallmark of NF1, in which they are associated with pigmented cutaneous macules (café-au-lait spots) as well as 'freckling', often axillary in location (see NF1 in Chapter 14).

Macroscopy
Cutaneous neurofibromas are either nodular to polypoid and rather circumscribed, or are diffuse and involve skin and subcutaneous tissue. On cut surface, each is firm, glistening and grey-tan. Those confined to nerves are fusiform and well-circumscribed on sectioning. Plexiform neurofibromas are elongate multinodular lesions formed when tumour involves either multiple trunks of a plexus or multiple fascicles of a large nerve, such as the sciatic {1977, 1640}. Some plexiform neurofibromas have the appearance of a bag of worms. Others, such as those affecting the sciatic, produce a massive ropy enlargement of the nerve.

Histopathology
A tumour composed of neoplastic Schwann cells, perineurial-like cells and fibroblasts in a matrix of collagen fibers and mucosubstances.

Cell nuclei are characteristically ovoid-to-spindle, often curved, and smaller than those of schwannomas. Neurofibromas may also exhibit scattered atypical nuclei (atypical neurofibroma) or increased cellularity (cellular neurofibroma). Mitotic figures are rare. Cell processes are thin and are generally not visible on routine light microscopy. Typically, the cells are surrounded by collagen fibers and an Alcian

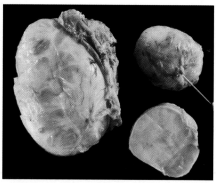

Fig. 10.8 Neurofibroma of a spinal root, with a firm consistency and homogeneous cut surface.

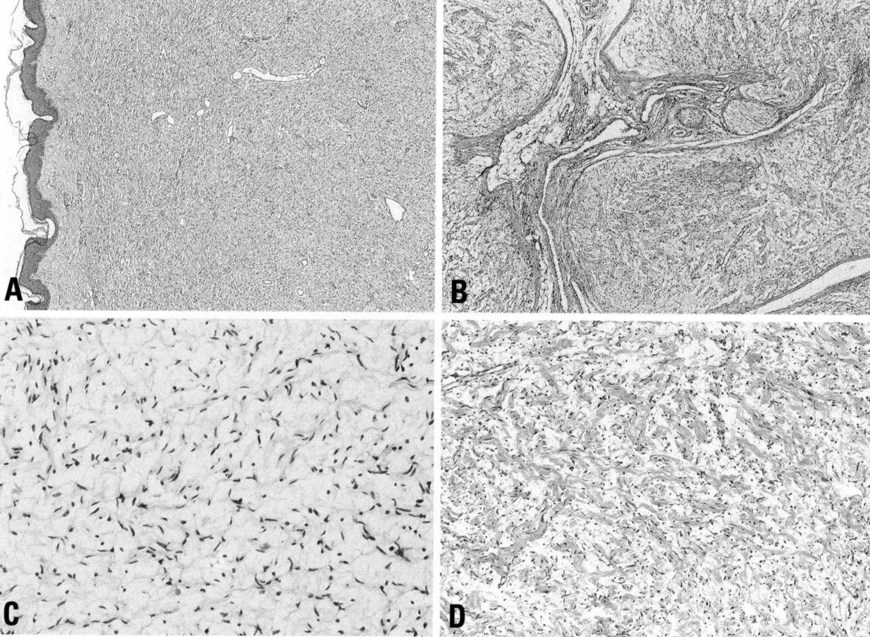

Fig. 10.7 A Cutaneous neurofibroma diffusely infiltrating the dermis and encasing skin adnexae. **B** Plexiform neurofibroma involving small skin nerves. **C** Histopathology of neurofibroma with small ovoid nuclei lacking obvious cell processes. The eosinophilic curved strands are collagen fibers produced by tumour cells. **D** Extensive collagen formation may cause a 'shredded carrots' appearance.

blue-positive myxoid matrix. Marked collagen formation may take the form of characteristic bundles resembling "shredded carrots". Growth of neurofibroma cells is initially along the course of nerve fibers, which become encased by tumour. If arising from a medium size or large nerve, the tumour may remain confined to the nerve but enclosed by its thickened epineurium. Commonly, tumours arising in small nerves spread diffusely into the surrounding dermis and soft tissues. Large diffuse neurofibromas often contain highly characteristic tactile-like structures referred to as Wagner-Meissner-like corpuscles, and may also contain melanotic cells. The multiple nerves or fascicles constituting plexiform neurofibromas are expanded by tumour cells and collagen, and commonly demonstrate residual string-like nerve fibers at their centers. Unlike schwannomas, blood vessels of neurofibromas generally lack hyalinization.

Immunohistochemistry

Staining for S-100 protein is invariably seen, but the proportion of reactive cells is less than in schwannomas. In contrast to perineurioma, the tumour lacks EMA staining in all but residual perineurium {1977}.

Electron microscopy

Electron microscopy shows a mixture of cell types, the two most diagnostically important being the Schwann cell, whether associated or unassociated with axons, and the perineurial-like cell {382, 1977, 1640}. The latter features long, attenuated cell processes, pinocytotic vesicles, and interrupted basement membrane.

Flow cytometry

In a study of 26 neurofibromas, 66% were found to be diploid and 34% aneuploid {1335}.

Genetic susceptibility

The occurrence of multiple neurofibromas is a hallmark of neurofibromatosis 1 (see NF1 in Chapter 14).

Genetics

Given their mixed cellular composition, it has been questioned whether neurofibromas are monoclonal. Early studies suggested that neurofibromas may be polyclonal lesions, but a more recent molecular genetic investigation indicates that NF1-associated neurofibromas are monoclonal in nature {1426}. As sporadic neurofibromas are histologically identical to those occurring in NF1, it seems likely that they too are monoclonal. This remains to be confirmed.

In view of the association of neurofibromas with NF1, investigations of the genetic basis of sporadic tumours have focused on the *NF1* gene. In NF1 patients harbouring germline *NF1* mutations, loss of the remaining wild-type *NF1* allele within their neurofibromas {1973, 1425} confirms the two-hit hypothesis for the genesis of these lesions {267, 1330}. The situation in sporadic tumors has yet to be elucidated, but the morphologic similarity between sporadic and inherited neurofibromas, as well as the clear involvement of the *NF1* gene in sporadic MPNSTs, suggest that *NF1* alterations may also be involved in the genesis of sporadic neurofibromas.

Prognosis

Plexiform neurofibromas and neurofibromas of major nerves are considered a precursor lesion to the majority of malignant peripheral nerve sheath tumours. Malignant transformation is a rare event in other forms of neurofibroma. A patient with a plexiform neurofibroma probably has NF1 and should be investigated for other evidence of the disorder.

Perineurioma

B.W. Scheithauer
C. Giannini
J.M. Woodruff

Definition

A benign tumour composed entirely of neoplastic perineurial cells. Intraneural perineuriomas exhibit proliferating perineurial cells throughout the endoneurium, with formation of characteristic pseudo-onion bulbs. Soft tissue perineuriomas are unassociated with nerve.

ICD-O code:

The provisional code proposed for the third edition of ICD-O is 9571/0.

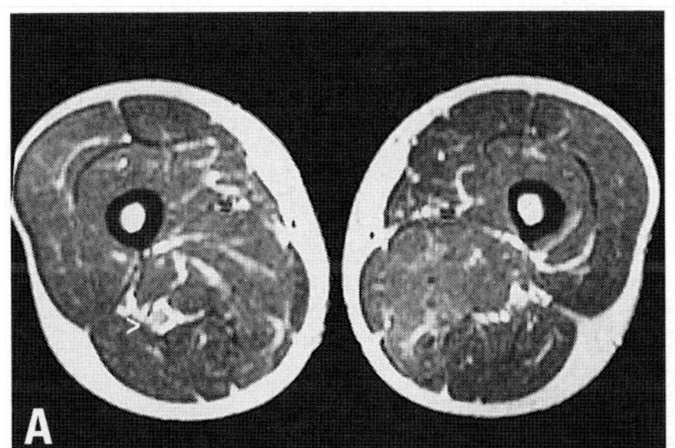

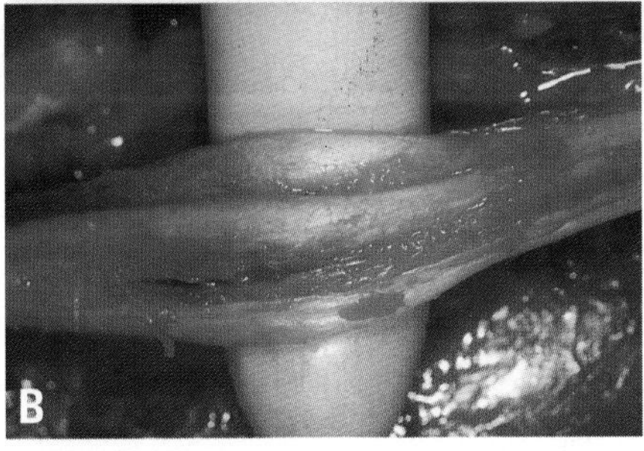

Fig. 10.9 Intraneural perineurioma. **A** MRI of midthigh showing enlarged sciatic nerve (arrow) on one side. **B** Segmental enlargement of the affected nerve.

Grading

Perineuriomas correspond histologically to WHO grade I.

Synonyms and historical annotation

Intraneural perineurioma, long mistakenly considered a form of hypertrophic neuropathy, is now recognised as a neoplasm {1856}. Over 30 cases have been reported to date. Such tumours should be distinguished from malignant peripheral nerve sheath tumours showing perineurial differentiation {1858}.

Soft tissue perineurioma is a morphologically distinctive tumour of superficial or less often deep soft tissue, and is unassociated with nerve. Approximately 15 cases have been described {1861}. Visceral involvement is rare. One example involving the central nervous system arose within a lateral ventricle {1857}.

Incidence

Both variants of perineurioma are exceedingly rare and represent less than 1 percent of nerve sheath and soft tissue neoplasms, respectively.

Clinical features

Intraneural perineuriomas typically present in adolescence or early adulthood and show no sex predilection. Progressive muscle weakness with or without obvious atrophy is more frequent than are sensory disturbances. Peripheral nerves of the extremities are primarily affected; cranial nerve lesions are rare. Soft tissue perineuriomas occur in adults of all ages, predominantly females (2:1), and present with non-specific mass effects.

Macroscopy

Intraneural perineuriomas produce segmental, tubular, several-fold enlargement of the affected nerve. Individual nerve fascicles appear coarse and pale. Most lesions are less than 10 cm in length but one 40 cm long sciatic nerve example has been reported {1856}. Although multiple fascicles are often involved, a "bag of worms" plexiform growth is not seen. Involvement of two neighbouring spinal nerves has been reported {1856}.

Soft tissue perineuriomas are solitary, generally small (1.5-7 cm) and well-circumscribed but not encapsulated. Only a single large example (12 cm) has been reported {1862}. On cut surface they are firm and grey-white to infrequently focally myxoid.

Histopathology

Intraneural perineurioma consists of neoplastic perineurial cells proliferating throughout the endoneurium, forming concentric layers around nerve fibers and characteristic pseudo-onion bulbs.

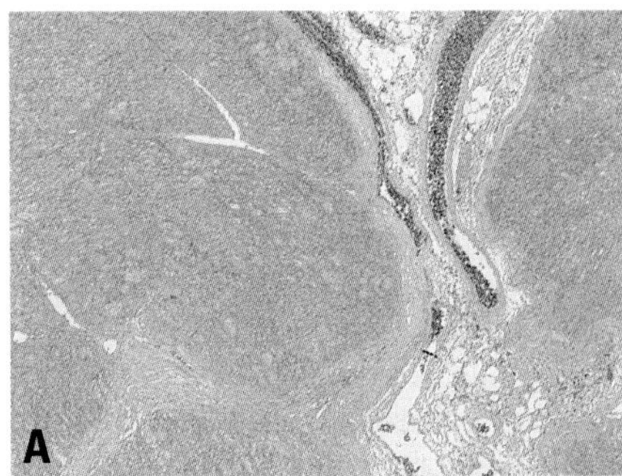

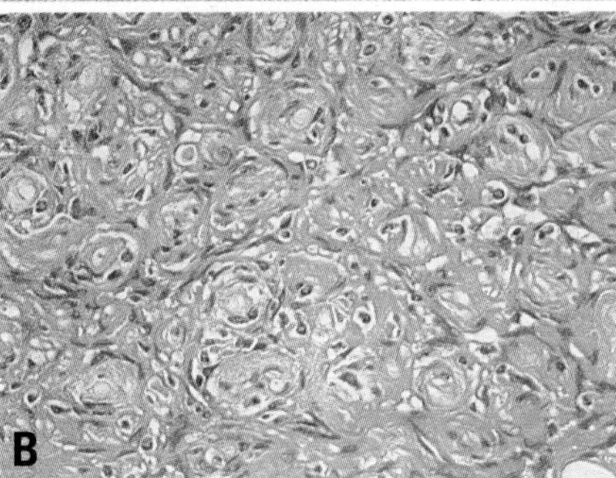

Fig. 10.10 Intraneural perineurioma. **A** Nerve enlargement involves individual fascicles. **B** Cross section of typical pseudo-onion bulbs formed by tumour cells.

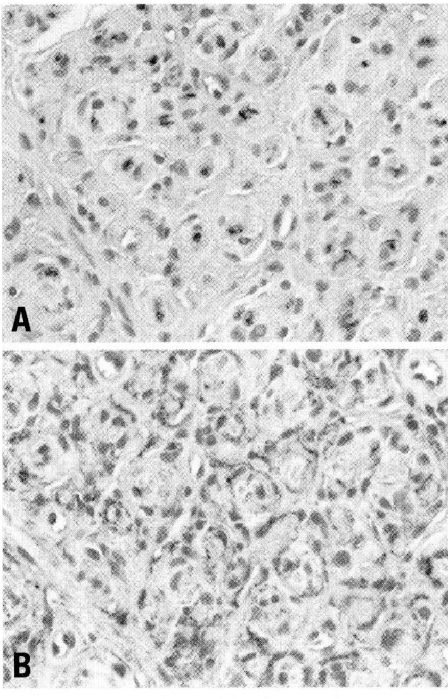

Fig. 10.11 Intraneural perineurioma. **A** S100 protein, labeling centrally situated residual Schwann cells. **B** EMA immunoreactivity in concentrically arranged tumour cells.

Microscopically, the nerve enlargement seen grossly in intraneural perineurioma involves fascicles. A characteristic finding at higher magnification are "pseudo-onion bulbs". This distinctive architectural feature is best seen on cross section, wherein fascicles vary in cellularity. Proliferation of perineurial cells largely takes place within endoneurium but perineurium is often affected as well. Numerous perineurial cells, most of which appear cytologically normal, are concentrically disposed in multiple layers around nerve fibers (Fig. 10.13 D). Particularly large whorls may envelop numerous nerve fibers. Occasionally, perineurial cells enclosing one axon will contribute to an adjacent onion bulb as well. Thus, pseudo-onion bulbs anastomose one with the other, forming a complex endoneurial network. Bielschowsky or Bodian stains often show one or several axons at the center of pseudo-onion bulbs. Luxol-fast blue preparations typically show myelin to be scant or absent. Even within a single fascicle, cell density and the complexity of the lesion may vary. Mitotic activity is rare. In early lesions, axonal density and myelination may be almost normal, whereas in fully developed lesions, when most fibers are singly surrounded by perineurial cells and therefore widely separated, myelin is often scant or absent on Luxol-fast blue stain. At late stages, only denervated Schwann cells may remain at the center of the perineurial whorls. Hyalinization may also be an impressive finding.

Soft tissue perineuriomas are composed of spindled, wavy cells with remarkably thin cytoplasmic processes arranged in wavy lamellae and embedded in collagen fibers. Partial whorls or storiform arrangements are commonly seen.

Aggregates of collagen fibers are often encircled by long tumour cell processes. Nuclei are elongate with tapered ends and often curved or wrinkled. Nucleoli are inconspicuous. Mitoses are generally rare, and necrosis is lacking. Degenerative atypia (nuclear pleomorphism and hyperchromasia) is seen primarily in long-standing tumours {1862}.

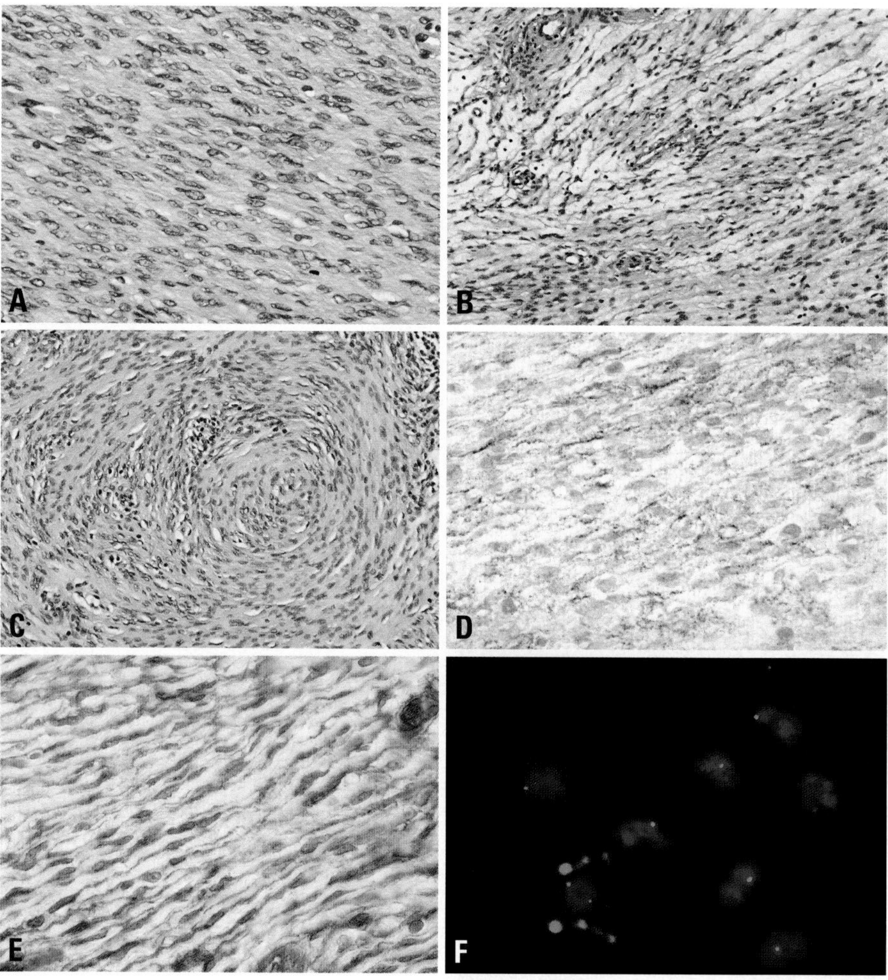

Fig. 10.13 Soft tissue perineurioma. **A** Tumour cells are layered, with nuclei and cell processes being typically curved. **B** Remarkably elongated tumour cell processes in less cellular areas. **C** Cell whorls. **D** EMA immunoreactivity. **E** Collagen IV immunoreactivity. **F** FISH using a probe for the M-ber locus on chromosome 22q11. Monosomy of 22 has been demonstrated in both intraneural and soft tissue perineuriomas.

Immunohistochemistry

Intraneural perineuriomas, like normal perineurial cells, are vimentin and epithelial membrane antigen (EMA)-immunoreactive. The pattern of EMA staining is membranous, as is that for collagen IV and laminin. Axon(s) at the center of pseudo-

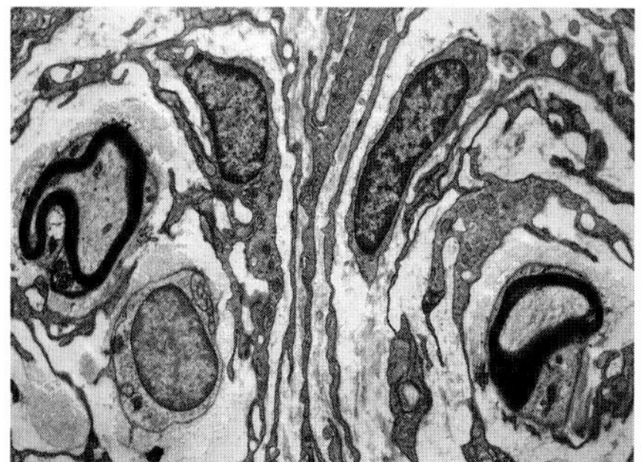

Fig. 10.12 Ultrastructure of an intraneural perineurioma showing the typical concentric arrangement of perineurial cells in pseudo-onion bulbs.

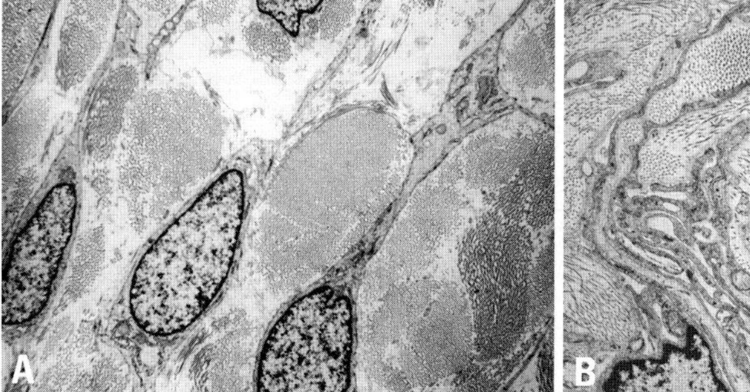

Fig. 10.14 **A** Ultrastructure of soft tissue perineurioma, showing thin, attenuated processes of perineurioma cells widely separated by collagen bundles. **B** Cell processes arranged in a whorl around collagen fibers. Tumour cells have numerous pinocytic vesicles and patches of basement membrane.

onion bulbs and residual Schwann cells stain for neurofilament protein and S-100 protein, respectively. Staining for p53 protein has also been reported {1856}. Soft tissue perineurioma features the same immunophenotype as the intraneural variant. Unlike various other soft tissue tumours, they lack reactivity for S-100 protein, desmin, muscle-specific actin, and CD34.

Proliferation
Despite a paucity of mitoses, MIB-1 labeling indices range from 5 to 15 percent {1856}.

Electron microscopy
Intraneural perineuriomas feature myelinated nerve fibers circumferentially surrounded by ultrastructurally normal-appearing perineurial cells. The cells have long, thin cytoplasmic processes bearing numerous pinocytotic vesicles and are lined by patchy surface basement membrane. Stromal collagen may be abundant. Soft tissue perineuriomas typically consist of spindle-shaped cells with long, exceedingly thin cytoplasmic processes embedded in an abundant collagenous stroma. Cytoplasm is scant and contains sparse profiles of rough endoplasmic reticulum, occasional mitochondria and a few randomly distributed immediate filaments. The processes exhibit numerous pinocytotic vesicles and a patchy lining of basement membrane. Intracellular junctions (poorly formed desmosomes) are relatively frequent.

Cytogenetics
Both intraneural and soft tissue perineuriomas feature the same cytogenetic abnormality, monosomy of chromosome 22 {1856, 1861}.

Prognosis
Intraneural perineuriomas are benign. Long-term follow-up indicates that they show neither a tendency to recurrence nor metastasis. Biopsy alone is sufficient for diagnosis. Resection of affected nerves should be avoided in order to retain neurologic function as long as possible. Even after excision and nerve graft reconstruction, recovery of nerve function may not occur. Soft tissue perineuriomas are usually amenable to gross total removal; no recurrences have been reported.

Malignant peripheral nerve sheath tumour (MPNST)

J.M. Woodruff
H.P. Kourea
D.N. Louis
B.W. Scheithauer

Definition
Any malignant tumour arising from a peripheral nerve or showing nerve sheath differentiation, with the exception of tumours originating from epineurium or the peripheral nerve vasculature. Approximately 50% of cases are associated with neurofibromatosis 1 (NF1).

ICD-O code:
The provisional code proposed for the third edition of ICD-O is 9540/3.

Grading
Histologically, this tumour corresponds to WHO grades III or IV.

Synonyms
Equivalent, although misleading, terms include neurogenic sarcoma, neurofibrosarcoma and malignant schwannoma.

Incidence
MPNSTs are uncommon neoplasms, accounting for nearly 5% of malignant tumours of soft tissue {886}. Almost two-thirds arise from neurofibromas {353, 625, 1969}, often of the plexiform type and in the setting of NF1. Second in frequency are MPNSTs arising *de novo* from peripheral nerves {1977, 1640}. Only rare examples also develop from conventional schwannoma {1646}, ganglioneuroblastoma/ganglioneuroma {1259, 1977} and phaeochromocytoma {1972}.

Age and sex distribution
MPNSTs primarily occur in adults in the third to the sixth decades of life. The mean age of patients with NF1-associated MPNSTs is approximately a decade younger (28-36 years) than that of sporadic cases (40-44 years) {353, 625}. Childhood and adolescent cases are uncommon {352, 986} and are rare in children under the age of six years. MPNSTs are slightly more frequent in females.

Localization
Large and medium nerves are distinctly more prone to involvement than are small nerves. The most common sites are the buttock and thigh, the brachial plexus and upper arm, and the paraspinal region. The sciatic nerve is most frequently affected. Cranial nerve MPNSTs are very uncommon, with the fifth cranial nerve being more often involved than the eighth nerve {102, 534, 833, 980, 1044, 1655}. With the exception of one trigeminal nerve example having its origin in a schwannoma {428, 1646}, MPNSTs of cranial nerves appear to arise *de novo* from the nerve. Only a single example of intracerebral MPNST has been reported {1454}.

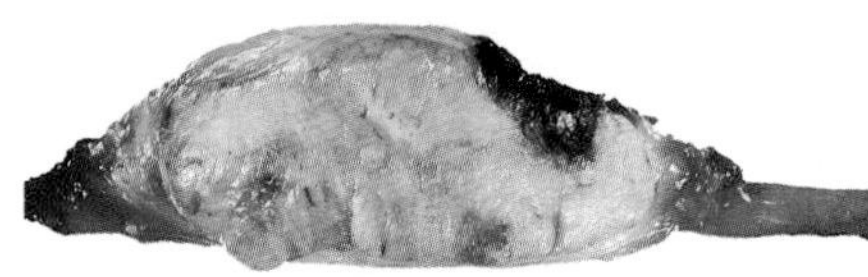

Fig. 10.15 Fusiform MPNST of the sciatic nerve with a partially trimmed pseudocapsule. The cut surface is firm, cream-tan and focally necrotic.

Clinical features
Symptoms and signs
About half of MPNSTs occur in the clinical setting of NF1. Roughly another 10% develop at the site of prior irradiation {350, 418}. The most common presentation of tumours of the extremities is a progressively enlarging mass with or without neurological symptoms {625}. Spinal tumours often present with radicular pain.

Neuroimaging
Findings correspond to those of a soft tissue sarcoma. Inhomogeneous contrast enhancement and irregularity of contour, a reflection of invasion, are commonly seen. However, some MPNSTs are indistinguishable from benign nerve sheath tumours {1977}.

Macroscopy
The gross appearance of MPNSTs is that of a globoid or fusiform, pseudoencapsulated tumour which is firm to hard in consistency. An attached large or medium sized nerve is often evident. The cut surface is typically cream coloured or grey, with foci of necrosis and haemorrhage that are sometimes extensive. The vast majority of tumours are larger than 5 cm and examples over 10 cm in diameter size are common.

Histopathology
MPNSTs typically feature a fibrosarcoma-like fasciculated growth of tightly packed, hyperchromatic spindle cells with abundant, faintly eosinophilic cytoplasm. Nuclei are elongate, and in contrast to those of smooth muscle, have tapered ends. Most tumours show a diffuse growth pattern or have alternating loose and densely cellular areas, as well as increased perivascular cellularity. Although unusual growth patterns may be seen, including haemangiopericytoma-like areas, nuclear palisading is not a feature. Three-quarters of tumours have geographic necrosis and mitotic activity; at least 4 mitotic figures per high power field are common. The above features are those of conventional MPNSTs. Uncommonly, cells of a MPNST have features of perineurial cells {1858}. About 15% of cases exhibit unusual histological features such as epithelioid morphology and divergent differentiation {351, 1977}.
Growth pattern. MPNSTs grow within nerve fascicles but commonly invade through perineurium and epineurium into the adjacent soft tissues. Commonly surrounding the tumour is a pseudocapsule of variable thickness comprised of tumour-invaded soft tissue and reactive fibrous tissue.

Epithelioid MPNST
This variant is defined as MPNST with a predominance of epithelioid cells.
Fewer than 5% of MPNSTs are either partially or purely epithelioid {334, 861, 907}. They show no association with NF1. Both superficial (above the fascia) and deep-seated examples are recognized. The superficial tumours carry a better prognosis {861}.

Glandular MPNST

This variant is defined as MPNST containing gland-forming epithelium.

Such divergent differentiation consists of intestinal-appearing, keratin- and CEA-positive glands, often with intra- and extracellular mucin. Neuroendocrine cells immunoreactive for chromogranin, somatostatin and serotonin are common. Ultrastructural studies have also shown luminal microvilli and dense core neurosecretory type granules {246, 1642}. Squamous differentiation is less common. Three-quarters of the patients have NF1 and mortality is high (79%) {1642}.

Malignant Triton tumour.

This term refers to MPNSTs showing rhabdomyosarcomatous differentiation.

Their incidence is 3- to 4-fold that of glandular MPNSTs. There are now at least 100 reported cases of this quintessential example of divergent mesenchymal differentiation {1645}. Often accompanying such myoid growth are areas of chondrosarcoma, osteosarcoma or epithelial glands (pluridirectional differentiation). Nearly 60% of the patients have NF1. Few cranial nerve examples have been reported {102, 534}. The prognosis of malignant Triton tumours is poor, with 2- and 5-year survival rates of approximately 33 and 12%, respectively {161}.

Immunohistochemistry

In 50-70% of MPNSTs, scattered tumour cells express S-100 protein {1597}. Immunostaining for p53 is present in a majority of tumours, in contrast to the infrequent staining seen in neurofibromas {530}. Conversely, immunostaining for other selected cell cycle regulatory proteins is common in neurofibromas but uncommon in MPNSTs. These include p27 {1974}, and p16 {1976}.

Electron microscopy

Given the poor differentiation of most MPNSTs, electron microscopy is usually of little diagnostic utility, short of excluding other histologically similar sarcomas such as leiomyosarcoma, synovial sarcoma and fibrosarcoma.

Proliferation

In the majority of MPNSTs, the growth fraction, as determined by Ki-67/MIB-1 immunoreactivity, ranges from 5 to 65%, in contrast to values often below 1% in schwannomas and neurofibromas {775}.

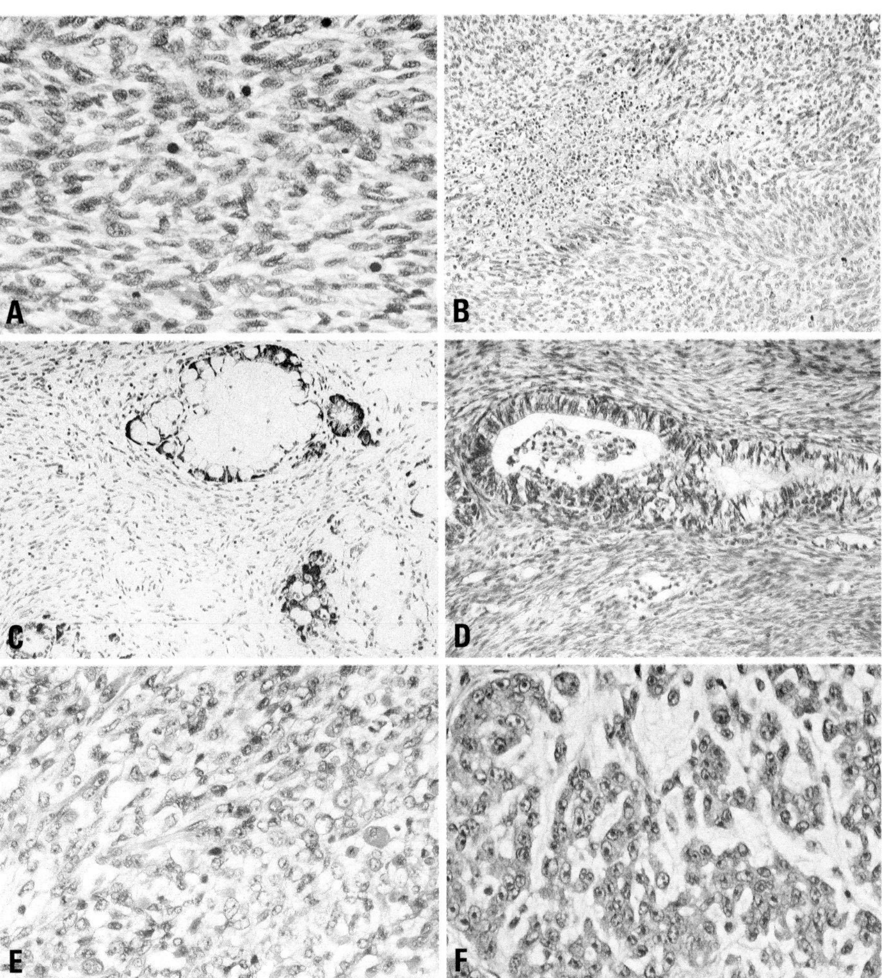

Fig. 10.16 A MPNST with brisk mitotic activity (commonly four or more mitoses per high-power field). **B** MPNST with a well-delineated geographic necrosis. **C** Benign glandular PNST containing neuroendocrine cells immunoreactive to chromogranin. **D** Formation of glands in an MPNST is interpreted as aberrant differentiation and considered as a sign of malignancy. **E** Malignant Triton tumour arising in a plexiform neurofibroma. Note strap-shaped and round rhabdomyoblasts on the background of anaplastic MPNST cells. **F** Epithelial MPNST. Tumour cells are embedded in a mucinous matrix and show abundant cytoplasm and prominent nucleoli.

Genetic susceptibility

Approximately one-half of MPNSTs manifest in patients with neurofibromatosis 1 (see NF1 in Chapter 14). This association is particularly strong in the glandular variant of MPNST.

Cytogenetics

Sporadic and NF1-associated MPNSTs typically have complex karyotypic abnormalities that are both numerical and structural. Although no consistent karyotypic pattern is seen, often observed abnormalities include near-triploid or hypodiploid chromosome numbers {998}, chromosomal losses, loss of genetic material related to structural aberrations {701} and recombinations that involve almost all chromosomes {998}. In one study of 10 tumours, structural abnormalities of chromosome 17 involving the *NF1* and *TP53* loci were common {701}. Chromosome 22 loss has also been noted somewhat frequently {701, 1971}. No cytogenetic differences have been noted between sporadic and NF1-associated tumours.

Molecular genetics

In MPNSTs of patients with NF1, inactivation of both *NF1* alleles has been demonstrated {872} implicating this gene in their formation (see NF1 in Chapter 14). Furthermore, sporadic MPNSTs also show alterations at the *NF1* locus. However, such *NF1* gene alterations are more likely to be involved in the early stages of nerve sheath tumorigenesis, i.e., in the formation of neurofibromas, rather than in the malignant progression to MPNST. There is now evidence that malignant progression is related to alterations of genes controlling cell cycle regulation. A clearly implicated gene is *TP53* {871, 914, 993}. Both *TP53* gene mutations and alterations of protein expression have been found in MPNSTs. In addition, homozygous deletions of the *CDKN2A* gene, which encodes the p16 cell cycle inhibitory molecule, occur in the progression of neurofibromas to MPNSTs, being found in 50% of MPNSTs but not in neurofibromas {1975, 1976}. It appears likely that additional oncogenes and tumour suppressor genes play a role in malignant transformation. The karyotypic complexity seen in these tumours lends support to this notion {998}.

Prognosis and predictive factors

Except those with perineurial cell differentiation {1858}, MPNSTs are highly aggressive tumours with a poor prognosis. About 60% of patients die of the disease {353}, with an even higher mortality (80%) in individuals with paraspinal lesions {1969} and those (100%) with divergent angiosarcoma {1977}. Overall 5- and 10-year survival rates are 34% and 23% {353}. MPNSPTs vary from low grade lesions to a vast majority of high grade tumours featuring high cellularity, brisk mitotic activity and necrosis. No firm association has been established between histologic grade and survival.

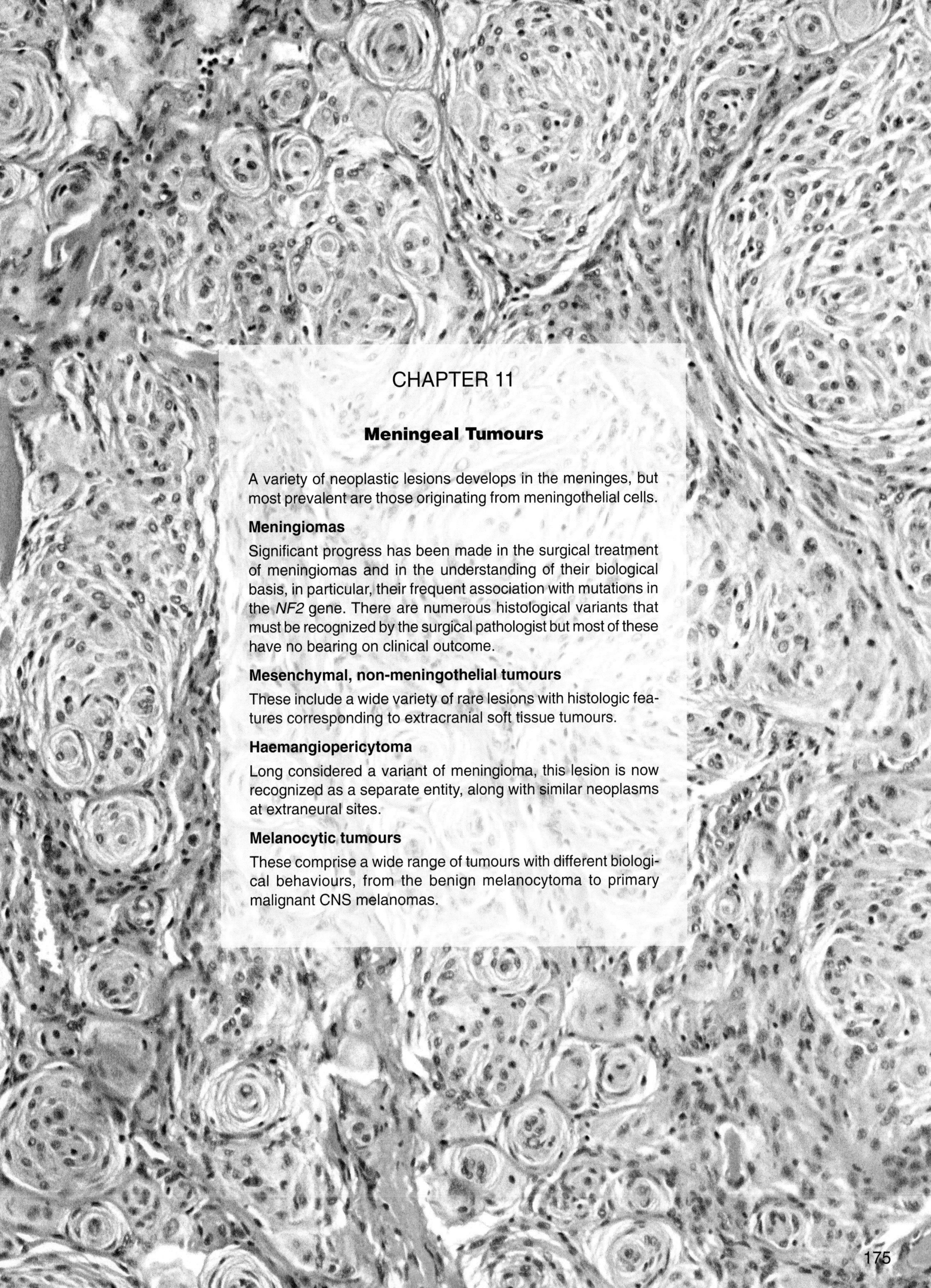

CHAPTER 11

Meningeal Tumours

A variety of neoplastic lesions develops in the meninges, but most prevalent are those originating from meningothelial cells.

Meningiomas

Significant progress has been made in the surgical treatment of meningiomas and in the understanding of their biological basis, in particular, their frequent association with mutations in the *NF2* gene. There are numerous histological variants that must be recognized by the surgical pathologist but most of these have no bearing on clinical outcome.

Mesenchymal, non-meningothelial tumours

These include a wide variety of rare lesions with histologic features corresponding to extracranial soft tissue tumours.

Haemangiopericytoma

Long considered a variant of meningioma, this lesion is now recognized as a separate entity, along with similar neoplasms at extraneural sites.

Melanocytic tumours

These comprise a wide range of tumours with different biological behaviours, from the benign melanocytoma to primary malignant CNS melanomas.

Meningiomas

D.N. Louis
B.W. Scheithauer
H. Budka
A. von Deimling
J.J. Kepes

Definition

Meningiomas are generally slowly growing, benign tumours attached to the dura mater and composed of neoplastic meningothelial (arachnoidal) cells. They typically manifest in adults and show a predominance for women.

ICD-O code: 9530/0

Grading

Most meningiomas are benign and can be graded into WHO grade I. Certain histological subtypes are associated with a less favourable clinical outcome and correspond to WHO grades II and III (Table 11.1).

Incidence

Meningiomas are estimated to constitute between 13% and 26% of primary intracranial tumours, with an annual incidence rate of approximately 6 per 100'000 population {859}. Many small meningiomas go unnoticed during life, but may be found incidentally at autopsy at a frequency of 1.4% {1235}. Such incidental meningiomas are being found increasingly because of the advent of CT and MRI. Meningiomas are often multiple in patients with neurofibromatosis 2 (NF2) and in other, non-NF2 families with a hereditary predisposition to meningioma {919}. Sporadic meningiomas may also be multiple; such multiple tumours occur in less than 10% of cases. Atypical meningiomas constitute between 4.7% and 7.2% of meningiomas, while anaplastic (malignant) meningiomas are less common, accounting for between 1.0% and 2.8% of meningiomas {661, 942, 943, 2165,2166}. An incidence for anaplastic (malignant) meningiomas of 0.17 per 100'000 persons has been reported {1276}.

Age and sex distribution

Meningiomas are most common in middle-aged and elderly patients, with a peak occurrence during the sixth and seventh decades of life, although these tumours can also occur both in children and in the very old. In children, there is a tendency towards more aggressive forms of meningioma. Among middle-aged patients, there is a marked female bias, with a female: male ratio of approximately 3:2, or even 2:1. In particular, spinal meningiomas show a marked predominance in women. Meningiomas associated with hereditary tumour syndromes generally occur in younger patients, and equally in men and women. Atypical and anaplastic meningiomas, on the other hand, may show a conspicuous predominance in

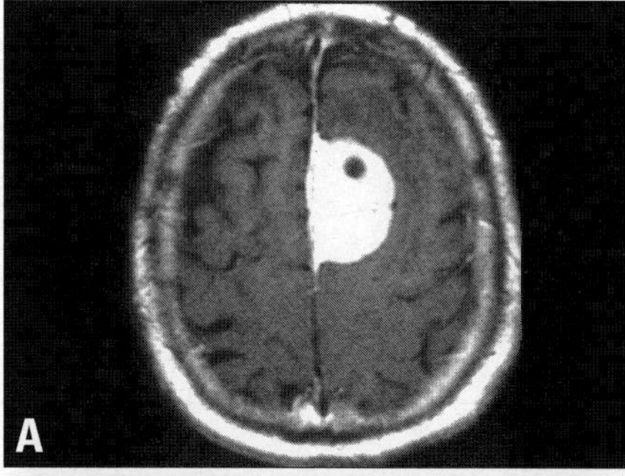

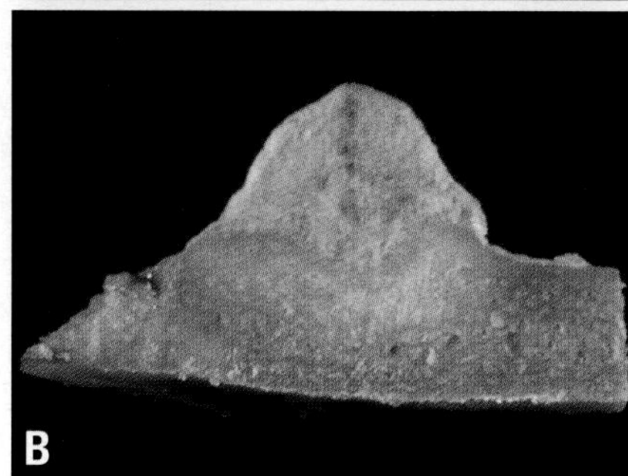

Fig. 11.1 A Large meningioma of the falx, presenting as contrast-enhanced mass with a central cyst. Note the tailing along the dura at either side of the neoplasm. **B** Ossifying meningioma inducing hyperostosis in the overlying skull.

Table 11.1
Meningiomas grouped by likelihood of recurrence and grade.

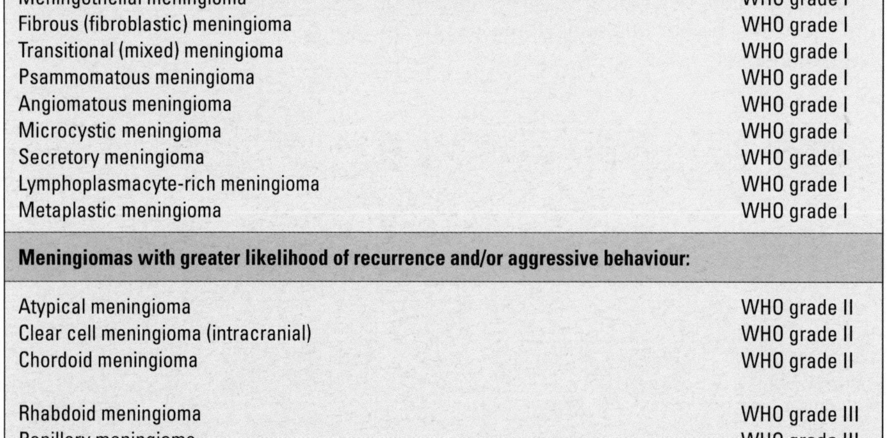

Meningiomas with low risk of recurrence and aggressive growth:	
Meningothelial meningioma	WHO grade I
Fibrous (fibroblastic) meningioma	WHO grade I
Transitional (mixed) meningioma	WHO grade I
Psammomatous meningioma	WHO grade I
Angiomatous meningioma	WHO grade I
Microcystic meningioma	WHO grade I
Secretory meningioma	WHO grade I
Lymphoplasmacyte-rich meningioma	WHO grade I
Metaplastic meningioma	WHO grade I
Meningiomas with greater likelihood of recurrence and/or aggressive behaviour:	
Atypical meningioma	WHO grade II
Clear cell meningioma (intracranial)	WHO grade II
Chordoid meningioma	WHO grade II
Rhabdoid meningioma	WHO grade III
Papillary meningioma	WHO grade III
Anaplastic (malignant) meningioma	WHO grade III
Meningiomas of any subtype or grade with high proliferation index and/or brain invasion	

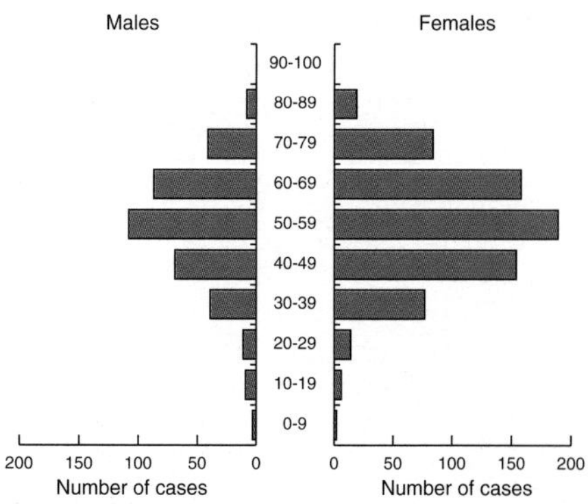

Fig. 11.2 Age and sex distribution of meningiomas, based on 1078 cases treated at the University Hospital, Zurich.

males {661}. Furthermore, proliferation indices tend to be higher in meningiomas occurring in male patients {971}.

Localization

The vast majority of meningiomas arise within the intracranial, orbital and intravertebral cavities, although rare meningiomas have been reported in almost all organs. Within the intracranial cavity, most meningiomas occur over the cerebral convexities, often closely associated with the falx cerebri {180, 181, 859, 1306}. Other common sites include the olfactory grooves, sphenoid ridges, parasellar regions, optic nerve, petrous ridges, tentorium cerebelli, posterior fossa and within the ventricles. Spinal meningiomas are most common in the thoracic region. Atypical and anaplastic meningiomas are more common on the falx and the lateral convexities than elsewhere {943}. With malignant meningiomas, metastatic deposits most often occur in the lung, pleura, bone, and liver, among other sites.

Clinical features

Symptoms and signs

Meningiomas are generally slow-growing masses that elicit neurological signs and symptoms by compression of adjacent structures; the specific deficits depend on the location of the tumour. Headache and seizures may also herald the presence of a meningioma.

Neuroimaging

On MRI, meningiomas are typically isodense dural masses which may be calcified and which show contrast enhancement. A characteristic feature is the presence of a so-called 'dural tail' adjacent to the main mass, which may or may not indicate dural spread. Peritumoural cerebral oedema is occasionally prominent, particularly in secretory variants {24} and in meningothelial tumours with so-called pericytosis {1266}. Findings on neuroimaging have not always been reliable in predicting tumour behaviour. Microcystic meningiomas may show poor enhancement on CT and MR imaging {2548}.

Macroscopy

Most meningiomas are rubbery or firm, well-demarcated, sometimes lobulated, rounded masses that have a broad dural attachment {180, 181, 859, 1306}. They often compress the adjacent brain, but rarely show overt attachment or invasion of the brain. However, invasion of the dura and of nearby dural sinuses is quite common. Occasional meningiomas invade through dura to involve the skull, where they may induce characteristic hyperostosis: such bony changes are highly indicative of skull invasion. Meningiomas may attach to or encase cerebral arteries, but only rarely do they infiltrate arterial walls. They may also infiltrate the skin and

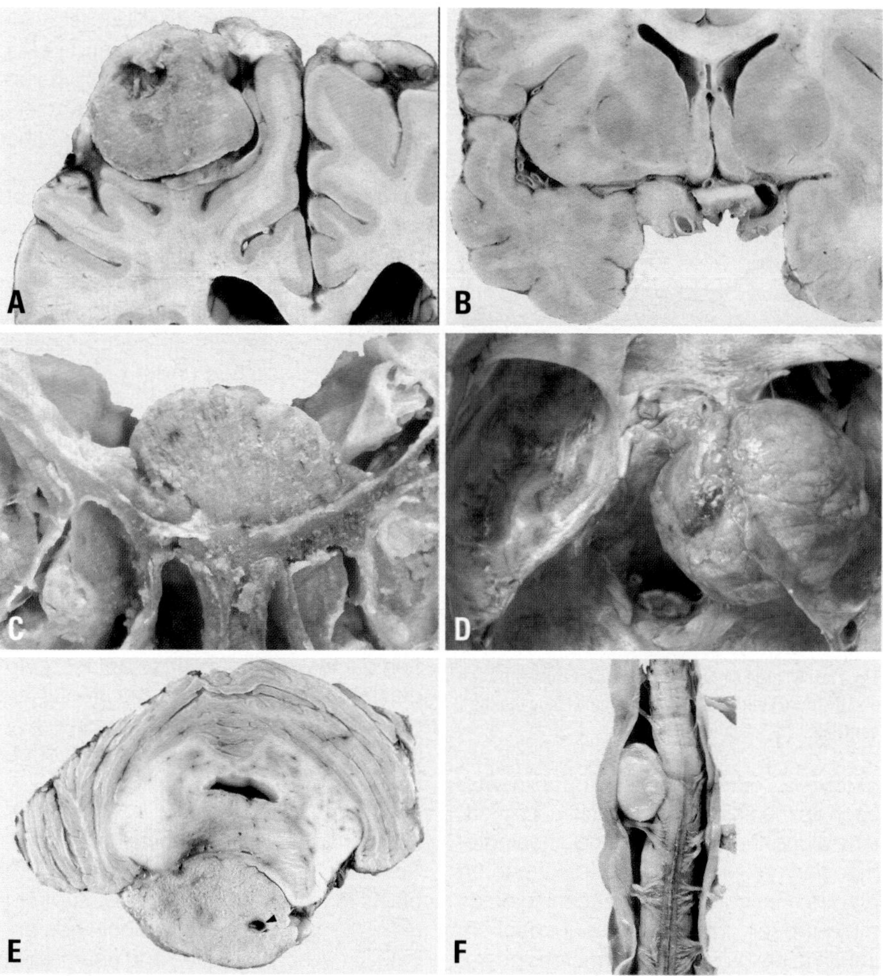

Fig. 11.3 Macroscopic features of meningioma. **A** Large parasaggital meningioma compressing the adjacent parietal lobe. **B** Meningioma of the medial sphenoid wing encasing the carotid artery. **C** Coronal section through the anterior cranial fossa showing a meningioma of the olfactory groove. **D** Meningioma of the sphenoid wing. E Large meningioma of the clivus compressing the brain stem. F Spinal meningioma compressing the spinal cord.

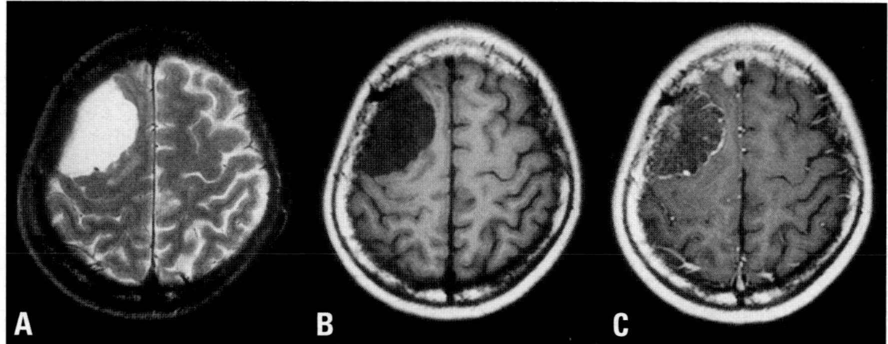

Fig. 11.4 MRI of a microcystic meningioma which presents as (**A**) hyperintense mass on T2-weighted MRI, and (**B**) as hypointense lesion on T1-weighted image. **C** Faint reticular pattern after Gd enhancement. From Shimoji *et al.* {2548}.

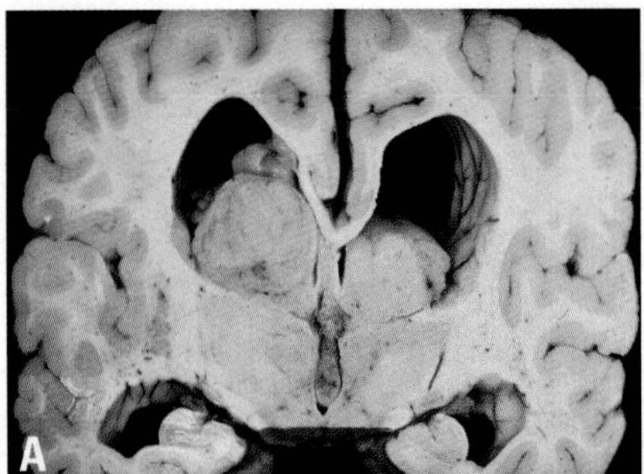
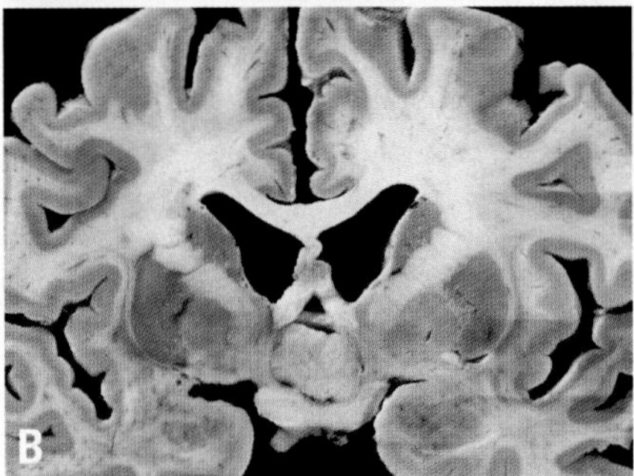

Fig. 11.5 **A** Large meningioma of the lateral ventricles and the third ventricle. **B** Meningioma filling the third ventricle.

extend to extracranial compartments, such as the orbit. In certain sites, particularly along the sphenoid wing, meningiomas may grow as a flat mass, termed en plaque meningioma. Some meningiomas may appear gritty on gross inspection, implying the presence of numerous psammoma bodies. Atypical and anaplastic meningiomas tend to be larger at operation than classical meningiomas {943}.

Histopathology

Meningiomas have a wide range of histopathological appearances {180, 181, 859, 1306, 2173}. Of the various subtypes, meningothelial, fibrous and transitional meningiomas are by far the most common. Most subtypes share a common clinical behaviour, although some subtypes are more likely to recur and follow a more aggressive clinical course (see below and Table 11.1). Pleomorphic nuclei and occasional mitoses may be noted in any of these variants without necessarily connoting more aggressive behaviour; furthermore, the criteria used to diagnose atypical meningioma are independent of meningioma subtype.

Meningothelial meningioma

In this classic and common variant, tumour cells form lobules which are surrounded by thin collagenous septae. Like normal arachnoid, tumour cells are largely uniform, with oval nuclei that on occasion show central clearing. Whorls and psammoma bodies are not common in meningothelial meningioma and, when present, tend to be less-well formed than in other subtypes.

Larger lobules should not be confused with the 'sheeting', or loss of architectural pattern, seen in atypical meningioma. Within the lobules, tumour cells appear to form a syncytium, as the delicate, intricately interwoven tumour cell processes cannot be discerned under light microscopy. The tumour cells closely resemble those of the normal arachnoid, and florid arachnoidal hyperplasia may simulate meningioma in small biopsy specimens; this phenomenon has most often been observed near optic nerve gliomas. Like the normal arachnoidal cells, meningothelial tumour cells feature oval nuclei and a delicate, even chromatin pattern.

Sometimes, rounded eosinophilic cytoplasmic protrusions into the nuclei are prominent. Other nuclei show central clearing, presumably secondary to glycogenation.

Fibrous (fibroblastic) meningioma

Spindle-shaped cells resembling fibroblasts form parallel and interlacing bundles on a matrix abundant in collagen and reticulin. Whorl formation and psammoma bodies are infrequent.

In this classic and common variant, tumour cells are predominantly spindle-shaped, appearing fibroblastic. However, cells with nuclear features characteristic of meningothelial meningioma are often found as well; these can be helpful in distinguishing fibrous meningiomas from other spindle cell tumours such as schwannoma. In fibrous meningioma, the tumour cells form wide fascicles, with varying amounts of either interfascicular or intrafascicular intercellular collagen and reticulin. In some cases, the amount of collagen may be striking.

Transitional (mixed) meningioma

These common tumours have features transitional between those of meningothelial and fibrous meningioma.

Lobular and fascicular arrangements are present and regions of cytologically typical meningothelial cells are common. Whorls are often conspicuous in this subtype, and are often tight. Psammoma bodies are also frequent, and are typically found in the center of cellular whorls.

Psammomatous meningioma

This designation may be used for meningiomas with abundant psammoma bodies. that may become confluent, forming irregular calcified and occasionally ossified masses.

Typically, the neoplastic cells in these tumours have a transitional appearance with whorls, although some tumours are almost replaced by psammoma bodies, and require careful examination to identify intervening meningothelial cells. These tumours characteristically occur in the thoracic spinal region, usually in middle-aged women.

Angiomatous meningioma

A meningioma in which numerous blood vessels prevail on the background of a typical meningioma.

The vascular channels may be small- or medium-sized and may be thin-walled or have hyalinized, thickened walls. Most often, the vessels are small with hyalinized walls. Differential diagnoses include vascular malformations and capillary haemangioblastoma, depending on the size of the

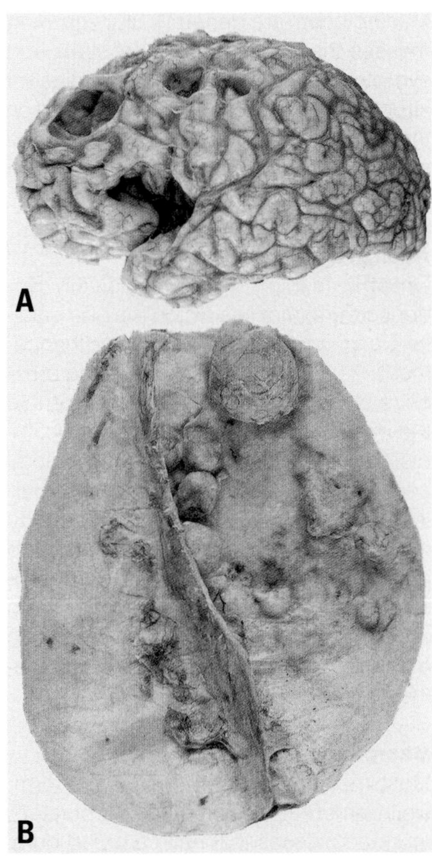

Fig. 11.6 Multiple meningiomas (**B**) of the hemispheric convexity and (**A**) the impressions caused in the left cerebral hemisphere.

meningiomatous vessels. This designation should not be equated with the obsolete term 'angioblastic meningioma' (see section on haemangiopericytoma), as angiomatous meningiomas do not display aggressive clinical behaviour.

Microcystic meningioma

This variant is characterized by cells with elongated processes and by a loose, mucinous background, giving the appearance of many small cysts. Pleomorphic cells may be numerous.

Secretory meningioma

The hallmark of this subtype is the presence of focal epithelial differentiation, in the form of intracellular lumina containing PAS-positive, eosinophilic material.

These structures are known as pseudopsammoma bodies {2172, 2173}, which stain immunohistochemically for carcinoembryonic antigen (CEA) and a variety of other epithelial and secretory markers, while the surrounding tumour cells are cytokeratin-positive. These tumours may be associated with elevated levels of circulating CEA {918}, which may be clinically significant in patients who also have breast carcinoma. In addition, secretory meningiomas may present with prominent peritumoural cerebral oedema {24}.

Lymphoplasmacyte-rich meningioma

A meningioma with extensive chronic inflammatory infiltrates, often relegating the meningothelial component to the background.

Care must be taken to avoid missing diagnoses of other meningeal-based haematological conditions, particularly as lymphoplasmacyte-rich meningiomas may be associated with haematological abnormalities {779}.

Metaplastic meningioma

A meningioma with striking focal mesenchymal differentiation.

Meningothelial, fibrous or transitional tumours may display osseous, cartilaginous, lipomatous, myxoid or xanthomatous changes. The clinical significance of these alterations is not clear.

While the above mentioned meningiomas correspond to WHO grade I, some histological variants of meningioma discussed below are often associated with more frequent recurrences and/or more aggressive behaviour (Table 11.1).

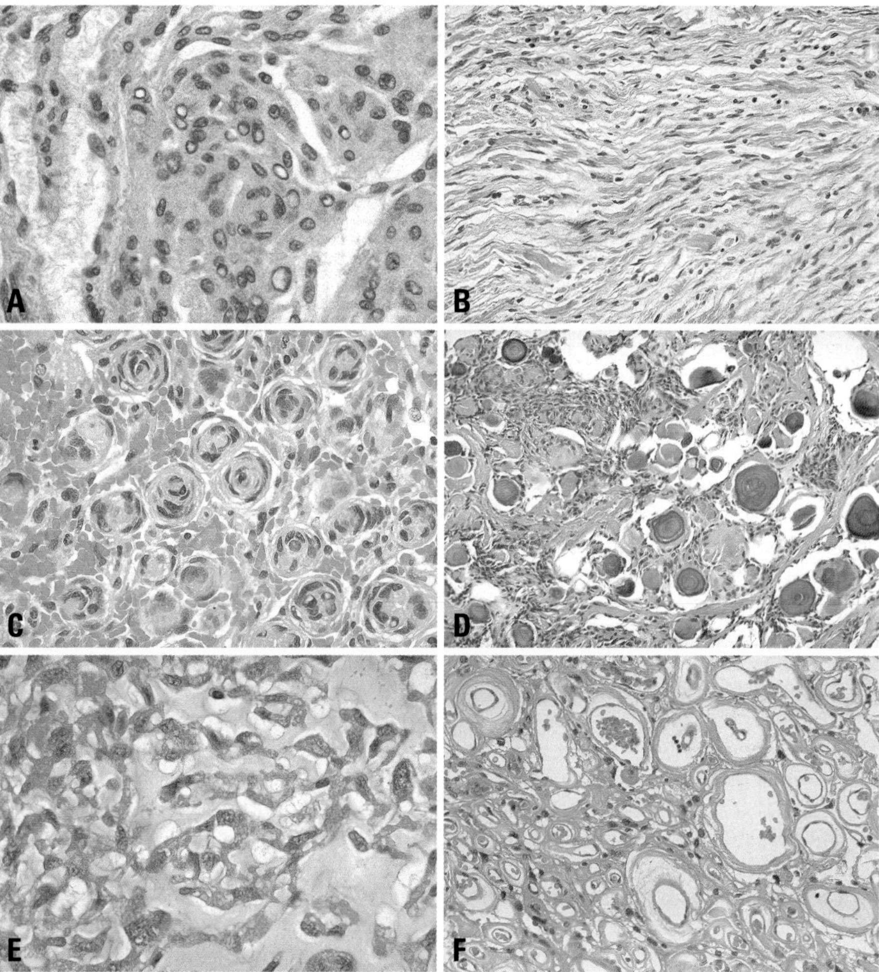

Fig. 11.7 Histological features of meningioma. **A** Meningothelial meningioma with typical intranuclear inclusions. **B** Fibrous meningioma characterized by parallel fascicles of fibroblastic cells. **C** Transitional meningioma with numerous, concentric, onion-bulb structures **D** Psammomatous meningioma with numerous calcified psammoma bodies and inconspicuous meningothelial component. **E** Chordoid meningioma with eosinophilic tumour cells in a mucous-rich matrix. **F** Angiomatous meningioma dominated by excessive vascularization interspersed with small meningothelial tumour cells.

Chordoid meningioma

A meningioma containing regions that are histologically similar to chordoma, with trabeculae of eosinophilic, vacuolated cells in a myxoid background.

Such chordoid areas are interspersed with typical regions of meningioma. Chronic inflammatory cell infiltrates may be prominent, and a few of affected patients have haematological conditions, such as Castleman's disease {755}. Chordoid meningiomas exhibit a high rate of recurrence following subtotal resection (WHO grade II).

Clear cell meningioma

An often patternless meningioma composed of polygonal cells with a clear, glycogen-rich cytoplasm.

This rare variant shows prominent PAS-positive cytoplasmic clearing. Classic features of meningioma may be few. There is a proclivity for the cerebellopontine angle and the cauda equina. Some of these tumours, particularly intracranial clear cell meningiomas, may be associated with a more aggressive behaviour (WHO grade II) {1680}.

Atypical meningioma

A meningioma with increased mitotic activity or three or more of the following features: increased cellularity, small cells with high nucleus: cytoplasm ratio, prominent nucleoli, uninterrupted patternless or sheet-like growth, and foci of 'spontaneous' or 'geographic necrosis'.

For this variant, increased mitotic activity has been defined as 4 or more mitoses per 10 high-power fields (defined as

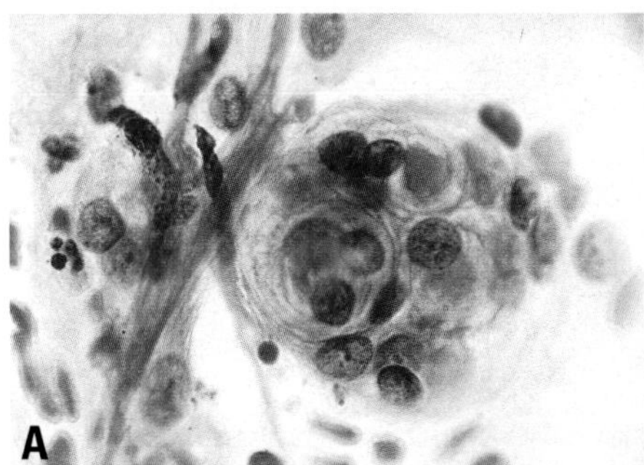

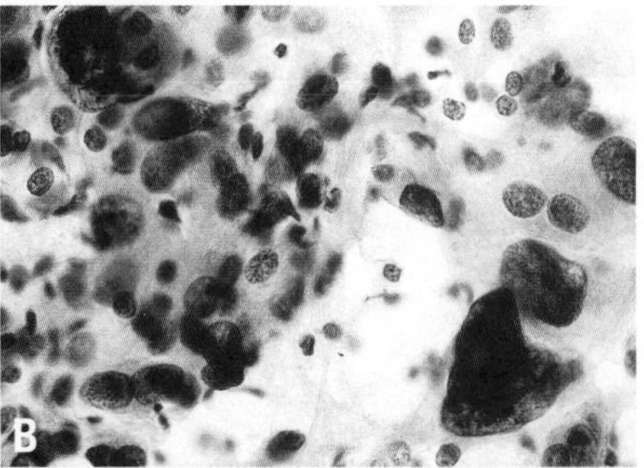

Fig. 11.8 A Squash preparation of a meningothelial meningioma showing the typical whorl formation. **B** Squash preparation showing prominent nuclear pleomorphism in a benign meningioma.

0.16 mm^2) {2166}, The above criteria have been shown to correlate with higher recurrence rates {2166}, as have criteria that have individually scored parameters to arrive at a sum {661}, or have simply combined hypercellularity with 5 or more mitoses per 10 high power fields {943}. Atypical meningiomas often have moderately high MIB-1 labelling indices and correspond histologically to WHO grade II.

Papillary meningioma

A rare meningioma variant defined by the presence of a perivascular pseudopapillary pattern in at least part of the tumour. Papillary meningiomas tend to occur in children {927}. Local invasion and invasion of the brain have been noted in 75% of these lesions, recurrence in 55%, and metastasis in 20% {1136}. Because of their aggressive clinical behaviour {927}, these tumours have been graded as WHO grade III.

Rhabdoid meningioma

An uncommon tumour containing patches or extensive sheets of rhabdoid cells, which are rounded tumour cells with eccentric nuclei, often with a prominent nucleolus, and prominent inclusion-like eosinophilic cytoplasm comprised of whorled intermediate filaments.

These rhabdoid cells resemble those described in tumours in other sites (e.g., kidney). Rhabdoid cells may be present only at the time of recurrence. Most rhabdoid meningiomas have high proliferative indices and additional histological features of malignancy. They typically display aggressive clinical course and correspond to WHO grade III {2167, 2168}. A minority of rhabdoid meningiomas have only focal rhabdoid features and lack other histological features of malignancy; the behaviour of these tumours remains to be determined.

Anaplastic (malignant) meningioma

A meningioma exhibiting histological features of frank malignancy far in excess of the abnormalities present in atypical meningioma.

Such features include either obviously malignant cytology (e.g., having an appearance similar to sarcoma, carcinoma or melanoma) or a high mitotic index (20 or more mitoses per ten high-power fields (defined as 0.16 mm2) {2165}. Tumors that meet the above criteria correspond to WHO grade III and are usually fatal, with median survivals of less than 2 years {2165}.

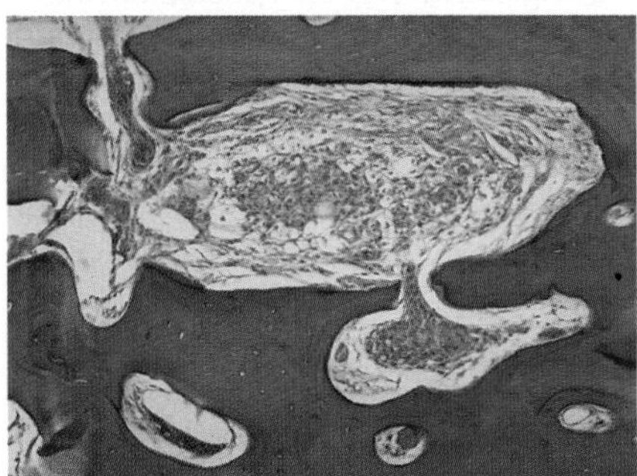

Fig. 11.9 Invasion of bones by meningiomas through osseous caniculi is not a sign of malignancy.

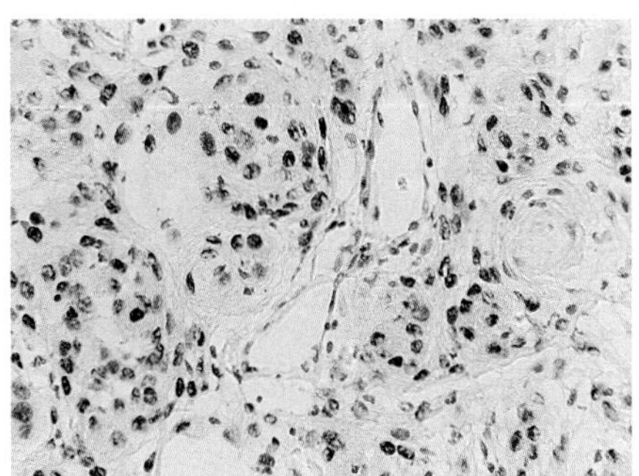

Fig. 11.10 Meningioma with marked immunoreactivity for progesterone receptor. Endothelial cells are negative.

Invasion of the brain alone is not sufficient for a diagnosis of anaplastic meningioma {2165}. Caution must also be taken in the setting of prior therapeutic embolization, since such therapy may cause extensive necrosis as well as increased perinecrotic proliferation {2169}.

Brain invasion and metastasis

Invasion of the brain by meningioma is characterized by irregular groups of tumour cells infiltrating the adjacent cerebral parenchyma, without an intervening layer of leptomeninges, often causing reactive astrocytosis. Brain invasion may occur in histologically benign, atypical or anaplastic (malignant) meningiomas.

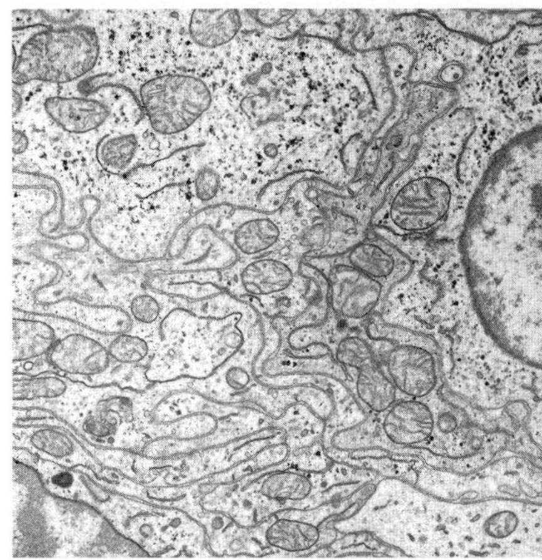

Fig. 11.11 Electron micrograph of a meningioma showing numerous interdigitated cellular processes and occasional desmosomal junctions.

The presence of brain invasion connotes a greater likelihood of recurrence (Table 11.1), with brain-invasive histologically benign meningiomas having clinical courses similar to atypical meningiomas {2166}. The genetic changes that characterize higher-grade meningiomas (see below) have not been found in brain-invasive, histologically benign meningiomas {1247, 1422, 2170}. Anaplastic (malignant) meningiomas may metastasize; the rare metastases of histologically benign meningiomas typically occur following surgery.

Immunohistochemistry and electron microscopy

The vast majority of meningiomas stain for epithelial membrane antigen (EMA), although EMA immunoreactivity is less consistent in atypical and malignant lesions. Vimentin positivity is found in all meningiomas. Immunohistochemical studies of S-100 protein have found varying positiv-

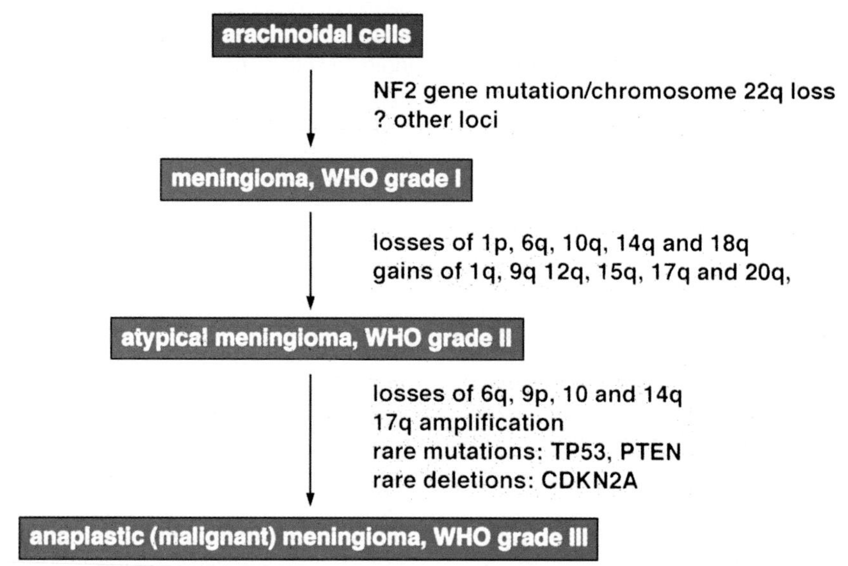

Fig. 11.12 Genetic changes associated with meningioma progression.

ity in meningiomas, but such staining is not usually prominent. Secretory meningiomas characteristically show strong positive staining for CEA in the pseudopsammoma bodies, and for cytokeratins in the cells surrounding the pseudopsammoma bodies. Diagnostic ultrastructural features of meningiomas include copious intermediate (vimentin) filaments, complex interdigitating cell processes (particularly in meningothelial variants), and desmosomal intercellular junctions.

Proliferation

In general, cellular proliferation increases from benign to atypical to anaplastic (malignant) meningioma. Mitotic index and the absence of calcification on CT correlate strongly with volume growth rate {661}. There are significant differences in mitotic indices (total counts per ten high-power fields) between tumour grades: 0.08 ± 0.05 for benign, 4.75 ± 0.91 for atypical, and 19.00 ± 4.07 for malignant variants. Tumour doubling times also show a close inverse correlation with BUdR labelling indices {234}. BUdR indices are low in benign meningiomas, and generally increase with grade, but malignant meningiomas may also show low BUdR incorporation {1404}.

MIB-1/Ki-67 indices also show a highly significant increase from benign (mean, 3.8%), to atypical (mean 7.2%), and anaplastic meningioma (mean 14.7%) {944}. MIB-1 indices may vary considerably among anaplastic meningiomas (1.3-24.2%; mean, 11.7%) {1201}. One study found that the Ki-67 proliferation index was the most important criterion for distinguishing anaplastic meningioma (mean, 11%) from atypical meningioma (mean, 2.1%) and from classical type with a mean Ki-67 index of 0.7% {795}.

Flow cytometric studies have demonstrated approximately equal numbers of diploid and aneuploid meningiomas, and have shown significant correlations between aneuploid tumours and features such as recurrence, pleomorphism, high cellular density, mitotic activity and infiltration of brain and soft tissue {290}.

Aetiology

Meningiomas are known to be induced by low-, moderate-, and high-dose radiation, with an average time interval to tumour appearance of 35, 26 and 19-24 years, respectively {786}. The majority of patients with radiation-induced meningiomas have a history of low-dose irradiation (800 rad) to the scalp for tinea capitis. The second largest group of patients with radiation-induced meningiomas received high-dose irradiation (>2000 rad) for primary brain tumours {543}. Radiation-induced meningiomas are more commonly atypical or aggressive, and multifocal, show higher proliferation indices and generally occur in younger age groups {543, 935, 1049}.

The role of sex hormones in the genesis of meningiomas is less clear. The overrepresentation of women among meningioma patients suggests an aetiological role for sex hormones in these tumours. While expression of oestrogen receptor is very low or undetectable in the majority of meningiomas, approximately two-thirds of meningiomas express progesterone receptors {203}, with a higher fraction in

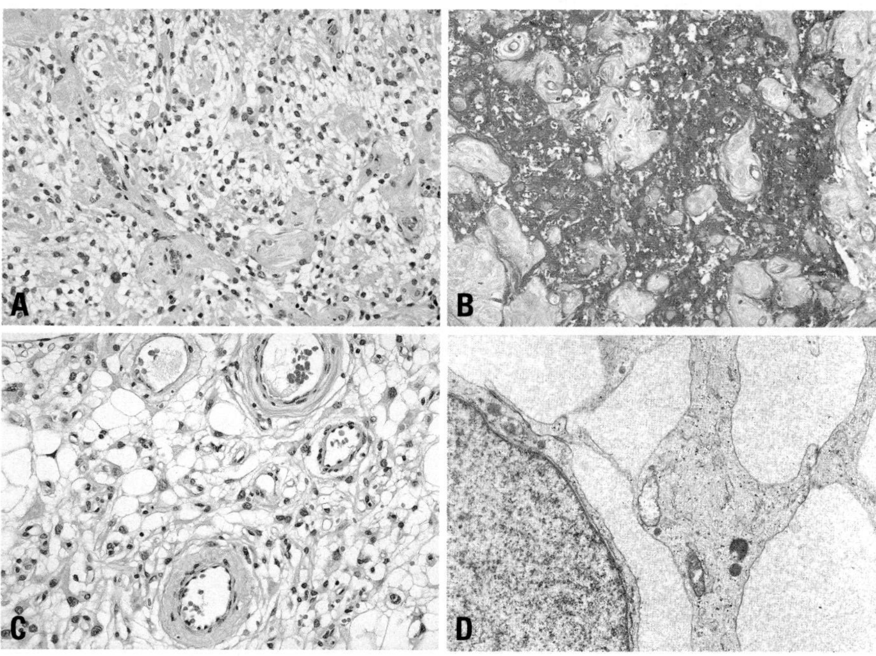

Fig. 11.13 Histogical variants of meningioma. Clear cell meningioma showing (**A**) a patternless neoplasm dominated by clear, (**B**) glycogen-rich cytoplasm (PAS staining). **C, D** Microcystic meningioma characterized by large intracellular cysts.

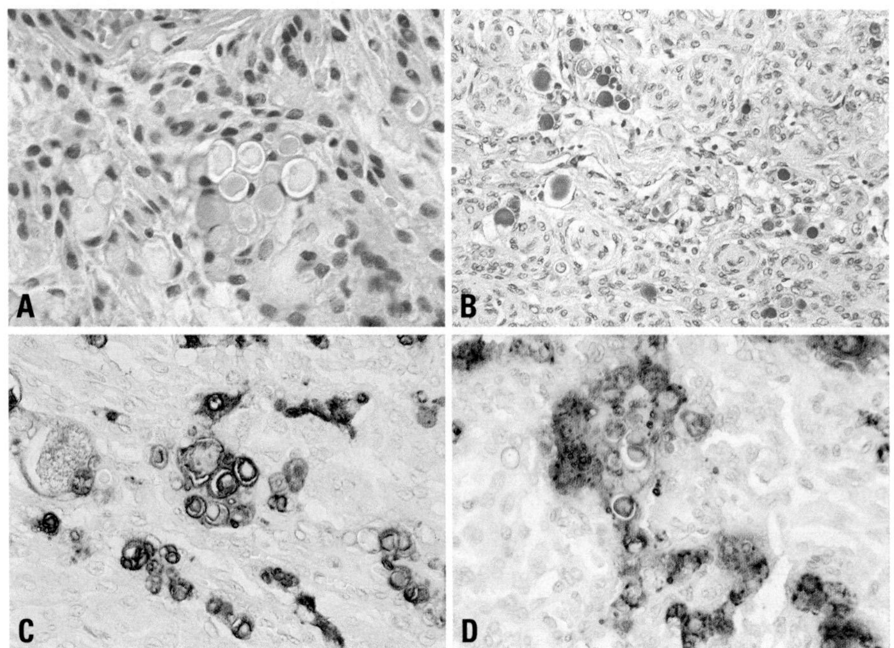

Fig. 11.14 A Secretory meningioma with numerous pseudopsammoma bodies rich in glycogen (**B**) and marked immunoreactivity for (**C**) epithelial membrane antigen (EMA) and (**D**) carcino-embryonic antigen (CEA).

meningiomas from female patients. However, it remains to be determined whether the expression of these receptors is integral to meningioma formation and growth, and whether hormonal therapy may have a role.

Genetic susceptibility

Meningiomas are a hallmark of neurofibromatosis type 2 (see NF2 in Chapter 14). However, a number of families with an increased susceptibility to meningiomas, but without NF2, have been reported {919}; in at least one of these families, the disease did not show linkage to the *NF2* locus on chromosome 22q {1212}, suggesting that there may be a second meningioma predisposition locus. The possible relationship of meningioma to other rare inherited tumour syndromes, such as Gorlin or Cowden syndrome, is less-well defined {922}.

Cytogenetics

Meningiomas were among the first solid tumours recognized as having cytogenetic alterations {1671}, the most consistent change being deletion of chromosome 22 {1670}. Loss of chromosome 22 also occurs in recurrent and atypical meningiomas {44}. In general, karyotypic abnormalities are more extensive in atypical and anaplastic (malignant) meningiomas {1168}. Among the other cytogenetic changes associated with meningioma, deletion of the short arm of chromosome 1 {795} and loss of chromosome 14 {1369} have been observed most frequently.

Molecular genetics

Allelic losses and chromosomal gains

Molecular genetic findings have demonstrated that approximately half of meningiomas have allelic losses that involve band q12 on chromosome 22 {357, 358, 899, 983, 1308}. In addition, atypical meningiomas often show allelic losses of chromosomal arms 1p, 6q, 9q, 10q, 14q, 17p and 18q, suggesting that progression-associated genes may lie at these loci {899, 994, 1247, 1421, 1422, 2170, 2488}. These alterations, with more frequent losses of chromosomes 6q, 9p, 10 and 14q, also occur in anaplastic meningiomas {2170}. Chromosomal gains have been noted in higher-grade meningiomas, with gains of chromosomes 20q, 12q, 15q, 1q, 9q and 17q most commonly observed {2170}. Significantly, of the above chromosomal loci, only the *NF2* gene on chromosome 22q has been implicated as a specific tumour suppressor; the responsible genes on the other frequently involved chromosomes remain to be identified. Furthermore, it is likely that genes other than *NF2* are involved in the formation of a substantial percentage of benign meningiomas, but it remains unclear whether these genes reside on the long arm of chromosome 22 or on other chromosomes, such as chromosomes 1p and 3p {2171}.

NF2 gene

Mutations in the *NF2* gene are detected in up to 60% of sporadic meningiomas {875, 1129, 1514, 1600}. The majority of the mutations are small insertions or deletions, or nonsense mutations that affect

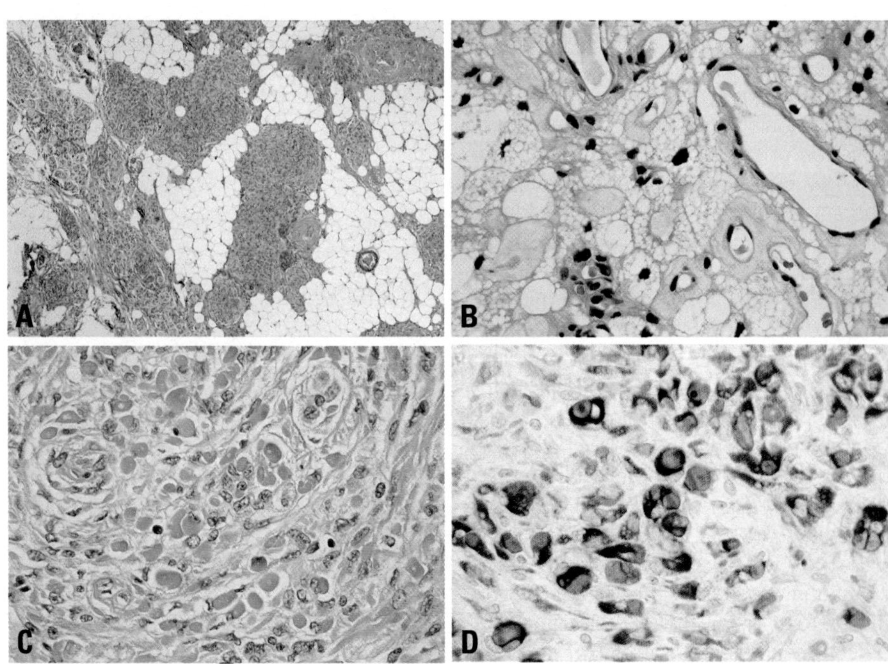

Fig. 11.15 A, B Metaplastic / lipomatous meningioma. **C** Meningioma with granular filamentous inclusions that stain strongly with antibodies to vimentin (**D**).

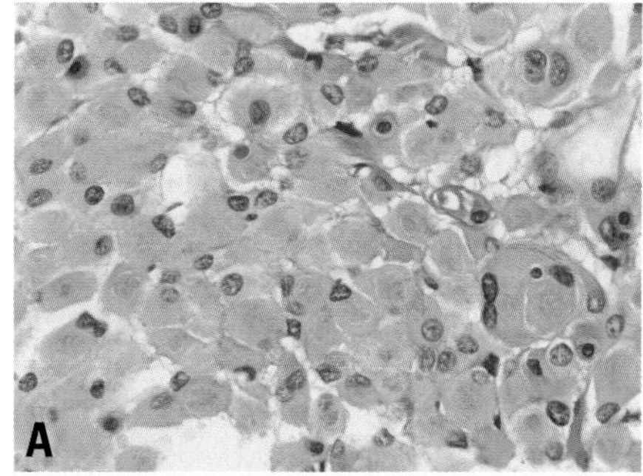

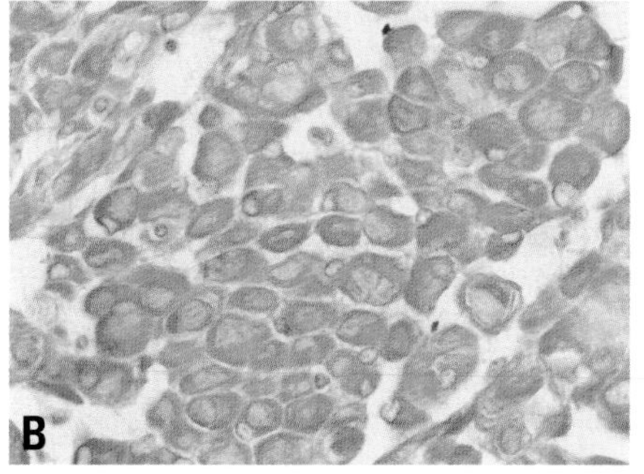

Fig. 11.16 Rhabdoid meningioma showing (**A**) typical large tumour cells with excentric nuclei and (**B**) cytoplasmic immunorectivity for vimentin.

splice sites, create stop codons or result in frameshifts and which occur predominantly in the most 5' two-thirds of the gene {919}. The predicted common effect of these mutations is a truncated, and presumably non-functional, merlin (schwannomin) protein. The frequency of *NF2* gene mutations varies among the three most frequent meningioma variants. Fibroblastic and transitional meningiomas carry *NF2* gene mutations in approximately 70-80% of cases. In contrast, meningothelial meningiomas harbour *NF2* gene mutations in only 25% of cases, suggesting that this variant has a genetic origin that is largely independent of *NF2* gene alterations {1600}. The observation of a close association between allelic loss on 22q and the fibroblastic meningiomas supports this hypothesis {1308}, as does the observation that most non-NF2 meningioma families develop meningothelial tumours {919}. Furthermore, reduced expression of merlin (schwannomin) has been observed in different histopathological variants of meningiomas, but appears to be rare in meningothelial tumours {867}. In atypical and anaplastic meningiomas, *NF2* gene mutations occur in approximately 70% of cases, matching the frequency of *NF2* mutations in benign fibroblastic and transitional meningiomas, suggesting that mutation of the *NF2* gene is not involved in progression to higher-grade meningiomas.

Other genes

The close association of *NF2* mutations in meningiomas with allelic loss on chromosome 22 suggests that *NF2* is the major meningioma tumour suppressor gene on chromosome 22 {1600}. Nonetheless, certain deletion studies of chromosome 22 have detected losses and translocations of genetic material outside the *NF2* region, raising the possibility that a second meningioma gene resides on chromosome 22. One candidate is the *adaptin* gene, which lies within a region that is homozygously deleted in a meningioma and shows reduced expression in some meningiomas; however, a partial mutational analysis of *adaptin* did not reveal mutations {1169}. Another candidate gene on chromosome 22q is *MN1*, which has been found to be disrupted by a translocation in a meningioma {876}. Although allelic losses of chromosome 17p have been noted in higher-grade meningiomas, studies of the *TP53* gene on chromosome 17p have not shown significant gene alterations in meningiomas. Nonetheless, immunohistochemical positivity for TP53 protein has been noted in some atypical meningiomas, and rare anaplastic meningiomas contain *TP53* gene mutations {1578}. Mutations and deletions of the *CDKN2A* gene are rare in meningiomas {1108}, as are alterations of the *PTEN* and *PTCH* genes.

Microsatellite instability

Microsatellite instability is thought to result from mutations in DNA mismatch repair genes. One study reported microsatellite instability in 4 of 16 meningiomas {1214}. A second, however, found no evidence of microsatellite instability in a series of 44 meningiomas {1421}.

Clonality of solitary, recurrent and multiple meningiomas

Studies of X-chromosome inactivation using Southern blot analysis have demonstrated that meningiomas are monoclonal tumours {668}, while PCR-based assays have hinted that a small fraction of meningiomas could be polyclonal {1676}. Nevertheless, both the Southern blot data {668} and the observation that the overwhelming majority of meningiomas with *NF2* mutations only have a single mutation {1600} argue that the origin of these lesions is clonal. Similarly, all recurrent meningiomas were found to be clonal with respect to the primary lesion {2572}.

The clonality of multiple meningiomas has also been analyzed using studies of X-chromosome inactivation and by mutational analysis of the *NF2* gene in multiple tumours from the same patient {860, 1448, 1562}. Lesions from patients with three or more meningiomas have been shown to have either the same copy of the

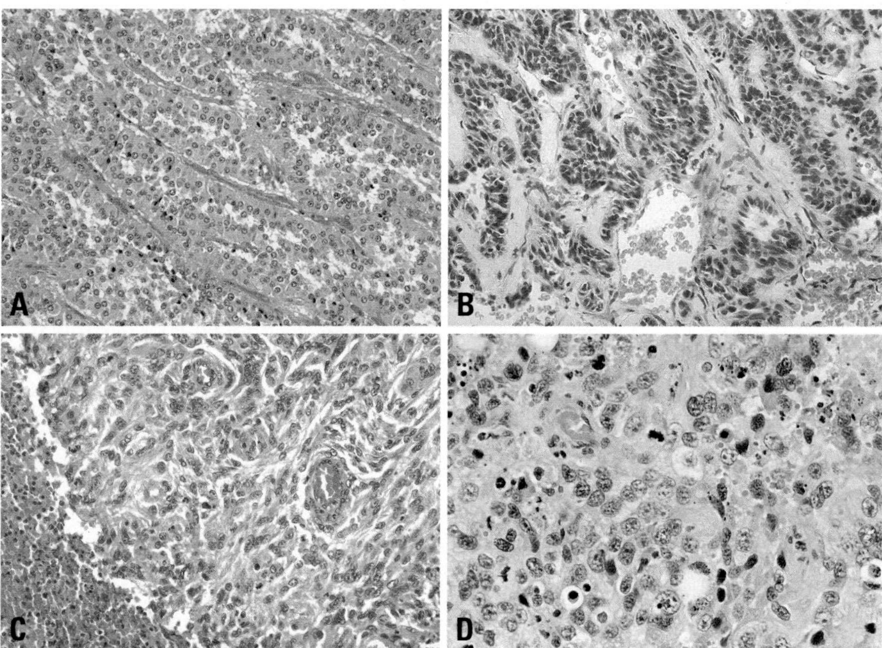

Fig. 11.17 Papillary meningioma with (**A**) papillary and (**B**) trabecular and papillary patterns on a collageneous stroma. **C** Anaplastic meningioma with nuclear polymorphism, numerous mitoses and geographic necrosis. **D** Anaplastic (malignant) meningioma WHO grade III, showing loss of meningiomatous tissue pattern and numerous typical and atypical mitoses.

X-chromosome inactivated, or to carry the same *NF2* mutation. These data provide strong evidence for a clonal origin of multiple meningiomas in patients with more than two lesions, suggesting that multiple lesions may arise through subarachnoid spread. Nevertheless, it remains possible that some of these cases represent genetic mosaics, with segmental, dural constitutional *NF2* mutations. Only about half of patients with two meningiomas have monoclonal tumours; the others have a variety of different *NF2* gene mutations in their tumours, indicating that these lesions have an independent origin {1448}. One study suggests that small meningothelial nests may surround some meningiomas and perhaps represent secondary tumours {149}.

Histogenesis
Meningiomas are considered to be derived from arachnoid cap cells.

Prognosis and predictive factors
The major prognostic questions regarding meningiomas are prediction of recurrence and, for malignant variants, prediction of survival.

Clinical factors
In most cases, meningiomas can be removed in a manner that seems complete, as assessed by microneurosurgical techniques. In one series, 20% of gross totally resected benign meningiomas recurred within 20 years {659}. The major clinical factor in recurrence is the extent of resection {660, 694} which is influenced by the site of occurrence, attachment to intracranial structures and the age of the patient. Other clinical factors have not proven particularly useful in assessing risk of recurrence.

Histopathology and grading
Some histological meningioma variants are more likely to recur {943}. Overall, tumour grade (e.g., benign, atypical, anaplastic) provides the most useful histological predictor of the likelihood of recurrence (Table 1). While benign meningiomas have recurrence rates of about 7-20%, atypical meningiomas recur in 29-40% of cases and anaplastic meningiomas have recurrence rates of 50-78% {660, 795, 943, 2165, 2166}. Malignant histological features are associated with shorter survival times {721}, with one series reporting median survival of under 2 years for malignant meningiomas {2165}.
There have been numerous attempts to correlate the likelihood of recurrence with specific histological features other than those formally used to establish grade and/or meningioma subtype {318, 694, 979}. Brain invasion suggests a greater likelihood of recurrence, with brain-invasive histologically benign meningiomas behaving similarly to atypical meningiomas in general {2166}.

Proliferation
Proliferation indices have also been used to predict recurrence and survival. Higher MIB-1 labelling indices correlate with increased risk of recurrence, but the specific cut-off levels and counting techniques have varied considerably between studies. High proliferative activity may also be focal within tumours, particularly in regions of high cellularity. Therefore, while it is not possible to establish universal values for determining recurrence risk, MIB-1 labeling indices above 5-10% suggest a greater likelihood of recurrence. Similarly, BudR labeling has been correlated with clinical behaviour {1404}, the mean BudR index of recurrent tumours being significantly higher than that of non-recurrent tumours (3.9% versus 1.9%)

Progesterone receptor status
The absence of progesterone receptors, a high mitotic index, and higher tumour grade were significant factors in shorter disease-free intervals in meningioma patients. Multivariate analysis showed that a three-factor interaction model, with a progesterone receptor score of 0, a mitotic index greater than 6, and malignant tumour grade, was a highly significant predictor for poor outcome {154, 627}. Atypical or anaplastic tumours more frequently lack progesterone receptors {443}, and progesterone-receptor-negative meningiomas tend to be larger than progesterone-receptor-positive tumours {154}.

Mesenchymal, non-meningothelial tumours

W. Paulus
B.W. Scheithauer

Definition

Benign and malignant mesenchymal tumours originating in the CNS or the meninges and showing fibrous, fibrohistiocytic, adipose, myoid, endothelial, chondroid or osseous, but not meningothelial differentiation.

Grading

According to their histological features and clinical behaviour, they vary greatly in grade, ranging from the benign neoplasms (WHO grade I) to highly malignant sarcomas (WHO grade IV).

Terminology and historical annotation

The histological features of mesenchymal tumours affecting the CNS are those of the corresponding extracranial soft tissue tumours {180, 378, 690}. Haemangiopericytoma, by far the most common mesenchymal, non-meningothelial neoplasm, is described separately (see next section). Gliosarcoma, a glial tumour with mesenchymal differentiation, is also discussed elsewhere (see Chapter 1). Antiquated nosologic terms, such as spindle-cell sarcoma, polymorphic cell sarcoma and myxosarcoma have been replaced by designations indicating specific differentiation {378}. The non-specific diagnostic term 'meningosarcoma' is also to be avoided since it has been used to denote both malignant meningioma and various types of sarcoma. Some non-mesenchymal tumours were previously classified as sarcomas; examples include CNS lymphoma ('reticulum cell sarcoma'), desmoplastic medulloblastoma ('cerebellar arachnoidal sarcoma') and giant cell glioblastoma ('monstrocellular sarcoma').

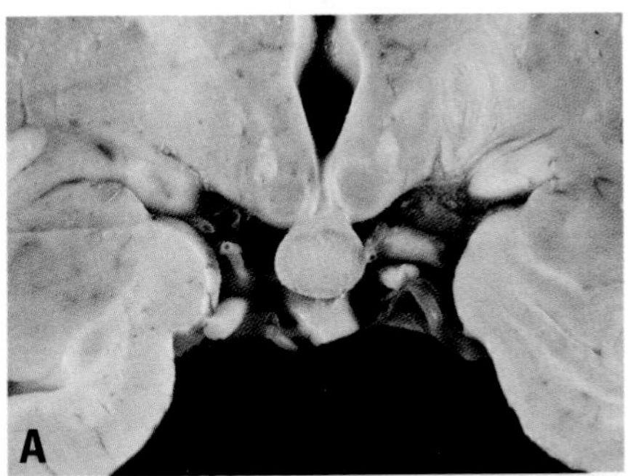

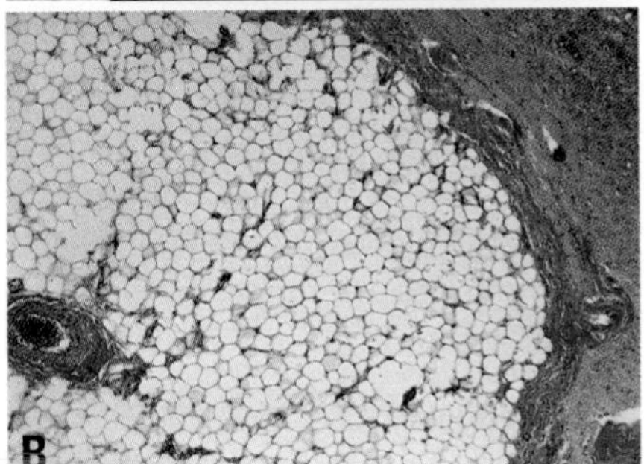

Fig. 11.18 A Lipoma beneath the mammillary bodies. **B** Histology of a cerebral lipoma composed of uniform fat cells sharply delineated from brain tissue.

Incidence

Whereas the various forms of lipoma represent 0.4 % of intracranial tumours, the other benign mesenchymal tumours are very rare, usually being the subject of single case reports. Sarcomas represent less than 0.1% of intracranial tumours, with malignant fibrous histiocytoma being the most common type {1155}. Reported higher values are a reflection of overdiagnosis related to historical classification schemes.

Age and sex distribution

Mesenchymal tumours may occur at any age. Rhabdomyosarcoma occurs preferentially in children, while malignant fibrous histiocytoma and chondrosarcoma usually manifest in adults. As a whole, sarcomas show no obvious gender predilection.

Localization

Tumours arising in meninges are more common than ones originating within CNS parenchyma or in choroid plexus. Whereas most mesenchymal tumours are supratentorial rather than infratentorial or spinal in location, rhabdomyosarcomas are more often infratentorial. Chondrosarcomas involving the brain arise most often in the skull base. Intracranial lipomas typically occur at midline sites, such as the anterior corpus callosum, quadrigeminal plate and cerebellopontine angle, intraventricular examples being rare. Osteolipomas prefer the suprasellar/interpeduncular region {2008}. Most spinal lipomas and angiolipomas arise in the epidural region; rare subpial examples occur in the thoracic region.

Clinical features

Symptoms and signs

Clinical symptoms and signs are variable, non-specific, and largely depend upon tumour location.

Neuroimaging

While the neuroradiological appearance of most mesenchymal tumours is non-specific, the neuroimaging characteristics of lipoma are usually diagnostic, as T1-weighted MRI images show fat having a high-signal intensity. Speckled calcifications are typical of chondroid and osseous tumours.

Macroscopy

The macroscopic appearance depends

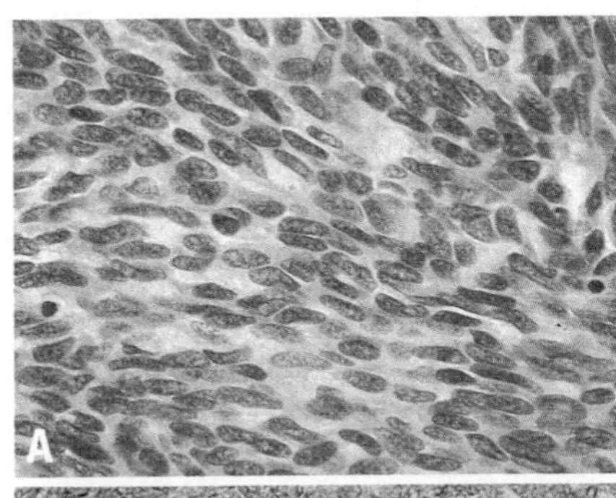

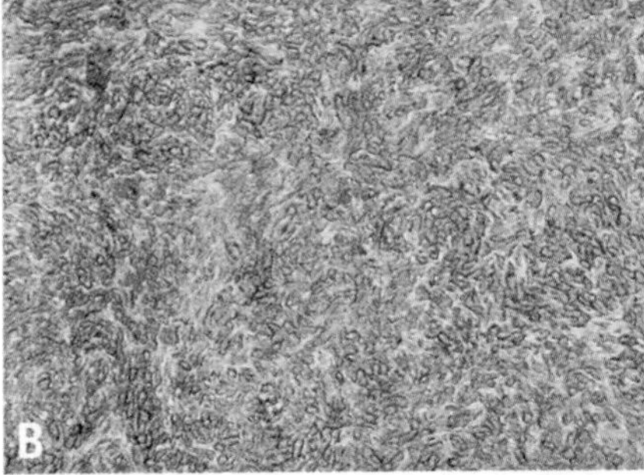

Fig. 11.19 A Primary CNS leiomyosarcoma, fasicles of spindle cells showing characteristic cigar-shaped nuclei and **(B)** strong immunoreactivity for desmin.

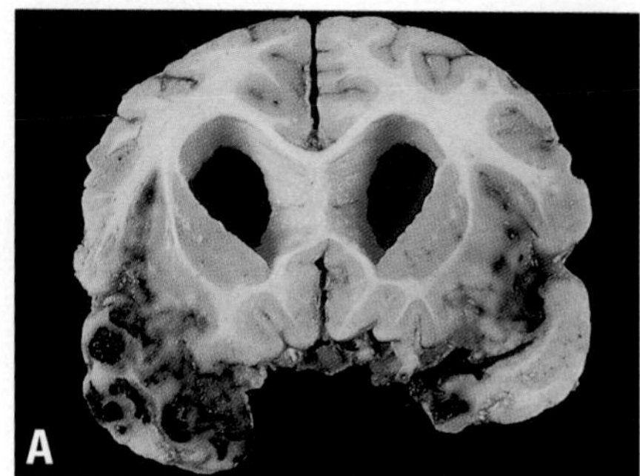

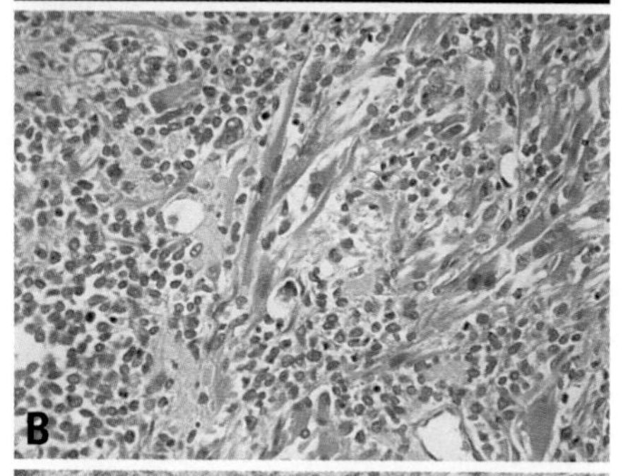

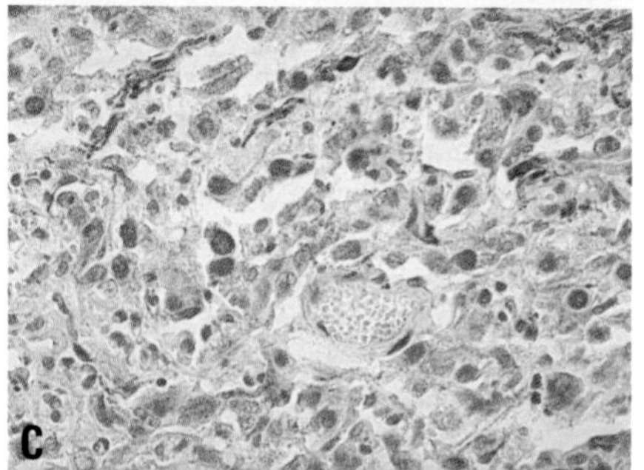

Fig. 11.20 Rhabdomyosarcoma. **A** Bilateral fronto-temporal lesion. **B** Small, non-differentiated cells intermingled with rhabdomyoblasts and strap-like cells. **C** Embryonal rhabdomyosarcoma showing strong desmin immunoreactivity.

on the type of differentiation and is similar to that of the corresponding extracranial soft tissue tumours. Lipomas are bright yellow, lobulated lesions. Lumbosacral lipomas (leptomyelolipomas) are comprised of subcutaneous and intradural components, the two being linked by a fibrolipomatous stalk that may attach to the dorsum of the cord, to the filum terminale, or to both. A "tethered cord" commonly results. Chondromas are solitary, grossly demarcated, grey-to-white, translucent, and typically form large, bosselated, dura-based masses indenting brain parenchyma. Meningeal sarcomas are firm in texture and tend to invade adjacent brain. Although intracerebral sarcomas appear well delineated, parenchymal invasion is also a feature. The cut surface of sarcomas is firm and fleshy; high grade lesions often show necrosis and haemorrhage.

Tumours of adipose tissue

Lipoma (ICD-O 8850/0)

This benign lesion does not differ significantly in appearance from normal adipose tissue {168}. Cells vary slightly in shape and size, measuring up to 200 microns, and show only occasional nuclear hyperchromasia. Whereas epidural lipomas are delicately encapsulated and discrete, intradural examples are often intimately attached to leptomeninges and CNS parenchyma.

Most lipomas show lobulation at low magnification. The ample capillary vasculature of even typical encapsulated lipomas is inconspicuous. Patchy hyalinization is a common feature, but calcification or myxoid stromal change is only occasionally seen. Osteolipomas are exceedingly rare and may show zonation with central adipose tissue and peripheral bone {2008}.

Angiolipoma (ICD-O 8861/0)

The proportion of adipose cells and vasculature varies {2007, 1208}. Vessels, by definition of capillary type, are generally most prominent beneath the tumour capsule. Fibrin thrombi are a common finding. With time, interstitial fibrosis may ensue. Angiolipomas may be overdiagnosed, since ordinary haemangiomas are often accompanied by fat.

Hibernoma (ICD-O 8880/0)

This lipoma originates from brown fat and is composed of uniform granular or multivacuolated cells with small, centrally placed nuclei {2004}.

Malformative variants

These vary considerably in terms of their histological composition. For example, lumbosacral lipomas (leptomyelolipomas) {595} consist of lobulated adipose tissue, often in association with fibrous tissue, vascular proliferation, smooth muscle elements, and neuroglial tissue, particularly ependyma ('fibrolipomatous hamartoma').

Lipomas of the cerebellopontine angle {1999}, an uncommonly affected off-midline site, may incorporate intradural portions of cranial nerve roots and their ganglia. Many also feature striated muscle or other mesenchymal tissues. It has even been suggested that intracranial lipomas containing various other tissue types represent a transition between lipoma and teratoma {1513}.

Intracranial liposarcoma

This neoplasm is extremely rare and may be associated with subdural haematoma {251}.

Epidural lipomatosis consists of diffuse hypertrophy of spinal epidural adipose tissue. This rare lesion represents not a neoplasm but a metabolic response, often to chronic administration of steroids {521}.

Fibrous tumours

Fibromatoses

These are locally infiltrative but cytologically benign, variably cellular lesions composed of elongate fibroblasts in an abundant stroma of broad collagen bundles {1018}. The condition must be differentiated from the pseudotumoural cranial fasciitis of childhood, a process closely histologically related to nodular fasciitis and featuring rapid growth within the deep scalp. As a rule, it lacks an intradural component and has no malignant potential {864}. Another pseudotumoural lesion, hypertrophic intracranial pachymeningitis, entails progressive dural thickening owing to pachymeningeal fibrosis and chronic inflammation often associated with autoimmune disorders {1484}.

Solitary fibrous tumour (ICD-O 8815/0)

This lesion occurs at cranial or spinal meninges of adults with variable invasion of CNS parenchyma or nerve roots {196}. Spindle cells are disposed in fascicles between prominent, eosinophilic bands of collagen. There is strong immunoreactivity for vimentin and CD34, but not EMA. The relation of solitary fibrous tumour with rare cases of intracranial fibroma and myxoma is unclear {1253}.

Fibrosarcoma (ICD-O 8810/3)

This rare, malignant tumour shows interlacing bundles of spindle cells disposed in a "herringbone" pattern. Fibrosarcomas are highly cellular and exhibit brisk mitotic activity and often necroses {458}.

Fibrohistiocytic tumours

Benign fibrous histiocytoma

This lesion is also termed fibrous xanthoma and is composed of a mixture of spindled (fibroblast-like) and rounded (histiocyte-like) cells arranged in a storiform pattern. Scattered giant cells and/or inflammatory cells are commonly seen. Many tumours initially published as fibrous xanthoma were subsequently shown to be GFAP-positive {751}, and thus were reclassified

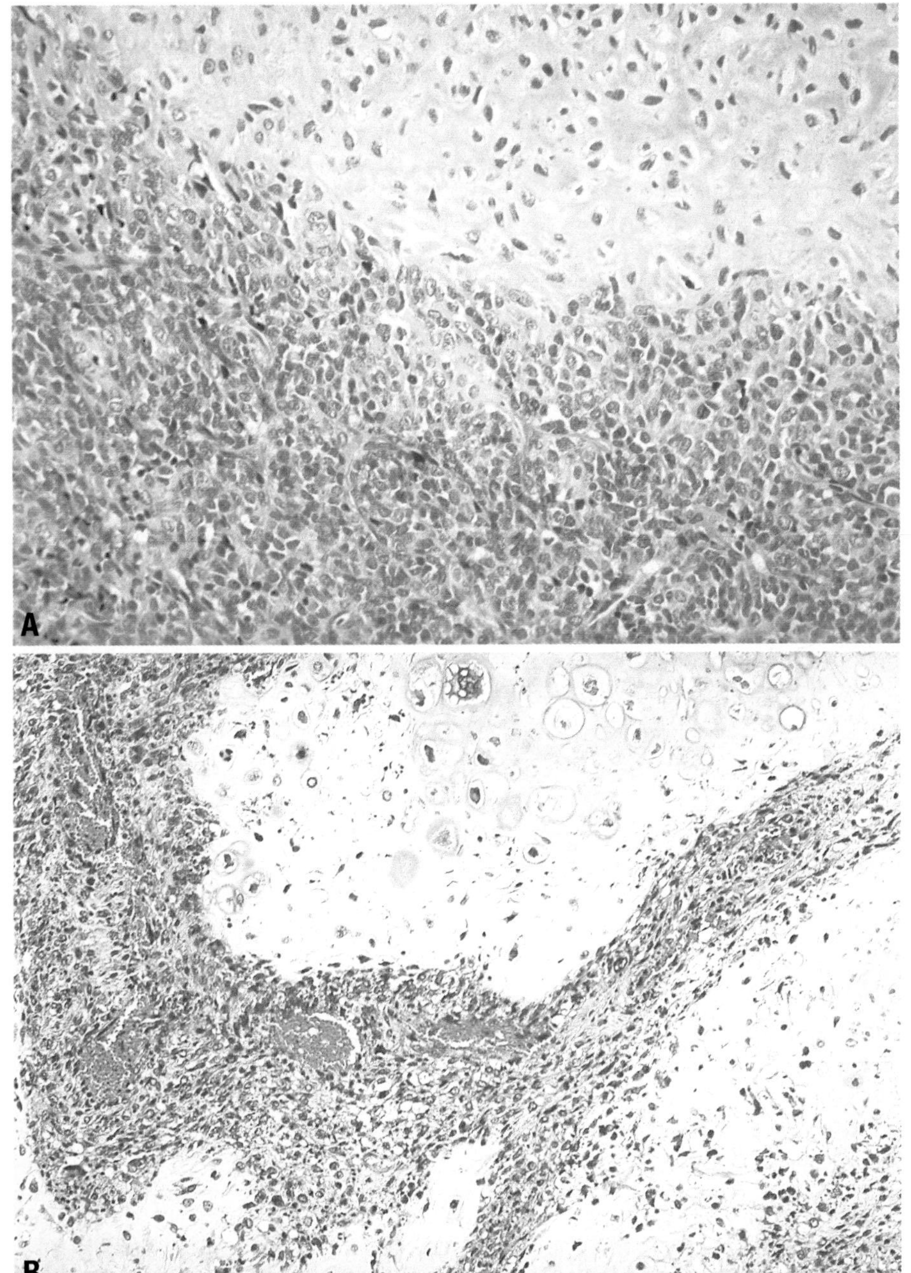

Fig. 11.21 A Mesenchymal chondrosarcoma with cellular portion resembling a haemangiopericytoma. **B** Biphasic pattern with well-differentiated cartilage alternating with highly cellular tumour areas.

as pleomorphic xanthoastrocytoma (see Chapter 1).

Malignant fibrous histiocytoma (MFH) (ICD-O 8830/3)

A neoplasm usually consisting of spindled, plump and pleomorphic giant cells also arranged in a storiform pattern (storiform-pleomorphic subtype). Most MFH are obviously malignant, featuring numerous mitoses as well as necrosis. Only isolated cases of the inflammatory variant of MFH have been described in the brain {967}.

Muscle tumours

Leiomyoma (ICD-O 8890/0)

These lesions are readily recognized by their pattern of intersecting fascicles composed of eosinophilic spindle cells with blunt-ended nuclei {897}. As a rule, they lack mitotic activity. Occasional tumours feature nuclear palisading and should not be mistaken for schwannoma. Diffuse leptomeningeal examples {678} as well as the angioleiomyomatous variant {847} have been described. Several AIDS-associated cases have been reported.

Leiomyosarcoma (ICD-O 8890/3)

Intracranial leiomyosarcomas {321} correspond histologically to their soft-tissue counterparts and express desmin and smooth muscle actin. Most arise in the dura, but one unique example originating in a pineal teratoma has been reported {1424}.

Rhabdomyoma (ICD-O 8900/0)

This lesion consists entirely of mature striated muscle, but one reported example associated with a cranial nerve featured a minor adipose tissue component {1544}. CNS rhabdomyoma must be distinguished from skeletal muscle heterotopias, most of which occur within prepontine leptomeninges {413}.

Rhabdomyosarcoma (ICD-O 8900/3)

Whether meningeal or parenchymal, nearly all CNS rhabdomyosarcomas are of the embryonal type {1227,1486}, while alveolar rhabdomyosarcoma has not been reported. Strap cells with cross striations may be observed. However, most tumours consist primarily of small cells that show little or no specific differentiation at the H&E level. Thus, immunohistochemistry and/or electron microscopy may be necessary for diagnosis. Immunostains for myoglobin, muscle-specific actin and desmin confirm the diagnosis. The ultrastructural findings of thick (myosin) and thin (actin) filaments arrayed in sarcomeres is also diagnostic. Rhabdomyosarcoma must be differentiated from other brain tumours that occasionally show skeletal muscle elements, such as medullomyoblastoma, gliosarcoma and germ-cell tumours. Malignant ectomesenchymoma, a mixed tumour composed of ganglion cells or neuroblasts and one or more mesenchymal elements, usually rhabdomyosarcoma, may also occur in the brain {1155}.

Osteocartilaginous tumours

Chondroma (ICD-O 9220/0)

Osteoma (ICD-O 9180/0)

Osteochondroma (ICD-O 9210/0)

These benign osteocartilaginous tumours are usually dura-based, whereas outside the CNS they often develop in the skull and only secondarily displace dura and brain {841}. Histologically, they correspond to similar tumours arising in bone, but are to be separated from asymptomatic dural calcification, ossification related to metabolic disease or trauma, and neuroecto-

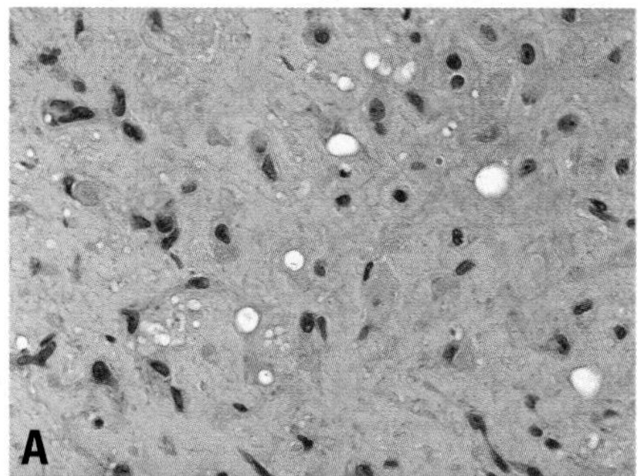

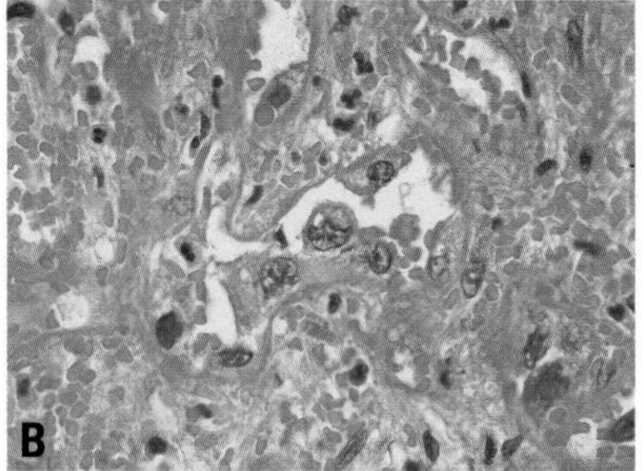

Fig. 11.22 A Epithelioid haemangioendothelioma with intracellular lumina and basophilic extracellular matrix. **B** Angiosarcoma showing abnormal vascular channels lined by atypical plump endothelial cells.

dermal tumours such as astrocytoma and gliosarcoma that occasionally show osseous or chondroid differentiation. Transition of CNS chondroma to chondrosarcoma has rarely been documented {1020}.

Mesenchymal chondrosarcoma (ICD-O 9220/3)
This neoplasm more often arises in bones of the skull or spine than within dura or brain parenchyma {1302, 1337}. Nonetheless, the CNS is the most common site of extraosseous examples. Some tumours consist primarily of the small-cell component punctuated by scant islands of atypical hyaline cartilage, whereas the cartilage predominates in others. The histological pattern of the small-cell element closely resembles haemangiopericytoma, replete with staghorn vascular spaces and an intercellular pattern of reticulin staining. Although the diagnosis of mesenchymal chondrosarcoma generally poses no problem, in the absence of cartilage, immunohistochemistry is of no particular benefit in distinguishing this lesion from haemangiopericytoma or other small-cell sarcomas {1473}. Even less frequent in the CNS are differentiated chondrosarcoma and myxoid chondrosarcoma {2005, 1155}. Chondrosarcomas arising in the skull base, particularly in the midline, should be distinguished from chondroid chordoma. Unlike chondroid chordoma, chondrosarcomas are non-reactive for keratin and epithelial membrane antigen {1019}.

Osteosarcoma (ICD-O 9180/3)
Preferred sites are the skull or spine and, more rarely, the meninges or the brain {2003, 77, 1320}. Direct formation of bone or osteoid by the proliferating tumour cells is requisite to the diagnosis. Osteosarcomatous elements may exceptionally be encountered in germ cell tumours and gliosarcomas.

Blood vessel tumours
Most vascular lesions of the central nervous system are malformative in nature and include arteriovenous malformation, cavernous angioma, venous angioma, and capillary teleangiectasis {688}. This discussion is limited to benign (haemangioma), intermediate grade (haemangioendothelioma), and malignant (angiosarcoma, Kaposi sarcoma) vascular neoplasms.

Haemangioma (ICD-O 9120/0)
These lesions vary in size from microscopic to massive. Depending upon their histological appearance, haemangiomas are classified as capillary or cavernous. Of those affecting the CNS, most are primary lesions of bone that impinge secondarily upon the CNS.

Epithelioid haemangioendothelioma (ICD-O 9133/1)
Skull base, dura or brain parenchyma are rare locations for this neoplasm {1088}. Its cells possess relatively abundant eosinophilic cytoplasm and may be vacuolated. In general, nuclei are round or occasionally indented, vesicular, and show only minor atypia. Mitoses and limited necrosis may be seen. Vascular lumens are often small and intracytoplasmic. Their somewhat nodular architecture often features chondroid or myxoid stromal change. Immunohistochemical (factor VIII-related antigen, *Ulex europeus* lectin, CD31) and ultrastructural studies (Weibel-Palade bodies) confirm the endothelial nature.

Angiosarcoma (ICD-O 9120/3)
The rare examples originating in brain or meninges {990} vary in differentiation from patently vascular tumours with anastomosing vascular channels lined by mitotically active, cytologically atypical endothelial cells, to poorly differentiated, often epithelioid lesions in which immunohistochemical and ultrastructural studies are required for a definitive diagnosis. Occasional cytokeratin reactivity poses a trap in distinguishing poorly differentiated angiosarcoma from metastatic carcinoma {1262}.

Kaposi sarcoma (ICD-O 9140/3)
This malignant neoplasm is characterized by spindle-shaped cells lining or forming slit-like blood vessels and is only exceptionally encountered as a parenchymal or meningeal tumour in the setting of AIDS {2002}. In such instances, it is often difficult to determine whether the lesion(s) is primary or secondary.
Blood vessel tumours are to be differentiated from intravascular papillary endothelial hyperplasia, a tumour-like, reactive papillary proliferation of endothelium associated with thrombosis, which may occur in brain or meninges {814}.

Meningeal sarcomatosis
Meningeal sarcomatosis is a diffuse leptomeningeal sarcoma lacking circumscribed masses. Strictly defined as a non-meningothelial mesenchymal tumour, most are poorly differentiated "spindle cell" sarcomas. Re-examination using immunohistochemistry has revealed that most published cases actually represented carcinoma, lymphoma, glioma, or primitive neuroectodermal tumours.

Aetiology
Intracranial fibrosarcoma, MFH, chondrosarcoma and osteosarcoma may occur several years after cranial irradiation, most commonly for sellar region tumours {2006, 180}. Single cases of intracranial and spinal fibrosarcoma, malignant fibrous histiocytoma (MFH) and angiosarcoma have also been related to previous trauma or surgery {599}, an aetiology which may be more common to fibromatoses {1018}. The Epstein-Barr virus probably plays a role in the development of intracranial leiomyosarcoma of immunocompromised patients {2000}.

Genetic susceptibility
Several associations with inherited disease are worth noting; intracranial cartilaginous tumours may be associated with Maffucci syndrome and Ollier disease, lipomas with encephalocraniocutaneous lipomatosis, and osteosarcoma with Paget disease.

Cytogenetics and molecular genetics

Although it can be expected that molecular genetic alterations of intracranial sarcomas correspond to those of corresponding soft tissue lesions {2001}, there are virtually no data so far. One case of cerebral malignant fibrous histiocytoma (MFH) showed a complex karyotype, similar to those reported for soft tissue MFH {107}.

Histogenesis

Mesenchymal tumours affecting the CNS are thought to arise from craniospinal meninges, vasculature and surrounding osseous structures. Osteocartilaginous and myoid tumours may arise: (i) from rarely occurring meningeal heterotopias, (ii) from multipotential mesenchymal cells, (iii) by acquisition of additional lines of mesenchymal differentiation in fibrous or fibrohistiocytic tumours, or (iv) within a teratoma {2003}. Since cranial and intracranial mesenchymal structures, such as bone, cartilage and muscle, are in part derived from the neuroectoderm (ectomesenchyme), the development of the corresponding sarcoma types could also represent reversion to a more primitive stage of differentiation. Lipomas arising within the CNS are often associated with developmental anomalies, particularly partial or complete agenesis of the corpus callosum and spinal dysraphism {1518}. Intracranial rhabdomyosarcoma may also be associated with malformations of the CNS {583}.

Prognostic factors

Whereas most benign mesenchymal tumours can be completely resected and carry a favourable prognosis, primary intracranial sarcomas are aggressive and associated with a poor outcome. Local recurrence and/or distant leptomeningeal seeding are typical. For example, despite aggressive radiation and chemotherapy, CNS rhabdomyosarcomas have been almost uniformly fatal within two years. Systemic metastases of intracranial sarcomas are relatively common.

Haemangiopericytoma

J. Jääskeläinen
D.N. Louis
W. Paulus
M.J. Haltia

Definition

Haemangiopericytoma (HPC) of the central nervous system is a highly cellular and richly vascularized tumour, almost always attached to the dura, and indistinguishable histologically from haemangiopericytomas occurring in somatic soft tissues, with a tendency to recur and to metastasize outside the CNS.

ICD-O code: 9150/1

Grading

Haemangiopericytomas correspond histologically to WHO grade II or III, but histological criteria for grading are not yet firmly established (see Predictive factors).

Synonyms and historical annotation

Haemangiopericytoma was named by Stout and Murray in 1942 {1461}, who also postulated that the lesion had a pericytic origin. In 1938, Cushing and Eisenhardt {294} had described 23 vascular meningeal tumours, 'angioblastic meningiomas', with three variants. In retrospect, variant 1 represented haemangiopericytoma and variant 3, haemangioblastoma {1306}. Their concept of a differentiating meningoblast was so sternly advocated by Russell and Rubinstein {616, 1306} that the 1979 WHO classification {1685} still contained the 'haemangiopericytic' variant of meningioma. However, haemangiopericytoma and meningioma are different entities, and the concept of 'angioblastic meningioma' is now considered obsolete.

Incidence

Meningeal haemangiopericytoma constitutes approximately 0.4% of all primary CNS tumours. In three large series of meningeal tumours, the ratio of meningeal haemangiopericytoma: meningioma was about 1:40 {515}, 1:50 {663} and 1:60 {694}.

Age and sex distribution

Meningeal haemangiopericytomas tend to occur at a younger age than meningiomas, and more often in men than in women. In three large clinical series of 66 men and 47 women (M/F ratio, 1.4:1), the mean age at diagnosis was 43 years {515, 663, 691}.

Localization

Primary haemangiopericytoma of the CNS is almost invariably a single tumour {1375} attached to the cranial or spinal dura. In four large series {515, 616, 691, 1179} of 153 meningeal haemangiopericytomas, only two were intraparenchymal, and the proportion of spinal tumours was 8%. Within the skull, haemangiopericytoma occurs somewhat more often in the occipital region, around the confluens sinuum, and attached to the venous sinuses {294, 664, 1179}.

Clinical features

Symptoms and signs

As suggested by their location, the symptoms of meningeal haemangiopericytoma are indistinguishable from those caused by meningiomas.

Neuroimaging

Plain films and angiography may distinguish haemangiopericytoma from meningioma. A well-demarcated, lytic destruction of the adjacent bone supports meningeal haemangiopericytoma, whereas hyperostosis, a typical feature of meningioma, is absent {515, 664}. Angiography may warn of the tendency to bleed, and typically shows a dual blood supply from meningeal and cortical arteries to many small, corkscrew-like vessels in a densely stained tumour {664}. CT and MRI show a sharply demarcated tumour with dural attachment, smooth or nodular margin, and intense contrast enhancement, but unlike meningiomas, meningeal haemangiopericytomas typically lack calcification.

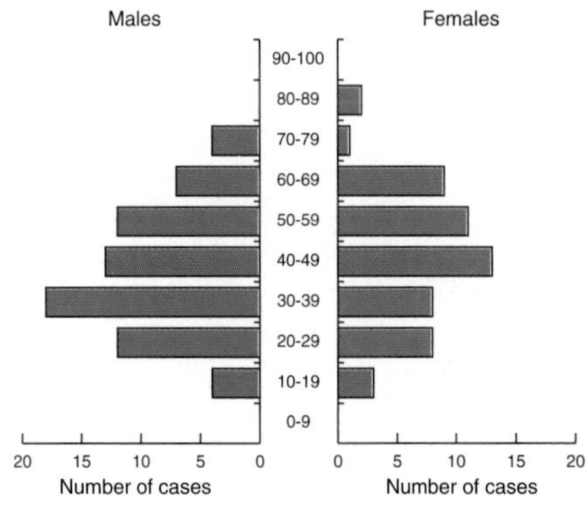

Fig. 11.23 Age and sex distribution of 125 haemangiopericytomas, based on 31 published cases from Vuorinen *et al.* {1571} and 94 cases from Mena *et al.* {991}.

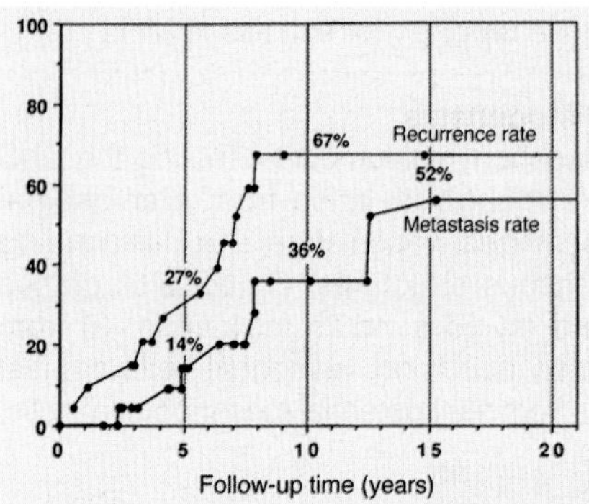

Fig. 11.24 Recurrence rate after seemingly complete removal and the overall metastatic rate of primary intracranial haemangiopericytoma. Modified from Jaaskelainen *et al.* {663}.

Macroscopy

At operation, meningeal haemangiopericytoma is a solid tumour, well-demarcated from the adjacent brain tissue, and thus may be regarded as meningioma until histological examination. Haemangiopericytoma has a tendency to bleed during removal, sometimes profusely, as there are multiple feeding arteries from the cortex and diffuse bleeding from the cut tumour surfaces {663}. Ex vivo, haemangiopericytoma is usually globoid, slightly lobulated and rather firm, and the cut surfaces are fleshy and greyish to red-brown, often with a number of visible vascular spaces.

Histopathology

Haemangiopericytomas are highly cellular, monotonous tumours composed of randomly oriented plump cells with scant, ill-defined cytoplasm, accompanied by numerous small vascular spaces and a dense network of reticulin fibres.

The nuclei are oval, occasionally elongated, with moderate chromatin density and inconspicuous nucleoli, and they lack the pseudo-inclusions characteristic of meningiomas {378, 691, 991}. Nuclear atypia may be seen, but varies from case to case. A rich network of reticulin fibres, typically investing individual cells, is one of the most characteristic, but not invariable, features of the neoplasm. The tumour cells grow as monotonous sheets, interrupted by numerous slit-like vascular spaces lined by flattened endothelial cells. When wide and branching, these vascular spaces may assume the appearance of so-called "staghorn sinusoids" and separate the tumour cells into small lobules. The uniform cellularity of the tumour may be relieved by 'geographic' areas of reduced cell density or perivascular fibrosis. Frank necrosis is uncommon, and calcification, including psammoma bodies, is not a feature. Although haemangiopericytomas generally form discrete masses, they may invade and destroy adjacent bone without, however, the hyperostotic reaction characteristic of meningiomas. Infiltration of the adjacent brain parenchyma may be observed.

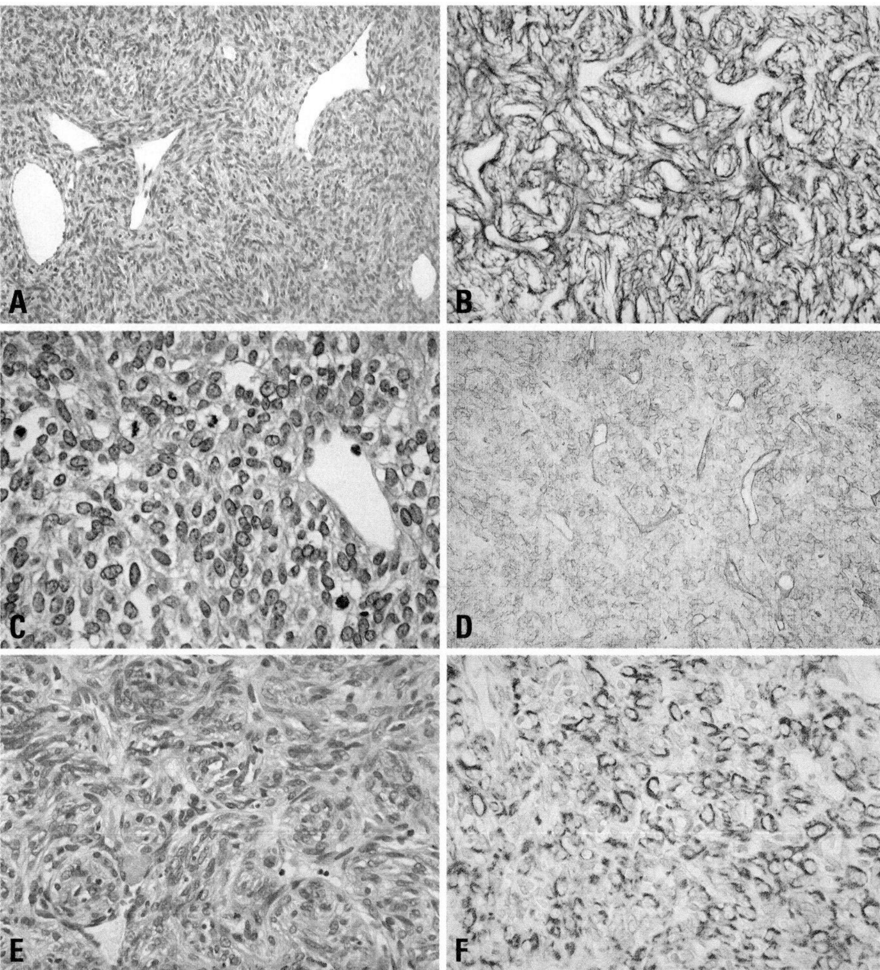

Fig. 11.26 Histological features of haemangiopericytoma. **A** Highly cellular tumour with dilated, staghorn-type vessels. **B** Dense reticulin network surrounding individual tumour cells. **C** High-power view showing tumour cells with indictinct borders and scattered mitotic figures. **D** Immunostaining for CD34 of tumour cells and endothelial cells. **E** Elongated tumour cells forming loose whorls separated by capillary vessels. **F** Perinuclear expression of vimentin by tumour cells.

Immunohistochemistry

The tumour cells are immunoreactive for vimentin (85%), factor XIIIa (80%) in individual scattered cells, Leu-7 (70%), and, in 33 -100% of cases, for CD34 {2015, 2013, 1250}. Focal positivity for desmin, smooth muscle actin, and cytokeratin may be occasionally encountered {2015, 378, 691, 1624}. In contrast to meningiomas, haemangiopericytomas lack epithelial membrane antigen {1250}. Tumour cells are also negative for S-100 protein, classical endothelial antigens such as factor VIII-related antigen and CD31 {2013}, as well as progesterone receptor {2011}. The extracellular matrix is immunoreactive for laminin and collagen IV {691}.

The vascular endothelial growth factor VEGF-A is upregulated in haemangiopericytoma tumour cells and the receptors VEGFR-1 and VEGFR-2 (but not VEGFR-3) in endothelial cells, suggesting a paracrine mode of interaction {552}. Endothelial cells also express Tie-1 {552}, a tyrosine kinase receptor associated with enhanced neovascularization.

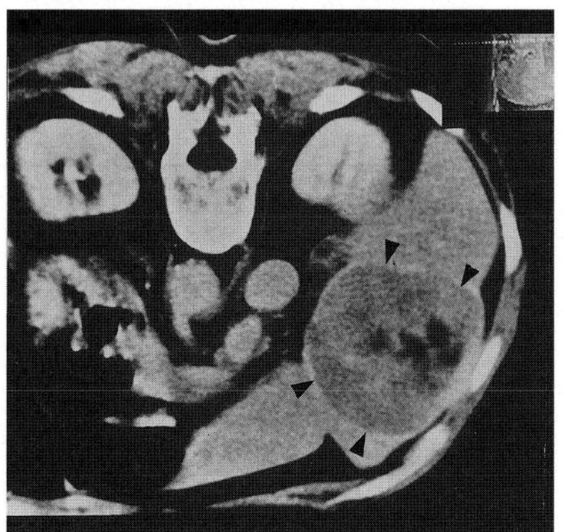

Fig. 11.25 Liver metastasis of a primary intracranial haemangiopericytoma seven and one half years after surgical resection (from Jääskeläinen *et al.*, ref. 663).

Electron microscopy

Neoplastic cells may contain small bundles of intermediate filaments, and are often surrounded by basal-lamina-like amorphous material. True desmosomes and gap junctions are absent {300, 691}.

Proliferation

The time to recurrence after seemingly complete removal, a rough indicator of the volume growth rate, varies remarkably, but the median time intervals of 40 {515} and 70 months {663} suggest that meningeal haemangiopericytomas tend to grow more rapidly than meningiomas {1375}. In most cases, mitotic activity is prominent. The median Ki-67 (MIB-1) labelling index was 10% (0.6 – 36%) in a series of 31 tumours {1571} and 5% (1.2 - 39 %) in another study of 62 tumours {2016}, i.e. values at the level of anaplastic (WHO grade III) meningiomas. The median S-phase fraction was 4% (1.6 –15%) in 31 tumours {1571}.

Genetic susceptibility

There is no evidence of familial clustering of meningeal haemangiopericytoma. One

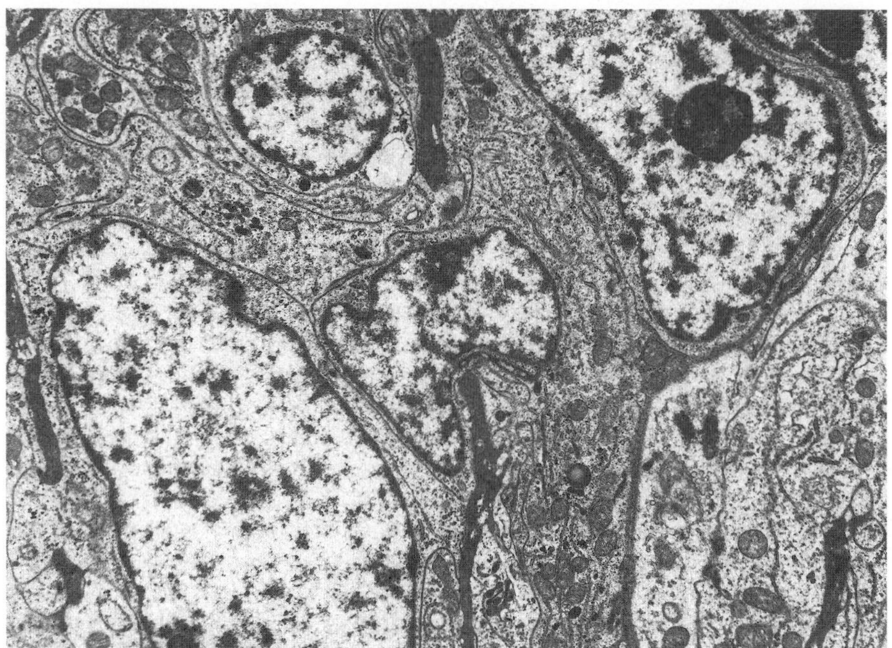

Fig. 11.27 Electron microscopy shows tumour cells lacking interdigitation of plasma membranes and the absence of desmosomes. Note the electron-dense material in the extracellular space.

report notes the occurrence of peripheral haemangiopericytoma in three members of one family {1189}

Cytogenetics and molecular genetics

Rearrangements of chromosome 12q13, a region that includes a number of oncogenes, and less consistently, alterations on 6p21, 7p15 and 19q13 have been reported {570, 573, 953}. However, no consistent chromosomal losses or gains were found in 11 peripheral haemangiopericytomas by comparative genomic hybridization {2014}. No allelic losses have been reported on 22q, the region harbouring the *NF2* gene, inactivation of which plays a causative role in meningiomas. Neither meningeal nor peripheral haemangiopericytomas contain *NF2* gene mutations (0/38), whereas 32% of meningiomas have such alterations {707}. Homozygous deletions of the *CDKN2A* gene on 9p were found in about 25% (7/28) of meningeal haemangiopericytomas but infrequently (1/26) in meningiomas {1108}. These data strongly suggest that haemangiopericytomas are distinct from meningiomas. No point mutations in *CDKN2A* nor *TP53* gene mutations are found in either tumour {1108}.

Histogenesis

The histogenesis of haemangiopericytoma is uncertain, but its microscopic and ultrastructural features suggest pericytic differentiation, probably from undifferentiated mesenchymal cells {377, 378}.

Prognosis and predictive factors

Treatment and clinical factors

These tumours are typically treated by complete microsurgical removal, followed by local irradiation of the tumour bed {2009, 2011, 515, 991}. Stereotactic radiotherapy can be used to control small tumours, including residuals, recurrences and local metastases {2010, 2012}. The majority of tumours can be removed in a seemingly complete manner but, unlike with meningiomas, local recurrences are almost inevitable in the long run. In two series, they occurred in 91% {1571} and 85% of cases {515} after 15 years. Postoperative external irradiation of the tumour bed delays recurrence {2009, 2011, 515, 991}. Nine of 17 irradiated haemangiopericytomas recurred with a median of 58 months, but 13 of the 15 non-irradiated tumours recurred with a median of only 29 months {515}. The majority of meningeal haemangiopericytomas eventually metastasize elsewhere in the body. This occurred in 68% {1571} and 64% {515} at 15 years, most frequently to the bones, lungs and liver, and the mean survival time after diagnosis of metastasis was 2 years {515}. In a series of 28 patients who had survived the primary removal, the probability of tumour-related death was 61% at 15 years {1571}.

Proliferation

If the tumour bed is not irradiated, meningeal haemangiopericytomas will recur, irrespective of their predicted proliferation potential. However, lower than average values for the Ki-67 (MIB-1) index {1571, 2016} and S-phase fraction {1571} are marginally associated with better prognosis in terms of longer time to recurrence, lower metastasis rate and extended survival. Such lesions may correspond histologically to WHO grade II.

In 94 CNS haemangiopericytomas {991}, decreased survival was associated with increased mitotic rate (five or more mitotic figures per 10 high-power fields), high cellularity, nuclear pleomorphism, haemorrhage and necrosis, in accordance with observations on peripheral haemangiopericytomas {377, 378}. These lesions may correspond histologically to WHO grade III.

Melanocytic lesions

K. Jellinger
P. Chou
W. Paulus

Definition

Diffuse or circumscribed, benign or malignant tumours arising from melanocytes of the leptomeninges. This group includes (1) diffuse melanocytosis (diffuse melanosis) and neurocutaneous melanosis, (2) melanocytoma, and (3) malignant melanoma, but intermediate or mixed cases may occur.

Incidence

Melanocytoma accounts for 0.06-0.1% of brain tumours, the other melanocytic lesions being even rarer. The annual incidence is approximately 1 per 10 million population {669}.

Age and sex distribution

Melanocytoma may occur at all ages (range 9-71 years), typically in the fifth decade, with a female: male-ratio of 2:1 {2017}, Caucasians being more frequently involved {904}. Diffuse melanocytosis usually manifests in children.

Localization

Diffuse melanocytosis involves the supra- and infratentorial leptomeninges. Melanocytomas occur as solid masses in the cranial and spinal compartments, mainly in the posterior fossa adjacent to the foramen magnum, in Meckel's cave, and within the thoracic spinal canal, where dumb-bell lesions may occur. They are often attached to the dura or are located near spinal root exit zones {1301, 1527}.

Clinical features

Symptoms and signs

Neurological manifestations of diffuse melanocytosis include seizures, psychiatric disturbances, and signs of raised intracranial pressure due to hydrocephalus {25}, although adult asymptomatic patients have been described. Melanocytomas and malignant melanomas present with signs of increased intracranial pressure or compression of the spinal cord by an extraaxial mass {2021}, with local neurological signs, depending on the location.

Neuroimaging

CT and MRI of diffuse melanocytosis show diffuse thickening and enhancement of the leptomeninges. Melanocytoma appears isodense with grey matter or hyperintense on T1-weighted MRI, but hypointense on T2-weighted MRI with homogeneous enhancement on postcontrast images depending on the amount of melanin pigment {296, 2021}, whereas the MRI appearance of intracranial malignant melanoma varies, depending on the degree of haemorrhage {1527}. In general, hyperintensity on short-repetition-time/short-echo-time MRI sequences is suggestive of melanin deposits {330}.

Macroscopy

Diffuse melanocytic lesions may appear as dense black replacement of the subarachnoid space or as a dusky clouding of the meninges. Involvement of the basal cisterns by diffuse melanocytosis is apt to cause internal hydrocephalus. Melanocytoma and malignant melanoma are single, often encapsulated lesions that may appear black, red-brown, blue or macroscopically non-pigmented.

Histopathology

Although identification of the type of melanocytic lesion typically requires histopathological examination, the diagnosis has occasionally been made by CSF cytology {215, 1252, 2018}.

A

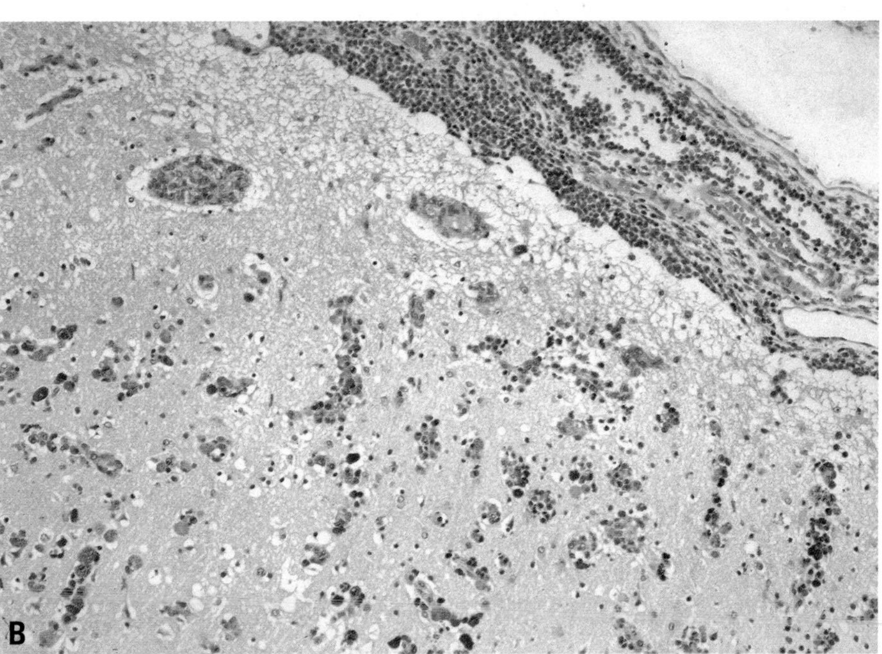

Fig. 11.28 Diffuse melanocytosis with invasion of the subarachnoid space and the cerebral cortex.

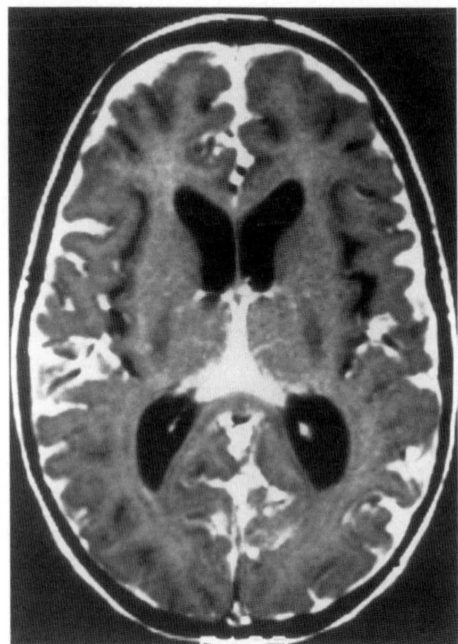

Fig. 11.29 T1-weighted MRI of diffuse melanocytosis, showing Gd enhancement of the infiltrated meninges.

Diffuse melanocytosis (ICD-O *8728/0*)
Diffuse or multifocal proliferation of uniform nevoid polygonal cells in the leptomeninges. Cells may spread into the Virchow-Robin spaces without frank invasion of the brain.

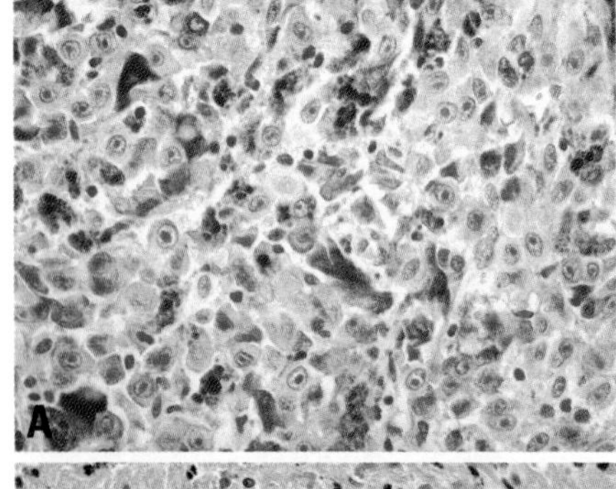

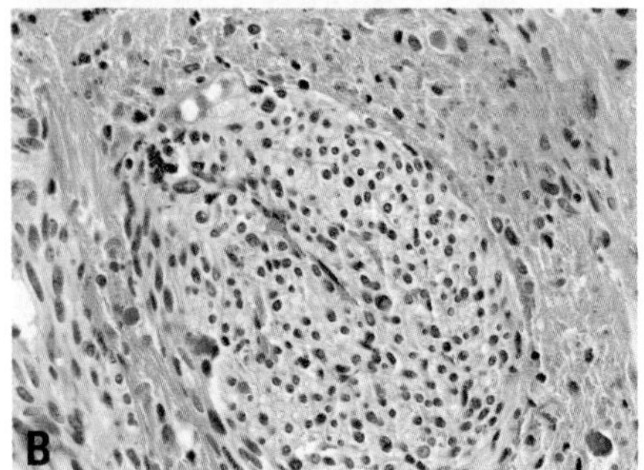

Fig. 11.30 A Histology of a melanocytoma, with densely packed, often melanin-laden cells and prominent nucleoli. **B** Melanocytoma of the spinal cord showing well defined, partly pigmented tumour cells. Note the Rosenthal fibres in the adjacent brain tissue.

Melanocytoma (ICD-O *8728/1*)
A tumour composed of monomorphic spindle, fusiform, epithelioid or polyhedral cells with round vesicular nuclei, prominent nucleoli, and a cytoplasm usually rich in melanin.
Scant iron-positive pigment may also occur. Arrangements include whorls, sheets, nests, and interlacing bundles with a focal storiform configuration. Mitotic activity is low, necrosis and haemorrhage are minimal. Meningeal melanocytoma histologically resembles melanocytoma of the optic nerve head and the uveal tract {2018}.

Malignant melanoma (ICD-O 8720/3)
Primary meningeal malignant melanomas show considerable pleomorphism, with large, and bizarre tumour cells, including multinucleated giant cells, and a variable amount of melanin pigment.
High mitotic rate, necroses, haemorrhage and invasion of brain or spinal cord parenchyma are common. In amelanotic variants, the eosinophilic cytoplasm is devoid of melanin. A malignant meningeal melanoma with secondary diffuse meningeal spread is referred to as meningeal melanomatosis.

Immunohistochemistry
Most tumours react with the anti-melanosomal antibody HMB-45. Melanocytic lesions usually express S-100 protein. Staining for vimentin and neuron-specific enolase are variable. There is no expression of GFAP, neurofilament proteins, cytokeratins and EMA {1091,1252}.

Electron microscopy
The cells of melanocytoma lack junctions and contain melanosomes at varying stages of development. In contrast to Schwann cell tumours, a well-formed pericellular basal lamina is lacking, but groups of melanocytoma cells may be ensheathed {1091}. In contrast to meningioma, no desmosomes and no interdigitating cytoplasmic processes are encountered {689, 1738}.

Differential diagnosis
Melanocytic lesions of the nervous system are to be distinguished from metastatic malignant melanoma and from histogenetically different nervous system tumours undergoing melaninization, such as schwannoma, medulloblastoma, paraganglioma and various gliomas {689, 725, 2023}. Whether melanotic meningiomas really exist remains to be determined. Melanotic neuroectodermal tumour of infancy (retinal anlage tumour) has been reported at intracranial locations {726}. Diffuse melanocytosis, melanocytoma, and malignant melanoma may constitute a spectrum of "naevomelanocytic neurocristopathies" {1252, 2020}.

Genetic susceptibility
Neurocutaneous melanosis (neurocutaneous melanocytosis) is a combination of diffuse melanocytosis with giant or numerous congenital melanocytic nevi of the skin, usually involving midline, head and neck, and with various malformative lesions, e.g. syringomyelia, lipomas, etc. {2018, 2022}. A genetic trait has not been

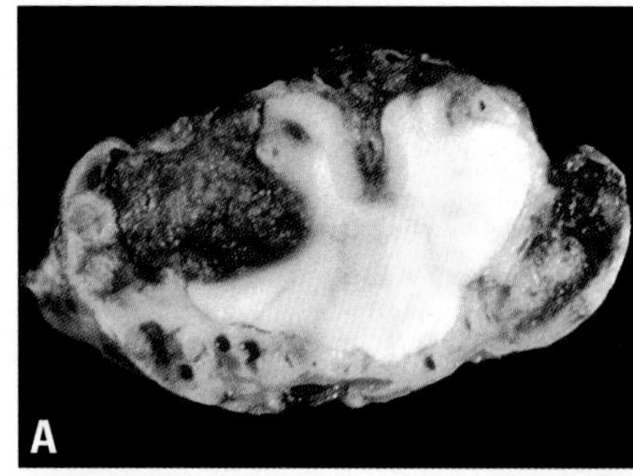

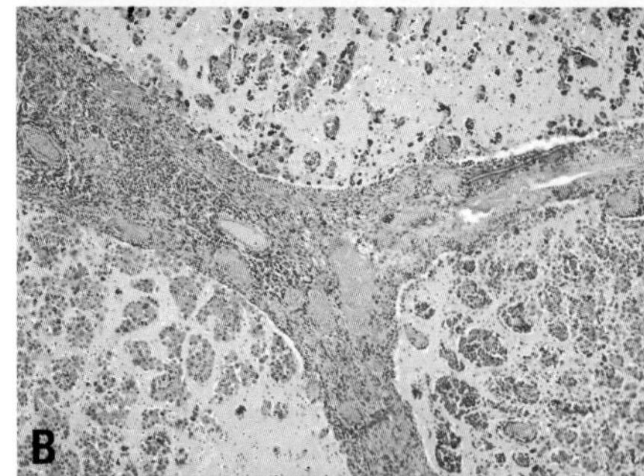

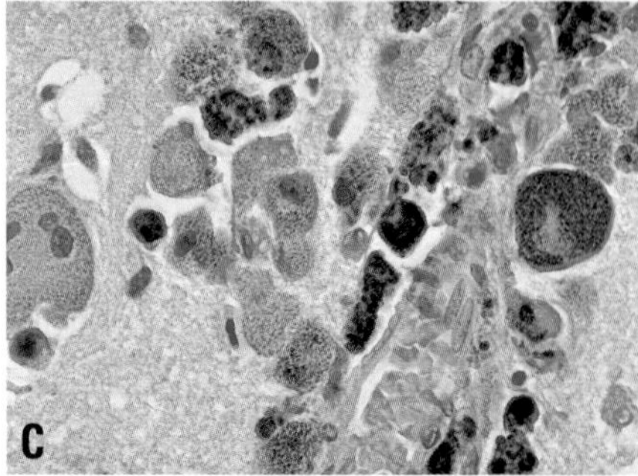

Fig. 11.31 A Primary spinal melanoma originating from the spinal cord and invading the subarachnoid space. **B** Primary malignant CNS melanoma showing extensive invasion of the cerebral cortex and subarachnoid space. **C** Highly polymorphic melanin-laden cells of a malignant melanoma invading the cerebral cortex.

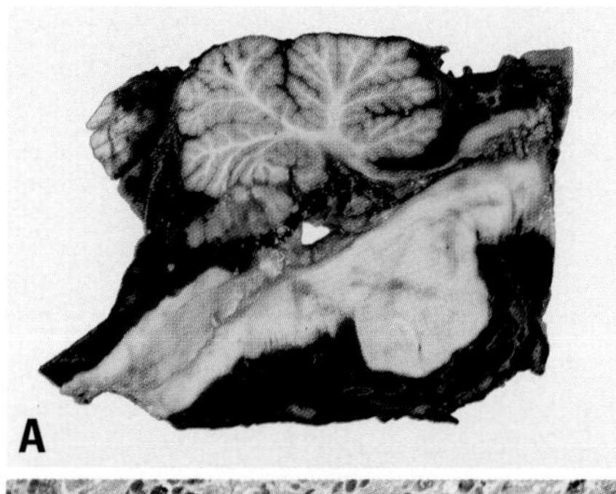

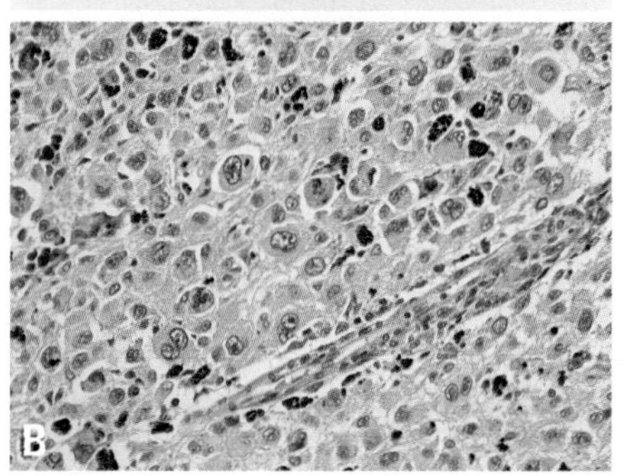

Fig. 11.32 **A** Malignant melanoma infiltrating the meninges around brain stem and cerebellum. **B** Histology shows partly pigmented, highly anaplastic melanoma cells. Note pigment uptake by histiocytes.

unequivocally established. Approximately 25% of patients with diffuse meningeal melanocytosis have significant concomitant cutaneous lesions. On the other hand, about 10% of patients with large congenital melanocytic nevi of the skin clinically present with CNS melanocytosis {325}, although radiologic evidence of CNS involvement may be more common {66}. Diffuse melanocytosis may also be associated with congenital naevus of Ota {62}.

Histogenesis

Melanocytic lesions of the nervous system and its coverings are thought to arise from leptomeningeal melanocytes that are derived from the neural crest. In the normal CNS, melanocytes are preferentially localised at the base of the brain, around the ventral medulla oblongata, and along the upper cervical spinal cord.

Prognosis and predictive factors

Diffuse melanosis carries a poor prognosis even in the absence of histologic malignancy {1252}. Melanocytoma lacks anaplastic features, but it is prone to undergo multiple local recurrences and to invade adjacent structures such as bone {689, 1738}. Melanocytomas are usually diploid; the presence of a significant aneuploid cell population increases the risk of aggressive growth {1958}. Malignant melanoma is a highly aggressive and radioresistant tumour with poor prognosis and may metastasize to remote organs {26}. The prognostic significance of a histologic pattern intermediate between melanocytoma and malignant melanoma is uncertain {2017}.

CHAPTER 12

Tumours of the Haemopoietic System

The incidence of malignant lymphomas of the CNS has continuously increased during the past two decades. In part, this can be explained by the HIV-1 epidemic since up to 10% of terminal AIDS patients develop an Epstein-Barr virus (EBV) associated malignant cerebral B-cell lymphoma. Lymphomas may originate in the CNS (primary CNS lymphoma) or systemic disease may spread to the CNS (secondary CNS lymphoma).

The vast majority of primary CNS lymphomas are malignant B-cell lymphomas which, unlike their systemic counterparts, carry a poor prognosis. Rare lymphomas involving the nervous system include T-cell lymphomas, plasmacytoma, angiotropic lymphoma and Hodgkin disease.

A variety of histiocytic tumours and histiocytoses, more commonly encountered at extracranial locations, may also arise within the CNS.

Malignant lymphomas

W. Paulus
K. Jellinger
S. Morgello
M. Deckert-Schlüter

Definition

Primary CNS lymphomas are extranodal malignant lymphomas arising in the CNS in the absence of obvious lymphoma outside the nervous system at the time of diagnosis. They are to be differentiated from secondary involvement of the nervous system in systemic lymphomas.

ICD-O code: 9590/3

Synonyms and historical annotation

CNS lymphomas were first described by Bailey in 1929 as "perithelial sarcoma". Until their lymphoid lineage and correct designation as lymphoma were generally accepted {693}, at least 12 synonyms have been used, including adventitial sarcoma, reticulum cell sarcoma and microglioma.

Incidence

The incidence of primary CNS lymphomas has recently increased markedly worldwide: from 0.8–1.5% up to 6.6% of primary intracranial neoplasms in several neuropathological series {1007}, which is mainly the consequence of the AIDS epidemic. Analysis from the updated Surveillance, Epidemiology, and End Results (SEER) database revealed an increase in the U.S. by more than 10-fold, from 2.5 cases per 10 million population in 1973 to 30 in 1991-1992 {1985}. In immunocompetent patients, the incidence has increased in some but not all series and populations {1988}. In AIDS patients, the incidence of 4.7 per 1000 person-years is about 3600-fold higher than in the general population {283}, with 2–12% of AIDS patients developing primary CNS lymphomas, mainly during late-stage AIDS {190}. CNS involvement occurs in 22% of post-transplant lymphomas, about 55% being confined to the CNS {1164}.

Age and sex distribution

Primary CNS lymphomas affect all ages, with a peak incidence in immunocompetent subjects during the sixth and seventh decade of life and a male: female ratio of 3:2. In immunocompromised patients, the age at manifestation is lowest in individuals who have an inherited immunodeficiency (10 years), followed by transplant recipients (37 years) and AIDS patients (39 years, 90% males).

Localization

About 60% of primary CNS lymphomas involve the supratentorial space, including the frontal (15%), temporal (8%), parietal (7%) and occipital (3%) lobes, basal ganglia/ periventricular regions (10%) and corpus callosum (5%), the posterior fossa (13%), and the spinal cord (1%). Approximately 25–50% are multiple (60–85% in AIDS and post-transplant subjects). Secondary meningeal spread is seen in 30–40% of primary CNS lymphomas, while primary leptomeningeal lymphoma may account for up to 8% of these tumours {512}. Primary dural and epidural malignant lymphomas appear to be very rare {1016}. Ocular disease (which may antedate intracranial lesions) is present in 15-20% of cases, and distant metastases in 6–10%, with a range from 3 to 27% {163}. Complete staging of malignant lymphomas presenting as a cerebral mass lesion is controversial, as some patients initially considered having primary CNS lymphomas may subsequently show disseminated malignant lymphoma {405}. Secondary CNS malignant lymphomas prefer the dura and leptomeninges, but parenchymal lesions may also occur. Rare instances of extracranial lymphoma restricted to peripheral nerve may be designated as neurolymphomatosis.

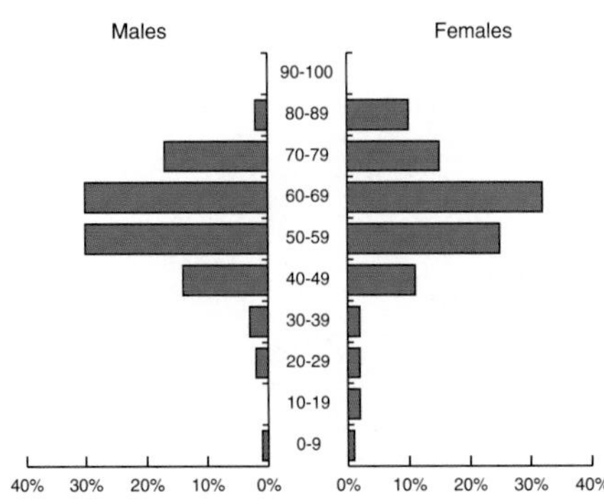

Fig. 12.1 Age and sex distribution of primary CNS lymphomas in immunocompetent patients.

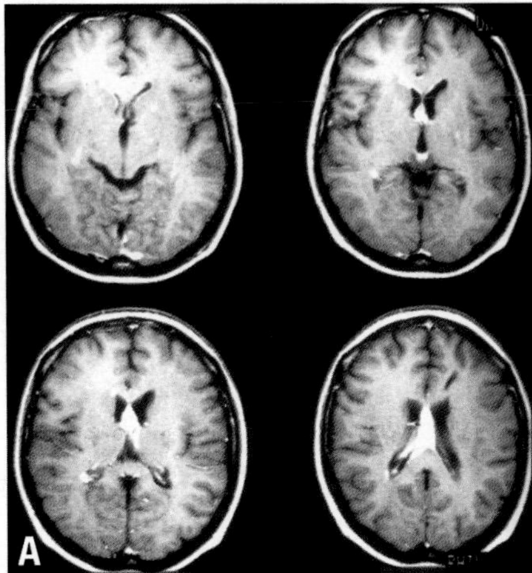

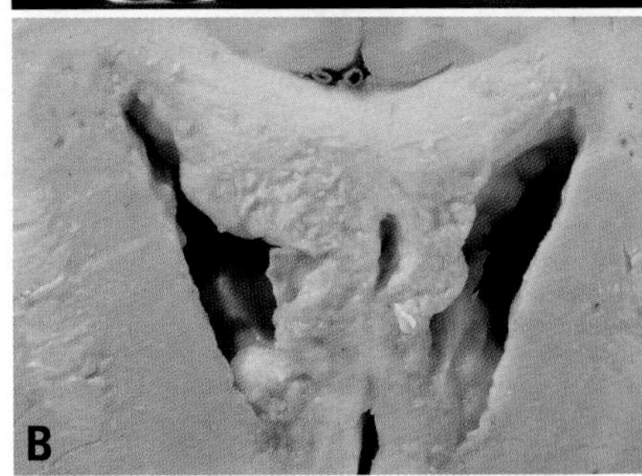

Fig. 12.2 T1-weighted MRI and macroscopic appearance of malignant lymphoma with diffuse infiltration of the ventricular walls.

Clinical features

Symptoms and signs

Symptoms and clinical presentation are non-specific. Around 50–80% of primary CNS lymphoma patients present with focal neurological deficits, 20–30% with neuropsychiatric symptoms, 10–30% with signs of increased intracranial pressure, and 5–20% with seizures. Cerebellar, brainstem and spinal cord symptoms are rare. Eye symptoms resulting from uveitis or vitrous lymphoma are seen in 5–20% of cases. For primary CNS lymphomas, the interval between initial symptoms and diagnosis ranges from days to two years, with an average of two months. Angiotropic lymphoma often manifests as rapidly progressing dementia with multifocal neurological deficits {224, 903}. Common features of CNS involvement in systemic malignant lymphoma include signs of increased intracranial pressure and nonspecific neuropsychiatric symptoms. About 50% of transplantation-associated primary CNS lymphomas appear within a year after transplantation (average, 32 months) {1164}.

Neuroimaging

Cranial CT and MRI of primary CNS lymphomas show solitary or multiple, hyperdense or isodense lesions, often solid and rarely cystic, typically with diffuse, rarely ring-like enhancement or lacking enhancement. Bilateral symmetrical subependymal high-signal foci are suggestive of primary CNS lymphomas. Peritumoural oedema is less severe than in malignant gliomas and metastases. FDG-PET scan {605} or Thallium-201-SPECT {1980} are helpful in the differential diagnosis of ring-enhancing mass lesions that are frequently seen in AIDS-related primary CNS lymphomas and which are difficult to distinguish from toxoplasmosis and other non-neoplastic conditions by CT or MRI. Meningeal infiltration may present as hyperdense corticomeningeal structures, but CT and MRI can fail to detect meningeal or eye lesions.

CSF cytology

Pleocytosis is found in 35–60% of primary CNS lymphoma patients, but despite the presence of tumour cells in the CSF, cell counts can be normal. Cytology is of diagnostic value in 5–30% of primary CNS lymphomas and in 70–95% of metastatic malignant lymphomas, particularly if immunocytochemistry is used to determine monoclonality {408}. The combination of flow cytometry and morphologic examination may enhance the detection of lymphoma cells in the CSF {1987}.

Stereotactic biopsy

In establishing the histological diagnosis of primary CNS lymphoma, stereotactic biopsy is currently the method of choice, since the tumour is often located deeply and gross surgical resection is not beneficial. Unless herniation is imminent, corticosteroids should be withheld before biopsy.

Macroscopy

Primary CNS lymphomas occur as single or multiple masses in the cerebral hemispheres. While they are often deep-seated and adjacent to the ventricular system, superficial tumours may also be encountered. The tumours can be firm, friable, granular, centrally necrotic, focally haemorrhagic, grey-tan, yellow, or virtually indistinguishable from the adjacent neuropil. Demarcation from surrounding parenchyma is variable. Some tumours appear well-delineated, like a metastasis. When diffuse borders and architectural effacement are present, the lesions resemble gliomas. Diffusely infiltrating forms without evidence of a mass lesion have been referred to as "lymphomatosis cerebri" {1982}. AIDS patients tend to have more necrotic areas, which may simulate necrotizing cerebral toxoplasmosis {1031}. Meningeal lymphoma mimics meningioma or meningitis, or appears macroscopically normal.

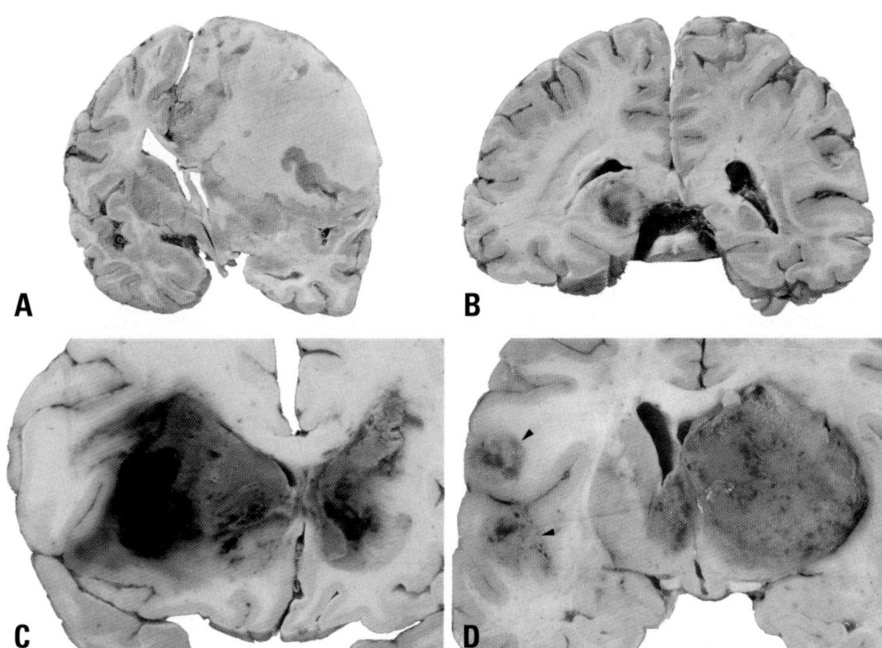

Fig. 12.3 Macroscopic features of primary malignant CNS lymphomas. **A** Large, necrotizing B-cell lymphoma in an HIV-1-infected seven-month-old infant. **B** B-cell lymphoma involving the medial temporo-occipital lobe. **C, D** Primary malignant CNS lymphomas of the basal ganglia with extension into the contralateral hemisphere. **D** Note the additional foci in the left insular region (arrows).

Classification systems and their relevance to primary CNS lymphomas

There is no universally accepted classification scheme for primary CNS lymphomas. The Working Formulation of non-Hodgkin Lymphomas for Clinical Usage is largely based on clinical correlations and classifies both B- and T-cell neoplasms together in ten categories that reflect three prognostic levels (low, intermediate, and high grade) and one miscellaneous category {1497}. The revised Kiel classification is based on morphological differentiation of lymphocytes with less regard to clinical outcome and considers B- and T-cell lesions separately, placing them in two cytologically defined categories (low and high grade) {878}. The third and most recent system is the Revised European-American Lymphoma (REAL) classification and the very similar WHO classification, which define entities on the basis of morphological, immunological, genetic and clinical information {1998}. The result is a system that segregates lymphomas into the categories of B-cell, T/NK-cell and Hodgkin diseases, the B- and T/NK-cell categories being divided into precursor and peripheral neoplasms. None of these classifications, however, specifically includes primary CNS lymphomas.

Histopathology

A malignant lymphoma that diffusely infiltrates brain parenchyma in an angiocentric pattern forming collars of tumour cells within concentric perivascular reticulin deposits.

Low-power microscopy of primary CNS lymphoma at the periphery demonstrates this angiocentric infiltration pattern best. From these perivascular cuffs, tumour cells invade neural parenchyma, either with compact cellular aggregates and a well-delineated invasion front resembling metastatic carcinoma, or with single diffusely infiltrating tumour cells resembling encephalitis. Virtually all primary CNS lymphomas show a diffuse growth pattern, while a follicular growth pattern has not been described. When tumours become confluent, geographic necrosis may be seen, with perivascular islands of viable tumour cells surrounded by large regions of coagulative necrosis. A focally prominent astrocytic and microglial response, large CD68-positive macrophages, and reactive lymphocytic infiltrates with a predominance of small CD4-positive T-cells are common. High-power microscopy of primary CNS lymphoma shows lymphoid cells with a variable appearance. Their ultrastructure does not differ from that seen in systemic malignant lymphoma.

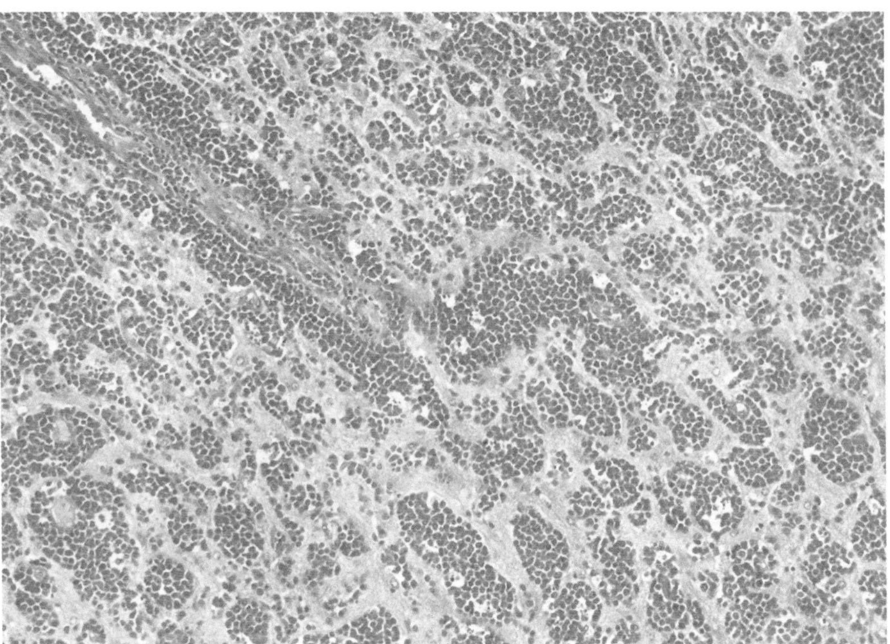

Fig. 12.5 Primary malignant CNS lymphoma, with characteristic perivascular spread of tumour cells.

B-cell lymphomas

Approximately 98% of primary CNS lymphomas are B-cell lymphomas with immunohistochemical expression of pan-B markers such as CD20 and CD79a. The majority of tumours express monoclonal surface or cytoplasmic immunoglobulins, the most frequent combination being IgM/kappa.

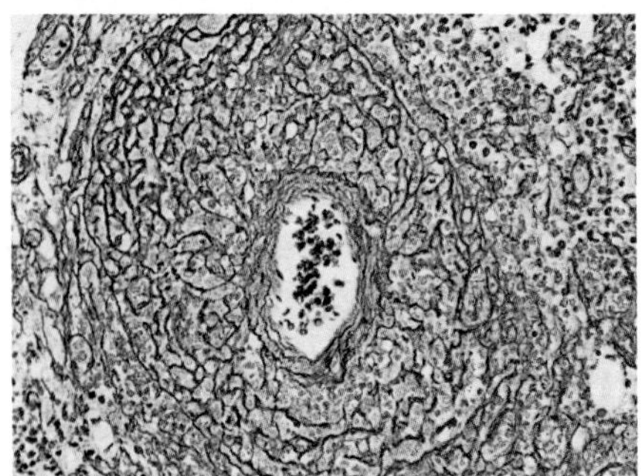

Fig. 12.4 Perivascular accumulation of lymphoma cells embedded in a concentric network of reticulin fibres.

Individual studies differ as to which histological subtypes of lymphoma predominate in the CNS. According to a meta-analysis {695}, subtypes of 590 sporadic primary CNS lymphomas, classified according to the Working Formulation, included diffuse large cell (43.4%), diffuse large cell immunoblastic (19.7%), diffuse small cleaved cell (9.5%), small non-cleaved cell/non-Burkitt (8.8%), atypical/unclassified (7.1%), diffuse mixed small and large cell (7.1%), lymphoblastic (2.9%) and small lymphocytic (1.5%). A total of 1068 sporadic primary CNS lymphomas were Kiel classified as immunoblastic (25.5%), centroblastic (19.3%), lymphoblastic (17.6%), immunocytic (13.5%), high-grade unclassified (13.3%), centroblastic/centrocytic (8.0%), centrocytic (1.3%) and T-cell lymphoma (1.5%). However, in different series the percentage of low-grade primary CNS lymphomas ranged from 0 to 75%, that of centroblastomas from 0 to 60%, and that of unclassified tumours from 0 to 90%. These discrepancies may reflect changes in the prevalence of lymphoma subtypes or, more likely, in the diagnostic approach taken {695}.

Major subtypes of HIV-associated primary CNS lymphomas have been diffuse large cell immunoblastic (33.6%), diffuse large cell (32.7%) and small non-cleaved cell (21.6%), but these tumours often show atypical features that do not readily fall into any classification scheme, including striking polymorphous components and cells that resemble Burkitt cells but which lack appropriate morphological features {1029}. This distribution contrasts to that in AIDS-related systemic NHL {190}. These difficulties of reconciling tumour histology to classification schemes that were not intended to evaluate CNS neoplasia, compounded by the failure to deal with prognostic significance (see below), may suggest that subtyping using the Kiel classification or the Working Formulation is of limited relevance. Applying the REAL classification or the WHO classification has greatly simplified CNS lymphoma subtying, since the great majority of tumours can be classified as diffuse large B-cell lymphoma, but it is debatable whether that simplification represents a progress. At present, subtyping of primary CNS B-cell lymphomas has to be considered as having little or no clinical relevance.

T-cell lymphomas

T-cell lymphomas constitute about 2% of all primary CNS lymphomas, are peripheral (also known as post-thymic or mature) T-cell lymphomas, and have been seen mainly in the immunocompetent {1030, 1085}, although single cases in AIDS patients are on record {126}. They occur as solitary or multiple intraparenchymal masses with a higher male: female ratio, a more frequent posterior fossa localization, particularly in the cerebellum {126}, and a propensity to arise in the leptomeninges {512}. A subset of Ki-1 lymphomas and lymphomatoid granulomatosis belongs into the T-cell lymphoma category {531,1152}. T-cell lymphoma must be distinguished from T-cell rich B-cell lymphoma.

Plasmacytoma

In its purely extraosseous form, intracranial plasmacytoma most often appears as a nodular or plaque-like dural mass, with variable infiltration of the underlying brain {87}. Although rare, exclusively intraparenchymal tumours have also been described {1626}. Some authors have suggested that intracranial plasma cell lesions may be categorised along a continuum ranging from polyclonal plasma cell granuloma to atypical monoclonal plasma cell hyperplasia, a precursor to plasmacytoma {626}.

Angiotropic lymphoma
Angiotropic lymphoma, also known as intravascular lymphoma, affects multiple organ systems. The CNS, including the entire neuraxis, is involved in more than 30% of cases. When specific lymphoid markers were not yet available, angiotropic lymphomas were regarded as malignant angioendotheliomatosis, because the origin of the tumour cells had been misinterpreted as being endothelial. Accumulations of large B-cells within small and medium vessels lead to vascular occlusion and disseminated small infarcts {903, 1996}. Absent or reduced expression of beta-2 integrins on tumour cells may contribute to an impaired capability for extravasation {672}.

Hodgkin disease
The diagnosis of Hodgkin disease rests upon the identification of Reed-Sternberg cells or their variants in the appropriate background of non-neoplastic haematopoietic cells (lymphocytes, plasma cells, histiocytes, eosinophils). The entity is rare in the CNS, and is most often seen in the setting of grade III or IV systemic disease {1323} but primary CNS presentation has also been described. Lesions are typically dural-based, but firm and well-demarcated intraparenchymal tumours do occur {1991}. Many series on "primary intraparenchymal Hodgkin disease" that predate immunohistochemical techniques have probably reported large cell anaplastic or pleomorphic lymphomas with atypical immunoblasts that resemble Reed-Sternberg cells. Currently, the diagnosis should only be made if immunohistochemistry confirms the identity of the Reed-Sternberg cell, *i.e.* immunoreactivity to CD30 (Ber-H2 or Ki-1) and CD15 (Leu-M1), and usually lack of CD45RB. Epstein-Barr virus genes and proteins may occur even in tumours of immunocompetent patients {1991}.

MALT lymphoma of the dura
Low-grade B-cell lymphoma of mucosa-associated lymphoid tissue (MALT) type may arise in the intracranial dura {1990, 1992}. Cytologically, they correspond to MALT lymphomas arising at other more typical sites and are composed of small lymphocytes with plasmacytoid differentiation and centrocyte-like cells. The tumour cells express CD20 and CD79a but not CD5, CD10 or CD23. In contrast to other types of primary intracranial lymphomas, a follicular growth pattern with germinal centre formation is usually present.

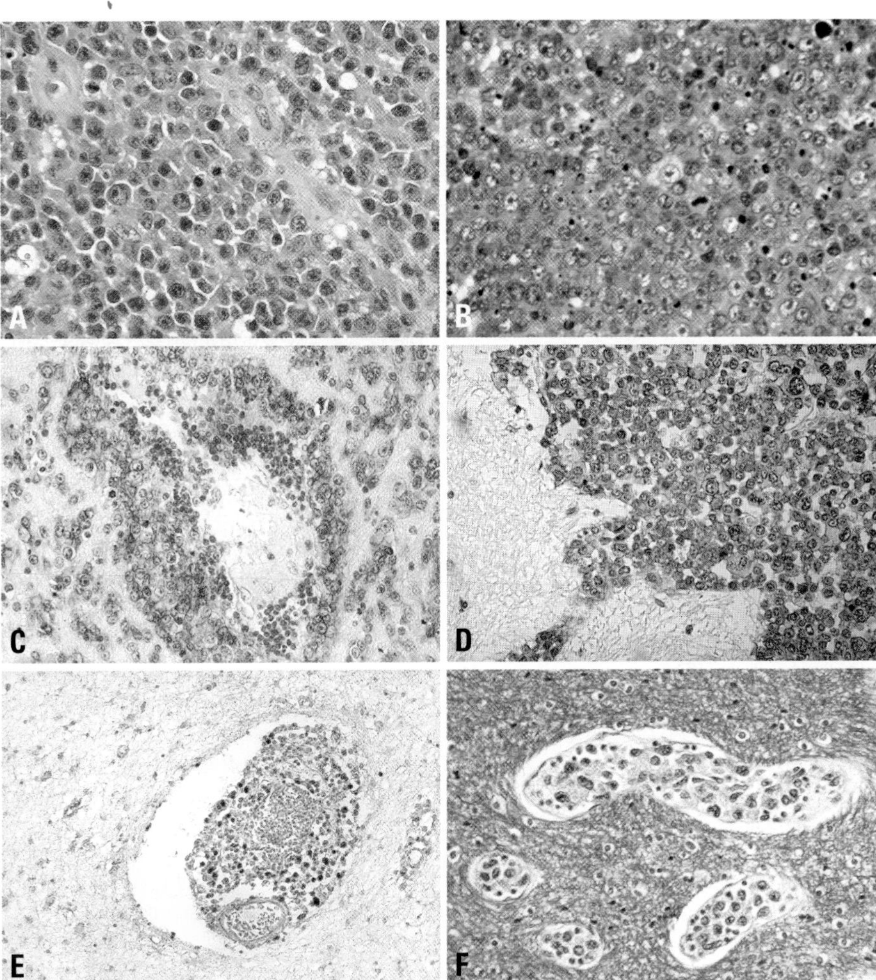

Fig. 12.6 **A** Malignant, diffuse large B-cell lymphoma. **B** Highly anaplastic malignant lymphoma with numerous mitotic figures and extensive apoptosis. **C** Tumour cells express the B-cell marker CD20, while small, predominantly perivascular reactive T-cell infiltrates remain unstained. **D** Immunostaining with UCHL1 of a malignant T-cell lymphoma invading the brain. **E** Malignant CNS B-cell lymphoma. *In situ* hybridization shows the presence of Epstein-Barr virus (EBV) in perivascular tumour cells. Reactive lymphocytes and glial cells remain unstained. **F** Angiotropic lymphoma showing small brain capillaries filled with lymphoblastoid cells.

Proliferation and apoptosis
Mean Ki-67/MIB-1 labelling indices are 19-24% in low-grade, 31–47% in high-grade Kiel types, and may even exceed 90% in individual high-grade tumours {9, 1984, 1986}. A variable number of TUNEL-positive apoptotic cells was detected in 27 of 35 (77%) of tumours, usually in less than 20% of cells, while the apoptotic fraction may exceed 50% after corticosteroid therapy {1986}. Expression of the apoptosis-inhibiting Bcl-2 but not the pro-apoptotic Bak protein in most tumours suggests that apoptosis is inhibited {1986}.

Aetiology
Inherited or acquired immunodeficiency predisposes to development of primary CNS lymphoma. This includes immunodeficiency produced by Wiskott-Aldrich syndrome, AIDS and immunosuppressive therapy following organ transplantation and, to a lesser degree, therapy of Hodgkin disease and autoimmune disorders such as rheumatoid arthritis and Sjögren syndrome.
The Epstein-Barr virus (EBV) appears to play a major role in immunocompromised patients with primary CNS lymphoma: the

EBV genome is present in tumour cells in more than 95% of immunocompromised patients, but in only 0–20% of immunocompetent patients {190,1029}. Lymphoma cells that are latently infected with EBV variably express six EBV-encoded nuclear antigens (EBNA 1–6, also called EBNA 1, 2, 3a, 3b, 3c and leader protein), several latent membrane proteins (LMP1, 2a, 2b), and two extraordinarily abundant, small non-polyadenylated nuclear RNAs, EBER1 and EBER2. Expression of these proteins has a wide variety of effects, including mimicking of CD4 and B-cell receptor engagement, activation of NF-kb and protein kinases, upregulation of adhesion molecules, upregulation of the BCL2 proto-oncogene, and inactivation of the *TP53* and *RB* tumour suppressor genes. More than half of AIDS-related primary CNS lymphomas examined so far express at least EBNA2, LMPs and EBERs {49,190}, a pattern referred to as type 3 latency which closely resembles that seen in B-cells transformed into lymphoblastoid cell lines by EBV infection *in vitro* {1277}. From the diagnostic viewpoint, PCR assay for EBV DNA in cerebrospinal fluid has been described as being highly specific (up to 100%) and sensitive (80%) for the detection of primary CNS lymphomas in AIDS patients {1983}.
Genomic DNA of herpes viruses (HHV-6 or HHV-8) has been identified in a few cases of primary CNS lymphomas {1032, 1150}. However, a comprehensive serologic evaluation coupled with tumour analysis for viral nucleic acids has conclusively ruled out a role for HHV-8 in AIDS-related CNS lymphomas {1981}. Similarly, no definite aetiological factors have been identified that could be held responsible for the development of primary CNS lymphomas in immunocompetent subjects.

Genetic susceptibility

With the exception for inherited immunodeficiency, no genetic predisposition to primary CNS lymphoma has been described to date. A previous or concomitant malignant neoplasm is present in about 8% of immunocompetent primary CNS lymphoma patients, most commonly leukaemia or adenocarcinoma. However, it is not known whether this is coincidental or reflects a genetic predisposition, prolonged survival in cancer patients, immunological impairment, or the effects of therapy with carcinogenic cytostatic agents {1249}. Associations of primary CNS lymphoma with other brain tumours such as meningioma and glioma in individual patients are likely to be coincidental {1428}.

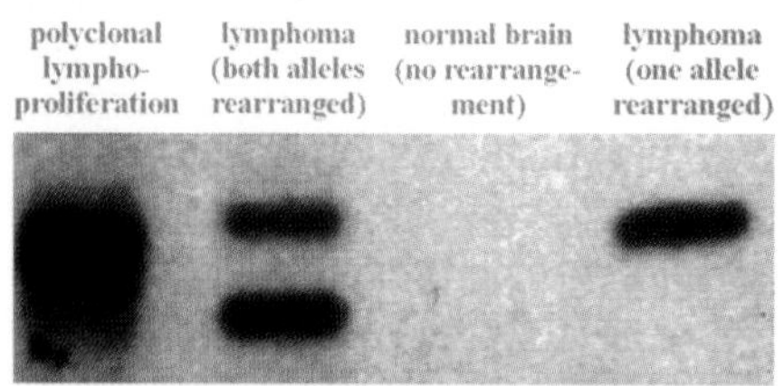

Fig. 12.7 PCR assay for immunoglobin gene rearrangement.

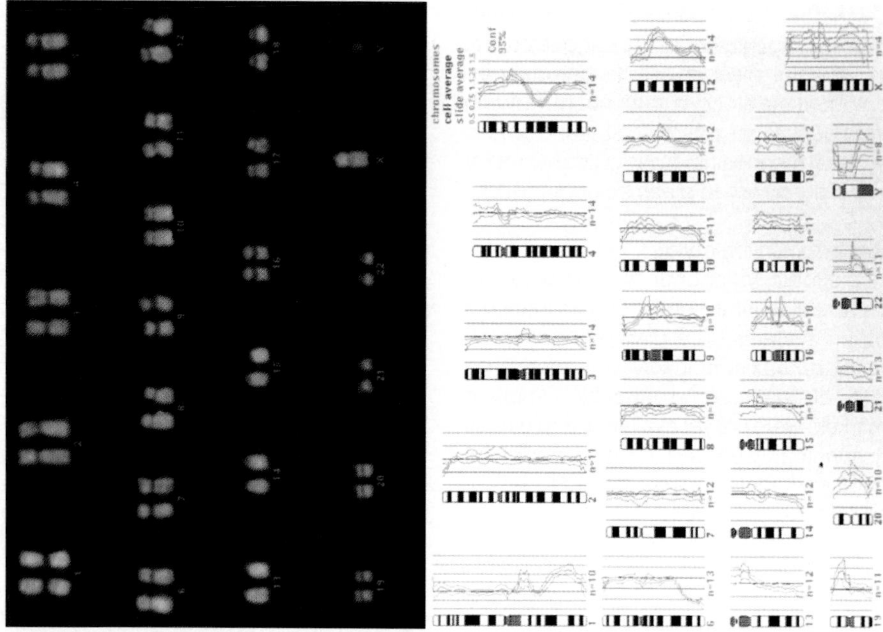

Fig. 12.8 Comparative genomic hybridization (CGH), showing chromosomal gains (green) on 1q, 12q, 22q and losses (red) on 5q and 6q. The fluorescence image is shown on the left, the CGH profile on the right.

Cytogenetics

Cytogenetic analyses of single cases of primary CNS lymphoma in non-AIDS patients revealed clonal abnormalities of chromosomes 1, 6, 7 and 14, as well as translocations (1;14), (6;14), (13;18) and (14;21), findings similar to those observed in nodal B-cell lymphoma {654}.

Molecular genetics

Development of B-cells is characterized by imprecise rearrangement of variable (V), diversity (D) and joining (J) segments of immunoglobulin (Ig) genes, leading to B-cells with uniquely rearranged Ig genes, and resulting in vast immunological diversity {506}. When encountering antigen, B-cells proliferate in the microenvironment of the germinal centre (GC) of secondary lymphoid organs, where somatic mutations are introduced into rearranged V region genes. Normally, during immune reactions, a polyclonal or oligoclonal lymphoproliferation is generated, whereas a clonal population indicates autonomous growth of tumour cells. From the diagnostic viewpoint, PCR performed on samples of CSF or on small specimens from brain biopsy can demonstrate lymphocyte clonality and is a valuable technique for corroborating the histological or cytological diagnosis of malignant lymphoma, even in archival material {1255}. Molecular analysis of rearranged V region genes of primary CNS lymphomas demonstrated clonally rearranged Ig genes with somatic mutations which were more frequent than in other lymphoma types; thus, primary CNS lymphomas correspond to GC B-cells. The GC origin of these tumours is also reflected by mutations of the 5′ non-coding regions of the BCL6 gene and expression of the bcl-6 protein {1993}. Furthermore, the mutation pattern of the rearranged Ig genes suggested that the tumour cells or their precursors may recognise a shared antigen or superantigen {2432}. Primary CNS lymphomas of HIV-negative, but not of HIV-positive patients show a biased usage of V region genes, suggesting different pathogenetic pathways in immunocompetent and immunodeficient patients {1989, 2599}.
Two series on chromosomal imbalances of 22 and 19 brain lymphomas of the dif-

fuse large B-cell type using comparative genomic hybridization revealed an average of 5.5 and 6.8 chromosomal changes per tumor, respectively, gains being more common than losses {2432, 2571}. The most common loss involved 6q (50% and 47%) and the most common gains involved 12q (41% and 63%) and 18q (36% and 37%) {2432, 2571}.

Common molecular genetic aberrations seen in nodal (extracerebral) diffuse large cell lymphomas, which resemble cytologically the majority of primary CNS lymphomas, include point mutations in *RAS* genes (*NRAS*, *KRAS2*) in 15%, deletions of *CDKN2A* and *CDKN2B* in 15%, amplifications of *REL* in 25%, and rearrangements of *BCL2* [associated with the t(14;18) translocation] in 20%, of BCL6 (BCL5, LAZ3) in 35%, and of MYCC in 25%. The mutational spectrum of primary CNS lymphoma is still being elaborated, but appears to differ from systemic tumours with regard to mutational frequencies. For example, inactivation of CDKN2A by either homozygous deletion or DNA hypermethylation appears to be particularly common in primary CNS lymphomas and has been found in 23 of 30 (77%) cases {1984,1997}. In contrast, aberrations of various oncogenes have not been detected and thus appear to be unimportant in primary CNS lymphomas, including *BCL2* and *CCND1* rearrangements and amplifications of *MYCC*, *REL*, *MDM2*, *CDK4* and *CCND1* {190, 982, 1984}. *TP53* mutations were found in 6 of 35 sporadic cases {793, 1984, 1995}, most of the mutated cases being from Japan (5 of 15).

Histogenesis

It is not known whether primary CNS lymphomas arise within or outside the brain and why they manifest in an organ that lacks a regular lymphatic system. Three hypotheses have been put forward. (i) B-cells may be transformed at a site elsewhere in the body and then develop adhesion molecules specific for cerebral endothelia. However, one study found that the expression pattern of a number of integrin and immunoglobulin adhesion molecules by tumour cells did not differ between primary CNS lymphoma and cytologically similar nodal lymphomas {1149}. It is possible that the responsible adhesion molecule(s) may have been missed in this study, or they may be down-regulated by lymphoma cells once they have entered the brain. (ii) Lymphoma cells may be systematically eradicated by an intact immune system but may be relatively protected within the CNS. (iii) A polyclonal intracerebral inflammatory lesion may expand clonally within the brain and progress to the monoclonal neoplastic state, a scenario that resembles the development of gastric MALT lymphoma from gastritis induced by *H. pylori*. Evidence in support of this idea includes the demonstration in a few patients of transient symptomatic contrast-enhancing brain lesions ('sentinel lesions'), which regress spontaneously or with corticosteroid treatment and ultimately lead to primary CNS lymphoma within one year; histological features are non-specific and include inflammatory T-cell infiltrates, demyelination and gliosis {23}. Possibly, intracerebral antigens or superantigens may stimulate persistence and intracerebral expansion of B-cells. On the other hand, infectious or inflammatory CNS diseases have only exceptionally been described to antedate the development of primary CNS lymphoma {38}. It remains to be determined whether sentinel lesions represent non-neoplastic precursor lesions of primary CNS lymphoma or neoplastic foci that are temporarily kept dormant by host immunity.

Therapy, prognosis and predictive factors

Favourable prognostic factors include single intracranial lesions, absence of meningeal or periventricular tumours, absence of immunodeficiency, age under 60 years and a preoperative Karnofsky score of over 70. With current therapy, consisting of radiotherapy and chemotherapy, immunocompetent patients show response rates of 85% with a median survival of 17–45 months and an overall survival of 40–70% and 25–45% at 2 and 5 years, respectively {100,1090}. AIDS patients have a much poorer prognosis, with a median survival of 2–6 months {743} or 13.5 months when treated with multimodal therapy {220}. Radiation doses exceeding 50 Gy and a regimen of chemotherapy after radiotherapy are often associated with late neurological toxicity clinically corresponding to dementia. The typically dramatic response of primary CNS lymphomas to corticosteroids is usually temporary, but can occasionally be long-term {1178}. As rare enigmatic spontaneous remissions may occur, primary CNS lymphomas have been termed 'disappearing' or 'ghost' tumours.

Whereas most authors have found no correlation between histological type and survival in primary CNS lymphoma, others have maintained that histological subtypes have a direct correlation with survival. However, such correlations have not been uniform. In one series, a diffuse mixed histology (Working Formulation) was associated with decreased survival {567}. In another study, patients having tumours of this intermediate grade seemed to fare better than those with high-grade lesions {1007}. In this study, patients with large cell and small non-cleaved cell lymphomas did better than those with large cell immunoblastic and large cleaved or non-cleaved {1007}. In contrast, yet another study showed that patients with diffuse mixed and small cleaved cell lymphoma had better prognoses than those with large cell, large cell immunoblastic, polymorphous and small non-cleaved lymphomas {555}. Like histological types, proliferation markers do not show any correlation to survival. Given these negative findings and the current problems in subtyping primary CNS lymphoma, the statement "subclassification and analysis of proliferative activity appears to be of no practical importance" {9} cannot be refuted. Since a correlation between chromosomal loss on 6q and shorter survival was recently found in one study {2432}, it remains to be determined whether subtyping on a genetic basis might be clinically more relevant.

Histiocytic tumours

W. Paulus
J.J. Kepes
K. Jellinger

Definition

A heterogeneous group of tumours and tumour-like masses composed of histiocytes that are commonly associated with histologically identical extracranial lesions. Langerhans cell histiocytosis (LCH) shows features of dendritic Langerhans cells whereas the various types of non-LCH show macrophage differentiation.

Synonyms and historical annotation

In 1997, the WHO Committee on Histiocytic/Reticulum Cell Proliferations and the Reclassification Working Group of the Histiocyte Society proposed classifying histiocytic disorders as: (1) dendritic cell-related disorders of varied biological behaviour, such as LCH and juvenile xanthogranuloma; (2) macrophage-related disorders of varied biological behaviour, such as haemophagocytic lymphohistiocytosis and Rosai-Dorfman disease; and (3) malignant histiocytic disorders, such as monocytic leukaemia and histiocytic sarcoma {2048}.

LCH was previously referred to as histiocytosis X, a term embracing eosinophilic granuloma, Hand-Schüller-Christian disease and Abt-Letterer-Siwe disease, 'X' being the unknown aetiological factor {1719}. Because there is much overlap between these subgroups, LCH is currently classified on the basis of extent as unifocal, multifocal (usually polyostotic) and disseminated. Historical descriptions of cerebral LCH with principal involvement of the hypothalamus and posterior pituitary were made under terms such as hypothalamic granuloma, Gagel's granuloma and Ayala disease (reviewed in {751}).

A wide variety of neoplastic and non-neoplastic intracranial masses containing high numbers of macrophages or other foamy ('xanthomatous') cells have previously been referred to as 'xanthogranuloma' or 'xanthoma', including LCH, dural or osseous masses in hyperlipoproteinaemia and Weber-Christian panniculitis, degenerative processes in craniopharyngiomas and various cysts, pleomorphic xanthoastrocytoma ('fibroxanthoma') and inflammatory malignant fibrous histiocytoma

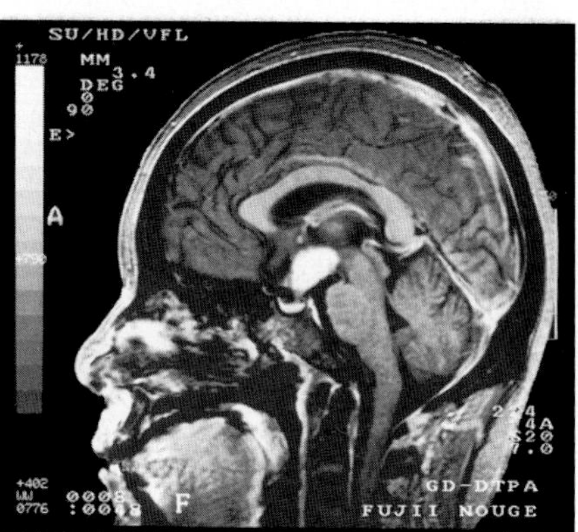

Fig. 12.9 Gadolinium enhanced MRI of a Langerhans cell histiocytosis in the hypothalamic region (Hand-Schüller-Christian disease).

('malignant xanthogranuloma') {751}. Benign and malignant fibrous histiocytomas are mesenchymal tumours and no longer regarded true histiocytic lesions (see Chapter 11).

Incidence

In children under 15 years of age, the incidence of LCH is estimated at 0.2 to 0.5 per 100'000 population per year {1733}. Non-LCH is even rarer. Xanthogranulomas and xanthomas of the choroid plexus are common incidental autopsy findings in 1.6 to 7% of cases {1724}.

Langerhans cell histiocytosis (LCH)

LCH typically occurs in children (mean, 12 years), without sex preference. The most common form of *LCH* is a solitary osteolytic lesion of the skull or spine (eosinophilic granuloma). Multifocal LCH lesions of the bone with hypothalamic involvement have been referred to as Hand-Schüller-Christian disease, while Abt-Letterer-Siwe disease involves skin, lymph nodes, viscera and rarely the CNS. Extension from osseous foci to hypothalamus and pituitary gland in multifocal or disseminated LCH is responsible for most cases with CNS involvement, but unifocal or multifocal infiltrates may occur primarily within or even restricted to the hypothalamus, infundibulum, optic chiasm, choroid plexus and cerebral hemispheres {1700, 1723, 1732}.

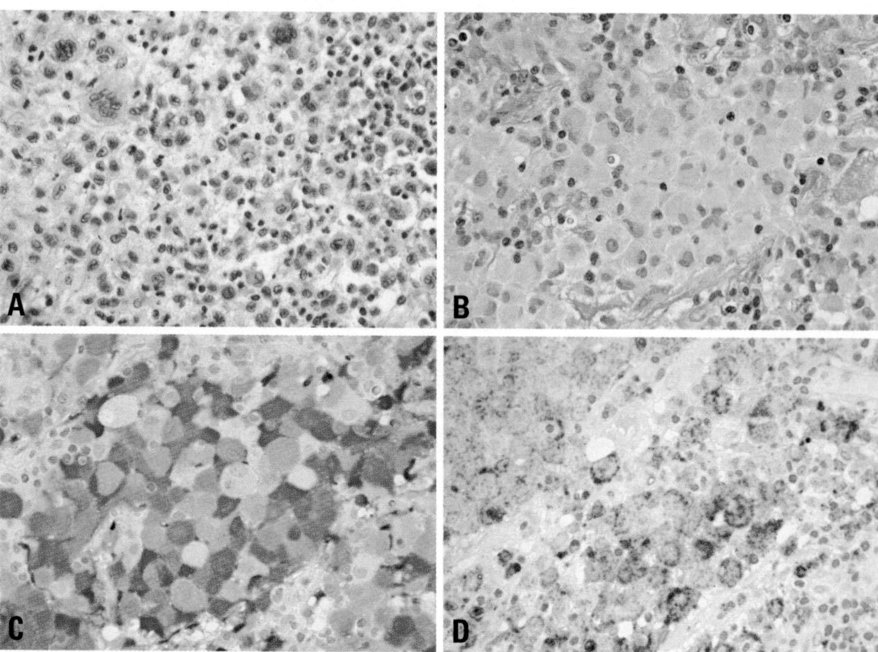

Fig. 12.10 Langerhans cell histiocytosis. **A** Mixed infiltrate composed of histiocytes, lymphocytes, eosinophils and multinucleated cells. **B** High-power view showing the typical grooving of nuclei. **C** Immunolabeling with S100 protein. **D** Expression of the macrophage marker CD 68.

Clinical features
The most common neurological signs of *LCH* are diabetes insipidus (25% of children with multifocal or disseminated disease) with or without associated signs of hypothalamic dysfunction (obesity, hypogonadism, growth retardation), signs of raised intracranial pressure, cranial nerve palsies, seizures, visual disturbances (visual field defect, optic atrophy), ataxia and rare progressive tetra- and paraparesis {1698}. On CCT and MRI, intracranial *LCH* may appear as (i) extraparenchymal solid mass, (ii) multiple well defined lesions in grey and white matter, (iii) poorly defined lesions in white matter, (iv) thickening of the pituitary stalk, or (v) demyelinating lesion of the cerebellum {1729, 2051}.

Macroscopy
Intracranial LCH lesions are often yellow or white and vary from discrete dural-based nodules to granular parenchymal infiltrates. CNS lesions may be well-delineated or ill-defined.

Histopathology
Massive granulomatous infiltrates composed of Langerhans cell histiocytes, macrophages, lymphocytes, plasma cells and a variable fraction of eosinophils.
The nuclei of Langerhans cells are typically slightly excentric, ovoid, reniform or convoluted with linear grooves and inconspicuous nucleoli. The cytoplasm is large (15 µm to 25 µm in diameter) and pale to eosinophilic. Touton giant cells may occur. Abundant deposition of collagen is often seen. LCH occasionally presents with demyelination and no or a sparse infiltration of Langerhans cells {1729, 2051}. Eosinophils may form into aggregates and undergo necrosis to produce granulomas or abscesses. Immunohistochemically, Langerhans cells consistently express S-100 protein, vimentin and certain histiocyte markers including HLA-DR, b_2 microglobulin and CD1a, variably CD68, rarely L1 antigen (clone MAC387) and almost never CD45, CD15 and lysozyme {1721}. CD1a expression, being very characteristic but not absolutely specific to LCH, can be demonstrated even on small and routinely processed materials {1721, 2048}. The ultrastructural hallmark and diagnostic "gold standard" of Langerhans cells are Birbeck granules (Langerhans cell granules), which are 34 nm wide rod-shaped or tennis-racket-shaped intracytoplasmic pentalaminar structures with cross-striation and a zipper-like central core, possibly originating from the cell membrane and/or Golgi apparatus {1704}. Either expression of CD1a or presence of Birbeck granules are currently required for definite diagnosis of LCH.
Proliferation. Immunohistochemical proliferation indices of neoplastic Langerhans cells are 4 to 16% using Ki-67, 8 to 12% using Ki-S1, and 6 to 15% using anti-PCNA {1708}.

Prognosis and predictive factors
The overall survival rates of all *LCH* patients at 5, 15, and 20 years are 88%, 88%, and 77%, with an event-free survival rate of only 30% at 15 years {1735}. While unifocal LCH may spontaneously recover or requires minimal treatment, *e.g.* surgical resection, multisystemic disease with organ dysfunction may resist systemic chemotherapy. The mortality rate in this latter subgroup of LCH reaches 40%. Of all patients with LCH, late sequelae are seen in 64%, including skeletal defects in 42%, diabetes insipidus in 25%, growth failure in 20%, hearing loss in 16%, and other CNS dysfunction in 14% {1735}. Concerning histopathologic features of LCH, no prognostic significance of cytologic atypia and mitotic activity was found in most studies {1731, 2048}, whereas it was also suggested that a distinct clinical entity of malignant LCH, characterized morphologically by malignant-appearing Langerhans cells and clinically by male predominance, atypical organ involvement, and an aggressive clinical course, does exist {1699}.

Non-Langerhans cell histiocytoses
This group of diseases differs from LCH by macrophage differentiation and the absence of features of dendritic Langerhans cells.

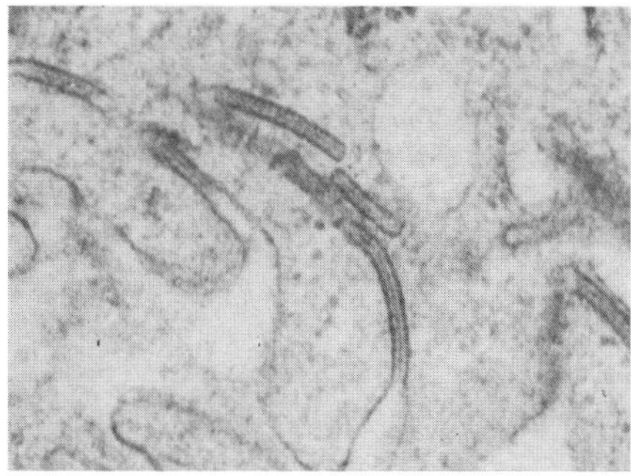

Fig. 12.11 Electron microscopy of Langerhans cell histiocytosis showing several Birbeck granules, apparently originating from cell membrane.

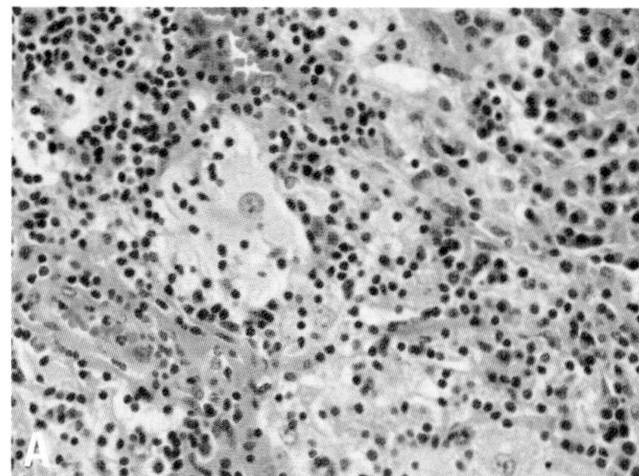

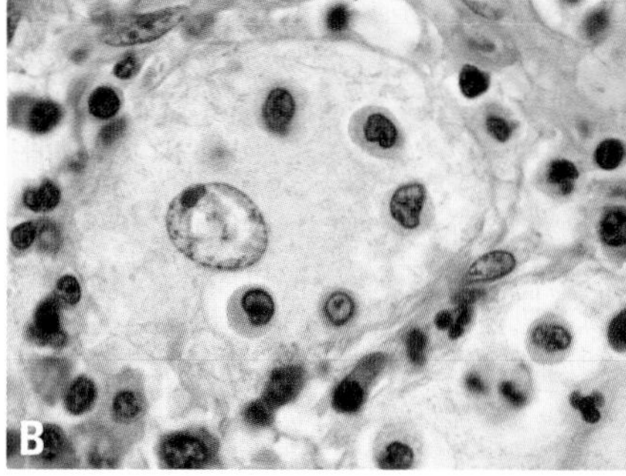

Fig. 12.12 Rosai-Dorfman disease. **A** Heterogeneous cellular infiltrate composed of lymphocytes, plasma cells and large histiocyte with emperipolesis. **B** Histiocyte with emperipolesis of lymphocytes and plasma cells.

Rosai-Dorfman disease
Rosai-Dorfman disease of lymph nodes is most common in children and young adults, but intracranial disease is usually seen in adults. Intracranially, it typically shows dural-based solitary or multiple masses {1717}; intrasellar lesions, meningeal masses and intracranial extension from an orbital mass may also occur. Clinically, the disease most often presents as an intracranial space-occupying mass (headaches, seizures); the 'classical' signs cervical lymphadenopathy, fever and weight loss (sinus histiocytosis with massive lymphadenopathy) are absent in 67% of these patients {1717, 1730}. The radiological appearance of intracranial *Rosai-Dorfman disease* usually mimics meningioma {1717} and carries a favourable prognosis after complete resection {1714, 1730}.
Histopathology shows sheets or nodules of histiocytes with vacuolated or eosinophilic cytoplasm (CD1a-, CD11c+, CD68+, MAC387+, lysozyme -/+, S-100 protein +), foci of lymphocytes and plasma cells, and fibrosis {1714, 1730}. Emperipolesis, *i.e.* well preserved lymphocytes and plasma cells within the cytoplasm of histiocytes, is typical, but may be inconspicuous.

Erdheim-Chester disease
The disease typically manifests in adults (mean, 55 years). Intracranial lesions may involve brain (preferably cerebellum), spinal cord, pituitary, meninges and orbit {1697, 2050}. Retention of MRI gadolinium enhancement for several days is typical {1697}. Patients may occasionally present with non-specific neurological signs without indication of systemic disease (bones, visceral organs, adipose tissue). Diabetes insipidus and progressive cerebellar dysfunction are common symptoms {1734, 2050}.
Histopathologically, lesions are composed of lipid-laden histiocytes (CD1a-, CD68+, S-100 protein -) with small nuclei, Touton-like multinucleated giant cells, a scant amount of lymphocytic infiltrates, a minimal number of eosinophils and fibrosis {1697, 2046}.

Haemophagocytic lymphohistiocytosis
This autosomal recessive systemic disease of early infancy (mean, 3 months) diffusely involves leptomeninges and, multifocally, the brain {1707}. Neuroimaging is characterized by focal hyperintense lesions in white and grey matter, diffuse abnormal T2 signal intensity in white matter, delayed myelination and parenchymal atrophy {1718}. Typical symptoms include fever, cytopenia, hypertriglyceridemia and hepatosplenomegaly. CNS involvement is seen in almost all patients, in 73% of patients already at time of diagnosis {1707}. Neurologic symptoms include irritability, bulging fontanelle, neck stiffness, seizures, cranial nerve palsies, ataxia and hemiplegia {1711, 1718}. The outcome is lethal without bone-marrow transplantation {1707, 1711}.
Histopathology shows non-malignant diffuse infiltrations of lymphocytes and macrophages with haemophagocytosis. The antigenic profile of the macrophages is CD11c+, CD68+, while staining for CD1a and S-100 protein is variable. Intracranial lesions consist of lymphohistiocytic meningeal and cerebral infiltrations and multifocal cerebral necroses {1707,1711}.

Juvenile xanthogranuloma (JXG) and xanthoma disseminatum
Juvenile xanthogranuloma preferentially manifests in young children as solitary cutaneous nodule, but may arise in the brain or the meninges, either with or without cutaneous lesions {1728}.
Xanthoma disseminatum occurs preferentially in young adults. Intracranial structures involved typically include hypothalamus, pituitary gland and dura mater {1709}. Pituitary and hypothalamic symptoms are most common (up to 40% of patients), while extracranial signs are related to involvement of skin, eyes, oral and respiratory mucosa {1725}.
Both lesions are composed of histiocytes (CD1a-, CD11c+, CD68+, factor XIIIa+, MAC387-/+, lysozyme -, S-100 protein -), scattered Touton giant cells, lymphocytes and eosinophils {1709, 1728}.

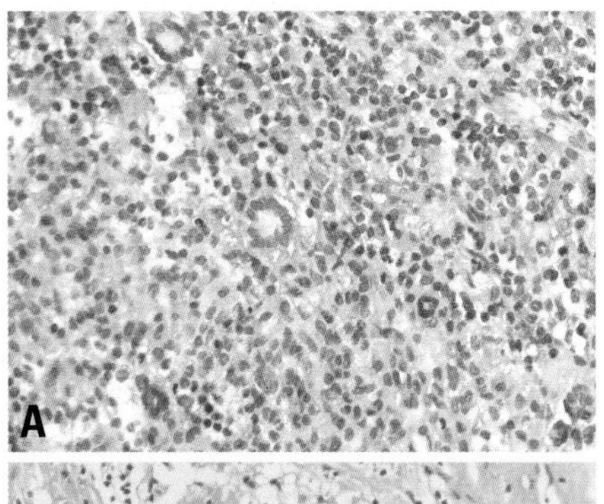

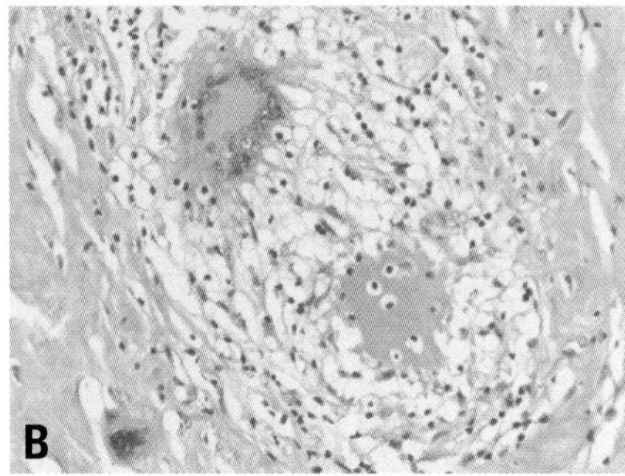

Fig. 12.13 **A** Juvenile xanthogranuloma composed of histiocytes, multinucleated Touton cells and lymphocytes. **B** Symptomatic choroid plexus xanthogranuloma with foreign body giant cells, chronic inflammatory infiltrates and calcification.

Choroid plexus xanthogranuloma
This lesion is localized in the lateral, rarely in the third ventricle; their incidence increases with age. Virtually all cases of *choroid plexus xanthoma* are non-symptomatic, whereas very rare symptomatic cases of *choroid plexus xanthogranuloma* present with sign of hydrocephalus due to obstruction of CSF pathways {1702, 1712}.
Xanthogranulomas are intraventricular, nodular, partly cystic grey masses with yellowish foci and a granular cut surface. Histopathology shows granulomatous nests of foamy histiocytes, foreign body giant cells, chronic inflammatory infiltrates composed of lymphocytes and plasma cells, cholesterol clefts, siderin, calcifications and trapped choroid plexus epithelium, while *choroid plexus xanthoma* is composed solely of aggregates of foamy histiocytes {1724}.

Aetiology
The aetiology of the histiocytic lesions is largely unknown. In the most patients with histiocytoses, there is no underlying defect in immunologic integrity. The presence as well as the etiologic and pathogenetic significance of human herpesvirus 6 DNA in LCH and Rosai-Dorfman disease is uncertain {1722}. Choroid plexus xanthomas and xanthogranulomas are regarded as non-pathologic ageing processes, xanthomas being correlated with hypercholesterolemia, atherosclerosis and diabetes mellitus {1724}.

Genetic susceptibility
Occurrence of multifocal LCH in monozygotic twins, in part with simultaneous onset of disease, has been repeatedly reported and suggests genetic susceptibility in at least some cases {1720}. Genes responsible for haemophagocytic lymphohistiocytosis may be located on chromosomes 9q21.3-22 and 10q21-22, the latter representing the *PERFORIN* gene {2047, 2600}.

Cytogenetics and molecular genetics
PCR-based X-chromosome inactivation assays of female tissues provided evidence in support of a clonal origin and a neoplastic nature of LCH {1736}, whereas Rosai-Dorfman disease was shown to be polyclonal {1727}. Monoclonal rearrangement of T-cell receptor genes was found in haemophagocytic lymphohistiocytosis {1726} but not in LCH {1736}. *TP53* mutations were not detected in LCH {2049}, while karyotypes and the involvement of oncogenes and tumour suppressor genes are virtually unknown in the histiocytic disorders described in this chapter.

Histogenesis
LCH is assumed to originate from dendritic Langerhans cells, whereas non-LCH is believed to arise from mononuclear phagocytes (macrophages). Microglial cells are the intrinsic histiocytes of the brain and although single tumours of possible microglial origin are on record {1713}, there is no indication that microglia might give rise to any one of the histiocytic disorders discussed in this chapter.

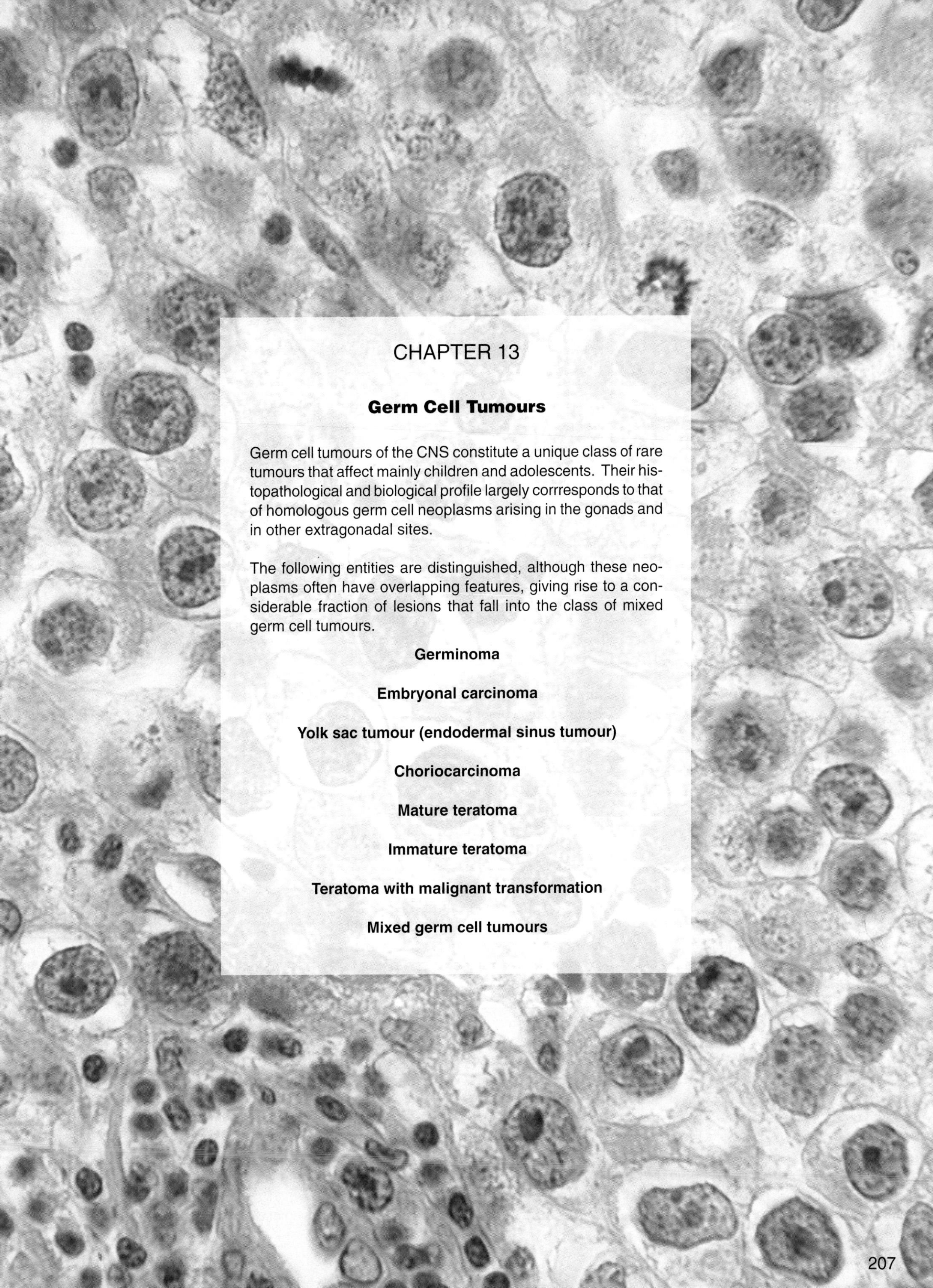

CHAPTER 13

Germ Cell Tumours

Germ cell tumours of the CNS constitute a unique class of rare tumours that affect mainly children and adolescents. Their histopathological and biological profile largely corrresponds to that of homologous germ cell neoplasms arising in the gonads and in other extragonadal sites.

The following entities are distinguished, although these neoplasms often have overlapping features, giving rise to a considerable fraction of lesions that fall into the class of mixed germ cell tumours.

Germinoma

Embryonal carcinoma

Yolk sac tumour (endodermal sinus tumour)

Choriocarcinoma

Mature teratoma

Immature teratoma

Teratoma with malignant transformation

Mixed germ cell tumours

CNS germ cell tumours

M.K. Rosenblum
M. Matsutani
E.G. Van Meir

Definition
Morphological homologues of germinal neoplasms arising in the gonads and in other extragonadal sites.

Incidence
CNS germ cell tumours (GCTs) vary considerably in their geographic incidence. In the West, they constitute only 0.3-0.5% of all primary intracranial neoplasms and approximately 3.0% of those encountered in children and adolescents, i.e., the cohorts at highest risk {129, 603, 699, 1300}. Far more prevalent in Asia, germ cell tumours account for at least 2.0% of all primary intracranial neoplasms, and for 9-15% of paediatric examples in series from Japan and Taiwan {597, 699, 972}.

Age and sex distribution
CNS germ cell tumours are primarily neoplasms of the young (Table 13.1): approximately 90% afflict those younger than 20 years {129, 597, 603, 699, 972, 1300, 1887}. Incidence peaks in 10-12 year olds, and 68% of histologically verified cases in a large retrospective review were found to occur in the second decade of life {699}. Congenital examples, usually teratomas or mixed tumours with prominent teratomatous components, are well recognized as are exceptional instances of late-adult onset. When the CNS as a whole is considered, the male: female ratio is 2-2.5:1; however, the regional distribution of these tumours varies according to sex. While the majority of examples arising in the pineal region affect boys, an excess of suprasellar germ cell tumours are encountered in girls. Sex differences are also apparent for germinomas versus germ cell tumours of other types {129, 597, 603, 699, 972}. Whereas the male: female case ratio for the former is approximately 1.5-2:1, it reaches over 3:1 when tumours of non-germinomatous histology are considered.

Localization
Like other extragonadal germ cell tumours, CNS variants hug the midline: 80% or more arise in structures about the third ventricle, with the region of the pineal gland being their most common site of origin, followed by the suprasellar compartment {129, 597, 603, 699, 972, 1300, 1887}. Intraventricular, basal ganglionic, thalamic, cerebral hemispheric, bulbar, intramedullary and intrasellar variants may be encountered, as may congenital holocranial examples (usually teratomas) and lesions that involve the brain extensively in complex with the orbit, cervical or cephalic soft tissues. Germinomas are the prevalent tumour type in the suprasellar compartment and basal ganglionic/thalamic regions, with non-germinomatous germ cell tumours dominating at other sites. Multifocal germ cell tumours usually involve the pineal region and suprasellar compartment simultaneously or sequentially {597, 603, 699, 972, 1523}. Bilateral basal ganglionic and thalamic lesions have also been recorded {790}.

Clinical features
Symptoms and Signs
The presenting clinical manifestations of CNS germ cell tumours and their duration vary with histological type and location {129, 597, 603, 699, 972, 1300}. Only the more common signs and symptoms are addressed here. In general, germinomas are associated with a more protracted symptomatic interval than other types. Tumours of the pineal region often compress and obstruct the cerebral aqueduct, resulting in progressive hydrocephalus with intracranial hypertension. Lesions so situated are also prone to compress and invade the tectal plate, producing a characteristic paralysis of upwards gaze and convergence known as Parinaud syndrome. Suprasellar germ cell tumours typically impinge on the optic chiasm, causing visual field deflects, and often disrupt the hypothalamo-hypophyseal axis as evidenced by the occurrence of diabetes insipidus and manifestations of pituitary failure which include retarded growth and sexual maturation. CNS germ cell tumours may also cause "precocious puberty" by pineal or hypothalamic destruction (which releases the immature gonads from tonic inhibitory controls) or by the elaboration of human chorionic gonadotropin (HCG), a stimulant of testosterone production that is secreted by neoplastic syncytiotrophoblasts . While the latter mechanism would suffice to account for cases of precocious sexual development encountered in boys (the overwhelming majority of those documented to date), the additional expression by the tumour of cytochrome P450 aromatase, which catalyzes the conversion of C19 steroids to oestrogens, has been suggested as an explanation of the rare accounts of precocious puberty affecting girls with HCG-producing intracranial germ cell neoplasms {1092}.

Table 13.1
Age distribution of CNS germ cell tumours

Age (years)	% of Cases
0-10	~25
11-20	~65
21-30	~8
31+	~2

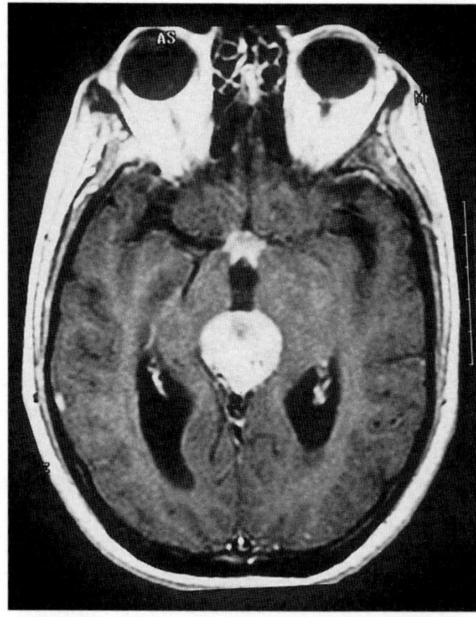

Fig. 13.1 MRI of a solid, contrast-enhancing germinoma of the pineal region, with a smaller CSF-borne metastasis in the suprachiasmatic cistern.

Neuroimaging
The neuroradiological profiles of CNS germ cell tumours are largely non-specific, and definitive histological subclassification requires tissue examination. Nevertheless, a few useful generalizations can be offered {2035, 1430}. On CT and magnetic resonance image (MRI), germ cell tumours other than teratomas usually appear as solid masses, that are iso- or hyperdense relative to grey matter and show prominent enhancement following the administration of contrast media (Fig. 13.1). The diagnosis of germinoma is especially suggested by demonstration on CT that a lesion with the foregoing characteristics contains an engulfed pineal gland, evidenced by a nodular cluster of small calcifications representing the native corpora arinacea of the gland. Pineal parenchymal tumours, by contrast, cause a dispersal ("explosion") of pineal calcifications as they expand and obliterate this structure. A diagnosis of teratoma should be considered for a lesion that can be shown to contain intratumoural cysts admixed with calcified regions and foci having the low signal-attenuation characteristics of fat. Intratumoral haemorrhage is particularly characteristic of choriocarcinoma and of mixed neoplasms with choriocarcinomatous elements. Finally, CT and MRI studies are of considerable value in demonstrating hydrocephalus, invasion of regional structures and CSF-borne metastases, the latter visualized as linear or nodular foci of contrast enhancement along ventricular surfaces or in the craniospinal subarachnoid space.

Cerebrospinal Fluid
Assay of serum and CSF for select oncoproteins has become standard practice in the pre-operative evaluation of patients suspected of harbouring CNS germ cell tumours and in monitoring the response of proven cases to treatment {597, 603, 699, 972}. The most useful markers are alpha-foetoprotein (AFP; normally synthesized by yolk sac endoderm, foetal hepatocytes and embryonic intestinal epithelium), beta-HCG (a glycoprotein normally secreted by syncytiotrophoblast) and placental alkaline phosphatase (PLAP; a cell-surface glycoprotein also elaborated by syncytiotrophoblast and produced by primordial germ cells as well). Elevation of levels of any of these markers constitutes compelling presumptive evidence that a CNS mass is a germ cell tumour, the pattern of marker elevation being somewhat predictive of tumour histology. As discussed below, expression of AFP at the immunohistochemically detectable level is generally restricted to yolk sac tumours and to the enteric-type glandular elements of teratomas, with these entities (or a mixed germ cell tumour containing such components) being the principal diagnostic considerations when this marker is elevated. Increased serum and CSF beta-HCG are particularly characteristic of germ cell tumours composed wholly, or in part, of choriocarcinoma, but can be associated with lesions, including the germinoma, that harbour HCG-producing syncytiotrophoblastic giant cells in the absence of the other defining characteristic of choriocarcinoma, the cytotrophoblast. The germinoma and other germ cell tumours share PLAP expression, but isolated elevation of this marker is most suggestive of pure germinomatous histology. The correlation of pre-operative marker status and tumour histology in neurosurgical material is potentially confounded by the difficulty of achieving complete resections of pineal, suprasellar and diencephalic lesions. Sampling artefact must be presumed to account for the scenario in which tissue morphology and immunohistochemical assay are at odds with serum and CSF profiles.

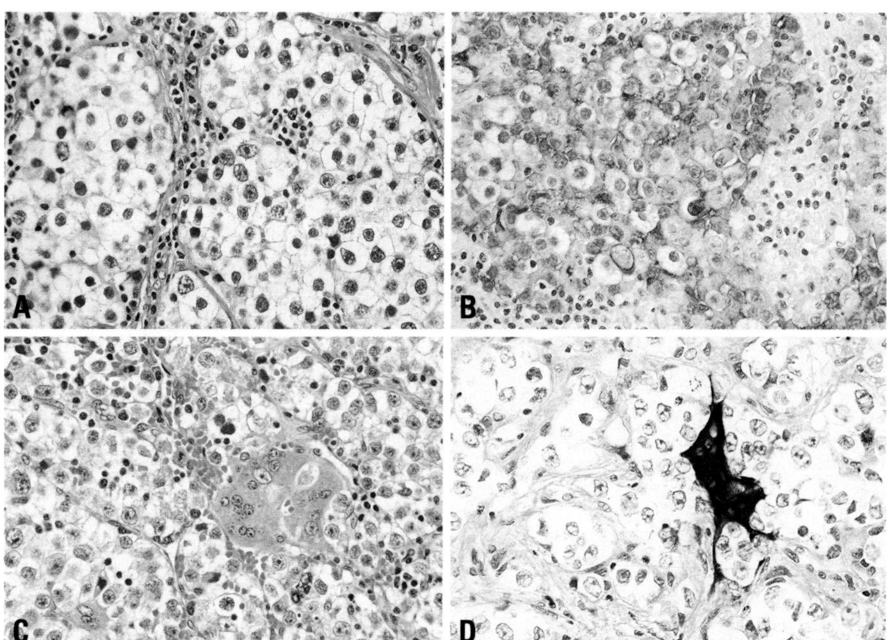

Fig. 13.2 Histological features of germinoma. **A** Tumour cells with abundant clear cytoplasm, round nuclei and prominent nucleoli. Note the lymphocytic infiltrates along fibrovascular septae. **B** Staining of the cytoplasm and cytoplasmic membrane with placental alkaline phosphatase (PLAP). **C** Syncytiotrophoblastic giant cell in an otherwise typical germinoma. **D** Immunostaining for human choriogonadotropic hormone (B-HCG).

Macroscopy
Germinoma is generally solid, although it may show small foci of cystic change and is composed of soft and friable, tan-white tissue. Conspicuous necrosis and haemorrhage are usually absent, but where present, these features suggest the presence of more virulent germinal components. Choriocarcinoma is especially prone to extensive haemorrhagic necrosis, while the accumulation of myxoid material lends a strikingly gelatinous appearance and consistency to some yolk sac tumours. Teratomatous elements manifest as mucous-laden cysts, fat, chondroid nodules, or bony spicules. Rarely, CNS teratomas contain teeth or well-formed hairs.

Histopathology
The accurate histological identification and subclassification of CNS germ cell tumours are critical to current treatment planning and prognostication. While the various entities collected under the generic designation of CNS germ cell tumour are here described in their unalloyed forms, intracranial germinal neoplasms are often of mixed histologic composition. In fact, only the germinoma and teratoma are likely to be encountered as pure tumour types {129, 597, 603, 699, 972, 1300, 1887}. The pathologist confronted by a

mixed CNS germ cell tumour is obliged to specifically enumerate its individual elements and should communicate the relative representation of each component present. As immunohistochemical studies may be required to delineate these entities {129, 400, 597, 1300}, the immunoprofiles of CNS germ cell tumours are summarized in Table 13.2.

Table 13.2
Immunohistochemical profiles of CNS germ cell tumours

	Alpha fetoprotein	Human chorionic gonadotropin	Human placental lactogen	Placental alkaline phosphatase	Cytokeratins
Germinoma	–	–[2]	–[2]	+	–[3]
Teratoma	+[1]	–	–	–	+[4]
Yolk sac tumour	+	–	–	+/–	+
Embryonal carcinoma	–	–	–	+	+
Choriocarcinoma	–	+	+	+/–	+[5]

[1] Alpha-fetoprotein is usually restricted to enteric-type glandular components.
[2] Syncytiotrophoblastic giant cells that may be found in otherwise pure germinomas (or in any of the other CNS GCT types) will be immunoreactive for human chorionic gonadotropin and human placental lactogen.
[3] A minority of germinomas exhibit cytokeratin reactivity that is usually distributed in patchy fashion.
[4] Cytokeratin reactivity is a feature of epithelial components.
[5] Immunoreactivity is a regular feature of syncytiophoblastic giant cells, while cytotrophphoblast is often negative.

Germinoma (ICD-O 9064/3)

This tumour is composed of uniform cells resembling primitive germ cells, with large, vesicular nuclei, prominent nucleoli and a clear, glycogen-rich cytoplasm. Additional features are lymphoid or lymphoplasmacellular infiltrates and, less frequently, scattered syncytiotrophoblastic giant cells.

The pure germinoma, the most common CNS germ cell tumour {129, 597, 603, 699, 972, 1887}, is populated by large cells that appear undifferentiated and that resemble primordial germinal elements (of which, in theory, they represent the neoplastic counterparts). These are disposed in monomorphous sheets, lobules or, in examples characterised by a desmoplastic stromal response, regimented cords and trabecula. Round, vesicular and centrally positioned nuclei, prominent nucleoli, discrete cell membranes and relatively abundant cytoplasm that is often strikingly clear because of the accumulation of glycogen typify promptly fixed specimens. These cytological features are basically retained in lumbar puncture or ventricular CSF samples that must be screened for tumour cells. Mitoses are usually identified without difficulty and may be conspicuous, but necrosis is uncommon. Delicate fibrovascular septa variably infiltrated by small lymphocytes - principally T cells of both helper/inducer and cytotoxic/suppressor types - are a usual feature {1312}. Some germinomas show a lymphoid or lymphoplasmacellular reaction so florid as to confound the identification of their neoplastic elements in biopsy material. The identification of a biphasic population of mature lymphocytes and larger germinoma cells permits cytological diagnosis of these tumours in smear preparations {1074}. Germinomas may also masquerade as sarcoidosis or tuberculosis by virtue of an obscuring granulomatous response {804}. Still other germinomas are extensively overgrown by fibrous tissue.

Immunohistochemistry of germinomas shows labelling for PLAP in a surface membrane or, somewhat less commonly, diffuse cytoplasmic distribution {129, 400, 597, 1300}. PLAP labelling is not a constant feature, however, and may be particularly difficult to demonstrate in inflammatory-looking examples and in specimens that were previously frozen. A minority of germinomas shows patchy foci of cytoplasmic labelling for cytokeratins {400, 597} or binding with the lectin *Dolichos biflorus* agglutinin {1078}. Together with demonstrations of intercellular junctional complex and true lumen formation at the ultrastructural level {1012}, this has been taken as evidence of differentiation along somatic epithelial lines or towards embryonal carcinoma. Such differentiation, to which no clinical significance has yet been attached, would appear to be a more frequent event in the germinoma than in its testicular counterpart, the seminoma. Otherwise typical germinomas may contain syncytiotrophoblastic giant cells that manifest cytoplasmic immunolabeling for beta-HCG as well as for human placental lactogen (HPL) and cytokeratins. Germinomas with syncytiotrophoblastic elements certainly do not manifest the virulence of choriocarcinomas and should not be confused with them, but emerge from some studies as more prone to recurrence than pure germinomas following radiation therapy (see below).

Teratoma (ICD-O 9080/1)

Teratomas differentiate along ectodermal, endodermal and mesodermal lines (*e.g.*, they recapitulate somatic development from the three embryonic germ layers). Mature and immature variants require distinction.

Mature teratoma (ICD-O 9080/1)

Mature teratomas are composed exclusively of fully differentiated, 'adult-type' tissue elements that are sometimes arranged in a pattern resembling normal tissue relationships. Mitotic activity is low or absent.

The more common ectodermal components encountered in such tumours include skin, brain and choroid plexus. Mesodermal representatives include cartilage, bone, fat and muscle (both smooth and striated). Cysts lined by epithelia of respiratory or enteric type are the usual endodermal participants, with some examples also containing pancreatic or hepatic tissue. Not infrequently, gut-like structures are formed, replete with mucosa and muscular coats. Advanced organogenesis and somatic organization may result in the phenomenon of intracranial foetus-in-foetu {1060}, though incorpora-

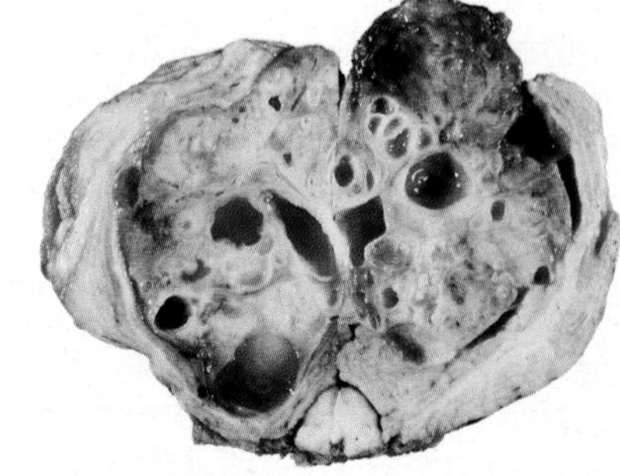

Fig. 13.3 Large teratoma of the cerebellum in a four-week-old infant, with characteristic cysts and chondroid nodules.

tion of a dizygotic twin via epithelial or neural tube defects that disrupt the amniotic septum has also been suggested to account for this pathological curiosity {1300}.

Immature teratoma (ICD-O 9080/3)

This teratoma variant is composed of incompletely differentiated components resembling foetal tissues.

Such incompletely differentiated areas mandate classification of the lesion as an immature teratoma even if they constitute only minor elements in an otherwise differentiated tumour. Particularly common are a hypercellular and mitotically active "stroma", reminiscent of embryonic mesenchyme and primitive neuroectodermal elements that may fashion neuroepithelial rosettes and canalicular arrays mimicking the developing neural tube. Clefts lined by melanotic neurepithelium are often encountered, these representing abortive retinal differentiation. Immature intracranial teratomas have been reported to undergo spontaneous differentiation into fully mature somatic-type tissues over time {1390}. However, re-resection specimens composed solely of mature teratoma are usually from patients whose immature teratomas or mixed germ cell tumours have been subjected to therapy {61, 2040}. The apparent tumour "maturation" in such cases presumably reflects the selective radio- or chemoablation of their more actively proliferating components.

Teratoma with malignant transformation (ICD-O 9084/3)

This is the generic designation for the occasional teratomatous neoplasm that contains as an additional malignant component a cancer of conventional somatic type.

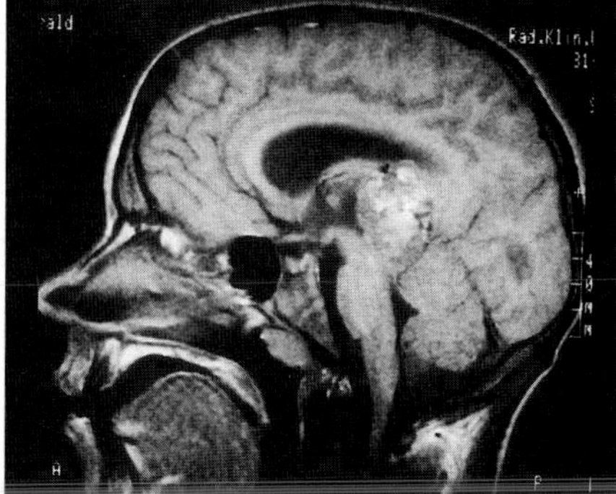

Fig. 13.4 Sagittal T1 weighted MRI of a teratoma in the pineal region, occupying the dorsal aspect of the third ventricle.

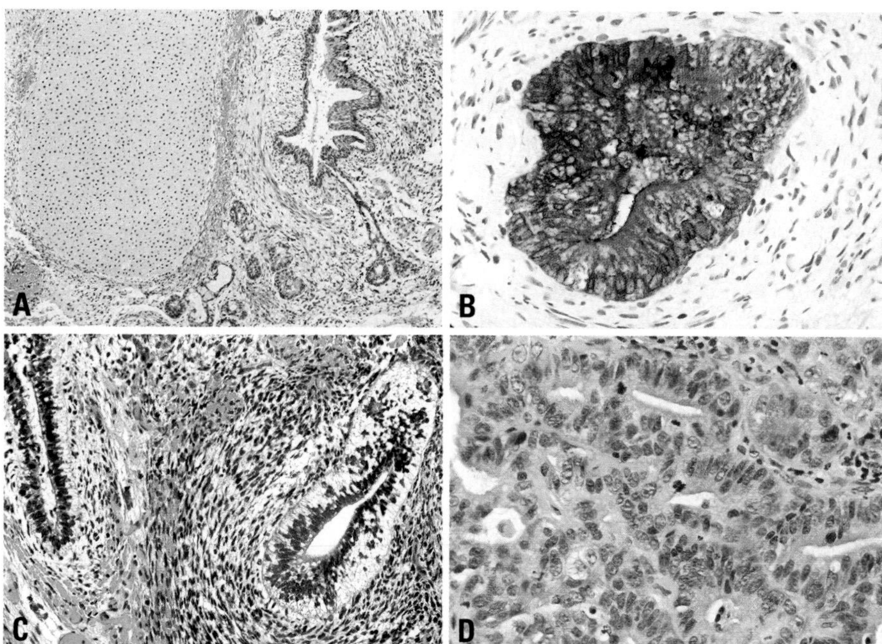

Fig. 13.5 A Mature teratoma with differentiated glands, smooth muscle bundles and a nodule of moderately hypercellular cartilage. **B** α–Fetoprotein (AFP) immunolabeling of enteric-like epithelium in a mature teratoma. **C** Immature teratoma with foetal-type glands and embyonic mesenchyme-like stroma. **D** Teratoma with malignant transformation into an enteric-type adenocarcinoma.

The latter is most often a rhabdomyosarcoma or undifferentiated sarcoma {129, 972, 1206, 1300}, less commonly a squamous cell carcinoma or enteric-type adenocarcinoma {429, 972}. Alternatively, yolk sac tumour elements have been put forward as the progenitors of select enteric-type adenocarcinomas arising from intracranial germ cell tumours {429}. A pineal germ cell tumour composed partly of immature teratoma has also been reported as the probable source of a systemic erythroleukemia {564}. The pathologist detecting evidence of "malignant transformation" within a germ cell tumour should state the specific histological form that this takes.

On immunohistochemical investigation, the constituent elements of the teratoma can be expected to express those antigens that are appropriate to their native somatic counterparts. Elaboration of AFP by teratomatous glandular epithelium may result in elevated levels of this important marker in the serum and CSF {129, 400, 597, 1300}.

Yolk Sac Tumour (ICD-O 9071/3)

This neoplasm is composed of primitive-appearing epithelial cells - putatively representing yolk sac endoderm - set in a loose, variably cellular and often conspicuously myxoid matrix resembling extra-embryonic mesoblast. Eosinophilic hyaline globules immunoreactive for AFP are a diagnostic feature.

The epithelial elements may proliferate in solid sheets but are more commonly disposed about an intervening meshwork of irregular tissue spaces ('reticular' pattern) or line anastomosing sinusoidal channels as a cuboidal epithelium draped, in some cases, over delicate fibrovascular projections to form distinctive papillae known as Schiller-Duval bodies. Yolk sac tumours may also contain eccentrically constricted cysts delimited by flattened epithelial elements ("polyvesicular vitelline" pattern), enteric-type glands lined partially by goblet cells, and foci of apparent hepatocellular differentiation ("hepatoid" variant). A diagnostically useful, though inconstant, feature of the yolk sac tumour is the presence of brightly eosinophilic, PAS-positive and diastase resistant hyaline globules that may appear to lie within the cytoplasm of epithelial cells or to be free in the adjoining stroma. Mitotic activity varies considerably and may be conspicuous, but necrosis in uncommon.

Cytoplasmic immunoreactivity for AFP of the epithelial component of the yolk sac tumour is characteristic {129, 400, 597, 1300} and may be of considerable value in distinguishing its solid variant from germinoma and embryonal carcinoma. The hyaline globules of the tumour are also AFP-immunoreactive.

Embryonal Carcinoma (ICD-O 9070/3)
The embryonal carcinoma is composed of large cells that proliferate in cohesive nests and sheets, form abortive papillae, or line irregular, gland-like spaces. Tumour cells may exceptionally replicate the structure of the early embryo, forming "embryoid bodies" replete with germ discs and miniature amniotic cavities. Arrestingly enlarged nucleoli, abundant clear to somewhat violet-hued cytoplasm, a high mitotic rate and zones of coagulative necrosis complete the histological picture.
The constituent cells uniformly show dense and diffuse cytoplasmic labelling for cytokeratins, attesting to their differentiation along epithelial lines and distinguishing these neoplasms from most germinomas (with which they share PLAP immunoreactivity) {400, 597}.

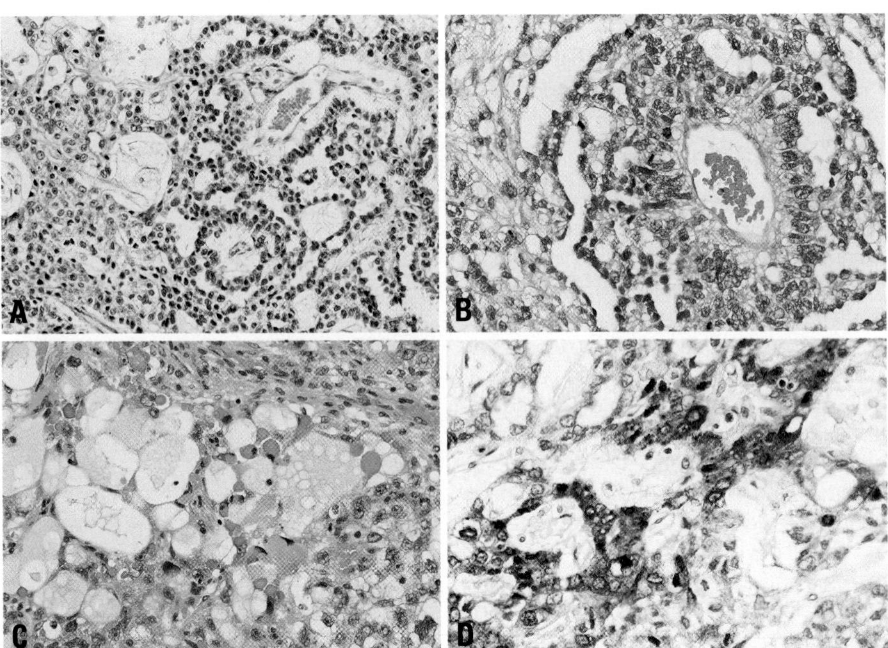

Fig. 13.6 Yolk sac tumour showing (**A**) typical sinusoidal growth pattern and numerous mitoses, (**B**) Schiller-Duval body, (**C**) reticular growth pattern with numerous hyaline globules, (**D**) alpha-foetoprotein immunolabelling.

Choriocarcinoma (ICD-O 9100/3)
The choriocarcinoma is characterized by extra-embryonic differentiation along trophoblastic lines. The diagnosis requires the identification of cytotrophoblastic elements, as well as syncytiotrophoblastic giant cells.
The latter may achieve enormous proportions and typically contain multiple, densely hyperchromatic nuclei, often clustered in a knot-like fashion, lying within a large expanse of basophilic or violaceous cytoplasm. The neoplastic syncytiotrophoblast surrounds or partially drapes cohesive masses of large mononucleated cells with vesicular nuclear features and clear or acidophilic cytoplasm, which represent the cytotrophoblastic component. Ectatic stromal vascular channels, blood lakes and extensive haemorrhagic necrosis are the rule. Cytoplasmic immunolabeling of syncytiotrophoblastic giant cells for beta-HCG and HPL are characteristic {129, 400, 597, 1300}.

Proliferation
Quantitative methods of assessing cell proliferation have not been systematically applied to these neoplasms and currently play no role in the assessment of prognosis or in tumour management. Similar considerations apply to automated ploidy analysis. In one study, mature and immature pineal teratomas were described as diploid or near diploid, while yolk sac tumours of the pineal region showed aneuploidy {1418}. Ploidy, as revealed in karyotypic analyses of CNS germ cell tumours, is addressed under Cytogenetics below.

Aetiology
Certain observations suggest that gonadotrophins play a role in the development or progression of CNS germ cell tumours {699}. These include the predilection of CNS germ cell tumours for peripubertal subjects, their tendency to arise in the vicinity of those diencephalic nuclei that regulate gonadotrophic activity, and their association with Klinefelter syndrome, a condition characterised by chronically elevated serum levels of gonadotrophins {2037, 699}.

Genetic susceptibility
CNS germ cell tumours typically afflict otherwise healthy individuals. An increased risk of intracranial germ cell neoplasia is associated with Klinefelter syndrome, which is characterised by a 47 XXY genotype and an array of anomalies that includes testicular atrophy, gynecomastia, eunuchoid habitus and elevated serum gonadotrophins {2037, 699}. Such patients are also predisposed to mediastinal germ cell tumours as well as mammary carcinoma. As discussed below, germ cell tumours commonly exhibit extranumerary X chromosomes. The susceptibility of Klinefelter syndrome patients to such tumours could reflect increased dosage of a chromosome X-associated gene. Noteworthy are descriptions of intracranial germ cell tumours affecting individuals with Down syndrome {2036, 548, 2031}, which has been associated with an increased risk of testicular germ cell tumorigenesis {2043}. Isolated accounts also document CNS germ cell tumours arising in the setting of neurofibromatosis type 1 {1638}, including siblings {1573}. Rarely, patients with germ cell tumours of the CNS have been reported to develop second gonadal germ cell tumours, suggesting that some individuals are at increased risk of germ cell neoplasia {1588, 548}. One such patient suffered from Down syndrome {548}.

Cytogenetics
Only eighteen CNS germ cell tumour karyotypes have been published to date. Three congenital intracranial examples studied - all immature teratomas of pure type - were diploid, two reportedly having normal karyotypes {1288} and the third a partial duplication of chromosome 1q {562}. As a lack of tumour cell-derived metaphases can result in a spuriously normal cytogenetic profile (requiring verification by ploidy analysis or *in situ* hybridization), these findings must be cautiously interpreted. It is noteworthy, however, that diploidy similarly characterises pure tera-

tomas (as well as yolk sac tumours) of the infantile testis and segregates these from other testicular germ cell tumour types [see {2031}]. Four intracranial teratomas arising later in childhood or adolescence were found to be near-diploid {206, 2038, 1667}, three exhibiting net gains of chromosome X, a relatively common finding in gonadal and other extragonadal germinal neoplasms. The remaining eleven cases studied - including examples of pure germinoma and tumours of mixed histology that, again, came mainly from older children - were predominantly aneuploid, with complex karyotypic alterations {15, 2033, 2034, 312, 564, 731, 2038, 2039, 2042, 1401}. Similar to cytogenetic abnormalities in morphologically homologous neoplasms of the testis and other extracranial sites are extranumerary X chromosomes, alterations of chromosome 1 (often resulting in additional copies of the 1q21–1qter region) and a high incidence of numerical and structural anomalies involving chromosome 12. The last included three neoplasms exhibiting chromosome 12p duplication ("isochromosome 12p"), a specific marker abnormality found in approximately 80% of testicular and mediastinal germ cell tumours {2034, 312, 2039}. Fluorescence *in situ* hybridisation has confirmed this finding {2034, 312, 2039, 2044}. More subtle, yet critical, alteration involving this chromosomal arm might well lie below the limited resolution of karyotypic analysis. The demonstration of isochromosome 12p in only a minority of these intracranial germ cell tumour types does, therefore, not exclude a common genetic or cellular origin for these neoplasms and their extracranial counterparts.

The comparative cytogenetic data summarized above suggest the existence of at least two fundamentally distinct classes of neoplasm - site of origin notwithstanding - within the germ cell tumour family {2031}. One would include the pure teratomas and yolk sac tumours of congenital/infantile onset, characterized by diploidy and normal chromosome 12 profiles. The second, characterized by aneuploidy, consistent over-representation of chromosome 12p and peri- or post-pubertal onset, would comprise those neoplasms harbouring primordial germ cell-like elements (*e.g.*, the germinoma/seminoma) or exhibiting mixed histology. The divergence of these tumour types could reflect their distinct cellular origins as well as initiating genetic events.

Molecular genetics

Molecular genomic analysis of intracranial germ cell neoplasms has been limited to investigation of the TP53 tumour suppressor gene. In one study, mutations of this gene were reportedly detected in one of seven germinomas and three of five yolk sac tumours assessed by single strand conformation polymorphism analysis (SSPA) and direct nucleotide sequencing {401}. These were principally of somatic, missense type and occurred mainly at, or in the vicinity of, hot spot codons 156, 176 and 273. Surprisingly, single tumours were described as harbouring as many as four distinct TP53 gene mutations and rare mutations involving codons 176 and 177 were found in two separate neoplasms. A second study, employing a yeast functional assay, however, failed to demonstrate TP53 gene mutations on assessment of seven germinomas, five teratomas (mature and immature) and two embryonal carcinomas {1995}. Further investigation, then, is required to determine whether TP53 mutations, uncommonly detected in testicular and other extracranial germ cell tumours {2031}], play a pathogenetic role, in germinal neoplasms of the CNS.

Histogenesis

Germ cell tumours of the central neuraxis have long been assumed to represent the neoplastic offspring of primordial germ cells that either migrate in aberrant fashion, or purposefully 'home', to the embryonic CNS rather than the developing genital ridges. Adduced in support of a germinal origin for these neoplasms is the fact that at least a subset, as described above, exhibit non-random genetic alterations comparable to those of their morphologic homologues in the gonads. However, studies of the human CNS, including the immunohistochemical screen of foetal pineal glands with antibodies to the primordial germ cell marker PLAP, have never shown it to harbour primitive germ cell elements {400}. Noteworthy in this regard is speculation that germ cells might differentiate into deceptively "somatic" forms on entering the CNS. Specifically, an enigmatic population of skeletal muscle-like cells native to the developing pineal gland has been proposed as possibly descending from primitive germinal elements attracted to this organ during neuroembryogenesis {1282}. Supporting this notion is the fact that striated muscle-type cells of unknown function also populate the thymus, another organ ostensibly devoid of germ cells yet a favoured site of extragonadal germ cell tumorigenesis {1282}.

An alternative to the unifying primordial germ cell hypothesis postulates an origin for CNS germ cell tumours in a variety of displaced embryonic tissues that presumably come to be misenfolded in the developing neural tube {2041}. In this scenario, only the germinoma would derive from misrouted primordial germ cells and so qualify as a true germ cell neoplasm, while intracranial choriocarcinomas would arise from misplaced trophoblast, yolk sac tumours from malpositioned elements of the secondary yolk sac proper, embryonal carcinomas from primitive constituents of the triploblastic embryo and teratomas from differentiating tissues of the later embryonic period. Like the primordial germ cell hypothesis, this theory is based on the existence of ectopic progenitors that have not been visualized in the developing human CNS. Furthermore, this scheme must postulate the co-ordinated neoplastic transformation of diverse cell types to account for mixed intracranial germ cell tumours and this is difficult to reconcile with the finding of similar genetic abnormalities in neoplasms of different histologic composition.

Another speculative proposal would impli-

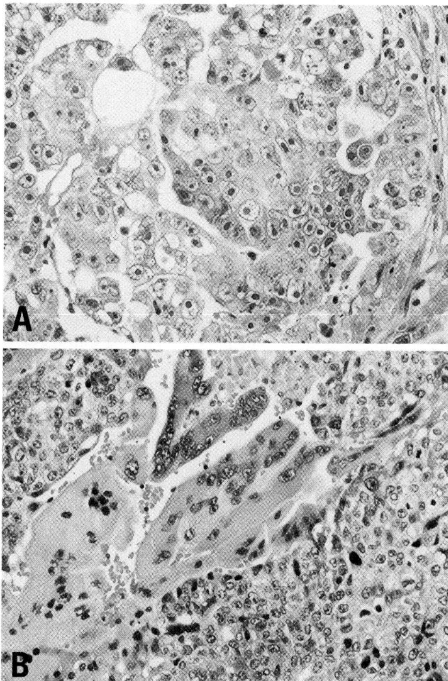

Fig. 13.7 A Embryonal carcimoma composed of large epithelial cells forming abortive papillae and glandular structures with macronuclei. **B** Choriocarcinoma with syncytiotrophoblastic giant cells and cytotrophoblasts.

cate toti- or pluri-potent stem cells in the histogenesis of CNS (and extracranial) germ cell tumours {2031}. As such cells are native to all three primitive embryonic layers, defective migration is not requisite to this hypothesis. Implicit, however, in this formulation is the selective genetic programming of uncommitted precursors along the germ cell differentiation pathway, as well as their neoplastic transformation. A modified version of this hypothesis suggests an embryonal stem cell origin for the pure, diploid teratomas and yolk sac tumours of congenital/infantile onset, reserving a primordial germ cell lineage for the peri- and post-pubertal neoplasms characterised by aneuploidy, over-representation of chromosome 12p and the presence of primitive germ cell-like or mixed histologic components {2031}. The differences in these tumour types could, however, reflect the mechanisms of their initiation rather than divergent cellular origins. Also invoked in the histogenesis of CNS teratomas are parthenogenetic mechanisms and the inclusion of blighted twins {1300}. Especially controversial is the nature of teratomatous tumours of the spinal cord. While some have viewed these as complex malformations, others contend that they are bona fide neoplasms of germ cell origin {2032}.

Treatment, prognosis and predictive factors

The single most predictive feature to have emerged from multivariant analyses of CNS germ cell tumour outcome is histological subtype {61, 699, 972, 2045, 1887}. The pure germinoma has an especially favourable prognosis owing to its remarkable radiosensitivity, a feature foreign to other germ cell tumours. Most patients with localized germinomas can be cured by radiation therapy alone, with 5-year survival rates ranging from 65-95%. The addition of chemotherapy to germinoma treatment regimens may effect comparable disease control at reduced radiation doses {2045}. Patients harbouring germ cell tumours of other histologic types do not fare as well - with the exception of those who can tolerate gross total resection of fully mature teratomas, which tend to be non-invasive and lend themselves to complete excision, though adjuvant chemotherapy has been shown to improve outcome {61, 2045, 1887}. Refinements in surgical technique have also permitted more radical extirpations of pineal region and other CNS germ cell tumours, which have been associated with increased disease-free survival for patients with non-germinomatous lesions {1887}. The presence of syncytiotrophoblastic giant cells in otherwise pure germinomas may be of biologic significance. While no dramatic differences in long-term outcome have been convincingly documented, some observers have noted an increased local recurrence rate and modest decrease in survival in the former group {972,1526}. In some studies, extent of disease at diagnosis has been shown to influence outcome {699}. In these analyses, infiltration of the hypothalamus, spread within the third ventricle and metastases to the spinal leptomeninges/subarachnoid space have all been found to augur poorly for patients with germ cell tumours. In exceptional instances, failure of treatment is due to blood-borne spread (principally pulmonary and osseous) or abdominal contamination via ventriculoperitoneal shunts {699}.

CHAPTER 14

Familial Tumour Syndromes Involving the Nervous System

Recent progess in the elucidation of the molecular basis of inherited cancer syndromes has greatly contributed to the understanding of carcinogenesis in general. The major syndromes with manifestations in the nervous system are listed below. All responsible genes have now been identified and sequenced.

Syndrome	Gene	Chromosome	Nervous system	Skin	Other tissues
Neurofibromatosis 1	*NF1*	17q11	Neurofibromas, MPNST, optic nerve gliomas, astrocytomas	Café-au-lait spots, axillary freckling	Iris hamartomas, osseous lesions, phaeochromocytoma, leukaemia
Neurofibromatosis 2	*NF2*	22q12	Bilateral vestibular schwannomas, peripheral schwannomas, meningiomas, meningioangiomatosis, spinal ependymomas, astrocytomas, glial hamartias, cerebral calcifications	–	Posterior lens opacities, retinal hamartoma
von Hippel-Lindau	*VHL*	3p25	Haemangioblastomas	–	Retinal haemangioblastomas, renal cell carcinoma, phaeochromocytoma, visceral cysts
Tuberous sclerosis	*TSC1* *TSC2*	9q34 16p13	Subependymal giant cell astrocytoma, cortical tubers	Cutaneous angiofibroma ('adenoma sebaceum'), *peau chagrin*, subungual fibromas	Cardiac rhabdomyomas, adenomatous polyps of the duodenum and the small intestine, cysts of the lung and kidney, lymphangioleiomyomatosis, renal angiomyolipoma
Li-Fraumeni	*TP53*	17p13	Astrocytomas, PNET	–	Breast carcinoma, bone and soft tissue sarcomas, adrenocortical carcinoma, leukaemia
Cowden	*PTEN (MMAC1)*	10q23	Dysplastic gangliocytoma of the cerebellum (Lhermitte-Duclos), megalencephaly	Multiple trichilemmomas, fibromas	Hamartomatous polyps of the colon, thyroid neoplasms, breast carcinoma
Turcot	*APC*	5q21	Medulloblastoma	-	Colorectal polyps
	hMLH1 *hPSM2*	3p21 7p22	Glioblastoma	Café-au-lait spots	Colorectal polyps
Naevoid basal cell carcinoma syndrome (Gorlin)	*PTCH*	9q31	Medulloblastoma	Multiple basal cell carcinomas, palmar and plantar pits	Jaw cysts, ovarian fibromas, skeletal abnormalities

Neurofibromatosis type 1

A. von Deimling
R. Foster
W. Krone

Definition

Neurofibromatosis type 1 (NF1) is an autosomal dominant disorder characterized by multiple neurofibromas, malignant peripheral nerve sheath tumours, optic nerve gliomas and other astrocytomas, multiple café-au-lait spots, axillary and inguinal freckling, iris hamartomas (Lisch nodules) and various osseous lesions.

MIM No. 162200 {978}.

Synonyms

Von Recklinghausen disease, von Recklinghausen neurofibromatosis, peripheral neurofibromatosis.

Incidence

Although the prevalence in most populations is estimated to be 1:4000, higher frequencies have been reported for Arab-Israeli subpopulations {456}. About 50% of patients have new germline mutations. With the exception of large deletions, these spontaneous mutations occur predominantly in the paternal germline.

Diagnostic criteria

The diagnostic criteria for NF1 are given in Table 14.1.

Table 14.1
Diagnostic criteria for NF1.

The presence of two or more of the following signs identify the NF1 patient:
1. Six or more café au lait patches, in diameter greater than 5 mm in prepubertal, and over 15 mm in postpubertal individuals
2. Two or more neurofibromas of any type or one plexiform neurofibroma
3. Axillary and/or inguinal freckling
4. Optic nerve glioma
5. A distinctive osseous lesion, such as dysplasia of the sphenoid wing, thinning of long bone cortex, with or without pseudoarthrosis
6. A first-degree relative (parent, sibling, or offspring) with NF1 according to the above criteria

From Stumpf *et al.* {1466}

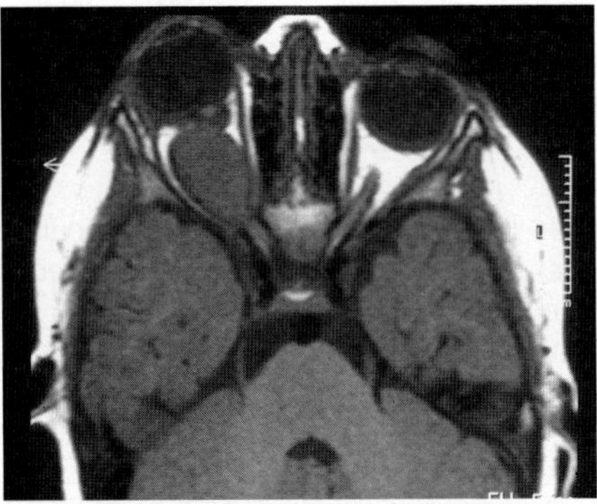

Fig. 14.1 Pilocytic astroytoma of the optic nerve (optic nerve glioma) in a NF1 patient.

Nervous system neoplasms

Neurofibromas

The neurofibromas that occur in NF1 patients show some features not commonly observed in their sporadic counterparts (see Chapter 10). Among the major subtypes of neurofibroma, the dermal and plexiform variants are characteristic of NF1.
Dermal neurofibroma is a well-circumscribed, non-encapsulated benign tumour variably composed of Schwann cells and fibroblast-like cells, with an admixture of endothelial cells, lymphocytes, and an unusually large number of mast cells. Deep-seated nodular neurofibromas arise less commonly {640}, have a more solid consistency, and may cause neurological symptoms.
Plexiform neurofibromas produce diffuse enlargement of major nerve trunks and their branches, sometimes yielding a rope-like mass and are almost pathognomonic of NF1. Plexiform neurofibromas may develop during the first one or two years of life as a single subcutaneous swelling with ill-defined margins. They may also cause severe disfigurement later in life, affecting large areas of the body. If these tumours arise in the head or neck region, they can impair vital functions. Plexiform neurofibromas have about a 5% risk of malignant progression. In contrast, malignant transformation is a very rare event for other neurofibromas.

Malignant peripheral nerve sheath tumours

The malignant peripheral nerve sheath tumours that arise in NF1 patients usually occur at a younger age and may include rhabdomyoblastic and other heterologous elements. Such lesions, referred to as malignant Triton tumours {1641}, are highly characteristic of NF1. In addition, the glandular variant of malignant peripheral nerve sheath tumour is also a lesion indicative of NF1.

Gliomas

The majority of gliomas in NF1 patients are pilocytic astrocytomas that are located

Table 14.2
Major manifestations of NF1.

Tumours	
Neurofibromas	Dermal Nodular Plexiform
Gliomas	Optic glioma Astrocytoma Glioblastoma multiforme
Sarcomas	Neurofibrosarcoma (MPNST) Rhabdomyosarcoma Triton tumour
Neuroendocrine tumours	Phaeochromocytoma Carcinoid tumour
Haematopoetic tumours	Juvenile chronic myeloid leukaemia
Other features	
Osseous lesions	Scoliosis Height reduction Macrocephaly Pseudoarthrosis Sphenoid wing dysplasia
Nervous system	Intellectual handicap Epilepsy Neuropathy Hydrocephalus (aqueduct stenosis)
Vascular lesions	Fibromuscular hyperplasia (renal artery)

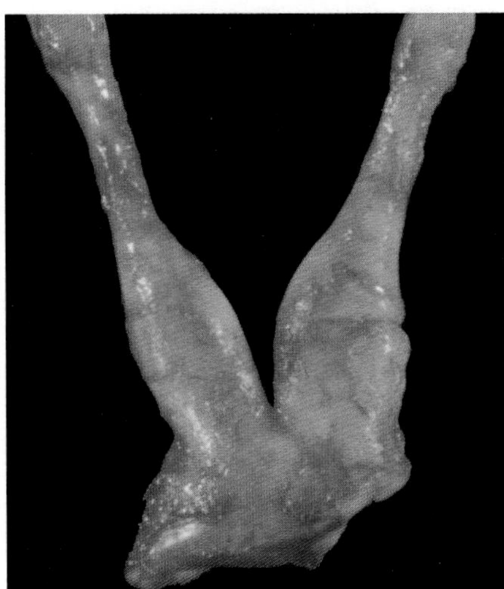

Fig. 14.2 Macroscopic preparation of a bilateral optic nerve glioma in a patient with NF1.

within the optic nerve {887}. Bilateral growth, when present, is characteristic of NF1. Optic nerve gliomas in NF1 patients may remain static for many years and some may regress. Other gliomas observed at an increased frequency in NF1 patients include diffuse astrocytomas and glioblastomas {600}.

Other CNS manifestations

The following features (Table 14.2) are more frequent in NF1 patients: macrocephaly {641}, intellectual handicap {147}, epilepsy {1257}, hydrocephalus, aqueductal stenosis, and neuropathy {150}.

Extraneural manifestations

Abnormalities of pigmentation

Café au lait spots, freckling and Lisch nodules all involve alterations of melanocytes. Café au lait spots are often the first manifestation of NF1 in the newborn child. Their number and size increase during infancy, but may remain stable or even decrease in adults (Table 14.1). Histopathologically, the ratio of melanocytes to keratinocytes is higher in the unaffected skin of NF1 patients, and this is more marked in the café au lait spots {430}. Axillary and/or inguinal freckling occurs in about two-thirds of NF1 patients, but may have a higher prevalence in young adults {640}. The histopathological features of these freckles are indistinguishable from those of café au lait spots. Lisch nodules are small, elevated pigmented hamartomas on the surface of the iris. The presence of Lisch nodules is a particularly useful diagnostic criterion, as they occur in nearly all adults with NF1.

Osseous and vascular lesions

In NF1, the orbits are often affected by sphenoid wing dysplasia. In addition, spinal deformities often result in severe scoliosis that may require surgical intervention. Thinning, bending and pseudoarthrosis may affect the long bones (predominantly tibial), and short stature may also be a component of NF1 {1258}. Fibromuscular dysplasia of the renal and other arteries, including the large cervical vessels, has also been reported as being associated with NF1.

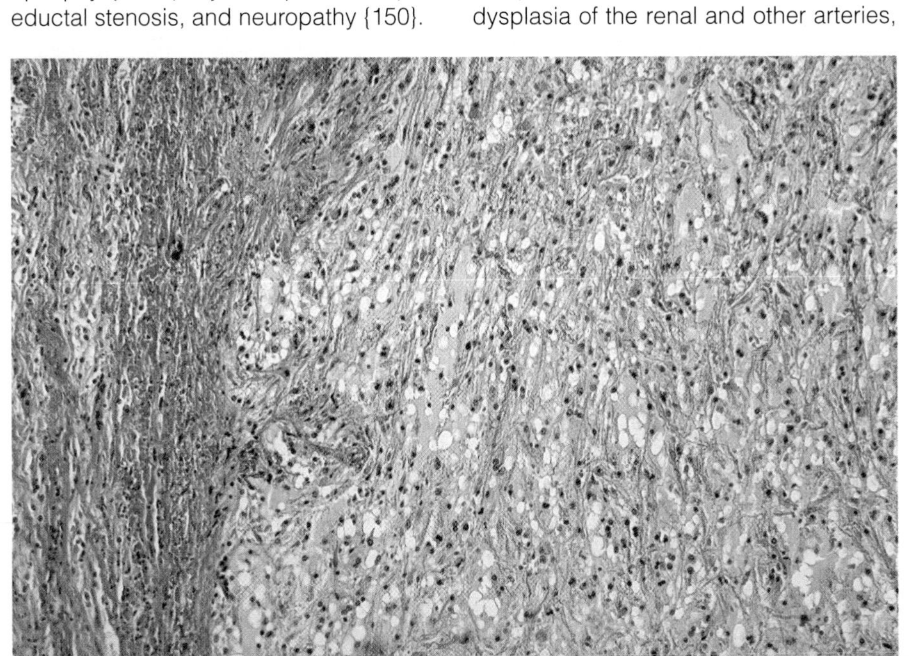

Fig. 14.3 Bilateral optic nerve glioma in a patient with NF1. The histology shows enlargement of the compartments of the optic nerves and collar-like extension into the subarachnoid space.

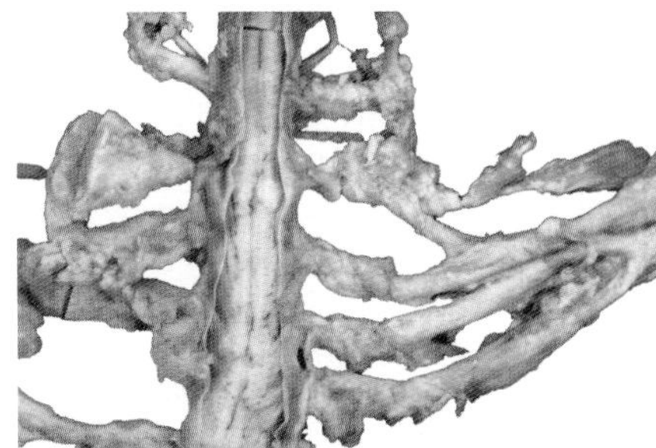

Fig. 14.4 Multiple neurofibromas of the spinal roots and the brachial cephalic plexus in a patient with NF1.

Tumours

NF1 patients have an increased risk of developing phaeochromocytoma {509}, duodenal carcinoid tumour {311}, rhabdomyosarcoma {641}, and childhood chronic myeloid leukemia {1034}, which are often associated with cutaneous xanthogranulomas.

Genetics

The NF1 locus is on chromosome 17q12 {1384}.

Gene structure

The NF1 gene is large, containing 60 exons and spanning at least 335 kb. One of the two extensive introns, 27b, includes coding sequences for three embedded genes that are transcribed in a reverse direction: EVI2A, EVI2B and OMGP (for review, see refs. {95,1400}). There are 12 non-processed NF1 pseudogenes localized on 8 chromosomes. None of these pseudogenes extends beyond exon 29.

Table 14.3
NF1 gene mutation types.

Mutation type	Number
Chromosome rearrangements	9
Deletion of the entire gene	38
Single- and multi-exon deletion	42
Small deletion	63
Large insertion	3
Small insertion	29
Direct stop mutation (nonsense)	51
Amino acid substitution (missense)	31
Mutations in introns	26
3'UTR mutations	4
Non-polymorphic silent base exchanges	4
Total	300

By the International NF1 Genetic Analysis Consortium of the National Neurofibromatosis Foundation (NNFF). Derived from data collected by Korf {1086}.

Gene expression

The NF1 gene gives rise to several alternatively spliced transcripts of 11-13 kb, the longest of which has an open reading frame of 8601 bp. Some of the different transcript isoforms are tissue- and cell-type-specific, and are expressed differentially in neurons and glia {95,1400}.

The product of the gene, neurofibromin, is a cytoplasmic protein that can be found in two major isoforms of 2818 amino acids (type 1) and 2839 amino acids (type 2) of 240-290 kD. The protein harbours a GAP-related domain (GRD) and thus belongs to the group of mammalian RasGTPase-activating proteins. In addition to the homology between the GAP domains, it has large segments that show moderate homology to the two Saccharomyces cerevisiae inhibitors of Ras protein, IRA1 and IRA2. While several features of these domains, including alternative splicing and the presence of mutations, suggest that they may be functionally important, their exact role is as yet unknown. Although neurofibromin is expressed almost ubiquitously in most mammalian tissues, the highest levels have been found in the central and peripheral nervous system and in the adrenal gland.

Gene mutations

Mutations in the NF1 gene do not appear to cluster in hot spots; the most frequent mutation in unrelated patients (R1947X) has been found in only 14 individuals. Of the 300 mutations reported, only 21 (7%) have been observed more than once {1086}. The mutations compiled by an international consortium are summarised in Table 14.3. More than 80% of mutations would be predicted to encode truncated proteins or none at all, However truncated neurofibromins have not been detected in cells derived from NF1 patients. Rapid degradation of the abnormal protein and a decreased amount of mRNA transcribed from the mutant allele may contribute to this failure {607}.

No convincing genotype-phenotype correlations have so far been established. Such correlations are complicated, however, by the unusually high degree of variable expressivity (intrafamilial variability of expression) within NF1 families. Evidence favouring a role for modifying non-allelic

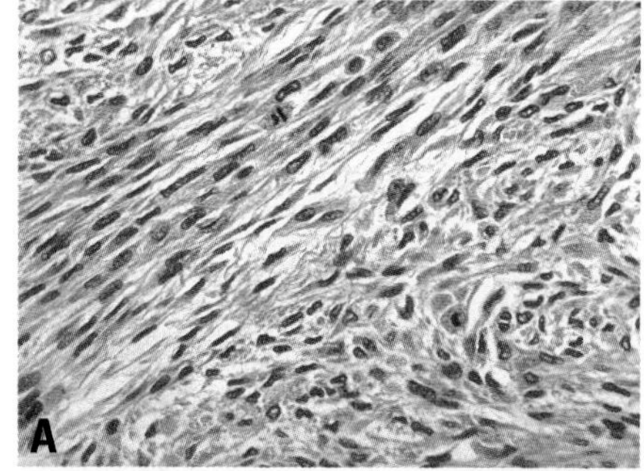

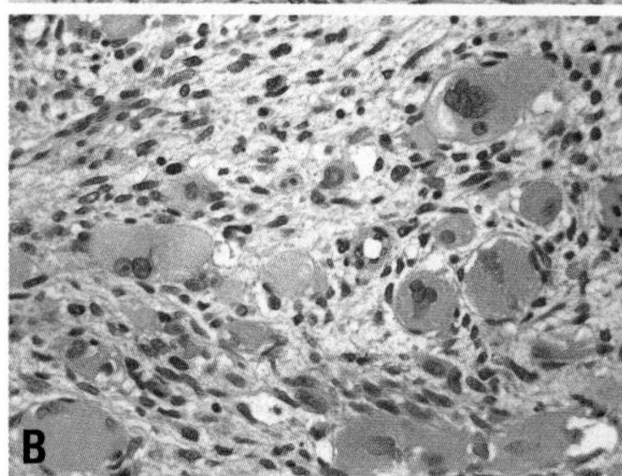

Fig. 14.5 Malignant Triton tumour. **A** Spindle-cell component with brisk mitotic activity. **B** Rhabdomyosarcomatous component.

genes has been provided by the correlation between clinical manifestations and the degree of relatedness of patients {360}. Several observations in sporadic and NF1-associated tumours indicate that neurofibromin acts as a tumour suppressor. Either loss of heterozygosity (LOH) or the presence of a mutation of the second allele has been demonstrated in neurofibrosarcomas {914, 872}, pheochromocytomas {2052}, in juvenile myelo-monocytic leukaemia {2060} and in neurofibromas {267, 1330}. Only the subpopulation of Schwann cells in a neurofibroma exhibited LOH at the NF1 gene {2064}, supporting the hypothesis that Schwann cells are the progenitor cells of neurofibromas.

NF1 variants

Variants of NF1 that do not co-segregate with the NF1 gene locus are known {800, 1648}. Even the autosomal dominant 'café-au-lait-spots only' variant exists as an NF1-gene-linked and as an unlinked entity {1, 2, 166}. Patients who meet diagnostic criteria for both NF1 and NF2 have occasionally been described, but it remains to be elucidated whether a 'mixed' form exists as a separate entity {1555}. The occurrence of a segmental form of NF1, caused by somatic mosaicism at the NF1 gene locus, further extends the range of variability {1555}. On the molecular level, somatic mosaicism was demonstrated in two sporadic patients heterozygous for two different large deletions in the majority of their cells {2056, 2059}. Germline mosaicism for a 12 kb deletion was found at the spermatozoa of the healthy father of two fully affected offspring {2055}.

Although some cell lines derived from malignant peripheral nerve sheath tumours respond to neurofibromin deficiency by dramatically increased levels of RasGTP, their tumorigenicity may depend at least as much on the inactivation of the *TP53* gene as on the loss of function of NF1 {993}. The generation of mice deficient in neurofibromin {2053, 2054} has aided the identification of potential cell-type specific functions of neurofibromin. Loss of the murine Nf1 gene product results in lethality at day 13.5 of embryogenesis due to abnormal cardiac development, a phenotype that has been linked to abnormal regulation of Ras activity {2062}. Mice heterozygous for the Nf1 knockout allele develop tumours associated with human NF1 {2054} and display learning and memory defects {2058}. Loss of heterozygosity at the Nf1 locus can be demonstrated in the observed tumours {2054}, indicating that the condition in heterozygous mice is similar to the human disease. Schwann cells derived from neurofibromin-deficient embryos are angiogenic, highly invasive, and hyperproliferative {2057}. Neurofibromin-deficient sensory neurons survive in the absence of neurotrophins via activation of a Ras-dependent pathway {2061}. Additionally, loss of neurofibromin in fetal liver cells renders the cells hypersensitive to the proliferative effects of multiple haematopoietic cytokines through constitutive activation of Ras signalling {2063}. Several instances in which biological responses to neurofibromin deficiency or overexpression are not accompanied by changes in the level of RasGTP suggest that neurofibromin may have additional functions that are independent of its RasGAP activity, and which may or may not depend on its interaction with the Ras proteins.

Neurofibromatosis type 2

D.N. Louis
A.O. Stemmer-Rachamimov
O.D. Wiestler

Definition

Neurofibromatosis type 2 (NF2) is an autosomal dominant disorder characterized by neoplastic and dysplastic lesions of Schwann cells (schwannomas and schwannosis), meningeal cells (meningiomas and meningioangiomatosis) and glial cells (gliomas and glial microhamartomas). Bilateral vestibular schwannomas are diagnostic. Additional lesions include posterior lens opacities and cerebral calcifications.

MIM No. 101000 {978}.

Synonyms

Central neurofibromatosis; bilateral acoustic neurofibromatosis. The term "von Recklinghausen neurofibromatosis" is associated with NF1 and should not be used for NF2.

Incidence

The incidence of the disease is 1 per 40,000 newborns. About half of all cases occurs in individuals with no previous family history of NF2, and are caused by newly acquired germline mutations.

Diagnostic criteria

The diagnostic criteria for neurofibromatosis 2 are given in Table 14.4.

Nervous system neoplasms

Meningiomas

Multiple meningiomas are the second hallmark of NF2 and occur in the majority of NF2 patients {919}. NF2 meningiomas occur earlier in life than sporadic meningiomas {385, 968, 1412}. These lesions are usually WHO grade I tumours; atypical or malignant meningiomas are not increased in NF2 patients. All major subtypes of meningioma occur in NF2 patients {919, 2065}.

Schwannoma

NF2-associated schwannomas are WHO grade I tumours that are comprised of neoplastic Schwann cells, but which differ from sporadic schwannomas in a number of ways. NF2 schwannomas present at an earlier age. Many NF2 patients develop the diagnostic hallmark of the disease, bilateral vestibular schwannomas, by their twenties {385, 968, 1412}. NF2 vestibular schwannomas may entrap seventh cranial nerve fibres {662} and have higher proliferative activity {35}, although these features do not necessarily connote more aggressive behaviour.
In addition to the vestibular division of the eighth cranial nerve, other sensory nerves may be affected, including the fifth cranial nerve and spinal dorsal roots. However, motor nerves such as the twelfth cranial nerve may also be involved {385, 919}. Cutaneous schwannomas occur, and may be plexiform {385, 968, 1412}. NF2 schwannomas may appear multilobular ("cluster of grapes") on both gross and microscopic examination {1616}, and multiple schwannomatous tumourlets may develop along individual nerves, particularly on spinal roots {919, 2074}.

Gliomas

Approximately 80% of gliomas in NF2 patients are spinal intramedullary or cauda equina tumours, with an additional 10% of gliomas occurring in the medulla {1268}. Ependymomas account for approximately 65-75% of all histologically diagnosed gliomas in NF2, and for almost all spinal gliomas {1268, 1306}. In most cases, NF2 spinal ependymomas are multiple intramedullary masses {1268, 1306}. Diffuse and pilocytic astrocytomas also occur in NF2, but are less common.

Neurofibromas

Cutaneous neurofibromas have been reported in NF2. On histological review, however, many 'neurofibromas' prove to be schwannomas, including plexiform schwannomas misdiagnosed as plexiform neurofibromas.

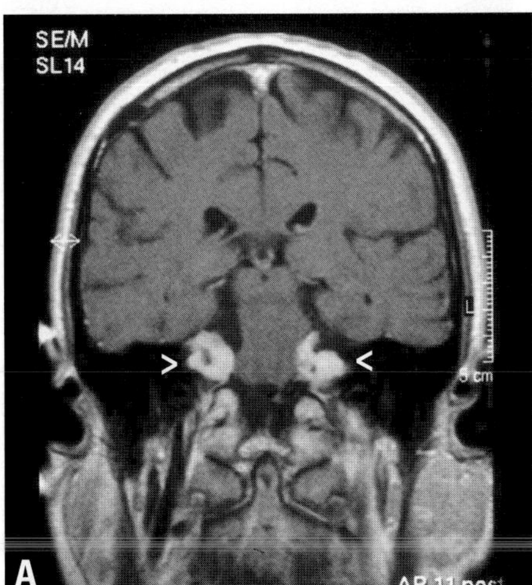

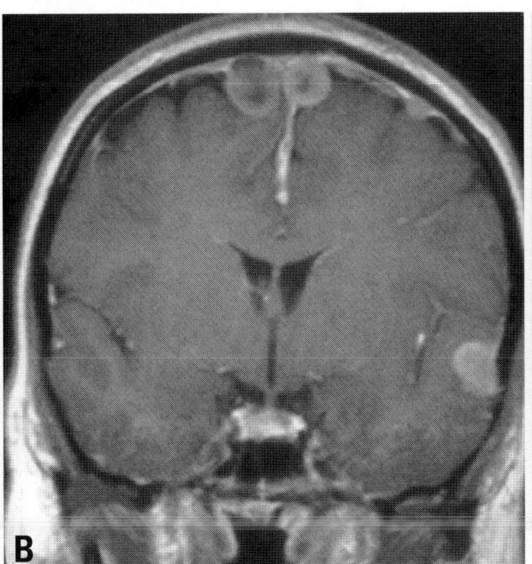

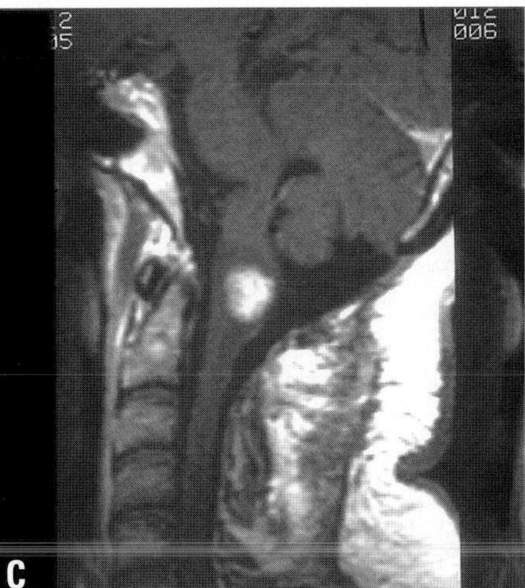

Fig. 14.6 T1-weighted, contrast-enhanced MR images from patients with NF2. **A** Bilateral acoustic schwannomas (arrows), the diagnostic hallmark of NF2. **B** Multiple meningiomas presenting as contrast-enhanced masses. **C** Ependymoma of the cervical spinal cord.

Table 14.4
Diagnostic criteria for NF2.

The following are diagnostic:
1. Bilateral vestibular schwannomas; or
2. A first-degree relative with NF2, and either
a. a unilateral vestibular schwannoma or
b. two of the following: meningioma, schwannoma, glioma, posterior subcapsular lens opacity, or cerebral calcification; *or*
3. Two of the following
a. unilateral vestibular schwannoma
b. multiple meningiomas
c. either schwannoma, glioma, neurofibroma, posterior subcapsular lens opacity, or cerebral calcification.

Other nervous system lesions

Schwannosis. This is a proliferation of Schwann cells, sometimes with entangled axons, but without frank tumour formation. In NF2 patients, schwannosis is often found in the spinal dorsal root entry zones, sometimes associated with a schwannoma of the dorsal root, or in the perivascular spaces of the central spinal cord, where the nodules appear more like small traumatic neuromas {1294, 1306}. Less robust, but otherwise identical, schwannosis has been reported in reactive conditions.

Meningioangiomatosis. This cortical lesion is characterized by a plaque-like proliferation of meningothelial and fibroblast-like cells surrounding small vessels, and occurs both sporadically and in NF2.

Meningioangiomatosis is usually a single, intracortical lesion, although multifocal examples, as well as non-cortical lesions, occur {1294, 1306}. It may be predominantly vascular, resembling a vascular malformation, or predominantly meningothelial, sometimes with an associated meningioma. Sporadic meningioangiomatosis is a single lesion that usually occurs in young adults or children who present with seizures or persistent headaches. In contrast, NF2-associated meningioangiomatosis may be multifocal and is often asymptomatic and diagnosed only at autopsy {1458}.

Glial hamartias. Glial hamartias (or microhamartomas) of the cerebral cortex are circumscribed clusters of cells with medium to large, atypical nuclei and scant, sometimes stellar, eosinophilic cytoplasm. The cells stain strongly for S-100 protein, but only focally for GFAP.

They are common in and pathognomonic of NF2 {1294, 1619}, but are not associated with mental retardation or astrocytomas. The hamartias are usually intracortical, with a predilection for the molecular and deeper cortical layers, but have also been observed in the basal ganglia, thalamus and cerebellum {1619}. Similar hamartomas occur in the dorsal horns of the spinal cord and are identical to so-called ependymal heterotopias {919}. Merlin expression is retained in glial hamartomas, raising the possibility that haploinsufficiency during development underlies these malformations {2073}.

Cerebral calcifications. Intracranial calcifications have been noted frequently in neuroimaging studies of patients with NF2. Preferred localizations are the cerebral and cerebellar cortices, periventricular areas and choroid plexus. The histopathological correlates remain unclear {1412}.

Peripheral neuropathy. Some NF2 patients develop a sensorimotor peripheral neuropathy {385, 1412}, which may be secondary to focal schwannomatous changes or onion-bulb-like Schwann cell or perineurial cell proliferation {1501}.

Table 14.5
Major manifestations of NF2.

Major manifestations
Schwann cells lesions:
Schwannomas (including bilateral vestibular)
Meningeal lesions:
Meningiomas
Meningioangiomatosis
Glial lesions:
Spinal ependymomas
Astrocytomas
Glial hamartias
Other lesions:
Posterior lens opacities
Cerebral calcifications

Extraneural manifestations

Posterior lens opacities are common and highly characteristic of NF2. Retinal hamartomas may also be found.

Genetics

The NF2 gene is located at chromosome 22q12 {1289, 1514}.

Gene structure

The *NF2* gene {1289, 1514} spans 110 kb, and comprises 17 exons. *NF2* mRNA transcripts encode at least two major protein forms generated by alternative splicing at the carboxyl terminus. Isoform 1, encoded by exons 1-15 and 17, has intramolecular interactions similar to the ERM proteins (see below); isoform 2, encoded by exons 1-16, exists only in an unfolded state {2072, 2071}.

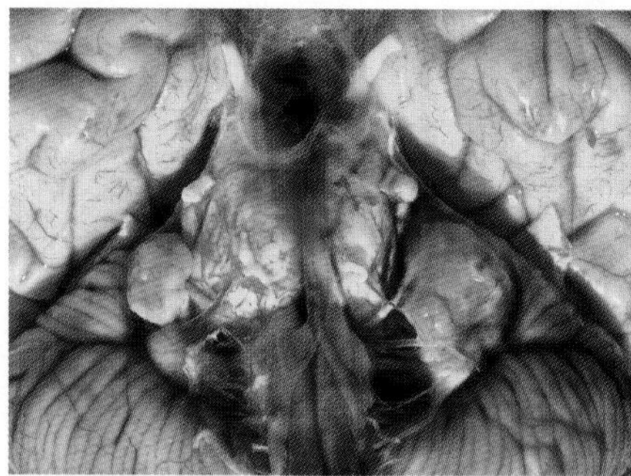

Fig. 14.7 Bilateral vestibular schwannomas, diagnostic for NF2.

Gene expression

The *NF2* gene is expressed in most normal human tissues studied, including brain {1289,1514}. The predicted protein product shows a strong similarity with the highly conserved protein 4.1 family of cytoskeleton-associated proteins, which includes protein 4.1, talin, moesin, ezrin, radixin, and protein tyrosine phosphatases. The similarity of the NF2-encoded protein to moesin, ezrin and radixin (ERM), resulted in the name merlin {1514}; the alternative name schwannomin has also been suggested {1289}. Members of the protein 4.1 family link the cell membrane to the actin

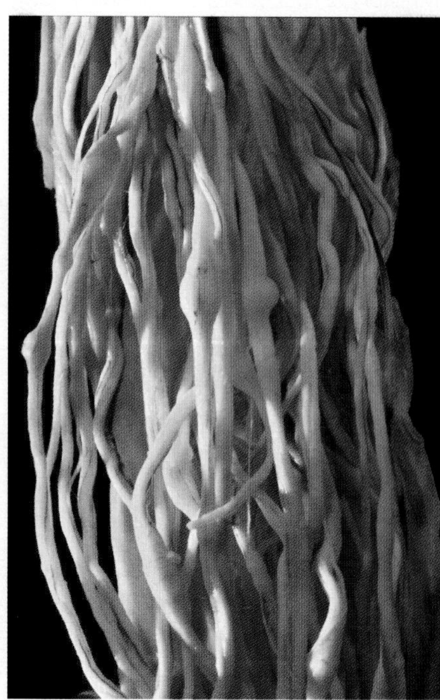

Fig. 14.8 Numerous schwannomas of the cauda equina in a patient with NF2.

cytoskeleton. These proteins consist of a globular amino terminal domain, an alpha-helical domain containing a praline rich region, and a charged carboxyl terminal domain. The amino terminus interacts with cell membrane proteins such as CD44, CD43, ICAM-1 and ICAM-2, while the carboxy terminal domain contains the actin binding site. The highest degree of structural similarity between merlin and the ERM proteins is in the amino terminal domain. Merlin lacks the actin binding site in the carboxy terminus but may have an alternative actin binding site {2072}. ERM proteins and merlin may be self regulated by head-to-tail intramolecular associations which result in folded and unfolded states. Some binding partners for merlin have been identified {2070}, including the regulatory cofactor of the Na^+-H^+exchange, hNHE-RF (EBP50). NHE-RF interacts with transmembrane proteins of ion channels and receptors and may therefore link merlin to intracellular signalling pathways. Other proteins that bind or interact with merlin include the other ERM proteins, spectrin, actin and CD44.

Gene mutations

Numerous germline and somatic *NF2* mutations have been detected, supporting the hypothesis that *NF2* functions as a tumour suppressor gene {514, 919}.

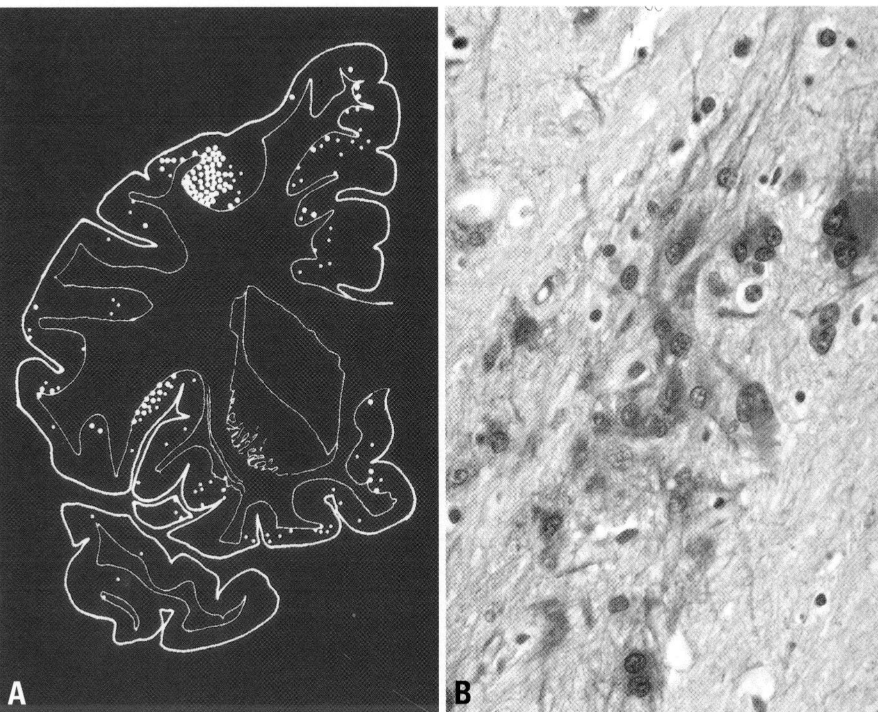

Fig. 14.10 Distribution of cerebral microhamartomas in a patient with NF2. These lesions are scattered throughout the cortex and basal ganglia and show strong immunoreactivity for S-100 (right). Reproduced from Wiestler *et al.* {1619}.

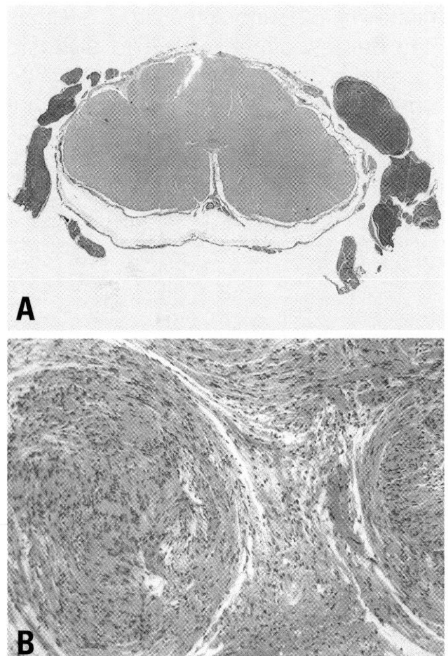

Fig. 14.9 A Multiple schwannomas of spinal roots. The histology (**B**) shows a nodular schwannoma in an NF2 patient.

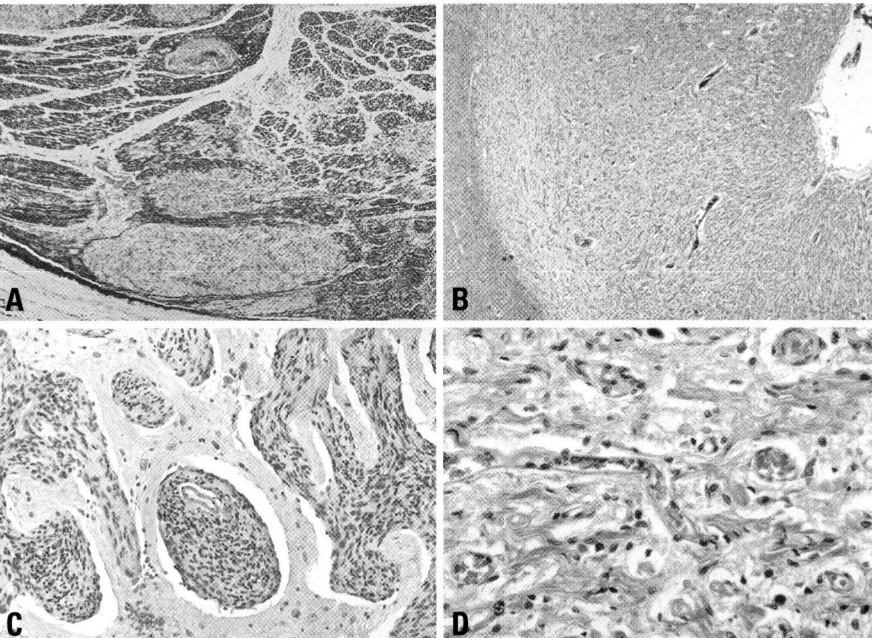

Fig. 14.11 Histological features of NF2. **A** Luxol fast blue staining of a section of the cauda equina with multiple early stages of schwannomas (tumourlets) and characteristic loss of myelin. **B** Diffuse cortical meningioangiomatosis (blue on trichrome staining). **C** Predominance of meningothelial cells in meningioangiomatosis. **D** High magnification of meningioangiomatosis (trichrome stain) with predominant vasculature.

Germline *NF2* mutations differ somewhat from somatic mutations identified in sporadic schwannomas (see Chapters 10) and meningiomas (see Chapters 11). The most frequent germline mutations are point mutations that alter splice junctions or create new stop codons {152, 514, 919, 931, 932, 996, 1289, 1310, 1514}. While germline mutations are found in all parts of the gene, with the exception of the alternatively spliced exons, they occur preferentially in exons 1 to 8 {996}. A possible hot spot for mutations appears to be position 169 in exon 2, in which a C to T transition at a CpG dinucleotide results in a stop at codon 57 {152, 996}; other CpG dinucleotides are also commonly targets for C to T transitions {1310}. *NF2* gene mutations also underlie some examples of schwannomatosis, a rare condition in which patients develop multiple peripheral schwannomas in the absence of vestibular schwannomas or other manifestations of NF2 {933}. The tumours may be limited to one side of the body or to one limb and are often painful. Molecular analysis of multiple tumours from affected patients have shown some *NF2* somatic mosaics and others with different somatic *NF2* mutations {2066}.

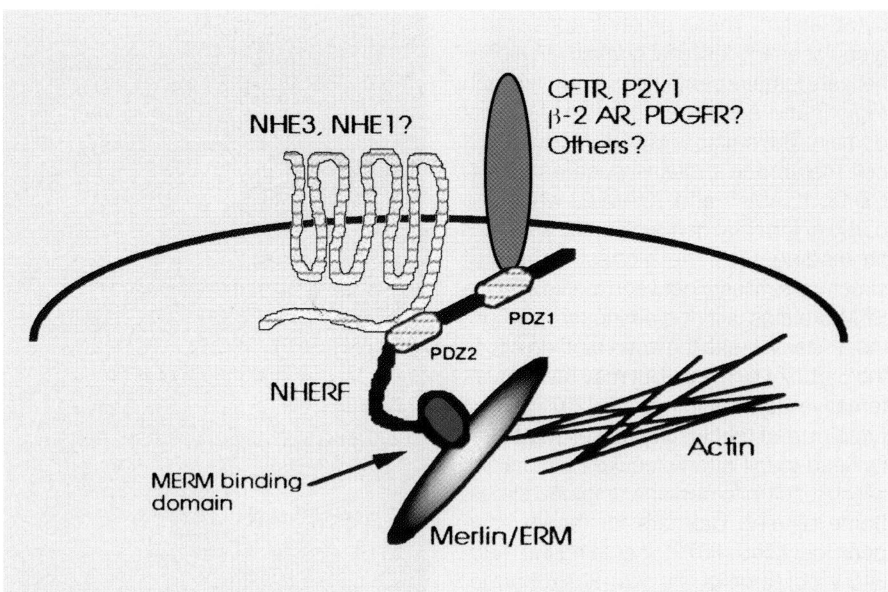

Fig. 14.12 A model connecting membrane receptors and ion channels to the actin cytoskeleton via merlin/ERM and NHERF.

Prognostic factors

The clinical course in patients with NF2 varies widely between families and, to a lesser extent, within families {385, 968, 1412}. Some families feature early onset with multiple diverse tumours (Wishart type), while others present later with only vestibular schwannomas (Gardner type). An effect of maternal inheritance on severity has been noted, as have families with genetic anticipation.

All families with NF2 show linkage of the disease to chromosome 22 {1059}, implying a single responsible gene, and correlations of genotype with phenotype have therefore attempted to predict clinical course on the basis of the type of the underlying *NF2* mutation. Nonsense and frameshift mutations are often associated with a more severe phenotype, regardless of their position in the gene, while missense mutations that preserve the carboxyl terminus of the protein result in milder phenotypes {996}. Phenotypic variability is observed in splice site mutations with more severe phenotypes observed in mutations upstream from exon 7 {2069}. Some mild phenotypes are associated with somatic mosaicism {2067, 2068}. On the other hand, two unrelated NF2 patients, one with the severe Wishart and the other with the mild Gardner phenotype, have been found to carry the same *NF2* mutation {152}, and some large deletions may be associated with mild disease. Therefore, additional factors appear to regulate phenotypic expression of mutant *NF2* genes.

Von Hippel-Lindau disease and capillary haemangioblastoma

T. Böhling
K.H. Plate
M.J. Haltia
K. Alitalo
H.P.H. Neumann

Definition

The von Hippel-Lindau (VHL) disease is inherited through an autosomal dominant trait and characterized by the development of capillary haemangioblastomas of the central nervous system and retina, clear cell renal carcinoma, phaeochromocytoma, pancreatic and inner ear tumours. The syndrome is caused by germline mutations of the *VHL* tumour suppressor gene, located on chromosome 3p25–26. The VHL protein is involved in cell cycle regulation and angiogenesis.

MIM No. 193300 {978}.

Synonyms and historical annotation

Lindau {898} described capillary haemangioblastoma, and also noted its association with retinal vascular tumours, previously described by von Hippel {1569}, and tumours of the visceral organs.

Incidence

Von Hippel-Lindau disease is estimated to occur at rates of 1: 36 000 {940} to 1: 45 500 population {937}.

Diagnostic criteria

The clinical diagnosis of von Hippel-Lindau disease is based on the presence of capillary haemangioblastoma in the CNS or retina, *and* the presence of one of the typical VHL-associated tumours, *or* a previous family history. In VHL disease germline VHL mutations can virtually always be identified {2085}

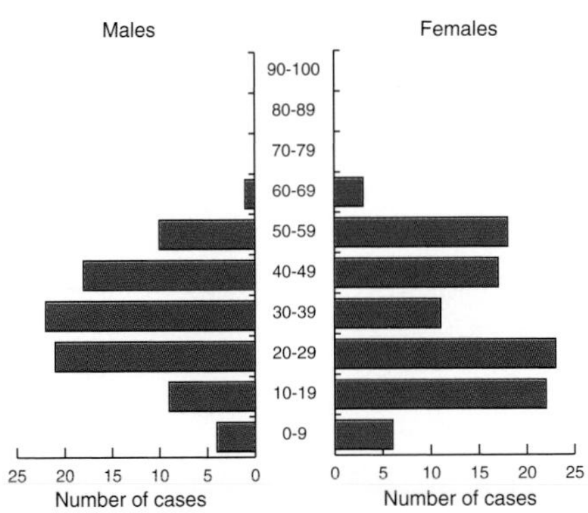

Fig. 14.13 Age and sex distribution of haemangioblastoma, based on 185 patients treated at the Universities of Freiburg (Germany) and Helsinki (Finland).

Capillary haemangioblastoma

Definition

A WHO grade I tumour of uncertain histogenesis, composed of stromal cells and abundant capillaries. Approximately 25% of haemangioblastomas are associated with VHL disease {1068}. The ICD-O code is 9161/1.

Age at clinical manifestation

Capillary haemangioblastomas usually occur in adults (see Fig. 14.13), with VHL-associated tumours occurring in significantly younger patients,with a mean age of 29 {941}.

Localization

Capillary haemangioblastomas may occur in any part of the CNS. Sporadic haemangioblastomas occur predominantly in the cerebellum, whereas VHL-associated haemangioblastomas are localized in the cerebellum, brain stem and spinal cord, while supratentorial lesions are rare. VHL patients often have multiple capillary haemangioblastomas at various sites; multiple tumours are almost exclusively found in VHL patients.

Clinical symptoms

Typically, capillary haemangioblastoma is a slowly growing mass frequently associated with cysts in the cerebellum or a syrinx in the brain stem or spinal cord. Symptoms generally arise from impaired CSF flow due to a cyst or solid tumour mass, resulting in an increase of intracranial pressure. These tumours produce erythropoietin, and this may cause secondary polycythaemia.

Neuroimaging

The diagnostic method of choice is gadolinium-enhanced MRI, which shows the tumour as a contrast-enhancing nodule and the associated cyst or syrinx. Both angiography and CT scan have been replaced by MRI.

Macroscopy

Macroscopically, capillary haemangioblastomas are seen as well-circumscribed, highly vascularized red nodules, often in the wall of large cysts. At places, the tumour may appear yellowish owing to its rich lipid content.

Histopathology

Capillary haemangioblastomas are characterized histologically by two main components, large vacuolated stromal cells and a rich capillary network. Cellular and reticular variants are distinguished on the basis of the abundance of the stromal cell component.

The stromal cells represent the neoplastic component of the tumour. Their nuclei may vary in size, with occasional atypical and hyperchromatic nuclei. However, their

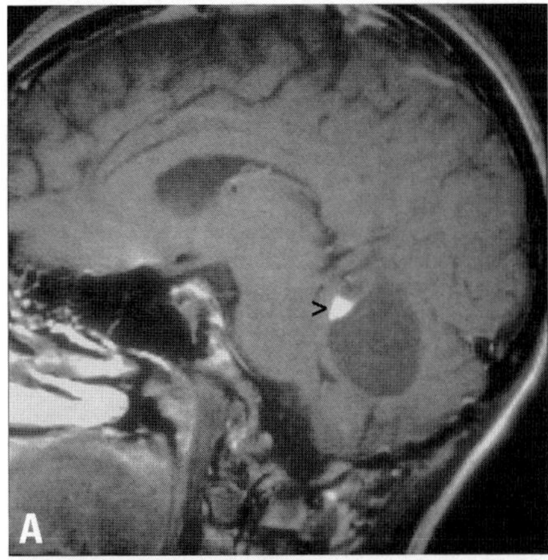

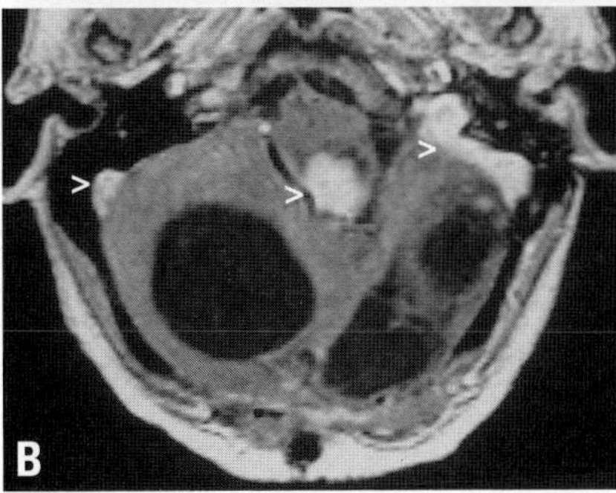

Fig. 14.14 A Lateral MRI view of a cerebellar haemangioblastoma showing the hyperdense tumour nodule (arrow) and a large adjacent cyst. **B** Multiple posterior fossa haemangioblastomas (arrows) and cerebellar cysts.

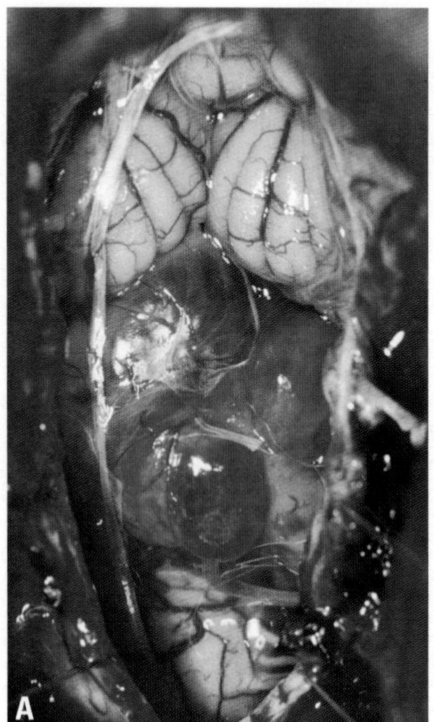

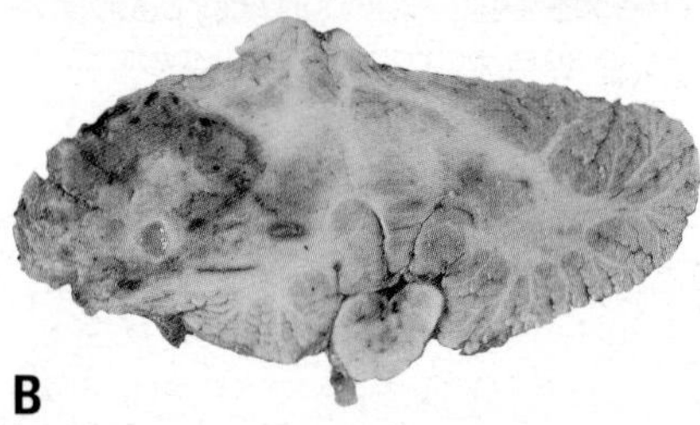

Fig. 14.15 A Intraoperative view of a cystic haemangioblastoma in the region of the fourth ventricle and dorsal medulla oblongata. **B** Well-delineated cerebellar haemangioblastoma with a haemorrhagic component and small cysts.

Table 14.6
Extracranial manifestations of VHL disease.

Organ	Lesion
Retina	Capillary haemangioblastoma
Kidney	Cysts Renal cell carcinoma
Pancreas	Cysts Islet cell tumours
Adrenal gland/ paraganglia	Phaeochromocytoma
Pancreas	Cysts Islet cell tumours
Inner ear	Endolymphatic sac tumour
Other organs	Visceral cysts Adenomas

most striking morphological feature is numerous lipid-containing vacuoles, resulting in the typical 'clear cell' morphology of capillary haemangioblastoma. This feature can sometimes lead to differential diagnostic problems between capillary haemangioblastoma and metastatic renal cell carcinoma. Immunohistochemistry for cytokeratin, EMA and pan-epithelial antigen facilitates this differential diagnosis, as capillary haemangioblastomas do not stain for these markers.

In accordance with the highly vascular nature of capillary haemangioblastoma, intratumoural haemorrhage may occur. Cystic changes are common, but necrosis is usually not seen. In adjacent reactive tissues, particularly the cyst walls, Rosenthal fibres may occur. The tumour edge is generally well-demarcated, and infiltration into surrounding neural tissues rarely occurs. The mitotic rate and the number of tumour cells entering the cell cycle are low, with a Ki67 index of less than 1%.

Ultrastructurally, the most prominent feature of the stromal cells is an abundant electron-lucent cytoplasm containing lipid droplets. Some studies have demonstrated electron-dense bodies, reminiscent of Weibel-Palade bodies, and small granules, reminiscent of neuroendocrine granules. Stromal cell histogenesis and differentiation remain unestablished {1628}.

The stromal and capillary endothelial cells differ significantly in their antigen expression patterns. Stromal cells lack endothelial cell markers, such as von Willebrand factor and CD34, and do not express endothelium-associated adhesion molecules, such as CD31 (PECAM) {140, 1628}. Unlike endothelial cells, stromal cells express neuron-specific enolase, neural cell adhesion molecule and ezrin {140, 142}. Vimentin is the major intermediate filament expressed by stromal cells. Stromal cells do not usually express glial fibrillary acidic protein {1628}.

The stromal cells express high levels of mRNA and protein for epidermal growth factor receptor (EGFR), but the *EGFR* gene is not amplified {139, 1240}. A subpopulation of the stromal cells also express transforming growth factor alpha (TGF-α), an EGFR ligand, which may suggest an autocrine or paracrine TGF-α-EGFR loop {1240}.

Vascular endothelial growth factor (VEGF), a prime regulator of physiological and pathological angiogenesis, is highly expressed in stromal cells, with corresponding endothelial expression of its receptors VEGFR-1 and -2 {1627}, and the endothelial cell receptor Tie-1 {552}. A subpopulation of stromal cells also expresses high levels of the endothelial receptors, suggesting paracrine and autocrine growth factor-receptor loops {552}. Most haemangioblastomas contain numerous mast cells, of interest as VEGF binds to heparin. The endothelial cells of haemangioblastomas also express receptors for other angiogenic growth factors, including platelet-derived growth factors {139}. In addition to VEGF, erythropoietin and the transcription factor HIF-2 alpha are upregulated in the stromal cells {2080, 2081}.

Other CNS manifestations

Capillary haemangioblastoma is the major CNS manifestation of VHL. Occasionally, cases of ependymoma, choroid plexus papilloma, and medulloblastoma have been observed in the setting of VHL disease.

Extraneural manifestations

A very common tumour in VHL patients is the retinal 'von Hippel tumour' or 'an-

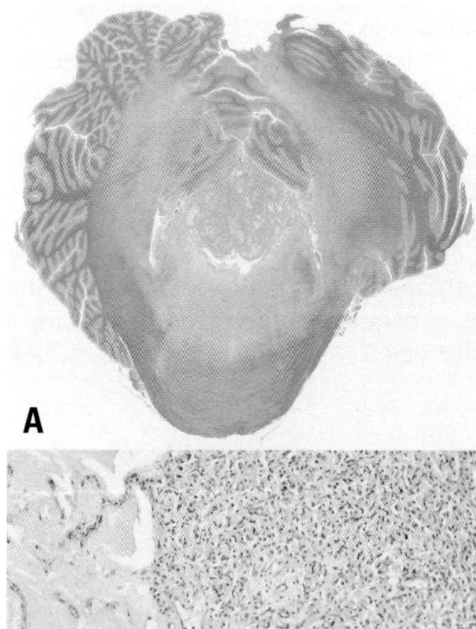

Fig. 14.16 Cerebellar section of a cerebellar haemangioblastoma extending into the fourth ventricle. Higher magnification shows the typical distribution of tumour cells within a network of small capillaries. Note the hyalinized vascular stroma (on the left).

gioma', which is histologically identical to capillary haemangioblastoma. Most other tumours and tumour-like lesions associated with VHL are concentrated in the visceral organs (Table 14.6), and no skin lesions are known. Of the visceral tumours, clear cell renal carcinomas and phaeochromocytomas are most common {1068}. A newly identified component of VHL disease is the endolymphatic sac tumour of the inner ear {2083}

Genetics

The VHL gene is located at chromosome 3p25–26 {863}. The VHL tumour suppressor gene has three exons and a coding sequence of 639 nucleotides {863} (see Fig. 14.18).

Gene expression

The VHL gene is expressed in a variety of human trissues, in particular epithelial cells of the skin, the gastrointestinal, respiratory and urogenital tract and endocrine and exocrine organs{2540, 2539}. In the CNS, immunoreactivity for pVHL is prominent in neurons, including Purkinje cells of the cerebellum {913, 2541}

Function of the VHL protein

Mutational inactivation of the VHL gene in affected family members is responsible for their genetic susceptibility to renal cell carcinoma and capillary haemangioblastoma but the mechanisms by which the suppressor gene product, the VHL protein (pVHL), causes neoplastic transformation, has remained enigmatic. Several signalling pathways appear to be involved {2538}, one of which points a role of pVHL in protein degradation and angiogenesis. The alpha domain of pVHL forms a complex with elongin B, elongin C, Cul-2 {1157, 2131, 2593} and Rbx1 {2586} which has ubiquitin ligase activity {2594}, thereby targeting cellular proteins for ubiquitination and proteasome-mediated degradation. The domain of the VHL gene involved in the binding to elongin is frequently mutated in VHL-associated neoplasms {2131}.

The beta-domain of pVHL interacts with the alpha subunits of hypoxia-inducible factor 1 (HIF-1) which mediates cellular responses to hypoxia. Under normoxic conditions and in the presence of functional pVHL, the alpha subunits are rapidly degraded. Under hypoxic conditions and in VHL deficient cells, the subunits are stabilised, with a concomitant induction of

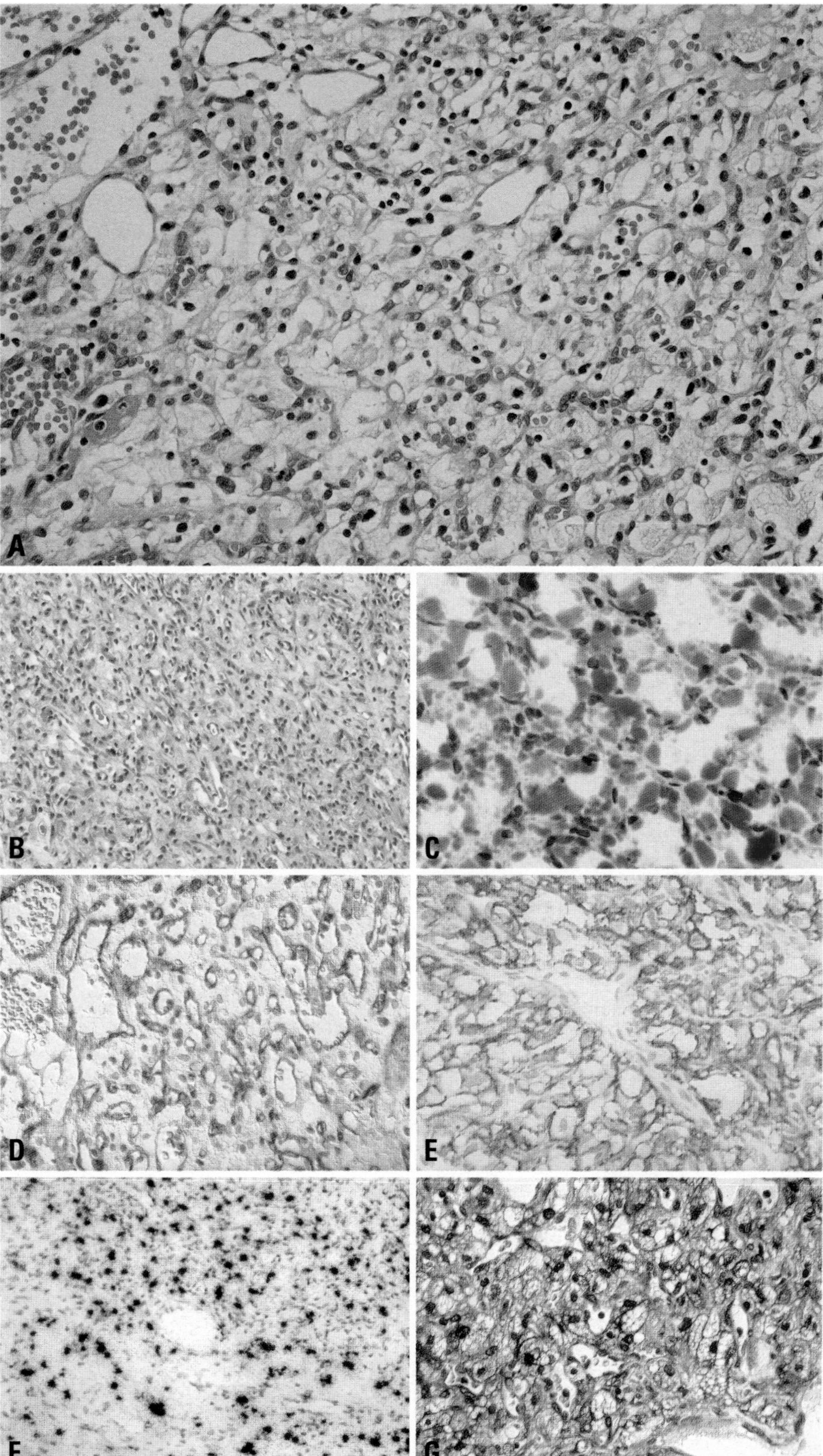

Fig. 14.17 Histopathological features of haemangioblastomas. **A** Accumulation of lipid droplets within stromal cells (**B**) Cellular variant showing densely packed tumour cells. **C** Semi-thin section (toluidine blue stain) showing stromal cells with lipid vacuoles. **D** Immunostaining of endothelial cells with anti-CD31 (PECAM-1), leaving the stromal cells unstained. **E** Membrane-bound expression of EGFR in stromal cells. **F** *In situ* hybridization showing expression of VEGF mRNA in stromal cells. **G** Immunostaining for VHL protein in stromal, but not in endothelial cells.

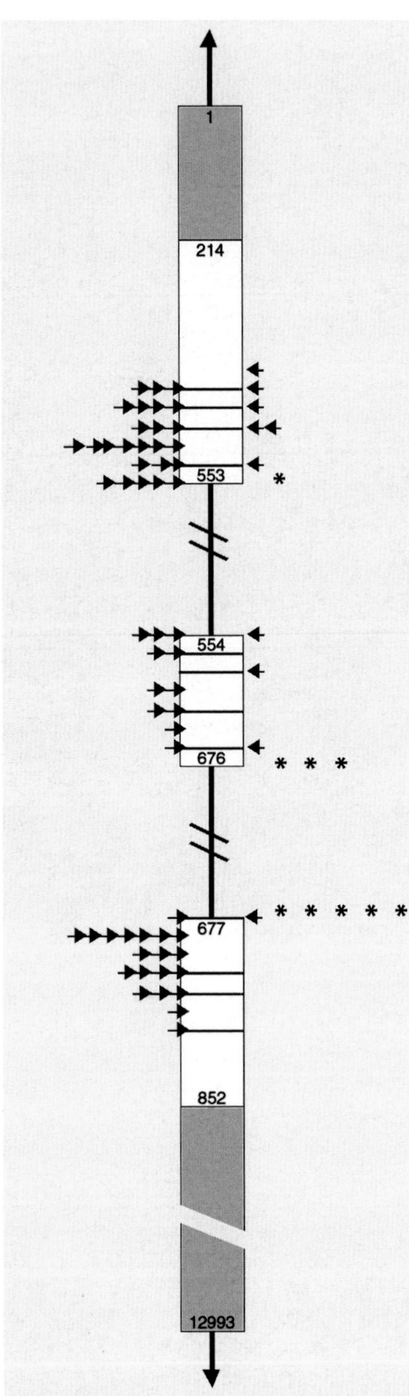

Fig. 14.18 Mutations of the *VHL* tumor suppressor gene detected in familial and sporadic haemangioblastomas of the CNS (from Neumann and Bender, 1998; updated). Untranslated regions are in grey. Arrows pointing to the right (->) indicate substitutions, arrows to the left (<-) insertions. Deletions are represented by a horizontal line and splice mutations by asterisks (*).

Table 14.7
Genotype – phenotype correlations in VHL patients.

VHL-type	Phenotype	Predisposing mutation
Type 1	Without phaeochromocytoma	686 T -> C Leu -> Pro
Type 2A	With phaeochromocytoma and renal cell carcinoma	712 C -> T Arg -> Trp
Type 2B	With phaeochromocytoma but without renal cell carcinoma	505 T -> C Tyr -> His 658 G -> T Ala -> Ser

hypoxia-regulated genes, including vascular endothelial growth factor (VEGF) {2132}. Constitutive overexpression of VEGF through this signalling pathway could explain the extraordinary capillary component of VHL associated neoplasms {2132}. The capillaries of CNS haemangioblastomas are known to be recruited through overexpression of VEGF and related angiogenic factors secreted by stromal cells and are considered non-neoplastic (see above).

Additional functions of the VHL protein may contribute to malignant transformation and the evolution of the phenotype of VHL associated lesions. Recent studies in renal cell carcinoma cell lines suggest that pVHL is involved in the control of cell cycle exit, i.e. the transition from the G_2 into quiescent G_0 phase, possibly by preventing accumulation of the cyclin-dependent kinase inhibitor p27 {2592}. Another study showed that only wild-type but not tumour-derived pVHL binds to fibronectin. As a consequence, VHL-/- renal cell carcinoma cells showed a defective assembly of an extracellular fibronectin matrix {2597}. Through a down-regulation of the response of cells to hepatocyte growth factor / scatter factor and reduced levels of tissue inhibitor of metalloproteinase 2 (TIMP-2), pVHL deficient tumours cells exhibit a significantly higher capacity for invasion {2589}. Further, inactivated pVHL causes an overexpression of transmembrane carbonic anhydrases that are involved in extracellular pH regulation {2598} but the biological significance of this dysregulation remains to be assessed.

Gene mutations and VHL subtypes

Germline mutations of the VHL gene are spread all over the three exons. Missense mutations are most common, but nonsense mutations, microdeletions/ insertions, splice site mutations and large deletions also occur {1673, 2082, 2084}. The spectrum of clinical manifestations of VHL reflects the type of germline mutation (Table 14.7). Phenotypes are based on the absence (type 1) or presence (type 2) of phaeochromocytoma. VHL type 2 is usually associated with missense mutations and subdivided on the presence (type 2A) or absence (type 2B) of renal cell carcinoma {2079, 226, 480, 1068}.

According to its function as a tumour suppressor gene, VHL gene mutations are also common in sporadic haemangioblastomas and renal cell carcinomas {724, 1094}.

Prognostic factors

The prognosis of CNS haemangioblastoma has been tremendously ameliorated with introduction of microsurgical techniques. Mortality is low and permanent neurological deficits are extremely rare in sporadic haemangioblastoma.

In VHL disease, CNS haemangioblastoma is the most common cause of death, followed by renal cell carcinoma. The median life expectancy of VHL patients was 49 years {732, 1068}. In order to detect VHL-associated hemangioblastomas in time, analyzes for germline mutations of the VHL gene has been recommended in every patient with CNS hemangioblastoma, particularly in those of younger age and with multiple lesions. Periodic screening of VHL patients by MRI should start after the age of ten years {2489}.

Tuberous sclerosis complex and subependymal giant cell astrocytoma

O.D. Wiestler
B.S. Lopes
A.J. Green
H.V. Vinters

Definition

Tuberous sclerosis complex (TSC) comprises a group of autosomal dominant disorders characterized by hamartomas and benign neoplastic lesions that affect the central nervous system as well as various non-neural tissues. Major CNS manifestations include cortical hamartomas (tubers), subcortical glioneuronal hamartomas, subependymal glial nodules and subependymal giant cell astrocytomas. Extraneural manifestations include cutaneous angiofibromas ('adenoma sebaceum'), peau chagrin, subungual fibromas, cardiac rhabdomyomas, intestinal polyps, visceral cysts, pulmonary lymphangio-leiomyomatosis and renal angiomyolipomas. The syndrome is caused by a germline mutation of the *TSC1 or TSC2* gene.

MIM No. TSC1: 191100; TSC2: 191092 {978}.

Synonyms

Tuberous sclerosis; Bourneville disease; Bourneville-Pringle disease.

Incidence

Variability of clinical manifestations previously led to underdiagnosis. Recent data indicate an incidence of between 1/5000 and 1/10000.

Diagnostic criteria

Clinical manifestations {1263} of TSC have been divided into definitive, provisional or suspect criteria {489}. Clinical symptoms of TSC relate to the appearance of hamartomas or slowly growing neoplasms in the central nervous system and retina, skin, heart and kidneys. Lesions involving these tissues are classified as definitive features. Major CNS manifestations include cortical tubers, subependymal nodules and white matter hamartomas in 90-100% of gene carriers. Skin involvement manifests as facial angiofibroma (adenoma sebaceum), hypomelanotic macules, shagreen patches and forehead plaques. The presence of multiple cutaneous angiofibromas, or their detection at an early age, is highly suggestive of TSC. Retinal hamartoma, retinal giant cell astrocytoma, renal angiomyolipoma and cardiac rhabdomyoma are commonly encountered. Other organs may also be affected, including the lungs, spleen, liver, pancreas, bones and teeth, gingiva and gastrointestinal tract. Most patients have manifestations of TSC before the age of 10 years {8}. The major features of TSC are summarized in Table 14.8.

Clinical features

Neurological symptoms are the most frequent and serious manifestations. In an epidemiological study in western Sweden, initial clinical signs in a majority of TSC patients were epilepsy and autistic withdrawal {8}. Mental retardation and behavioural abnormalities are usually present {489}. Infantile spasms represent another characteristic neurological deficit in TSC.

Subependymal giant cell astrocytoma

Definition

Subependymal giant cell astrocytoma (SEGA) is a benign, slowly growing tumour typically arising in the wall of the lateral ventricles and composed of large ganglioid astrocytes.

ICD-O code: 9348/1

Grading

Subependymal giant cell astrocytomas correspond to WHO grade I.

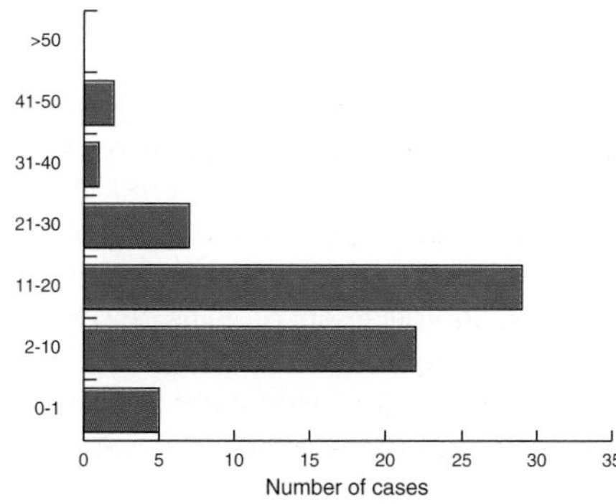

Fig. 14.19 Age distribution of subependymal giant cells astrocytomas (SEGA) at the time of clinical manifestation. Combined data for male and female patients.

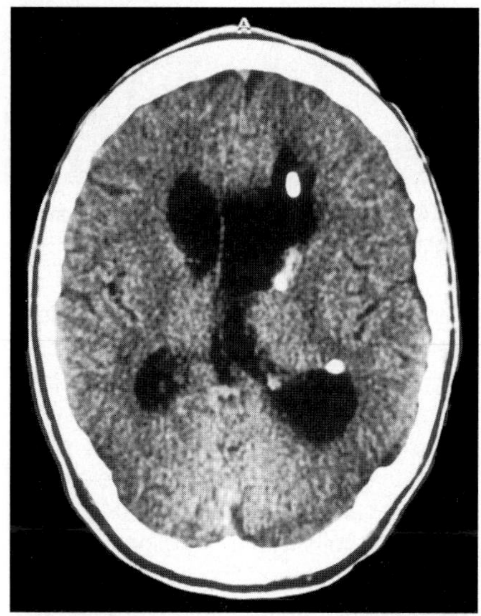

Fig. 14.20 CT of typical subependymal calcifications in a patient with tuberous sclerosis.

Incidence and clinical features

Although there is debate as to whether SEGA occurs outside the setting of TSC, it is the most common CNS neoplasm in TSC patients {8, 489, 1403}. Its incidence ranges from approximately 6% to 16% in patients with confirmed TSC {8, 1403}. This tumour typically occurs during the first two decades of life, although cases involving infants have been reported {240, 1100}. Most patients show either a worsening of epilepsy or present with symptoms of increased intracranial pressure. Extension of the tumours into the third ventricle region and obstruction of the foramen of Monro may cause blockage of CSF pathways and increased intracranial pressure. Calcifications and signs of previous haemorrhage may also be present. Massive spontaneous haemorrhage has occasionally been observed in these lesions.

Histopathology

A circumscribed, often calcified tumour composed mainly of large, plump, cells resembling astrocytes. Clustering of tumour cells and perivascular pseudopalisading are common features. Cellular pleomorphism and occasional mitoses do not indicate malignant behaviour.

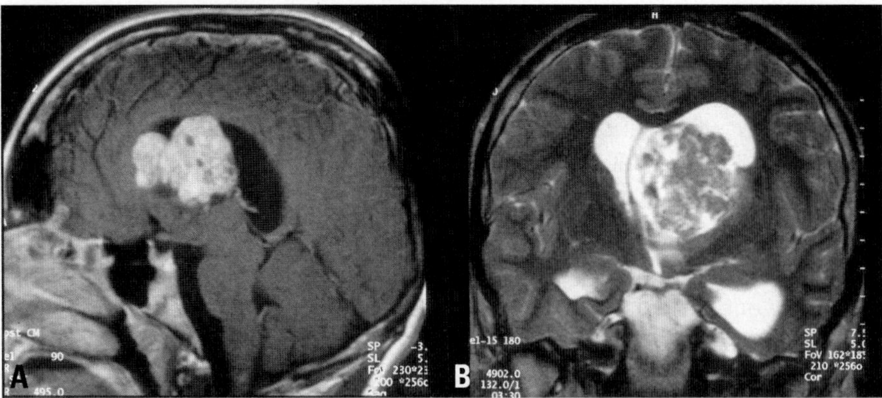

Fig. 14.21 Subependymal giant cell astrocytoma of the left lateral ventricle on (**A**) T1 weighted and (**B**) T2 weighted MRI.

The tumour cells composing these lesions show a wide spectrum of astroglial phenotypes. Typical appearances range from polygonal cells with abundant, glassy cytoplasm (resembling gemistocytic astrocytes) to smaller, more elongate elements within a variably fibrillated matrix. Giant pyramidal cells with a ganglionic appearance are common. The nuclei display a finely granular chromatin pattern with distinct nucleoli. Considerable nuclear pleomorphism and multinucleated cells are frequent. SEGAs may demonstrate increased mitotic activity. However, these features do not appear to denote an adverse clinical course. Similarly, the occasional presence of endothelial proliferation and necrosis are not indicative of anaplastic progression. The rare examples of SEGAs that recur have not been reported to show malignant transformation.

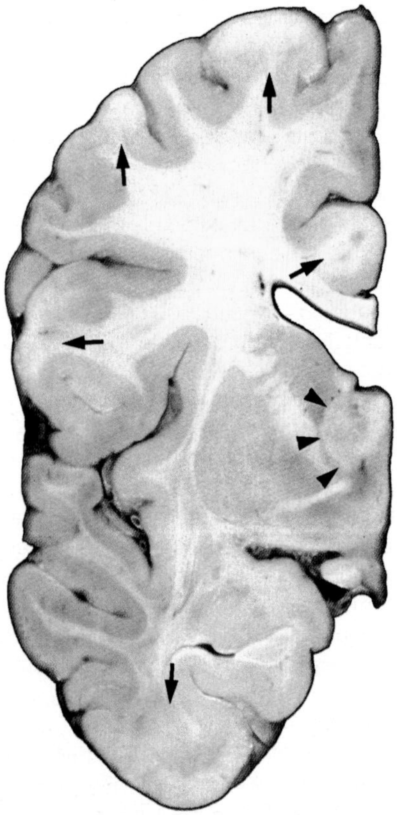

Fig. 14.22 Coronal section of the left hemisphere of a patient with tuberous sclerosis, showing a subependymal giant cell astrocytoma (arrowheads) and multiple cortical tubers.

Proliferation

Flow cytometric studies have demonstrated diploid patterns in most cases {1403}. Low Ki-67 (MIB-1) labelling indices provide further support for the benign nature of these neoplasms {517}.

Immunohistochemistry

SEGA has been designated as a distinctive type of well-circumscribed astrocytoma {779} but usually exhibits a mixed glioneuronal phenotype and so has also been termed subependymal giant cell tumour {859}. Tumour cells demonstrate variable immunoreactivity for GFAP and S-100 protein. Some neoplastic cells in SEGA express both glial and neuron-associated antigens. Neurofilament proteins and neuron-associated class III beta-tubulin are both demonstrated {1696}. Class III beta-tubulin appears more widespread in its distribution than any other neuronal epitope. Neurofilament proteins tend to be more restricted and mainly highlight cellular processes and a few large ganglionic cells. Variable immunoreactivity for a number of neuropeptides has also been detected. These findings suggest cellular lineages with a variable capacity for divergent phenotypes, including glial, neuronal and neuroendocrine differentiation in SEGAs. Ultrastructural features of neuronal differentiation, such as microtubules, occasional dense-core granules, and, rarely, synapse formation may be detectable {592}. Immunohistochemical and ultrastructural features are similar to those seen in the cortical tubers of TSC.

Other CNS manifestations

Cortical tubers in TSC may be detected by either CT or MRI {1402}. These malformative lesions have a strong association with the development of epilepsy, especially infantile spasms and generalized tonic-clonic seizures. On microscopical examination, they consist of giant cells (like those seen in SEGA), and show dysmorphic neurons (often with cytoskeletal disorganisation), disrupted cortical lamination, gliosis, calcification of blood-vessel walls and/or parenchyma, and myelin loss. As in other forms of focal cortical dysplasia, disrupted lamination, and possibly altered synaptic connectivity, may account for the intrinsic epileptogenicity of tubers. The surrounding cortex usually demonstrates a normal cytoarchitecture {642}.

Dysmorphic neurons and giant cells may be seen in all cortical layers as well as in the underlying white matter, where heterotopic clusters of abnormal neurons and giant cells can be found. Dysplastic neurons show altered radial orientation in the cortex, aberrant dendritic arborization, abnormal somatic morphology (loss of pyramidal shape), and accumulation of perikaryal fibrils {404, 592, 642}. Although affected neurons express proteins such as neurofilament subunits, MAPs, and class III beta-tubulin, they display cytoarchitectural features of immature or poorly differentiated neurons, such as reduced axonal projections and spine density {592, 642}. Giant cells in cortical tubers show a cellular and molecular heterogeneity similar to

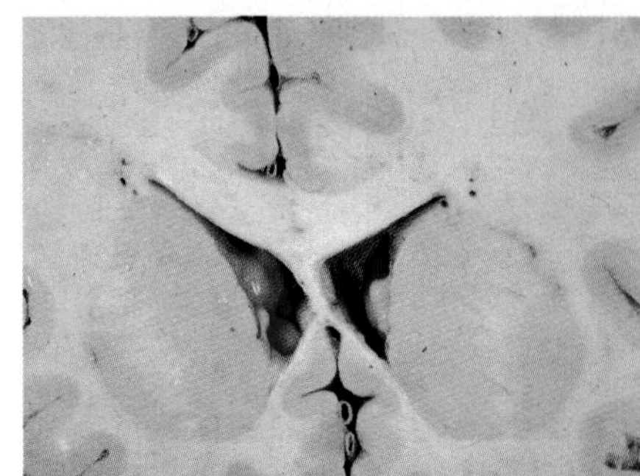

Fig. 14.23 Multiple small subependymal giant cell astrocytomas at the walls of the lateral ventricles.

that seen in SEGA. While the developmental lineage of giant cells in tubers remains to be determined, immunohistochemical markers characteristic of glial as well as neuronal phenotypes suggest a mixed glioneuronal origin. Many giant cells in tubers express both nestin mRNA and protein; nestin is an intermediate filament found in neuroepithelial glial and neuronal precursor cells {287}. Some giant cells demonstrate immunoreactivity for GFAP {592}. A subset of these cells with an identical morphological phenotype do not express GFAP mRNA or protein, or mRNA for the glial connexin 43 {287}. In contrast, mRNA and proteins of certain neuronal markers, such as the connexins 26 and 32, neurofilament, class III beta-tubulin, MAP2, and alpha-internexin can be found in many giant cells {287, 592}. However, formation of well-defined synapses between giant cells and adjacent neurons is not a consistent finding.

Cortical hamartomas morphologically indistinguishable from tubers may occur in chronic focal epilepsies without clinical evidence for an underlying TSC condition {2215}. The pathogenesis of these sporadic lesions is unresolved.

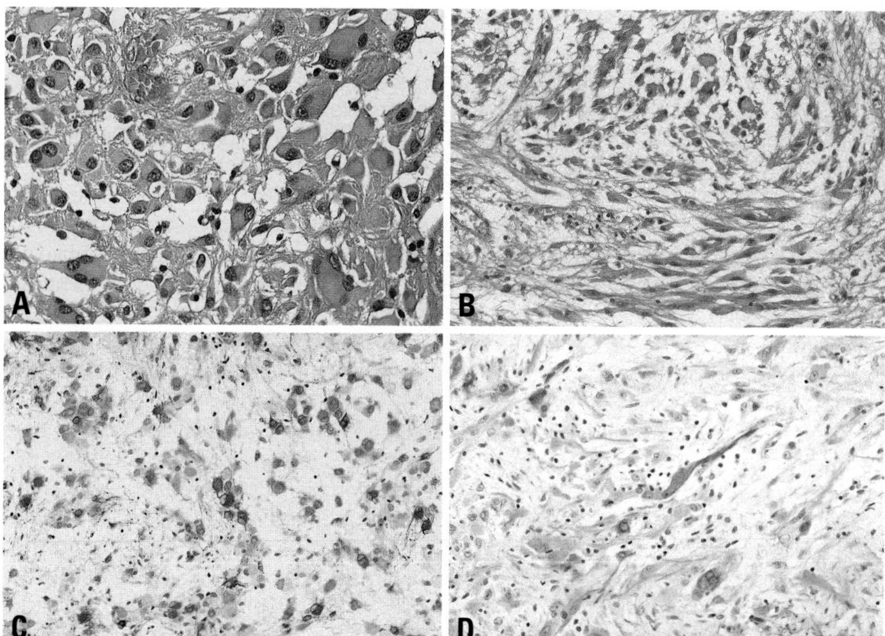

Fig. 14.24 Histopathological features of subependymal giant cell astrocytoma. **A** Pleomorphic multinucleated eosinophilic tumour cells. **B** Elongated tumour cells forming streams. **C** GFAP immunostaining of tumour cells. **D** Neuronal differentiation, demonstrated by immunoreactivity to class III beta-tubulin.

Table 14.8
Major Manifestations of the Tuberous Sclerosis Complex (TSC).

Manifestation	Frequency (%)
Central nervous system	
Cortical tuber	90-100
Subependymal nodule	90-100
White matter hamartoma	90-100
Subependymal giant cell astrocytoma	6-16
Skin	
Facial angiofibroma (adenoma sebaceum)	80-90
Hypomelanotic macule	80-90
Shagreen patch	20-40
Forehead plaque	20-30
Peri- and subungual fibroma	20-30
Eyes	
Retinal hamartoma	50
Retinal giant cell astocytoma	20-30
Hypopigmented iris spot	10-20
Kidney	
Angiomyolipoma	50
Heart	
Cardiac rhabdomyoma	50
Digestive system	
Microhamartomatous rectal polyp	70-80
Liver hamartoma	40-50

Extraneural manifestations

Extraneural manifestations of TSC and the frequencies at which they occur are summarized in Table 14.8.

Genetics

Inheritance and genetic heterogeneity

Approximately 50% of TSC patients have a positive family history, indicating a high rate of *de novo* mutations. In affected kindreds, the disease follows an autosomal dominant pattern of inheritance, with high penetrance, but considerable phenotypic variability {1413}. Neuroradiological observations suggest that first degree relatives of affected patients may have minor clinical signs or a forme fruste of the disease.

Molecular genetics

Genetic linkage studies have provided evidence for two distinct TSC loci on chromosome 9q (*TSC1*), and on chromosome 16p (*TSC2*) {270, 723}. These are likely tumour suppressor genes, as analyzes of TSC lesions from affected individuals have demonstrated loss of heterozygosity at both loci {192, 503}. It has not been possible to associate *TSC1* and *TSC2* with distinct clinical phenotypes, suggesting that both genes may be involved in the same regulatory pathway. Recent findings do indeed indicate that the products of the two TSC genes interact within the cell {2210}. Mutations in *TSC2* are much more common than those in *TSC1* {2490}.

The TSC1 gene

The *TSC1* gene maps to chromosome 9q34 {270}.

Gene structure. The *TSC1* gene contains 23 exons, spanning 45kb of genomic DNA {2213}. Of these, 21 appear to carry coding information.

Gene expression. *TSC1* encodes a 8.6 kb mRNA. Its gene product, hamartin, has a molecular weight of 130 kD. Studies in cultured cells have localized this protein to cytoplasmic vesicles without assigning a specific function to the molecule {2210}. Hamartin is strongly expressed in brain, kidney and heart, i.e. tissues frequently affected in TSC. Immunohistochemically, significant hamartin staining was reported in cortical neurons, kidney epithelia, pancreatic islets, bronchial epithelia and alveolar macrophages {2209}. Its pattern of expression overlaps with that of tuberin, the product of the *TSC2* gene. Recent data indicate that hamartin and tuberin interact within the cell {2210}. This property may explain the almost indistinguishable clinical manifestations of the two forms of TSC.

Gene mutations. Systematic screening in 225 unrelated patients yielded *TSC1* mutations in 29 cases (13 %). Virtually all mutations resulted in a truncated gene product and more than half of the changes affected exons 15 and 17 {2211}. Genotype-phenotype correlations were not apparent.

The TSC2 gene

The *TSC2* gene maps to chromosome 16p13.3 {723} and contains 40 exons.

Gene expression. *TSC2* encodes a large transcript of 5.5 kb which shows widespread expression in many tissues, including the brain and other organs affected in TSC. Alternatively spliced mRNAs have been reported {1649}. A portion of the 180 kD protein product, tuberin, bears significant homology with the catalytic domain of the GTPase-activating protein, Rap1-GAP, a member of the ras family. Studies in the Eker rat, a strain with hereditary kidney cancer, demonstrated mutations of the rat *TSC2* homologue, providing support for the hypothesis that *TSC2* acts as a tumour suppressor. Immunohistochemical and *in situ* localization studies of tuberin and *TSC2* mRNA revealed expression in normal neurons and glia. Some TSC lesions appear to express high levels of the gene and protein, while others are virtually devoid of immunoreactive tuberin {762}.

Gene mutations. While germline *TSC2* mutations have been described {1623}, genotype-phenotype correlations have not emerged. In sporadic tumours and hamartomas, *TSC2* alterations have been reported, although loss of the *TSC2* gene is less common in brain lesions than in kidney tumours {571}. Furthermore, neuroglial lesions that are almost indistinguishable from TSC hamartomas have been observed in the brains of patients with chronic focal epilepsies. A molecular analysis for LOH on chromosomes 9q and 16p failed to detect any involvement of the *TSC1* and *TSC2* loci in these sporadic malformative lesions {1630}. This finding appears to exclude the possibility that some of these patients are afflicted with a forme fruste of TSC.

Expression of the TSC1 and TSC2 gene products in TSC lesions

Using antipeptide antibodies, Johnson and co-workers {2208} have analyzed the immunohistochemical distribution of the *TSC1* and *TSC2* gene products in cortical tubers from TSC patients. Surprisingly, both hamartin and tuberin were strongly co-expressed in a subpopulation of dysmorphic neuroglial cells.

Li-Fraumeni syndrome and *TP53* germline mutations

H. Ohgaki
A. Vital
P. Kleihues
P. Hainaut

Definition

Li-Fraumeni syndrome (LFS) is a autosomal dominant disorder and is characterized by multiple primary neoplasms in children and young adults, with a predominance of soft tissue sarcomas, osteosarcomas, breast cancer, and an increased incidence of brain tumours, leukaemia and adrenocortical carcinoma. The majority of Li-Fraumeni cases is caused by a *TP53* germline mutation.

MIM No.

Li-Fraumeni syndrome: 151623;
TP53 mutations (germline and somatic): 191170 {978}.

Synonyms

Sarcoma family syndrome of Li and Fraumeni.

Incidence

From 1990 to 1998, a total of 143 families with a *TP53* germline mutation were reported {2570}. See IARC database http://www.iarc.fr/p53/germ.htm

Diagnostic criteria

The clinical criteria used to identify an affected individual in a Li-Fraumeni family are: (i) occurrence of sarcoma before the age of 45 and (ii) at least one first degree relative with any tumour before age 45 and (iii) a second (or first) degree relative with cancer before age 45 or a sarcoma at any age {128, 453, 889, 890}.

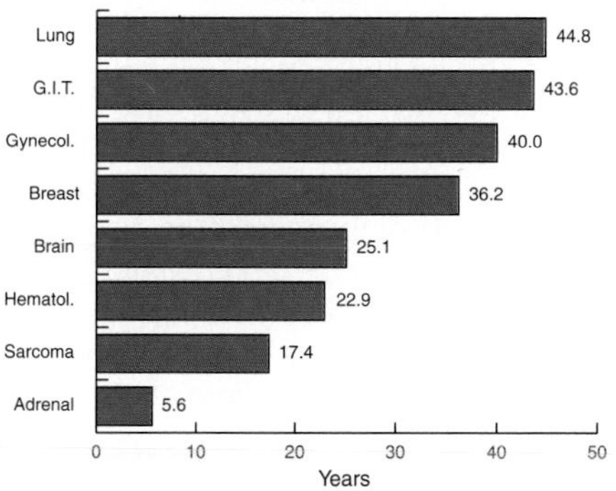

Fig. 14.25 Mean age of patients with tumours caused by a *TP53* germline mutation, according to organ site. From Ohgaki *et al.* {2570}, updated through 1998.

Table 14.9
Brain tumours associated with *TP53* germline mutations

Histology	No. of tumours	Mean age of patients (years)
Classified (61 cases)		
Astrocytic brain tumour	39 (35.8%)	32.4
Medulloblastoma/PNET	11 (5.2%)	5.2
Choroid plexus tumour	4 (3.7%)	1.3
Ependymoma	1 (0.9%)	8.0
Ganglioneuroma	1 (0.9%)	2.0
Meningioma	2 (1.8%)	37.5
Schwannoma	3 (1.5%)	41.0
Unclassified (27 cases)	48 (44.0%)	26.7
All (67 cases)	109 (100%)	25.5

The male/female ratio for all patients with nervous system tumours was 1.7.

Criteria for the diagnosis of LFS variant are somewhat less stringent: (i) three separate primary cancers, the first tumour diagnosed under the age of 45, or the combination of (i) childhood cancer or LFS-associated neoplasm under the age of 45, (ii) first or second degree relative with LFS-associated tumour at any age, (iii) first or second degree relative with any cancer diagnosed under age 60 {2575, 2573}.

Nervous system neoplasms

In the 143 families with a *TP53* germline mutation communicated during 1990-1998, a total of 805 tumours were reported; 109 of these (13.5%) were located in the nervous system (Table 14.10), and 69 kindred (48.3%) had at least one family member with a brain tumour.

Age and sex distribution

The male: female ratio of patients with brain tumours is 1.7, similar to that of sporadic brain tumours excluding meningiomas (1.6) {859}.

As with sporadic brain tumours, the age

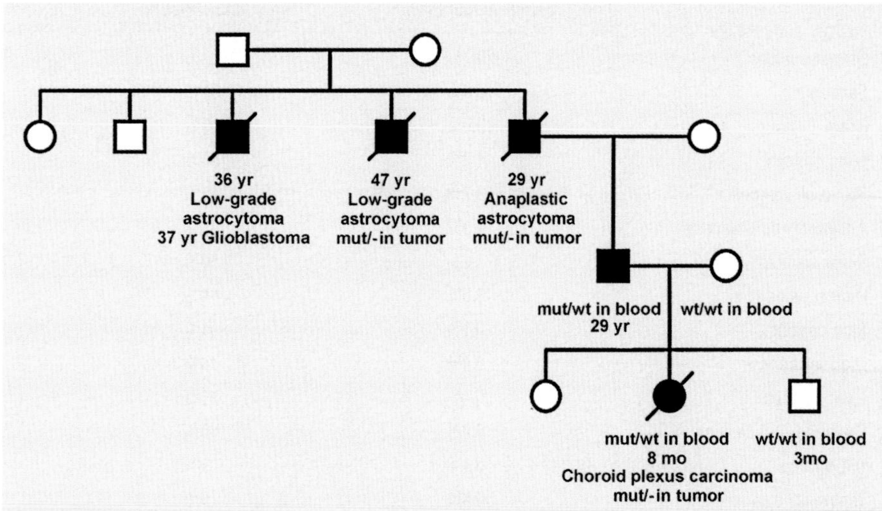

Fig. 14.26 Typical example of a pedigree of a family carrying a *TP53* germline mutation (codon 248, CGG -> TGG, Arg -> Trp), with remarkable clustering of brain tumours. Black gender symbols indicate carriers of gene mutations. From Vital *et al.* {2030}.

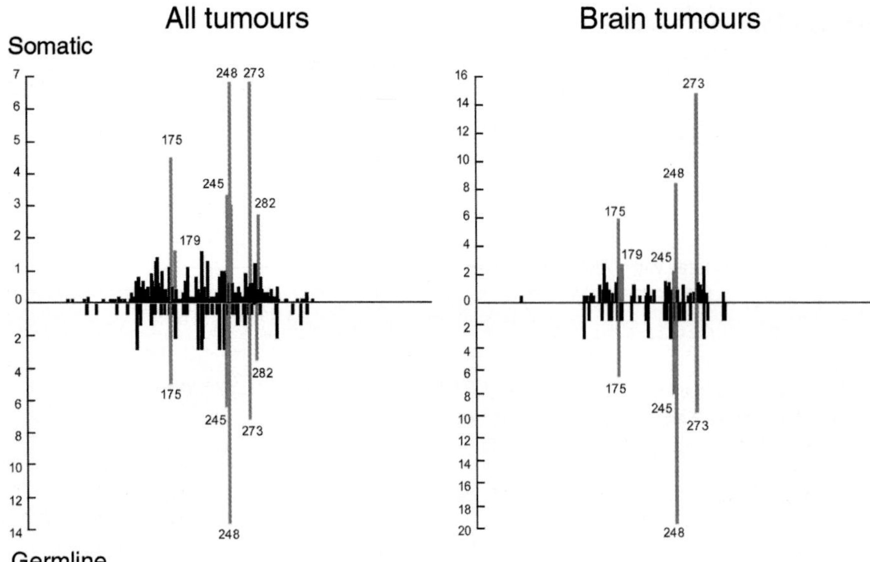

Fig. 14.27 Somatic and germline *TP53* mutations share the major hotspot codons 175, 248 and 273 within the DNA-binding domain (exons 5-8). Germline mutations prevail in codon 245 and 248. Based on 805 tumours in 143 reported families. See online IARC database on *TP53* mutations www.iarc.fr/p53/index.html

of patients with nervous system neoplasms associated with *TP53* germline mutations shows a bimodal distribution. The first peak of incidence is in children (representing mainly medulloblastomas and related primitive neuroectodermal and choroid plexus tumours), and the second (mainly astrocytic brain tumours) in the third and fourth decades of life (Table 14.9).

Familial clustering
Among families with at least one case of brain tumour, the mean number of CNS tumours per family is 1.6. Several reported families {925, 999, 2030, 2129, 2570} showed a remarkable clustering of brain tumours (Fig. 14.26). This raises the question of whether some mutations carry an organ- or cell-specific risk, but genetic analyzes have not revealed mutational hotspots for specific tumour types or target tissues {784}. An exception are choroid plexus tumours: of four lesions associated with a *TP53* germline mutation, three were located in codon 248 {2030}. Another possibility is that the familial clustering of certain tumour types is influenced by the genetic background of the affected family {784, 949}. Familial clustering due to gene-environment interactions, e.g., exposure of families to similar environmental carcinogens or life-style factors has been suggested for stomach and breast cancer {784}, but is considered to be less likely to play a role in the evolution of brain tumours associated with *TP53* germline mutations.

Histopathology of CNS tumours
Of the 109 brain tumours recorded, 61 (56%) had been classified histologically, and of these, 39 (64%) were of astrocytic origin, including low-grade astrocytoma, anaplastic astrocytoma, glioblastoma multiforme, oligoastrocytoma and gliosarcoma (Table 14.9). Paediatric brain tumours, including medulloblastomas and related primitive neuroectodermal tumours (PNETs; 11 cases) and choroid plexus tumours (4 cases) were less frequent (together 25%). This correlates with the occurrence of *TP53* mutations in sporadic brain tumours, which prevail in astrocytomas and are considerably less frequent in medulloblastomas {1096, 1097}. Histopathologically, CNS tumours associated with *TP53* germline mutations are indistinguishable from their sporadic counterparts, though one report suggests that inherited *TP53* mutations are more frequently associated with multifocal glioblastomas {844}.

Extraneural manifestations

Breast cancer and sarcomas (osteosarcomas and soft tissue sarcomas) are the most frequent manifestations and account for 40% of all tumours in affected family members (Table 14.10). The sporadic counterparts of these tumours also show a high frequency of *TP53* mutation, suggesting that in these neoplasms, *TP53* mutations are capable of initiating the process of malignant transformation (Table 14.10).

Age distribution
In general, tumours associated with a *TP53* germline mutation develop earlier

Table 14.10
Comparison of somatic vs. germline *TP53* mutations

Tumour	Fraction of tumours in families with a *TP53* germline mutation	Incidence of somatic *TP53* mutations in sporadic tumours
Breast cancer	20.7%	22%
Sarcoma	18.6%	31%
Brain Tumour	13.5%	25%
Lung cancer	4.2%	56%
Stomach cancer	3.2%	41%
Adrenocortical carcinoma	3.1%	23%
Colon cancer	1.2%	50%
Pancreas cancer	0.5%	44%
Skin cancer	0.1%	44%
Bladder cancer	0.4%	34%
Liver cancer	0.4%	29%
Oesophageal cancer	0.4%	45%
Melanoma	0.4%	9%
Testicular cancer	0.4%	0%
Neuroblastoma	0.2%	1%

Data for sporadic tumours are from Greenblatt *et al.* {504}. Data for *TP53* germline mutations are from Kleihues *et al.* {784}, updated with reports published in 1998.

Table 14.11
Types of somatic and germline *TP53* mutations in human neoplasms

		G:C				A:T			deletion/	Splicing
		->T:A	->C:G	->A:T (at CpG)	->A:T (not at CpG)	->T:A	->G:C	->C:G	insertion	
Brain tumour	Somatic	9%	6%	35%	18%	2%	13%	4%	13%	2%
	Germline	9%	6%	38%	16%	3%	7%	4%	12%	6%
Breast cancer	Somatic	10%	7%	20%	22%	6%	13%	5%	14%	2%
	Germline	1%	4%	42%	14%	3%	11%	3%	17%	6%
Sarcoma	Somatic	10%	6%	20%	30%	6%	14%	2%	10%	2%
	Germline	4%	5%	43%	15%	7%	8%	0%	15%	2%
All tumours	Somatic	15%	8%	23%	21%	5%	11%	4%	10%	2%
	Germline	7%	4%	38%	17%	6%	11%	2%	11%	3%

In all tumours, there is a tendency for G:C->A:T transitions at CpG sites to be more frequent in tumours associated with *TP53* germline mutations than in those with somatic *TP53* mutations. The pattern of somatic and germline *TP53* mutations are remarkably similar in brain tumours. Breast cancer and sarcomas in affected family members show a typical pattern of *TP53* germline mutations, while their respective sporadic counterparts show a lower frequency of G:C->A:T transition at CpG sites.

than their sporadic counterparts, but there are marked organ-specific differences (Fig. 14.25). Adrenocortical carcinomas associated with a *TP53* germline mutation develop almost exclusively in children, in contrast to sporadic adrenocortical carcinomas, which have a broad age distribution with a peak beyond age 40 {71}.

Genetics

In approximately 70% of Li-Fraumeni cases, affected family members carry a germline mutation of one allele of the *TP53* tumour suppressor gene {950, 1446}. Conversely, approximately 50% of families with *TP53* germline mutations meet the criteria of the Li-Fraumeni syndrome; however, the extent of the overlap may be greater, as in some families with *TP53* germline mutations only one tumour was analyzed or data were available for only one generation.
Some of the families classified as Li-Fraumeni or Li-Fraumeni variant that lack a *TP53* germline mutation have been reported to carry a heterozygous *hCHK2* germline mutation {2576}. This gene codes for a protein involved in G2 checkpoint control which prevents cells with damaged DNA to enter mitosis {2574}.

Gene

The *TP53* gene on chromosome 17p13 has 11 exons that span 20 kb. Exon 1 is non-coding, and exons 5 to 8 are remarkably conserved among vertebrates.

TP53 protein

The *TP53* gene encodes a 2.8 kb transcript encoding a 393 amino-acid protein which is widely expressed at low levels. This protein is a multi-functional transcription factor involved in the control of cell cycle progression, of DNA integrity and of the survival of cells exposed to DNA-damaging agents as well as several non-genotoxic stimuli such as hypoxia. DNA damage or hypoxia induces a transient nuclear accumulation and activation of the TP53 protein, with transcriptional activation of target genes that are responsible for induction of cell cycle arrest or apoptosis {789, 883}. A number of these properties are consistent with a tumour suppressor function (Fig.14.29).
TP53 mutant proteins differ from each other in the extent to which they have lost suppressor function and in their capacity to inhibit wild-type TP53 in a dominant-negative manner {422}. In addition, some TP53 mutants appear to exert an oncogenic activity of their own, but the molecular basis of this gain-of-function phenotype is still unclear. The functional characteris-

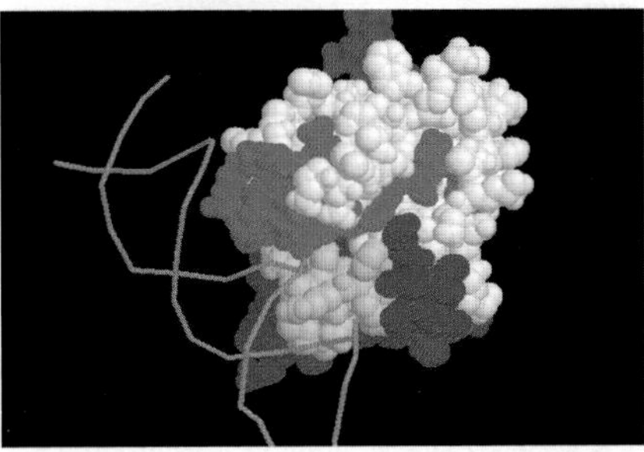

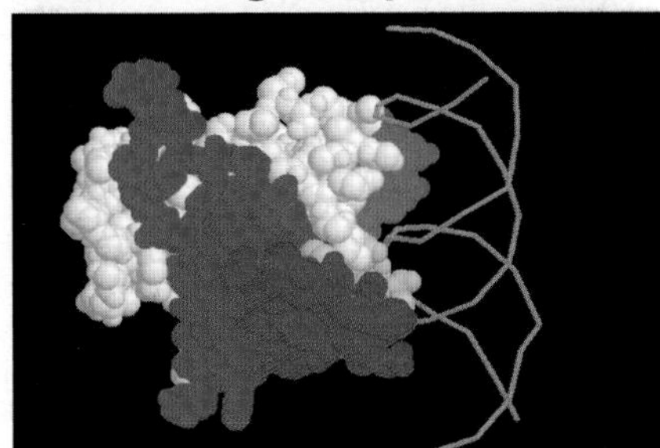

	Residues	Germline mutations	Somatic mutations
Domain I	164–194	11.2 %	16.3 %
Domain II	195–236	14.7 %	13.1 %
Domain III	237–249	25.2%	19.1 %
Domain IV	267–286	15.4 %	19.3 %

Fig.14.28 Models of the crystal structure of TP53 protein in complex with DNA. The distribution of somatic and germline mutations is similar in the four domains shown, with the exception of an excess of germline mutations in domain three. Protein structure data are from Cho *et al.* {236}.

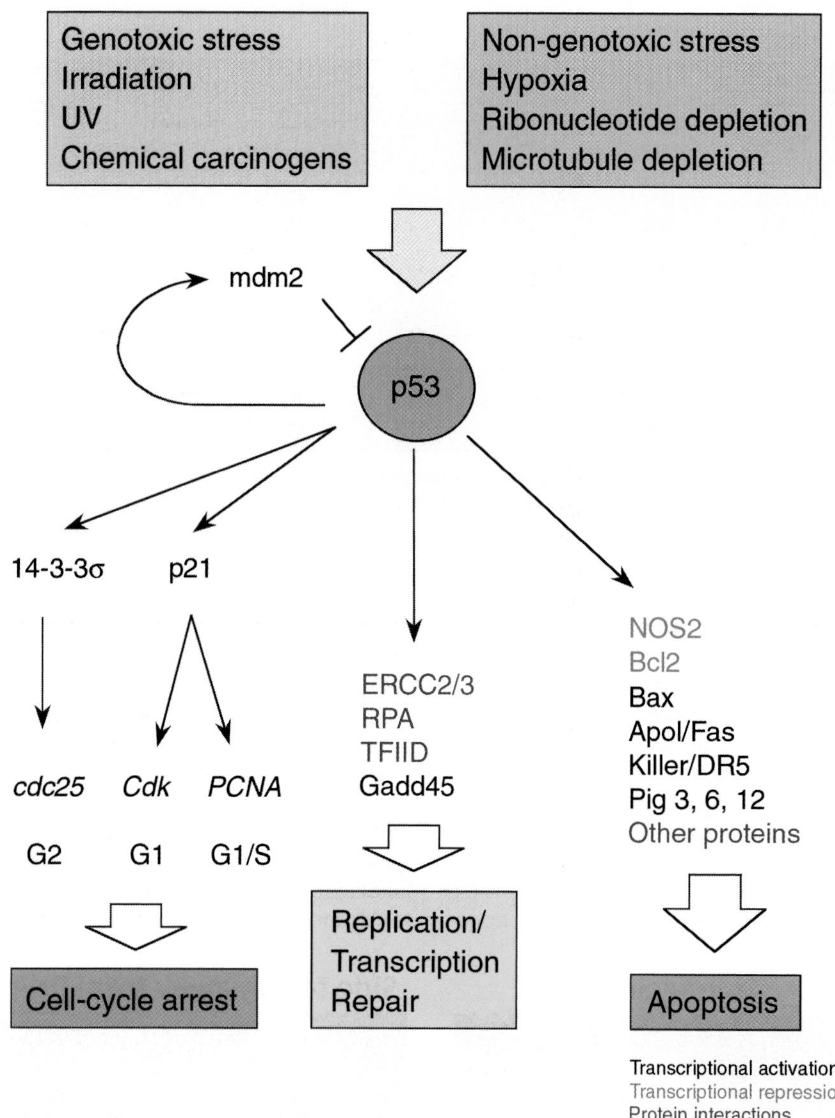

Fig. 14.29 A general view of the TP53 signalling pathway. The TP53 protein is activated and stabilised in response to several genotoxic and non-genotoxic forms of stress. Active TP53 acts on downstream effectors through transcriptional repression and protein-protein interactions. Several effectors of of TP53 are involved in the control of cell cycle progression in G1/S and in G2, in DNA replication, transcription and repair, and in the regulation of apoptosis. Together, this set of celular responses allows TP53 to act as an antiproliferative agent in cells exposed to various forms of stress. MDM2 is a transcriptional target of TP53 involved in a negative, feedback loop to control TP53 levels and activity. The extent and consequences of the biological response elicited by TP53 vary according to stress and cell type.

tics of each mutant TP53 protein may depend, at least in part, on the degree of structural perturbation that the mutation imposes on the protein.

Gene mutations

As with somatic *TP53* mutations {504}, *TP53* germline mutations are located in highly conserved regions of exons 5 to 8, with major hotspots at codons 175, 248, and 273. However, for germline mutations, there seems to be a preference for codons 245 and 248 (Fig. 14.27). Although most mutations at codons 248 and 273 may have a relatively mild phenotype, the substitution of Arg for His at codon 175 has been shown to have a strong dominant-negative phenotype in several experimental systems {1110}. This suggests that potential dominant-negative mutations may remain silent in normal cells for a long time and that expression of this phenotype is dependent upon a specific cellular context. The molecular architecture of the DNA-binding domain of TP53 consists of a scaffold of two beta-sheets that supports two distinct, flexible domains made up of non-contiguous loops and helixes that are in direct contact with DNA {236}. The distribution of mutations among these four domains is similar for both germline and somatic mutations, the only difference being an excess of mutations within domain 3 in germline mutations (Fig. 14.28). Three mutations, Cys 176, His 179 and Arg 249, which are commonly mutated in tumours with somatic *TP53* mutations, were not found in tumours associated with *TP53* germline mutations. Residues 176 (Cys) and 179 (His) are involved in the coordination of a zinc atom that forms a bridge between domain 1 and domain 3, and which is crucial in stabilizing the architecture of the whole DNA-binding domain. Residue 249 (Arg) makes essential contacts with several residues of the scaffold through hydrogen bridges {236}. These substitutions may thus result in mutant TP53 proteins that are not tolerated when present in the germline.

In the 143 families reported, point mutations (85.3%) are most frequent, followed by deletions (9.1%), splice mutations (3.5%) and insertions (2.1%). Among the point mutations, G:C->A:T transitions at CpG sites prevail (Table 14.11). A similar pattern is observed in sporadic brain tumours and in those associated with *TP53* germline mutations. The G:C->A:T transitions at CpG sites are considered to be endogenous, e.g., formed as a result of deamination of 5-methylcytosine, which occurs spontaneously in almost all cell types but which is usually corrected by DNA repair mechanisms {526}.

Cowden disease and dysplastic gangliocytoma of the cerebellum / Lhermitte-Duclos disease

O.D. Wiestler
G.W. Padberg
P.A. Steck

Definition

Cowden disease (CD) is an autosomal dominant condition that causes a variety of hamartomas and neoplasms. Dysplastic gangliocytoma of the cerebellum (Lhermitte-Duclos disease) is the major CNS manifestation. Peripheral lesions include verrucous skin changes, cobblestone-like papules and fibromas of the oral mucosa, multiple facial trichilemmomas, hamartomatous polyps of the colon, thyroid neoplasms, and breast cancer. The syndrome is frequently caused by a germline mutation of the *PTEN/MMAC1* gene.

MIM No. 158350 {978}.

Synonyms and historical annotation

The condition was originally described in 1963 by Lloyd & Dennis in the family of Rachel Cowden {906}. Weary *et al.* {1589} gave a more detailed description of clinical features and proposed the term multiple hamartoma syndrome.

Incidence

Reliable incidence figures for this rare disease are not available, as some patients show only mild mucocutaneous changes. A large number of small families have been reported, suggesting that the syndrome frequently arises from *de novo* mutations. This may obscure the hereditary pattern and, therefore, the proper diagnosis of Cowden disease.

Diagnostic criteria and clinical features

More than 100 patients with Cowden disease have been reported. Clinical manifestations of the disease include combinations of multiple trichilemmomas, i.e. benign skin appendage tumours, oral papillomatosis, cutaneous keratoses, gastrointestinal polyps, hamartomatous soft tissue lesions, thyroid tumours and both benign breast tumours and breast cancer {164, 461, 535, 1449, 1589}. At least one of the mucocutaneous manifestations can usually be found in carriers of the gene mutation. The incidence of trichilemmomas is approximately 85%, while 70% of those affected have thyroid disorders, 40 % have gastrointestinal polyps, and approximately 30% have breast cancer {536}. Breast carcinomas represent a major risk for females afflicted with Cowden disease {1577,1621}.

Dysplastic gangliocytoma of the cerebellum (Lhermitte-Duclos disease)

Definition

A benign cerebellar mass manifesting predominantly in young adults and composed of dysplastic ganglion cells.

ICD-O code:

The provisional code proposed for the third edition of ICD-O is 9493/0.

Grading

This lesion corresponds histologically to WHO grade I.

Synonyms and historical annotation

Dysplastic gangliocytoma of the cerebellum was first described in 1920 by Lhermitte and Duclos {888} and by Spiegel {1445}. The disease has also been termed cerebellar granule cell hypertrophy, diffuse hypertrophy of the cerebellar cortex and gangliomatosis of the cerebellum. More than 60 patients have been reported since. However, the association of Cowden disease with dysplastic gangliocytoma of the cerebellum has only recently been recognized {18, 374, 1120, 1553, 1556, 1604}. In a systematic survey of 72 reported cases of Lhermitte-Duclos disease, Vinchon *et al.* found evidence for Cowden disease in almost half of the patients {1553}.

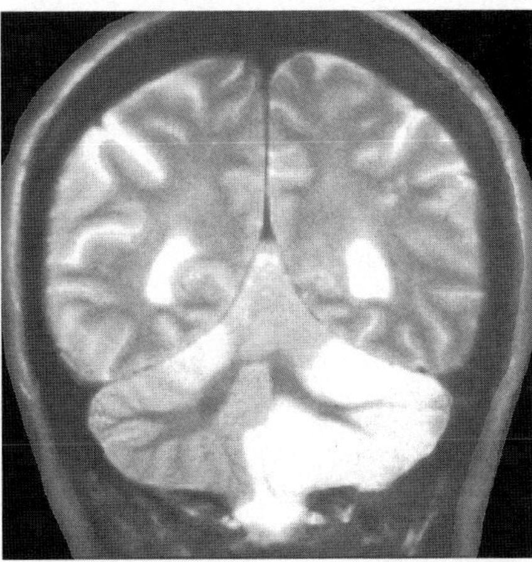

Fig. 14.30 T2-weighted MRI showing the characteristic broadening of the cerebellar cortex (hyperintense signal) on the right side, with a smaller focus in the left cerebellar hemisphere (from Sonier *et al.* {1437}).

Clinical features

Signs and symptoms. Lhermitte-Duclos disease presents as a cerebellar mass lesion, frequently associated with symptoms of ataxia and raised intracranial pressure. Variable periods of preoperative symptoms have been noted, with a mean interval of approximately 40 months {1553}. In a series published by Ambler *et al.* {30}, the average age at diagnosis was 34 years, with a broad range between the neonatal period and 74 years. As cerebellar lesions may develop before the appearance of other features of Cowden disease, patients with Lhermitte-Duclos should be monitored for the development of additional signs, including breast cancer in females.

Neuroimaging. Neuroradiological studies demonstrate a distorted architecture of the affected cerebellar hemisphere with enlarged cerebellar folia and cystic changes in some cases; MRI is particularly sensitive in depicting the enlarged folia {1002}.

Macroscopy

The affected cerebellum displays diffuse hypertrophy and a coarse gyral pattern that extends into deeper layers. Usually, the gangliocytoma is confined to one hemisphere.

Histopathology

A diffuse enlargement of a portion of the cerebellum, characterized by large neuronal cells that expand the granular and molecular layers.

The dysplastic gangliocytoma shows characteristic changes of the cerebellar architecture. The regular granular cell and Purkinje cell layers of the cerebellar cortex

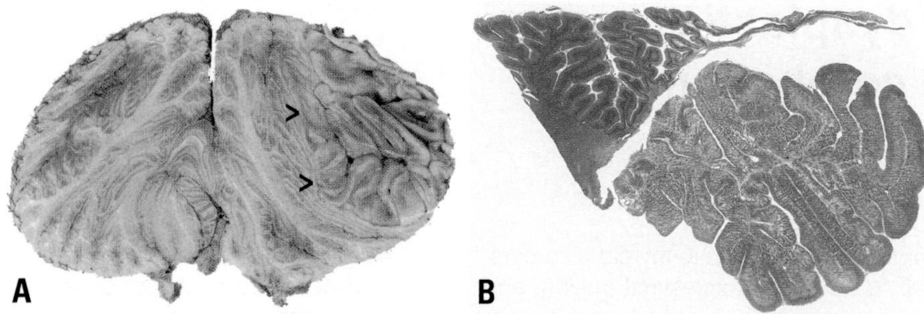

Fig. 14.31 **A** Macroscopic aspect of Llhermitte-Duclos disease (arrows). Note the well-delineated enlargement and coarsening of the cerebellar foliae. **B** Low-power view showing moderate distortion of the cerebellar cortex.

are replaced by an outer layer of abnormally myelinated axon bundles in parallel arrays, and by a widened inner layer composed of an accumulation of dysplastic and disorganized neurons. The resulting structure of these dysmorphic cerebellar folia has been referred to as inverted cerebellar cortex. Two populations of neurons can be distinguished in dysplastic gangliocytomas. A prominent component of small neuronal elements with hyperchromatic nuclei is usually predominant, whereas large polygonal neurons with prominent nucleoli occur in smaller numbers. In addition, abnormal subarachnoid vasculature may be observed, as well as calcification within the lesion.

Immunohistochemistry

Antibodies to synaptophysin can be used to demonstrate axosomatic synapses on a subpopulation of affected neurons. Antineurofilament reactions illustrate bundles of extended neurites in the outer layer of dysplastic folia. Antibodies to the Purkinje cell antigens Leu-4, L7, PEP19 and calbindin have been used to determine the cell of origin in dysplastic gangliocytomas {528, 1411}. These antibodies labelled a minor subpopulation of large atypical ganglion cells, but did not react with the majority of the neuronal elements. This indicates that only a small fraction of neurons are derived from a Purkinje cell source.

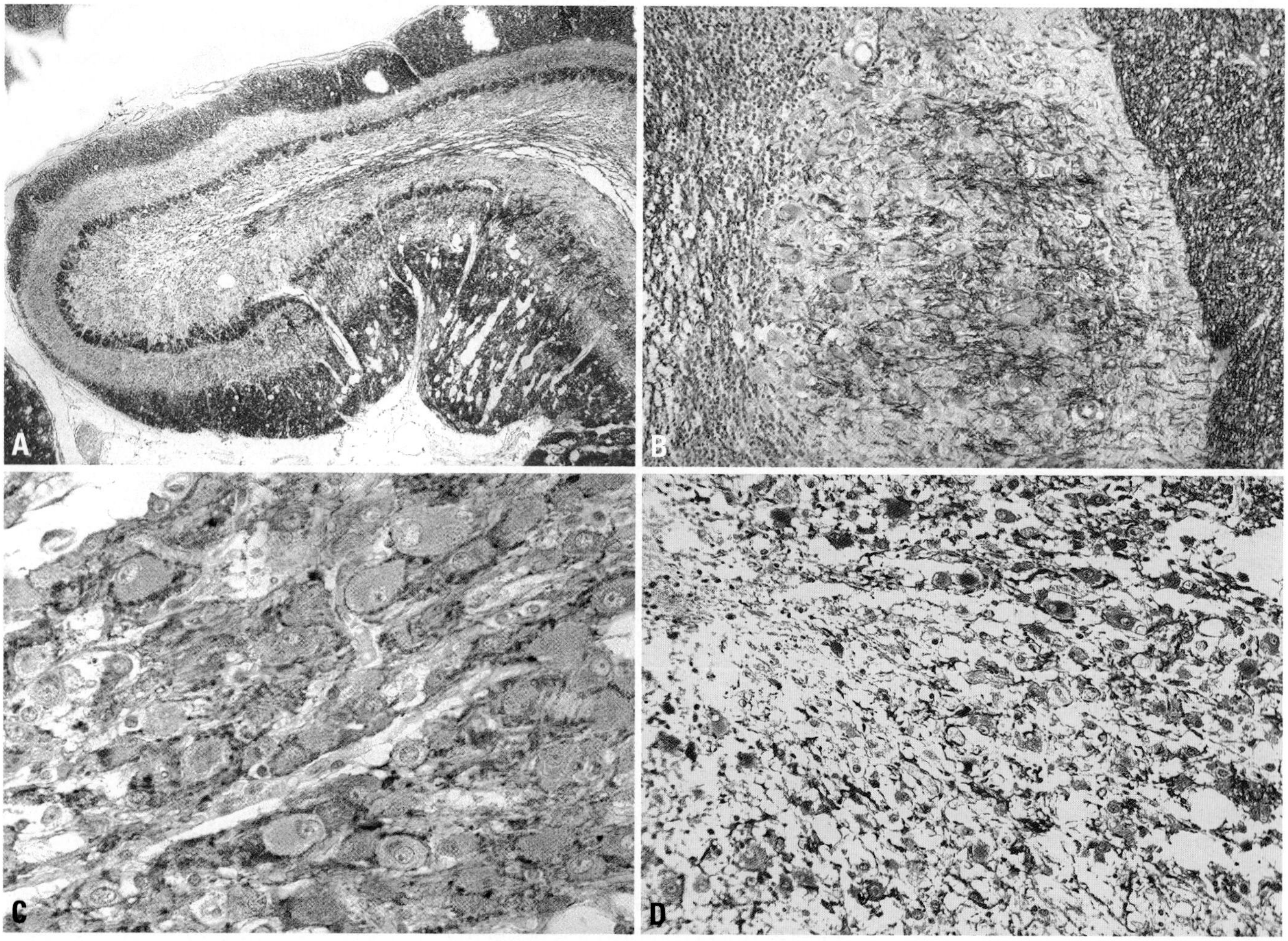

Fig. 14. 32 **A** Low magnification showing the anatomical rearrangement of the cerebellar cortex: the granular cell and Purkinje cell layers of the cerebellar cortex are, to a variable extent, replaced by an outer layer of abnormally myelinated axon bundles in parallel arrays, and by a widened inner layer of dysplastic neurons. **B** Junction between normal and dysplastic cerebellar cortex. **C** Marked synaptophysin immunostaining of dysplastic neurons, predominantly at the cytoplasmic membrane. **D** Neurofilament staining of dysplastic neurons.

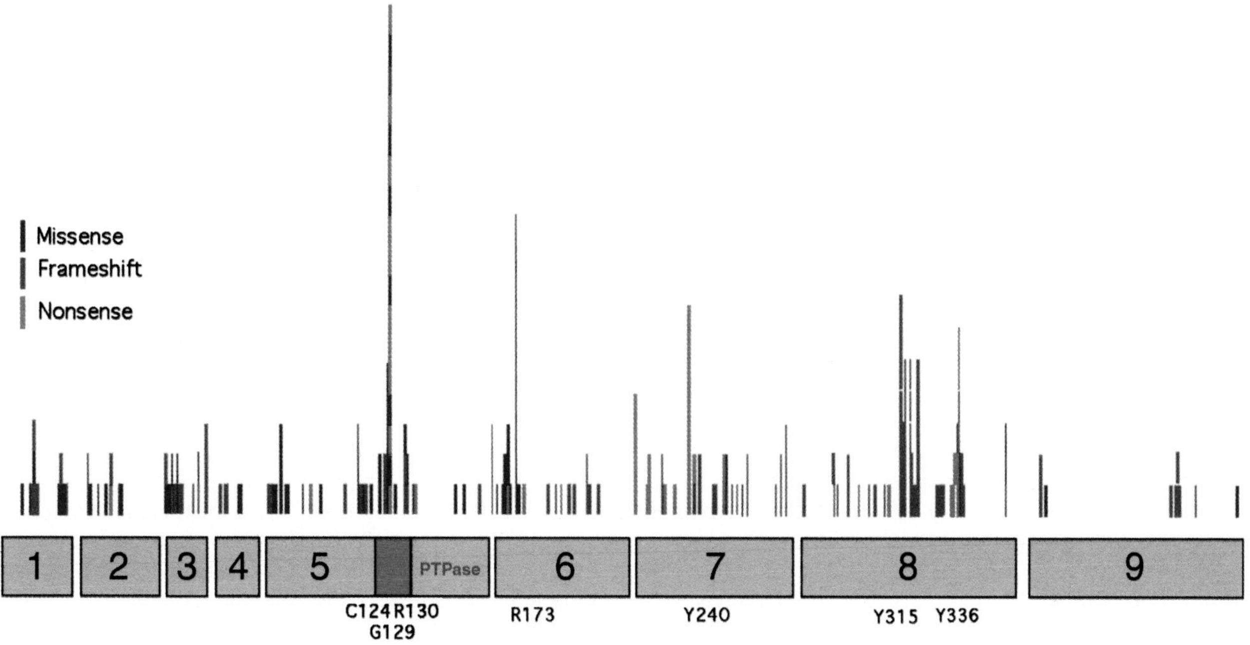

Fig. 14.33 Survey of germline and sporadic mutations detected in the *PTEN/MMAC1* gene. Mutational hot spots can be recognized in the phosphatase domain of exon 5 and a putative regulatory site in exon 8.

Proliferation

Undetectable or very low proliferative activity have been reported in the few cases analyzed with proliferation markers {528}.

Histogenesis

It remains unclear whether Lhermitte-Duclos is hamartomatous or neoplastic in nature. Malformative histopathological features, a very low proliferative activity and the absence of progression support a classification as hamartoma. However, recurrent growth has occasionally been noted and dysplastic gangliocytomas may develop in adult patients with previously normal MRI scans {528, 956}. The histogenesis and cellular origin of these unusual lesions are also a matter of debate. There is some evidence from ultrastructural and immunohistochemical studies that the larger cell type is derived from Purkinje cells. The predominating smaller class of dysplastic ganglion cells appears to originate from granular neurons of the cerebellum {528}.

Other CNS manifestations of Cowden disease

Additional cerebral manifestations include megalencephaly in 20-70% of cases, as well as heterotopic grey matter, hydrocephalus, mental retardation and seizures {536, 1120}. Few examples of meningiomas {929, 1589} and medulloblastomas {54} have been documented in individual cases of Cowden disease, but a specific association of these tumour entities with Cowden disease remains to be shown.

Genetics

This syndrome follows an autosomal dominant mode of inheritance with high penetrance in both sexes. Genetic anticipation in successive generations has been suggested, but there is insufficient information available to confirm this hypothesis {536}. Cowden disease is closely related to other inherited hamartoma syndromes {2156} such as the Bannayan-Zonana Syndrome (BZS [MIM 153480]). Characteristic features of BZS include macrocephaly, other CNS abnormalities associated with mild to severe mental retardation and seizures, and hamartomas. Both, Cowden disease (CD) and BZS appear to be caused by germline mutations of the *PTEN/MMAC1* gene {2157}.

Gene structure

The gene involved in Cowden disease, *PTEN/MMAC1*, is located at chromosome 10q23 {893, 1064, 1451, 1773}, contains 9 exons and has a coding sequence of approximately 3 kb {1451, 1611}.

Gene expression and function

The *PTEN/MMAC1* gene is widely expressed at relatively high levels {1451, 1611}. *PTEN/MMAC1* encodes a 403 amino acid protein that bears structural similarity to dual specificity protein phosphatases. Subsequent studies have documented that PTEN/MMAC1 serves as a major regulator of the phosphatidylinositol 3' kinase (PI3K) pathway by mediating the presence of a phosphate residue on the 3' position of phosphatidylinositol phosphates {1774}. The PI3K pathway is involved in a number of cellular functions including growth control, survival, migration, and calcium fluxes {2158}.

Gene mutations

Germline mutations of *PTEN/MMAC1* have been detected in four of five Cowden families, one of which also presented with Lhermitte-Duclos disease {895}. These mutations preferentially target the catalytic phosphatase motif (HCxxGxxRT) at amino acids 123-131, along with truncations involving the C-terminal portion of PTEN/MMAC1, suggesting that the phosphatase activity and a potential regulatory region at the C-terminus are of critical importance for the function of the protein. Mutations in *PTEN/MMAC1* are also observed in a number of sporadic cancers, including glioblastoma, breast, prostate, endometrial, thyroid, renal, bladder carcinoma, and melanoma. With the exception of endometrial cancer, the majority of sporadic mutations are found in the advanced forms of these cancers, suggesting that a loss of function of PTEN/MMAC1 is involved in tumour progression {893, 1451, 2155}.

Turcot syndrome

W.K. Cavenee
P.C. Burger
E.G. van Meir

Definition
Autosomal dominant disorders {2267} characterized by adenomatous colorectal polyps or colon carcinomas and by malignant neuroepithelial tumours, usually medulloblastomas or glioblastomas. Most cases of Turcot syndrome occur in the setting of the familial adenomatous polyposis (FAP) or hereditary non-polyposis colorectal carcinoma (HNPCC) syndromes.

MIM No. 276300 {978}.

Incidence
Approximately 160 cases of Turcot syndrome have been reported since 1949.

Diagnostic criteria
Turcot syndrome is heterogeneous, encompassing at least two syndromes {1130}. Turcot syndrome type 1 consists of glioblastoma in patients without FAP, some of whom have HNPCC and germline mutations of DNA mismatch repair genes such as *hPMS2, hMSH2* or *hMLH1*. Turcot syndrome type 2 consists of medulloblastoma in patients with FAP and germline mutations of the *APC* gene.

Nervous system neoplasms
Medulloblastoma, glioblastoma and anaplastic astrocytoma account for about 95% of brain tumours reported {1130}. Glioblastomas in Turcot syndrome generally occur in a younger age group than sporadic glioblastomas {2267}. It is unclear whether other patients with colonic polyposis and other CNS tumours (lymphoma, pituitary adenoma, meningioma, craniopharyngioma, ependymoma, cervical spinal astrocytoma, oligodendroglioma) are part of the heterogeneity.

Extraneural manifestations
There are two major variants of colorectal manifestations. Turcot type 1 presents with small numbers of large polyps and patients develop colorectal cancer at a young age in 56% of cases. Type 2 presents with innumerable adenomatous polyps and 21% of such cases will develop colorectal cancer. Skin lesions occur in approximately 50% of type 1 and 20% of type 2 Turcot patients. Café-au-lait spots occur in 38% of type 1 patients. Craniofacial exostosis and congenital hypertrophic retinal pigmented epithelium occur in a minority of patients.

Genetics
Genetic heterogeneity
The association of neuroepithelial neoplasms with colorectal polyps was first noted by Crail {286} and genetic predisposition was later suggested by Turcot {1524}. Lewis {885} proposed three groups: type (I) those with two or more siblings with multiple colonic polyps and a malignant brain tumour, with neither the parents nor other generations being affected; type (II) affected individuals having an autosomal dominant colonic polyposis and with polyps occurring in several generations of their family; and, type (III) isolated non-familial cases. This led to the proposal that Turcot syndrome was sometimes a variant of the FAP syndrome. Lasser {862} demonstrated genetic linkage to *APC*, the gene responsible for FAP, in a Turcot syndrome family with medulloblastomas. This was followed by the identification of germline *APC* mutations in three unrelated cases of Turcot syndrome {1033}, two of which presented with medulloblastoma, the other with a malignant astrocytoma. Hamilton {533} analyzed 14 Turcot syndrome families and found that 10 of the 14 families had germline *APC* mutations and that the predominant tumour was medulloblastoma.

Molecular genetics of mismatch repair associated Turcot syndrome (type 1)
Mismatch repair-associated Turcot syndrome is characterized by an inherited DNA replication error defect that leads to genomic instability. Several genes are now known to encode proteins involved in this process: *hMLH1* at chromosome 3p21, *hMSH2* at 2p16, *hMSH3* at 5q11-q13, *hMSH6/GTBP* at 2p16, *hPMS1* at 2q32 and *hPMS2* at 7p22.
Gene structure. The *hMLH1* gene resides at chromosome 3p21.3, where its 19 coding exons span 100 kb of DNA. It encodes an 85 kDa protein, which is part of the complex responsible for strand-specific DNA mismatch repair. The *hPMS2* gene at chromosome 7p22 has 15 coding exons encompassing 16 kb of DNA and encodes a 100 kDa protein that interacts with hMLH1 in the mismatch repair complex. The *hMSH2* gene resides at chromosome 2p22-p21, where its 16 coding exons span 73 kb of DNA. Its encoded product complexes with the hMSH6 protein to form a sliding clamp on DNA that recognizes mismatches.
Gene expression. Recognition and repair of basepair mismatches in human DNA is mainly mediated by heterodimers of hMSH2 and hMSH6. Cells that are deficient for hMSH2 or hMSH6 expression are defective in repair of mispaired bases and insertions/deletions of single nucleotides resulting in high mutation rates and microsatellite instability. The carboxy-terminal region of hPMS2 interacts with hMLH1 and this complex binds to hMSH2/hMSH6 heterodimers to form a functional mispair recognition complex. Substitution of hMSH3 for hMSH6 in this tetramer shifts its recognition of single base mispairs to insertion/deletion mispairs in yeast. Most HNPCC families have either *hMSH2* or *hMLH1* mutations. Interestingly, replication-error-driven microsatellite instability is rare in brain tumours in the absence of Turcot syndrome {2264, 2268}, although reduced expression of hMSH2, hMLH1 and hPMS1 in malignant astrocytomas has been reported {2266}. Screening for lack of expression of mismatch repair genes is possible by immunohistochemistry {2580}.
Gene mutations. So far, genetic alterations have been found in the germlines of Turcot syndrome families in *hPMS2* (three cases), *hMSH2* (three cases) and *hMLH1* (one case) {533, 2264, 2265}. The tumours found in these patients showed evidence of replication errors that lead to genomic instability. This mutator phenotype induces somatic mutations in gatekeeper genes *TP53* and *APC* in the tumours of these

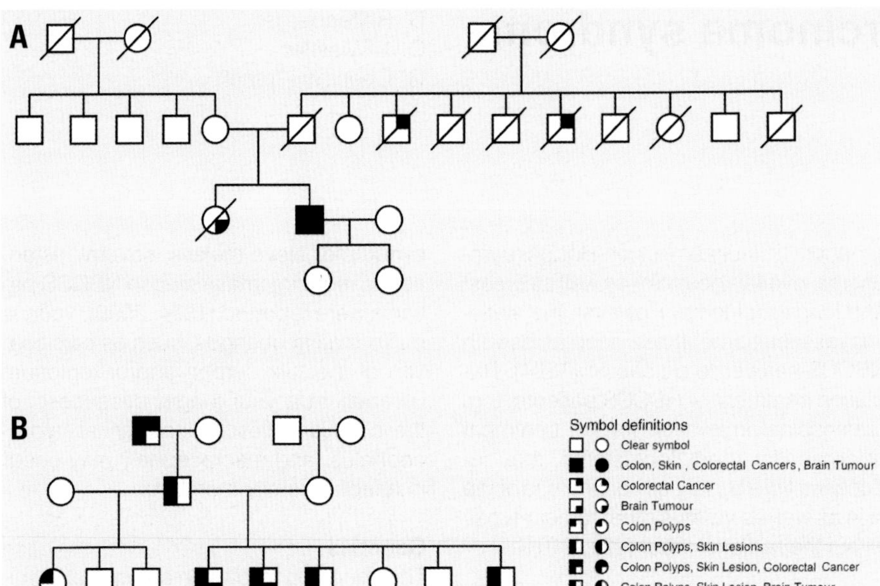

Fig. 14.34 Typical pedigrees of Turcot families. **A** Turcot type 1 (non-polyposis colon cancer and predominantly glioblastomas, frequently associated with mutations in DNA mismatch reair genes). **B** Turcot type 2, characterized by familial adenomatous polyposis, colon carcinomas, and medulloblastomas, caused by a *APC* germline mutation.

patients {2265}. Notably, these families each had astrocytoma or glioblastoma as the inclusive brain tumour.

Molecular genetics of FAP-associated Turcot syndrome (type 2)

The gene responsible for FAP-associated Turcot syndrome lies on chromosome 5q21.

Gene structure. The *APC* gene has an 8538 base-pair coding sequence, divided into 15 exons.

Gene expression. The *APC* gene encodes an ubiquitously expressed protein of about 300 kDa which interacts with the beta-catenin protein and mediates its degradation. Beta-catenin links the cytoplasmic tail of the cell-cell homotypic adhesion molecule cadherin to the actin cytoskeleton. Alteration of APC function may modify the movement/adhesion of epithelial stem cells in the colonic crypt. It is unclear whether it fulfils a similar function for cerebellar precursor cells, and in the absence of Turcot syndrome, the *APC* gene is rarely mutated in sporadic brain tumours { 533, 862}. About 10% of sporadic medulloblastomas show loss of heterozygosity or mutations in the beta-catenin gene {1928} and *APC* missense point mutations occur in less than 5% of cases {2552}. Beta-catenin has a role in signalling mediated by the nuclear translocation of transcription factors of the lymphoid enhancing factor (LEF-1) family. The loss of the *APC* gene product results in increased binding of beta-catenin to LEF-1 and an increase in the transcription of cyclin D1 and other genes which have not yet been characterized. Increased cyclin D1 expression then promotes cell division.

Gene mutations. A recent survey reported truncating germline *APC* mutations in all but one family with FAP-associated Turcot syndrome {1130}. The final family examined by Hamilton showed no mutations in the *APC* gene and had no evidence for DNA replication errors. Thus, there remains a fraction of Turcot families in which the disease has other underlying causes, adding to the aetiological heterogeneity of the syndrome. The association of brain tumours and colon cancer can also occur in the setting of germline *TP53* mutations {844}.

Prognostic factors

A recent survey established that the median age for occurrence of glioblastoma in Turcot syndrome type 1 was 18 years while the peak incidence in the general population is 40-70 years of age {2267}. These patients showed an average survival of over 27 months, which is remarkably longer than the 12 month survival for sporadic cases. In Turcot type 2, the median age for occurrence of medulloblastomas was 15 years which is later than the peak occurrence for sporadic medulloblastoma (7 years of age). In FAP families, the appearance of medulloblastoma at young age in patients having no evidence of polyps is of poor prognosis {2267}.

Naevoid basal cell carcinoma syndrome

G. Reifenberger
O.D. Wiestler
G. Chenevix-Trench

Definition
Naevoid basal cell carcinoma syndrome (NBCCS) is an autosomal dominant disease associated with a wide spectrum of developmental anomalies and a predisposition for benign and malignant neoplasms. The major clinical manifestations are multiple basal cell carcinomas of the skin, odontogenic keratocysts, and palmar and plantar dyskeratotic pits. CNS manifestations include intracranial calcifications, macrocephaly, and medulloblastoma. The syndrome is typically caused by a germline mutation of the *PTCH* gene.

MIM No. 109400 {978}.

Synonyms
Basal cell nevus syndrome; Gorlin-Goltz syndrome; Gorlin syndrome; fifth phacomatosis.

Incidence
A population-based study in the UK reported a prevalence of 1 case per 57.000 population {384}. Approximately 5% of mutation carriers develop medulloblastoma, while the prevalence of NBCCS in 173 consecutive cases of medulloblastoma was found to be 1-2 % {384}.

Diagnostic and clinical features
The key manifestations of NBCCS are multiple basal cell carcinomas and jaw keratocysts developing during the first decades of life {492, 1394, 2093}. A detailed analysis of 84 patients {386} found that both features were present in more than 90% of affected individuals by the age of 40 years. A significantly increased incidence of intracranial calcifications (most commonly calcification of the falx cerebri), palmar and plantar pits, abnormal ribs and other skeletal malformations, epidermal cysts, and ovarian fibromas has also been observed {386, 492, 1394, 2096}. Less common clinical signs include ophthalmic abnormalities, cleft palate, dysgenesis of the corpus callosum, and cardiac fibroma. Several other tumour types have been reported in individual NBCCS patients, including meningioma, melanoma, chronic lymphocytic leukaemia, non-Hodgkin lymphoma, ovarian dermoid, as well as breast and lung carcinoma. However, the statistical association of these neoplasms with NBCCS has yet to be shown {1394}. Radiation treatment of NBCCS patients, e.g. craniospinal irradiation for the treatment of cerebellar medulloblastoma, may induce multiple basal cell carcinomas of the skin as well as various other tumour types within the radiation field {221, 2101}.

NBCCS-associated medulloblastoma
At least 40 cases of medulloblastoma associated with NBCCS have been reported {384}. The majority of these tumours develop during the first three years of life and there is some evidence for a more favourable outcome of this rare group of medulloblastoma patients. The medulloblastomas in NBCCS patients have microscopic and immunohistochemical features that are identical to sporadic medulloblastomas. However, the majority of NBCCS associated medulloblastomas correspond to the desmoplastic variant (see Chapter 8) of medulloblastoma {1372}.

Other CNS manifestations
There is no statistically proven evidence for an increased risk of other CNS neoplasms in naevoid basal cell carcinoma syndrome. Nevertheless, several instances of meningioma arising in NBCCS patients were reported {1394, 2090}. Various malformative changes, such as calcification of the falx cerebri and/or tentorium cerebelli at a young age, dysgenesis of the corpus callosum, congenital hydrocephalus, and macrocephaly may occur in affected family members.

Genetics
The condition follows an autosomal dominant pattern of inheritance, with full penetrance but variable clinical expression. It has been estimated that at least 40% of the cases represent new mutations {2093, 1394}. Other investigators reported a considerably lower percentage of patients without a positive family history {386}.

Molecular genetics
NBCCS results from germline mutations in the human homologue of the Drosophila segment polarity gene patched (*PTCH*) {524, 705}. The *PTCH* gene maps to chromosome band 9q22.3 {705}.

Gene structure
The *PTCH* gene has at least 23 exons and spans approximately 34 kb of genomic distance {524, 705}.

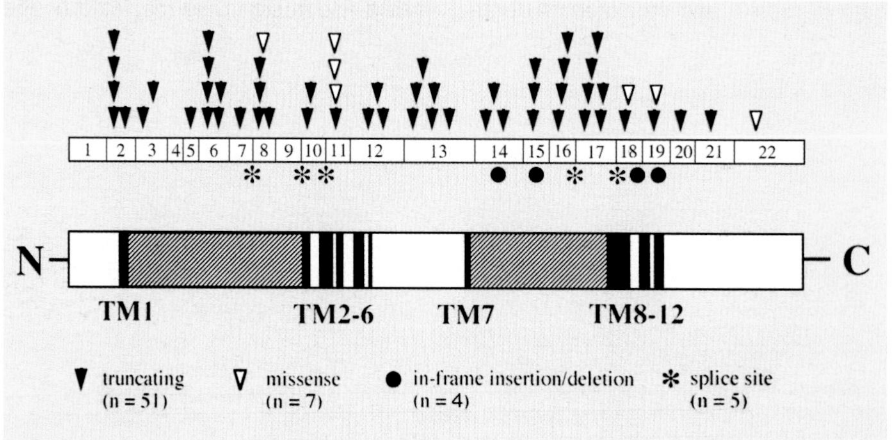

Fig. 14.35 Graphical presentation of 67 *PTCH* germline mutations associated with NBCCS. Note that more than 70% of the mutations are frameshift or nonsense mutations resulting in protein truncations. There are no mutational hot-spots. Modified, from Wicking *et al.* {1618}.

Gene expression

The *PTCH* gene codes for a multipass transmembrane protein (Ptch) that functions as receptor for members of the secreted hedgehog protein family of signalling molecules {960, 1460}. In humans, this family consists of three members designated as Sonic hedgehog (Shh), Indian hedgehog (Ihh), and Desert hedgehog (Dhh). The *PTCH* gene product forms a complex with another transmembrane protein, the human homologue of the Drosophila smoothened protein (Smoh) {1460, 2091}. In the absence of ligand, Ptch inhibits the activity of Smoh {1460, 2091}. Binding of hedgehog proteins to Ptch can relieve this inhibition of Smoh, which results in signal transduction and transcriptional activation of several genes coding for members of the TGFß, Gli and Wnt protein families, as well as Ptch itself {1460, 2091, 2095}. In Drosophila, the hedgehog signalling pathway is essential for correct segmentation and patterning during embryogenesis. In vertebrates, this pathway is critically involved in the development of various tissues and organ systems, such as limbs, gonads, bone, and CNS {2095, 1898}. Germline mutations in the Sonic hedgehog (*SHH*) and *PTCH* genes were found to cause holoprosencephaly {86, 1271, 2100}.

Gene mutations

So far, 67 different *PTCH* germline mutations associated with NBCCS have been reported {230, 524, 705, 1530, 1618, 2097, 2103, 2094, 2092}. The vast majority of these mutations are frameshift or nonsense mutations leading to the expression of truncated proteins. Mutations are distributed over the entire *PTCH* coding sequence without demonstrating any mutational hot spots and there appears to be no clear genotype-phenotype correlation {1618}. Somatic mutations of *PTCH* have been demonstrated in various sporadic human tumours, including basal cell carcinoma {445, 524, 705, 1634}, trichoepithelioma {2102}, oesophageal squamous cell carcinoma {2098}, invasive transitional cell carcinoma of the bladder {2099}, and medulloblastoma {1174, 1218, 1634, 1923}. Similar to the germline mutations in NBCCS, the vast majority of mutations detected in sporadic tumours result in truncations at the protein level. There is no obvious clustering of mutation sites. One study of 68 sporadic medulloblastomas detected *PTCH* mutations exclusively in the desmoplastic variant, but not in 57 tumours with classical morphology {1174}. In line with these data, LOH analyzes of sporadic medulloblastomas demonstrated frequent allelic loss at 9q22.3-q31 in desmoplastic medulloblastomas (up to 50%), but not in classical medulloblastomas {20, 1372}. These data would be consistent with the observation that medulloblastomas associated with NBCCS are predominantly of the desmoplastic variant. However, other studies also reported *PTCH* mutations in classical medulloblastomas {1218, 1634, 1923}. Recently, a novel *PTCH* homologue (*PTCH2*) has been cloned and mapped to chromosome band 1p32 {1918, 2104}. So far, *PTCH2* germline mutations have not been detected in NBCCS patients but single cases of medulloblastoma and basal cell carcinomas carrying somatic *PTCH2* mutations have been reported {1918}.

CHAPTER 15

Tumours of the Sellar Region

A variety of neoplasms arising from the skull base may affect the CNS, mainly by expansion, causing optic nerve and hypothalamic symptoms. Most frequent are pituitary adenomas, which are traditionally not grouped together with CNS tumours. Other, less frequent lesions in this region include granular cell tumours of the pituitary stalk and chordomas.

Craniopharyngioma affects mainly children and young adults. Recent studies indicate that the age distribution and, to some extent, prognosis are different between the adamantinomatous and the papillary variant.

Xanthogranulomas of the sellar region are now recognized as separate entity and not as a result of marked degeneration within an adamantinomatous craniopharyngioma.

Craniopharyngioma

R.C. Janzer
P.C. Burger
F. Giangaspero
W. Paulus

Definition

A benign, partly cystic epithelial tumour of the sellar region presumably derived from Rathke pouch epithelium. Two clinicopathological forms are distinguished, the adamantinomatous and the papillary craniopharyngioma. Xanthogranuloma of the sellar region is a related but distinct clinicopathological entity.

Grading

Craniopharyngiomas correspond histologically to WHO grade I.

ICD-O code: 9350/1

The provisional code proposed for the third edition of ICD-O is for adamantinomatous craniopharyngioma 9351/1 and for papillary craniopharyngioma 9352/1.

Incidence

Craniopharyngiomas account for 1.2% to 4.6% of all intracranial tumours, corresponding to 0.5-2.5 new cases per million population per year {2421}, being more frequent in Japanese children with an annual incidence of 5.25 cases per million in the paediatric population {2422}. They are the most common non-neuroepithelial intracerebral neoplasm in children, accounting for 5-10% of intracranial tumours in this age group {5}.

Age and sex distribution

A bimodal age distribution is observed {2421}, with peaks in children aged 5 - 14 years and adults aged >50 years (Fig. 15.1). Rare neonatal and intrauterine cases have been reported {835}. Papillary craniopharyngiomas occur almost exclusively in adults, at a mean age of 40-45 years {5, 288}, while xanthogranulomas preferentially manifest in adolescents and young adults {2425}. Craniopharyngiomas show no obvious sex predilection.

Localization

The most frequent localization is suprasellar with an intrasellar component. Cases restricted to the suprasellar region represent 20%, while only 5% are entirely intrasellar. They show a significant anterior extension in 30%, into the middle fossa in 23% and a retroclival extension in 20% {547}. Rare ectopic localizations include the optic nerves, the pineal region, sphenoid bone, pharynx and cerebellopontine angle {2429}. The papillary variant usually involves the third ventricle {5, 464, 2426}.

Clinical features

Symptoms and signs

Clinical features are non-specific and essentially include visual disturbances (observed in 62-84% of the patients, more frequently in adults than in children) and endocrine deficiencies (observed in 52-87% of patients, more frequently in children) and are more often associated with papillary craniopharyngioma than with the adamantinomatous type {1660}. Endocrine deficiencies include those for GH (75%), LH/FSH (40%), ACTH (25%) and TSH (25%). Diabetes insipidus is noted in up to 17% of children and up to 30% of adults. Cognitive impairment and personality changes are observed in about half of patients {1660}. Signs of increased intracranial pressure are frequent, especially in cases with compression or invasion of the third ventricle.

Neuroimaging

For adamantinomatous craniopharyngioma, radiography provides a most accurate depiction of the configuration of the sella and the typical calcifications. CTs show contrast enhancement of the solid portions and the cyst capsule, as well as the typical calcifications. On T1-weighted MRI, the cystic areas appear as well delineated homogeneous hyperintense structures, whereas the solid components and mural nodules are iso-intense, with a slightly heterogeneous aspect. In enhanced MRI images, the cystic portion is iso-intense with an enhancing ring, whereas the solid parts are hyperintense {547} (Fig. 15.2). The papillary craniopharyngioma is non-calcified and has a more uniform appearance in CT and MRI images {288, 2426}.

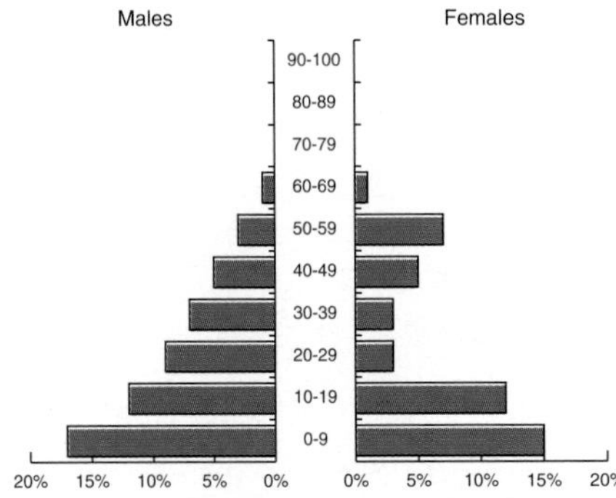

Fig. 15.1 Age and sex distribution of craniopharyngiomas, based on 144 published cases. Data from Adamson *et al.* {5} and Yasargil *et al.* {1660}.

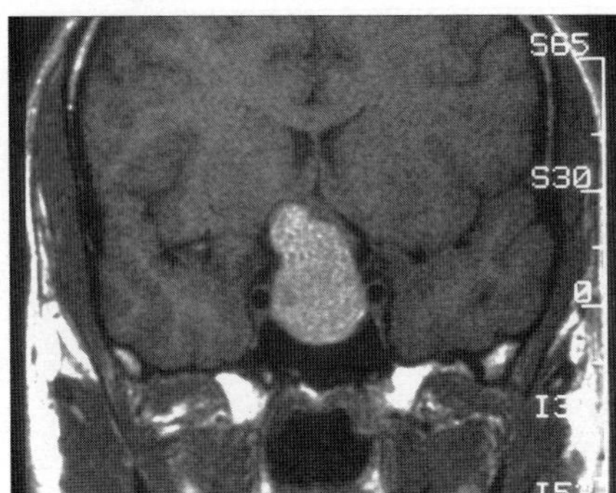

Fig. 15.2 T1-weighted MRI of a suprasellar craniopharyngioma containing a small cyst.

Macroscopy

Craniopharyngiomas are solid tumours with a variable, sometimes predominant cystic component (Fig. 15.4 A). They vary greatly in size and extension, are well delimited, with a smooth surface, but have an irregular lobulated or micronodular outline and are firmly attached to adjacent brain and vascular structures. The adamantinomatous type is frequently calcified (Fig. 15.4 B), the papillary variant only rarely. The cysts of the adamantinomatous type may contain a cholesterol-rich, machine oil-like, thick brownish-yellow fluid, sometimes with crumbly debris. The papillary type lacks the machine oil component.

Histopathology

Adamantinomatous craniopharyngiomas consist of broad strands, cords and bridges of a multistratified squamous epithelium with peripheral palisading of nuclei. Diagnostic features include nodules of compact 'wet' keratin and dystrophic calcification.

The squamous cells are columnar or polygonal at the periphery forming a palisade resting on a basement membrane. Towards the internal layers, the cells become loosely textured and form a spongy "reticulum". The lining of the cysts may have a simpler, sometimes flattened epithelium. Diagnostically relevant is the presence of compact "wet keratin", more nodular than lamellar and with a clearcut tendency to dystrophic calcification. This is in contrast to the flaky, lamellar keratin of epidermoid cysts. However, some authors emphasize that craniopharyngiomas and epidermoid cysts cannot always be distinguished on the basis of histology {2428}. The histopathology closely resembles either ameloblastoma or calcifying odontogenic cyst of the jaw {2424}. Circumscribed areas showing cholesterol clefts, xanthoma cells, fibrosis and chronic inflammation may occur, but they are more typical of the xanthogranuloma (see differential diagnosis).

Papillary craniopharyngioma is composed of sheets of squamous epithelium which separate to form pseudopapillae. This variant typically lacks nuclear palisading, wet keratin, calcification, and cholesterol deposits.

The solid portions do not have the columnar sheet at the periphery and do not typically form a spongy reticulum in the internal layers. The epithelial strands rest on a villous fibrovascular stroma forming papillae. The lining of the cystic parts may be composed of a simple squamous epithelium.

Immunohistochemistry

Craniopharyngiomas express high- and low-molecular weight keratins (Fig. 15.6 B). The biological significance of the reported expression of p-glycoprotein, somatostatin-receptors and oestrogen-receptors is uncertain {1496}.

Growth pattern

Craniopharygiomas are slowly growing tumours and the adjacent brain tissue reacts with an intense gliosis, including extensive formation of Rosenthal fibres. Finger-like protrusions of tumour into the brain parenchyma are characteristic of adamantinomatous craniopharygiomas.

Differential diagnosis

Xanthogranuloma of the sellar region {2425} is histologically composed of cholesterol clefts, macrophages (xanthoma cells), chronic inflammatory cellular reaction, necrotic debris and haemosiderin deposits (Fig. 15.7). Xanthogranulomatous aspects have been considered to be the result of marked degeneration within the adamantinomatous craniopharyngioma. However, recent clinico-pathological data indicate that xanthogranuloma of the sellar region is distinct from adamantinomatous craniopharyngioma with respect to preferential occurrence in adolescents and

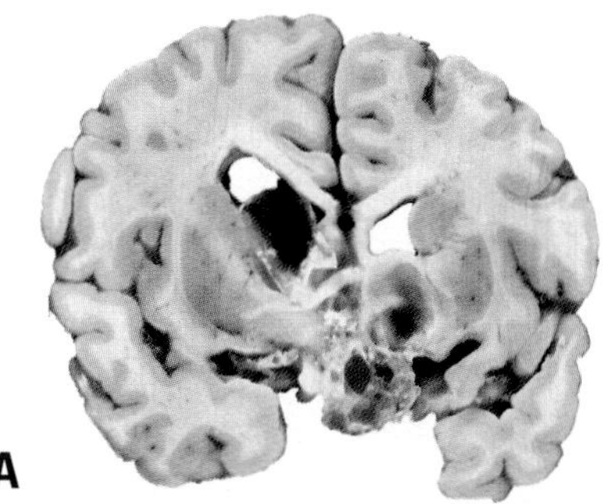
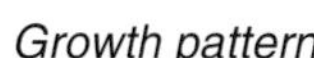

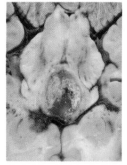

Fig. 15.4 A Cystic craniopharyngioma invading the third ventricle and the basal ganglia. B Adamantinomatous craniopharyngioma extending towards the cerebral peduncles. Note the colloid material and calcifications.

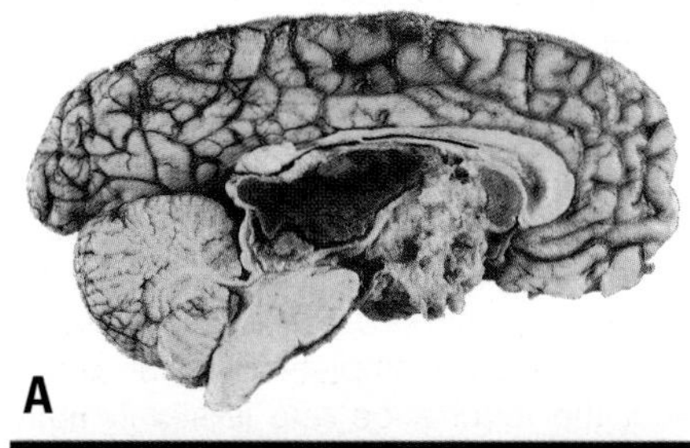
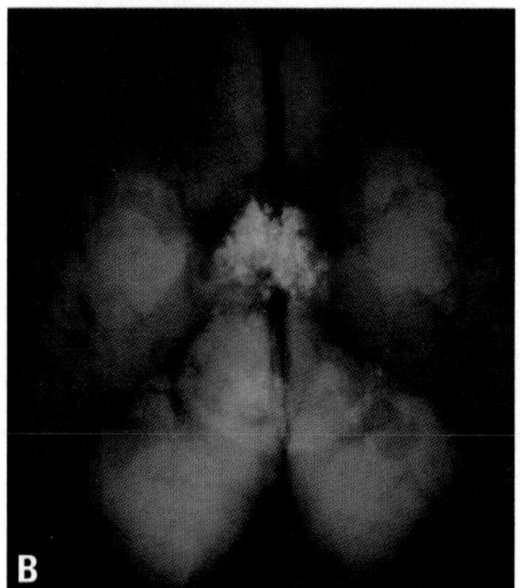

Fig. 15.3 Large adamantinomatous craniopharyngioma extending into the third ventricle. Note the dorsal portion resembling 'machine oil'. Postmortem X-ray showed extensive calcification.

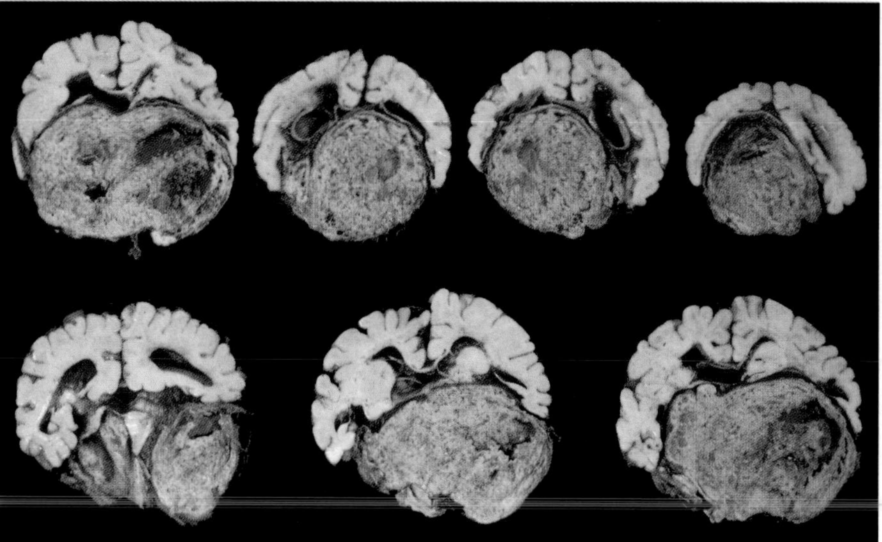

Fig. 15.5 Congenital case of an unusually large, partly cystic craniopharyngioma causing compression and shift of basal brain structures.

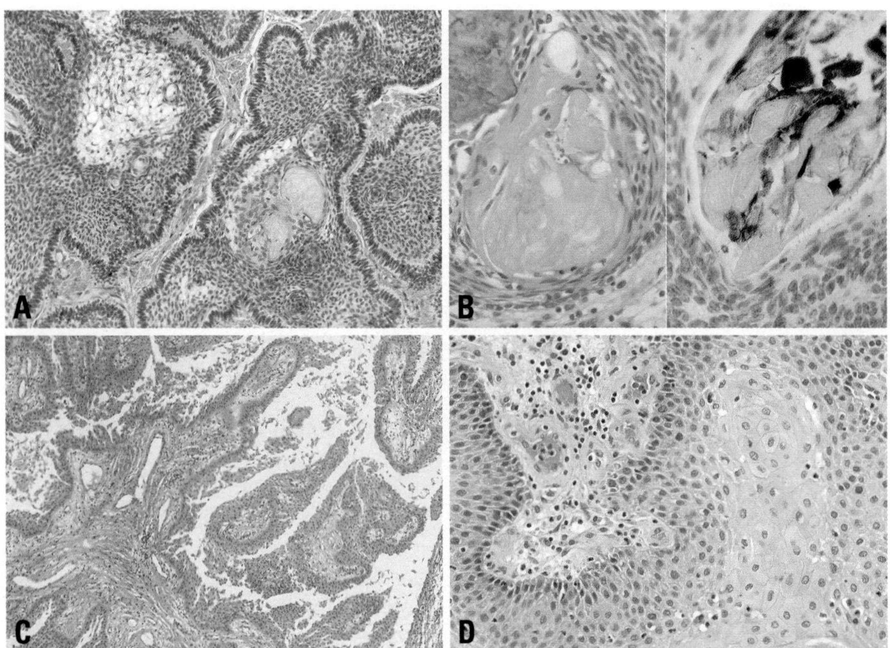

Fig. 15.6 A Adamantinomatous craniopharyngioma with focal keratinization. **B** Higher magnification shows keratin structure (left) and immunoreactivity for cytokeratin (right). **C** Papillary craniopharyngioma with well-differentiated epithelium and (**D**) differentiated squamous epithelium.

young adults, predominant intrasellar localization, smaller tumour size, more severe endocrinological deficits, longer preoperative history, better resectability and a more favourable outcome. Non-adamantinomatous squamous or cuboidal epithelium as well as small tubuli may be focally encountered, while typical adamantinomatous epithelium usually is absent or amounts to less than 10% of tissue {2425}.

Proliferation

In vivo cell kinetic studies with pre-operative intravenous infusion of bromodeoxyuridine (BrdU) {337} and tritiated thymidine {160} indicate a labelling index (LI) of <1% in the first biopsy. Non-recurrent craniopharyngiomas have a MIB-1-LI of 3.4% {2423}. In recurrent tumours a tritiated thymidine LI of 3.3% {160} and a MIB-1 LI of 13.2% {2423} have been reported. Other authors have not established a clear relationship between MIB-1 LI and clinical behaviour {2427}. The proliferating activity is regionally heterogeneous and most marked in the squamous cells lining the cyst walls.

Genetics

There is no known genetic susceptibility. Only one report describes the occurrence of craniopharyngiomas in consanguineous siblings {2420}. Multiple chromosomal abnormalities have been reported in two cases {493, 731}. Both tumours had abnormalities involving chromosomes 2 and 12. *TP53* mutations were not detected in four craniopharyngiomas {1995}.

Histogenesis

Several observations indicate that craniopharyngioma is derived from Rathke pouch epithelium. During embryonal development, the anterior wall of the pouch develops into a glandular, pseudostratified columnar epithelium, normally representing the primordium of the adenohypophysis. The remaining stomodeum develops into a non-keratinised squamous epithelium, which normally gives rise to the oral mucosa, and into the tooth primordia. If parts of the Rathke pouch fail to develop into the adenohypophysis as normal, they may differentiate into either tooth primordia (giving rise to adamantinomatous craniopharyngioma) or into oral mucosa (giving rise to papillary squamous craniopharyngioma). Further support for the assumption that craniopharyngiomas originate from the Rathke pouch is provided by the occasional occurrence of mixed tumours with characteristics of craniopharyngioma and Rathke cleft cyst, and by the report of a unique congenital craniopharyngioma {1653} with ameloblastic, as well as tooth bud and adenohypophyseal primordia components.

The hypothesis that craniopharyngiomas contain a neuroendocrine lineage is supported by the finding that scattered tumour cell groups may express one ore more pituitary hormones {1475}, chromogranin A {1653} and human chorionic gonadotropin {1478}. Also in support is the observation of a tumour that arose from a Rathke cleft cyst and contained cells that were transitional between squamous, mucus-producing and anterior pituitary lobe secretory cells {750}.

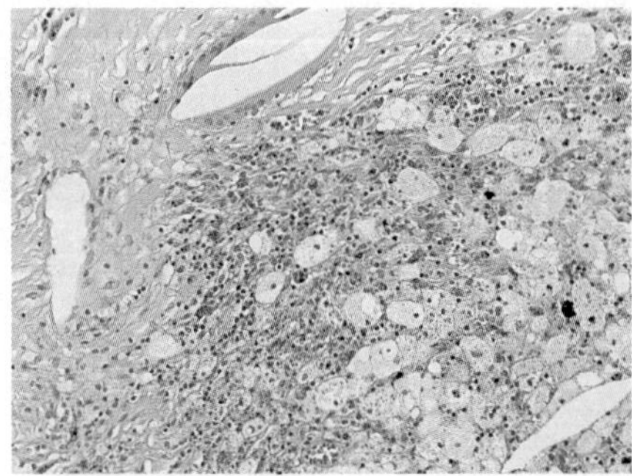

Fig. 15.7 Xanthogranuloma of the sellar region showing xanthoma cells, lymphocytic infiltrates, haemosiderin deposits, cholesterol clefts and occasional multinucleated giant cells

Prognosis and prognostic factors

In the large series, 60-93% of patients had 10-year recurrence-free survival and 64-96% an overall 10-year survival {288, 1224, 1660}. The most significant factor associated with craniopharyngioma recurrence is the extent of surgical resection {1322, 1594, 1660} with lesions >5cm in diameter carrying a markedly worse prognosis {1660}. After incomplete surgical resection, the recurrence rate is significantly higher {1594, 1660}. While some authors doubt its usefulness {1594}, others consider radiotherapy beneficial, particularly in incompletely resected craniopharyngiomas {288, 964, 1557}. Histological evidence for brain invasion, more frequently documented in the adamantinomatous than in the papillary type, is not correlated with a higher recurrence rate in cases with gross surgical resection {1594}.

Some authors have documented a better prognosis for the papillary than for the adamantinomatous type of craniopharyngioma {5, 464}, while others failed to demonstrate significant differences {288, 1594}. So far, only one study suggests that a MIB-1 LI >7% is a useful predictor of recurrence {2423}. Malignant transformation of craniopharyngioma to squamous carcinoma after irradiation may exceptionally occur {2430, 2483}.

Granular cell tumour of the neurohypophysis

R.W. Warzok
S. Vogelgesang
W. Feiden
S. Shuangshoti

Definition

An intrasellar and/or suprasellar mass arising from the neurohypophysis or infundibulum, composed of nests of large cells with granular, eosinophilic cytoplasm due to abundant intracytoplasmic lysosomes.

Grading

Granular cell tumours (GCTs) correspond histologically to WHO grade I.

ICD-O code:

The provisional code proposed for the third edition of ICD-O is 9582/0.

Synonyms

Granular cell myoblastoma, granular cell neuroma, choristoma, pituicytoma, Abrikossoff tumour.

Incidence

A total of 47 symptomatic cases have has reported in the literature. Most frequently the tumours are diagnosed in adults, twice as often in females as in males {2568, 2561}. In systematic postmortem histological studies, small aggregates and micronodules of granular cells (tumourettes) were found incidentally in up to 17% of unselected autopsy cases {2565, 2567, 2566}. Evidently, the vast majority of these never grow to sufficient size to become symptomatic.

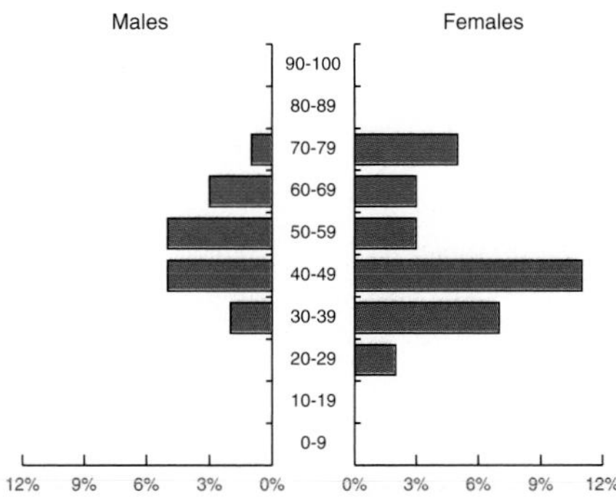

Fig. 15.8 Age and sex distribution of neurohypophyseal granullar cell tumours based on 47 published symptomatic cases.

Localization

Granular cell tumours (GCTs) arise from the neurohypophysis or infundibulum, and may be localized intrasellarly and/or suprasellarly.

Clinical features

The clinical symptomatology corresponds to that of hormonally inactive adenomas of the pituitary. Symptoms usually develop insidiously and include hormonal and visual disturbances with secondary amenorrhoea, galactorrhoea, decreased libido, infertility and diabetes insipidus as well as bitemporal hemianopia, headache and repeated vomiting. Rarely, clinical symptoms develop within a few weeks {2563, 2561, 2568}.

Neuroimaging

Skull X-ray may show either a normal or a ballooned sella turcica. Lack of calcification is characteristic and helps differentiate these lesions from craniopharyngioma {2562}. MRI shows sharply demarcated iso-intense masses with remarkable contrast enhancement due to rich vascularization. As a rule, the neoplasms measure less than 3 cm in diameter.

Macroscopy

The tumours are usually well circumscribed, with soft to medium consistency and with a grey to yellow homogeneous or granular cut surface. Necrosis and cystic degeneration are uncommon features. In rare cases, the neoplasm may infiltrate surrounding structures such as the optic chiasm and cavernous sinus.

Histopathology

Granular cell tumours consist of densely packed polygonal cells with abundant eosinophilic, granular, PAS-positive cytoplasm.

PAS staining of cytoplasmic granules is resistant to diastase digestion. Sometimes, small areas of foamy cells can be observed. Tumour cell nuclei are small, with inconspicuous nucleoli and evenly distributed karyoplasm. Perivascular lymphocytic aggregates are a common feature. Mitotic activity is absent. Some lesions are characterized by remarkable cellular and nuclear polymorphism, with irregular chromatin, prominent nucleoli and multinucleated cells.

Proliferative activity, as assessed by Ki-67/MIB-1 immunoreactivity, is usually very low but in rare cases some tumour areas showed up to 5% positive cells {2568}.

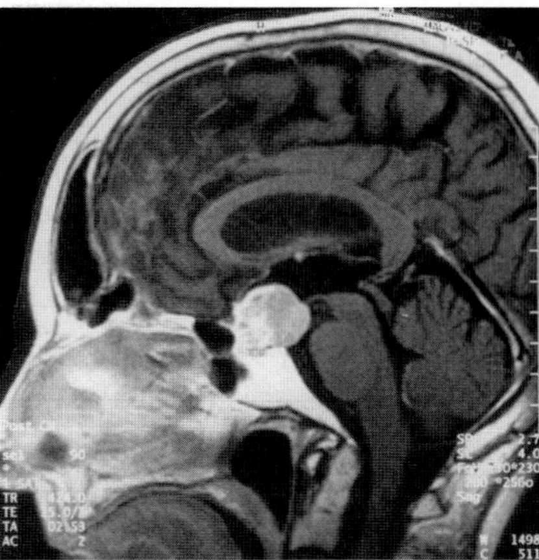

Fig. 15.9 T1-weighted MRI of a granular cell tumour with non-homogenous contrast enhancement and intra- and suprasellar extension.

Immunohistochemistry

Immunohistochemical data are still limited and conflicting. Usually the tumours are strongly positive for neuron-specific enolase, S-100 protein, α_1-antitrypsin and α_1-antichymotrypsin and negative for neurofilament proteins, cytokeratins, chromogranin A, synaptophysin, desmin, smooth muscle actin and hypophyseal hormones. Variable immunoreactivity to glial fibrillary acidic protein has been noted in a subset of GCTs.

Electron microscopy

The cytoplasm of granular cells is filled with abundant, membrane-bound, unevenly electron-dense material suggestive of autophagic vacuoles and heterolysosomes. A few mitochondria may be registered, but other organelles are rarely observed. In some cases, intracytoplasmic filaments have been described {2562}.

Histogenesis

GCT is a purely descriptive term of a histogenetically heterogeneous group of neoplasms. In the more frequent GCTs of extraneural tissues, a derivation from Schwann cells, myoblasts and macrophages has been postulated. Neurohypophyseal GCTs most likely arise from pituicytes, the glial element of the posterior lobe of the hypophysis. Taking into account the conflicting results of immunohistochemical studies, one possible explanation is that despite their homogenous appearance in conventional histology, pituitary GCTs are composed of heterogeneous cell populations.

Genetics

To date no cytogenetic data have been published. In one case of atypical GCT, 95% of the tumour cells showed nuclear accumulation of TP53, while 15% expressed the apoptosis-inhibiting protein bcl-2. No cells were positive for the apoptosis-inducing protein Bax or for EGFR {2568}.

Predictive factors

Most GCTs are benign, with slow progression and lack of invasive growth. Surgical removal is the therapy for larger tumours, as for other sellar lesions. In 7 out of 47 reported cases, a second surgical intervention was necessary due to tumour recurrence. There is no consensus with regard to postoperative radiotherapy. Some authors see no benefit {2562} while others report that it extends time to recurrence and survival {2564}.

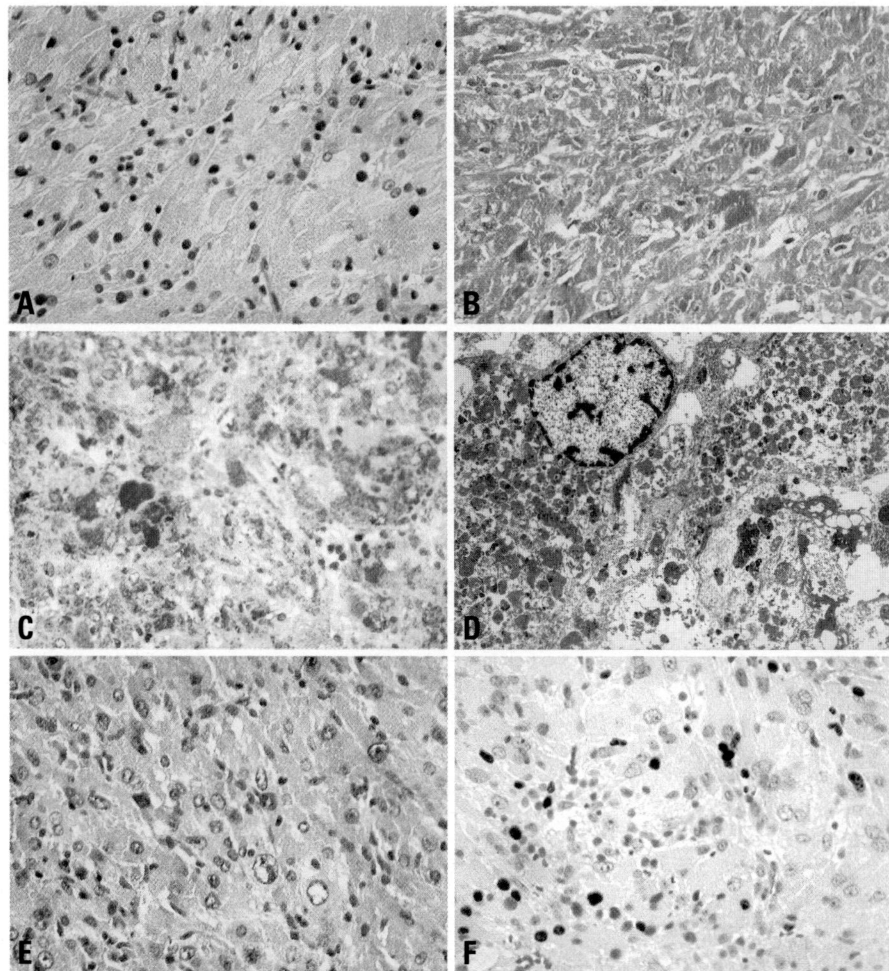

Fig. 15.10 **A** Isomorphic granular cell tumour (GCT) with abundant granular cytoplasm. **B** Strongly PAS-positive cytoplasmic granules. **C** GCT showing strong immunoreactivity to α_1-antichymotrypsin. **D** Electron microscopy, showing tumour cells filled with numerous lysosomes. **E** Atypical GCT with striking cellular and nuclear polymorphism and (**F**) focally high MIB-1 labeling index.

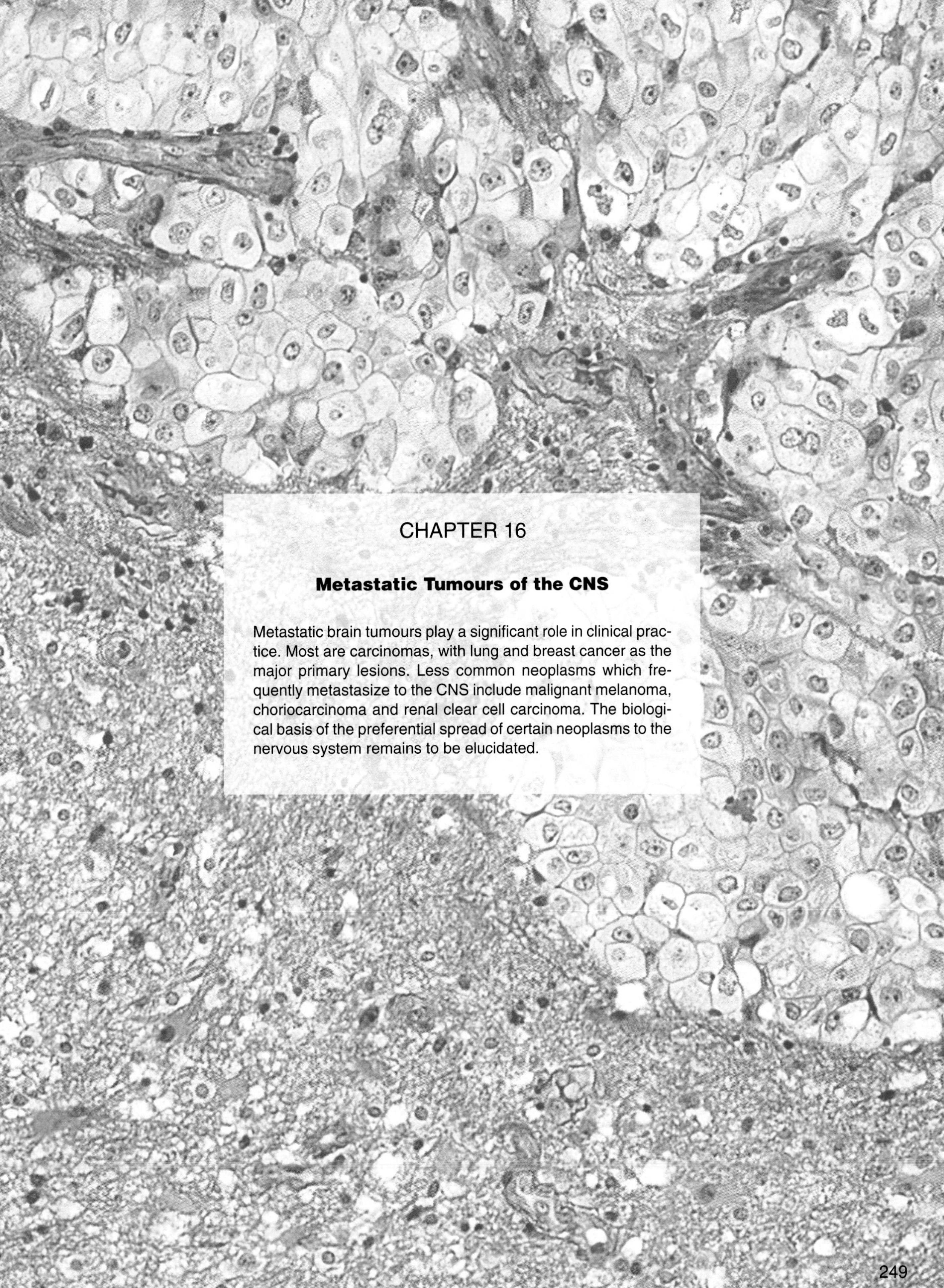

CHAPTER 16

Metastatic Tumours of the CNS

Metastatic brain tumours play a significant role in clinical practice. Most are carcinomas, with lung and breast cancer as the major primary lesions. Less common neoplasms which frequently metastasize to the CNS include malignant melanoma, choriocarcinoma and renal clear cell carcinoma. The biological basis of the preferential spread of certain neoplasms to the nervous system remains to be elucidated.

Metastatic tumours of the CNS

J.S. Nelson
A. von Deimling
I. Petersen
R.-C. Janzer

Definition

Tumours involving the CNS that originate from, but are discontinuous with, primary systemic neoplasms.

Incidence

Incidence data from two population-based studies and a probability sampling study are presented in Table1 {416, 1166, 1576}. Autopsy studies have revealed the presence of intracranial metastasis in 24% and of intraspinal metastasis in 5% of cancer patients {98, 1198}.

Age and sex distribution

The incidence of CNS metastases increases with age (Table 2 and ref. {1166}). The male: female ratio for cerebral metastasis is 1.36:1 {1576} while for intraspinal metastases a ratio of 1.16:1 has been reported {416}.

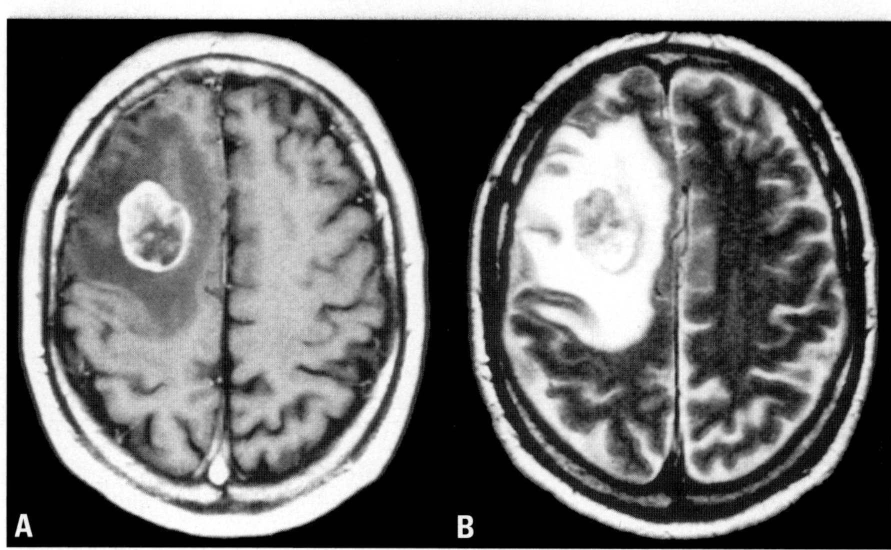

Fig. 16.1 Metastasis of an adenocarcinoma in the right frontal lobe. **A** Gadolinium enhanced T1-weighted MRI, showing a large area of hypointensity corresponding to a perifocal oedema that (**B**) shows bright hyperintensity on T2-weighted MRI.

Origin of CNS metastases

The frequencies of common brain metastases by primary tumour type and the common metastases causing epidural spinal cord compression (ESCC) are shown in Tables 16.3 and 16.4 {329,1197}. Additional sources of CNS metastases include primary tumours that occur less frequently but have a propensity for CNS metastasis, *e.g.* choriocarcinoma {1419} and clear cell carcinoma of the kidney. Up to 40–50% of intramedullary spinal cord metastases originate from primary neoplasms in the lung. Diffuse infiltration of the leptomeninges is most frequently associated with leukaemias, lymphomas, breast cancer, melanoma, lung cancer and carcinomas of the gastro-intestinal tract {1197}.

Table 16.1
Annual incidence of metastatic tumours (per 100'000 population).

CNS metastases	4.1–11.1
Intracranial metastases	3.4–8.3
Intraspinal metastases	0.7

Table 16.2
Age-specific incidence rate of CNS metastases (per 100'000 population and year).

Age (years)	Rate
0-24	0.6
25-44	5.3
45-64	31.1
65+	42.7

Localization

Intracranial metastases are most frequent in the brain and dura. Eighty percent of brain metastases are located in the arterial border zones of the cerebral hemispheres, 3% are found in the basal ganglia, and 15% in the cerebellum. In the cerebrum, metastases occur typically near the junction of cortex and white matter. In the cerebellum, they often lie in the border zone between the superior and inferior cerebellar arteries. Other intracranial sites include the leptomeninges, pituitary, pineal, choroid plexus, and pre-existing lesions such as tumours, infarcts, or vascular malformations.

Metastases affecting the spinal cord occur in the epidural space, leptomeninges, or spinal cord (intramedullary). Epidural metastases are the most common type, usually arising by extension from a metastatic deposit in the vertebral bodies or paravertebral tissues. Rarely, tumours may metastasise directly to the epidural space {329, 1197, 1198}.

Clinical features

Symptoms and signs

Intracranial metastases cause general and focal symptoms and signs which evolve over days or weeks, and include headache, focal weakness, mental disturbances, hemiparesis, ataxia, hemisensory loss, and papilloedema. Spinal metastases are most often associated with evidence of cord compression, such as back pain, weakness of the extremities, sensory disturbances, and incontinence. These symptoms may develop over hours, days or weeks {1197}.

Fig. 16.2 Macroscopic images of metastatic brain tumours. The primary neoplasms were as follows: **A, C, D, E, P, Q, S** lung carcinoma; **B, R** oesophageal carcinoma; **G, I** spinal metastases of malignant melanoma; **J, K** cerebral and dural metastasis of mammary carcinoma; **H** chorion carcinoma; **L** carcinoma of the nasal sinus; **M** carcinoma of the colon; **N** dural metastasis of an osteosarcoma; **O** malignant fibrous histiocytoma; **F, S** cystic metastases following therapeutic radiation.

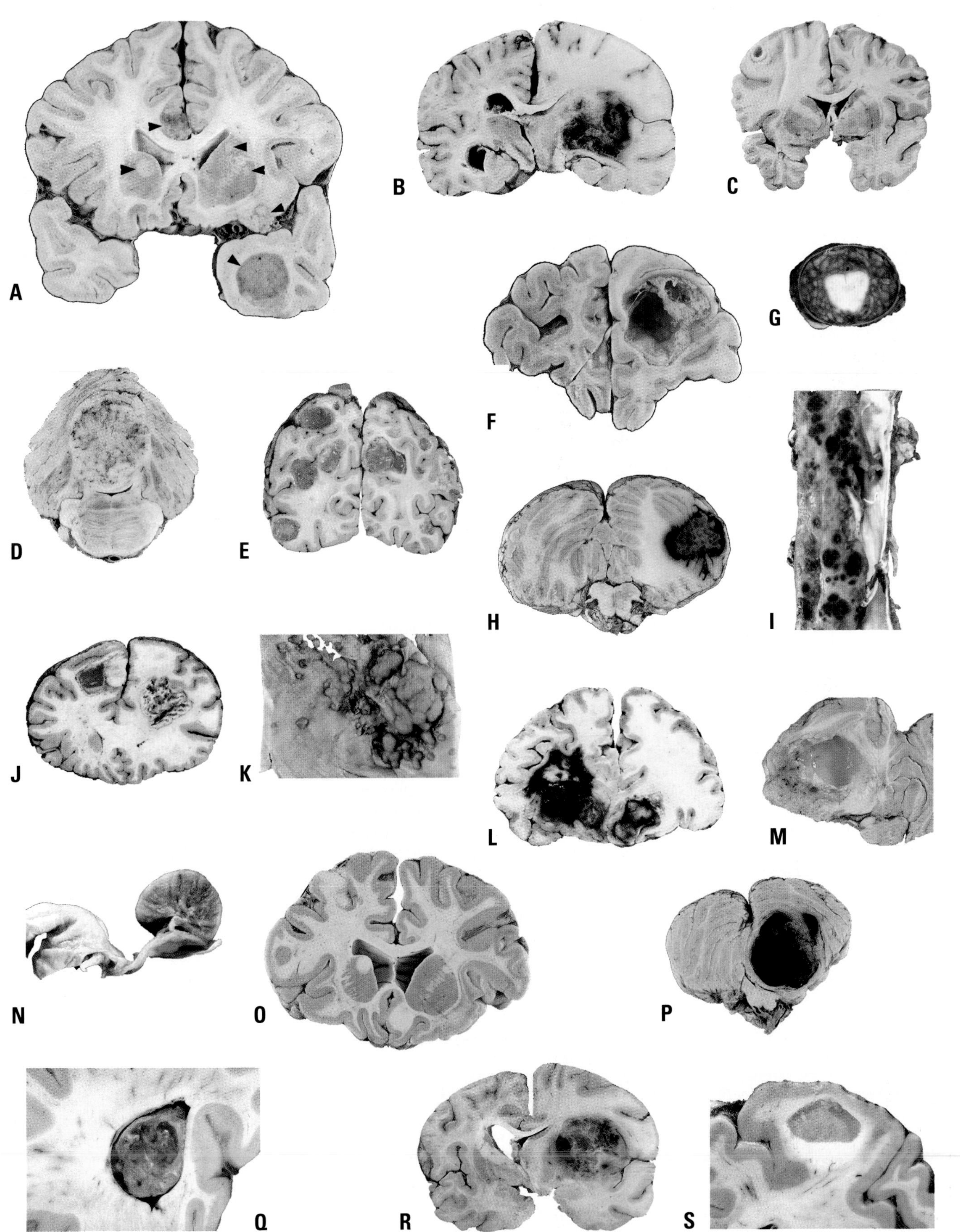
A
B
C
D
E
F
G
H
I
J
K
L
M
N
O
P
Q
R
S

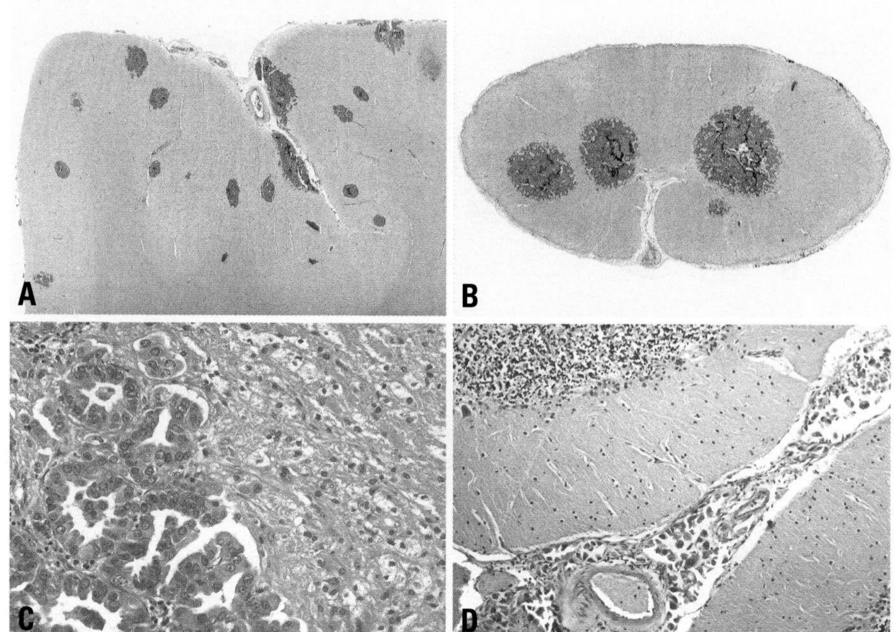

Fig. 16.3 **A** Multiple cortical micrometastases and (**B**) spinal metastases of a small cell lung carcinoma. **C** Well-delineated brain metastasis of an adenocarcinoma. **D** Cerebellar meningeal carcinomatosis.

Neuroimaging

Brain and intramedullary spinal cord metastases. On CT, these appear as discrete, rounded, iso- or hypodense masses with strong solid or ring enhancement and a surrounding zone of parenchymal oedema {511, 1111, 1226}. Approximately 50% of patients have one metastasis and an additional 20% have two metastases. Solitary metastases are often associated with primary carcinomas of the prostate, uterus, gastrointestinal tract and breast, while multiple metastases are most commonly associated with carcinoma of unknown primary site, melanoma and lung carcinoma. On MRI, metastases appear hypointense on T1-weighted, and as hyperintense mass with adjacent parenchymal oedema on T2- weighted imaging, typically with marked contrast enhancement {511, 1111, 1197, 1226}.

Dural, leptomeningeal, and vertebral metastases. MRI is the most sensitive method for detecting these lesions. With contrast enhanced MR imaging, dural and leptomeningeal metastases are recognisable as nodular or sheet-like areas of increased signal intensity around the brain or spinal cord. Metastases in vertebral bodies are visualised on T1-weighted images as discrete, confluent or diffuse areas of low signal intensity.

Table 16.3
Origin of brain metastases

Primary tumour site	% of brain metastases
Respiratory tract	50%
Breast	15%
Skin / melanoma	10.5%
Unknown primary site	11%

Macroscopy

Metastases to brain parenchyma form discrete round or confluent well circumscribed grey white or tan masses. Haemorrhagic deposits are characteristic of metastatic melanoma, choriocarcinoma and lung and renal cell carcinoma. Tumours attached to the dura or leptomeninges may form plaques or nodules.

Histopathology

The histological, ultrastructural and immunohistochemical phenotypes of CNS metastases are usually but not always similar to those of the primary tumour from which they arise. Vascular proliferation may be seen within and adjacent to the tumour, occasionally with formation of glomeruloid structures. Tumour necrosis is frequent and may be extensive, leaving recognisable tumour tissue only at the periphery of the lesion or around blood vessels. With the exception of small cell anaplastic tumours and some melanomas, parenchymal metastases have histologically well defined borders with the adjacent parenchyma, and displace rather than infiltrate tissue as they enlarge. Diffuse leptomeningeal infiltration may occur as sole manifestation or in conjunction with parenchymal metastasis.

Table 16.4
Origin of metastases causing epidural spinal cord compression (ESCC)

Primary tumour	Percentage
Breast	22%
Lung	15%
Prostate	10%
Malignant lymphoma	10%

Proliferation

Progressively enlarging or symptomatic CNS metastases are unequivocally malignant tumours with marked mitotic activity. The labelling index may be greater than in the primary neoplasm {235}.

Pathogenesis

The metastatic process involves haematogenic spread of tumour cells to the brain or spinal cord or bone, dura and meninges, with subsequent extension into the CNS. Secondary tumours of the CNS may also develop through invasion from primary tumours arising in adjacent anatomic structures, such as the paranasal sinuses or bone. These tumours are not considered metastases because they remain in continuity with the primary neoplasm.

Molecular genetics

Secondary tumours originate from a subpopulation of cells in the original neoplasm capable of metastasis. Investigation of the genetic control of metastasis is in its early stages and only limited information is available. Expression of some metastasis-related genes such as *EGFR*, *MMP-2*, *MDR-1* and *KAI-1* is regulated by the TP53 tumour suppressor protein {2108, 2111}. Expression or overexpression of CD44R1 in colon carcinoma and S100A4 (p9Ka) or c-erbB2 in breast carcinoma are associated with increased metastatic potential {2107, 1196, 2109}. In some tumours, decrease or loss of specific gene expression is associated with tumour progression. Examples include: *DCC* in endometrial carcinoma; *KAI-1* in prostate, lung, breast bladder, pancreatic, and hepatocellular cancers; and *BAI1* in colon cancer {1452, 2105, 2106, 2108, 2110}. Comparative

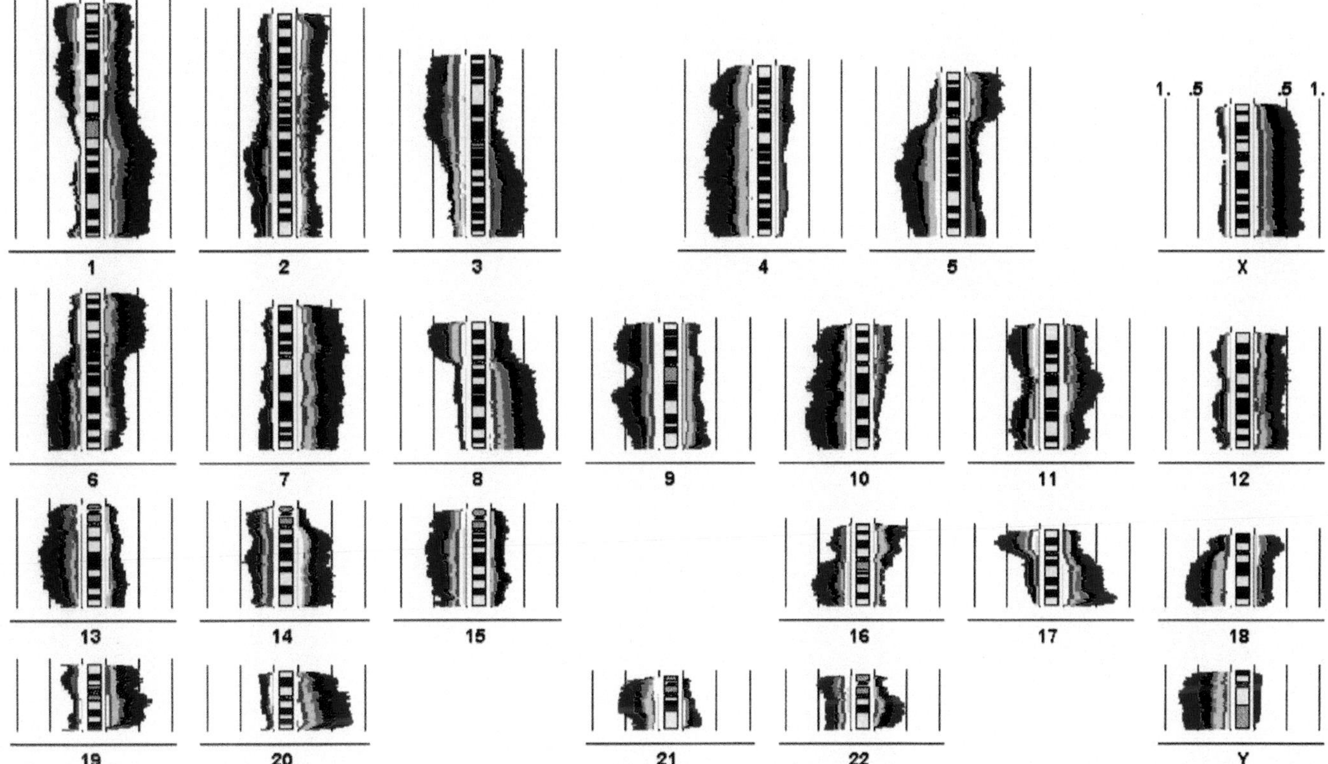

Fig. 16.4 Super histogram of the chromosomal imbalances in 40 brain metastases. DNA losses are indicated by the incidence curve on the left chromosome ideogram, DNA gains are shown on the right side. Each tumour type is indicated by a different colour: blue, lung carcinomas (n=14), black, melanomas (n=7), red, breast cancer (n=5), orange, colorectal cancer (n=5), green, kidney carcinomas (n=4), white, unknown primaries (n=3), yellow, thyroid carcinoma (n=1), magenta, adrenal gland carcinoma (n=1). A peak incidence is seen for the DNA gain on chromosome 17q24-q25.

genomic hybridisation studies revealed that CNS metastases have a characteristic though not specific pattern of chromosomal imbalances, with DNA gains on 1q23, 8q24, 17q24-25, and 20q13 being present in more than 80% of cases (Fig. 16.4). Comparison of primary tumours and their corresponding metastases indicated clonal relationship in every case {2579}.

Predictive factors

Younger age and high Karnofsky performance status are associated with longer survival. Other prognostic factors include the number and location of CNS metastases, sensitivity of the tumour to therapy, and progression of the primary neoplasm. Currently, the median survival for patients with multiple brain metastases treated with radiation is 3–6 months {1197}. Longer survival is seen in patients who undergo resection of a solitary brain metastasis.

Contributors

Dr Adriano AGUZZI
Institute of Neuropathology
University of Zurich
Schmelzbergstrasse 12
CH-8091 Zurich
SWITZERLAND
Tel: +41 1 255 2869/2107
Fax: +41 1 255 4402
adriano@pathol.unizh.ch

Dr Kari ALITALO
Molecular/Cancer Biology Lab.
University of Helsinki
Haartmaninkatu 3, POB 21
SF-00014 Helsinki
FINLAND
Tel: +358 9 191 26434
Fax: +358 9 191 26448
kari.alitalo@helsinki.fi

Dr Laurence E. BECKER *
Dept. of Pediatric Laboratory Medicine
Hospital for Sick Children, Univ. of Toronto
555 University Ave., Suite 3112
Toronto, Ontario M5G 1X8
CANADA
Tel: +1 416 813 5967
Fax: +1 416 813 5974
lebecker@sickkids.on.ca

Dr Michael E. BERENS
Neuro-Oncology Research Laboratory
Barrow Neurological Institute
350 W. Thomas Rd.
Phoenix, AZ 85013-4496
USA
Tel: +1 602 406 3648
Fax: +1 602 406 7172
mberens@chw.edu

* The asterisk indicates participation in the Working Group Meeting on the WHO Classification of Tumours of the Nervous System that was held in Lyon, France, July 27-30, 1999.

Dr Jaclyn A. BIEGEL
Division of Human Genetics
and Molecular Biology
Children's Hospital of Philadelphia
1002 Abramson, 3516 Civic Center Blvd.
Philadelphia, PA 19104
USA
Tel: +1 215 590 3856
Fax: +1 215 590 3764
biegel@mail.med.upenn.edu

Dr Wojciech BIERNAT *
Department of Oncology
Medical University of Lodz
4 Paderewski Str.
93-509 Lodz
POLAND
Tel: +48 42 681 1603
Fax: +48 42 681 1117
biernat@psk2.am.lodz.pl
wbier@poczta.onet.pl

Dr Darell D. BIGNER
Department of Pathology
Duke University Medical Center
Box 3156
Durham, NC 27710
USA
Tel: +1 919 684 5018
Fax: +1 919 684 5231
bigne001@mc.duke.edu

Dr Sandra H. BIGNER
Department of Pathology
Duke University Medical Center
Box 3712
Durham, NC 27710
USA
Tel: +1 919 684 5410
Fax: +1 919 684 8756
bigne002@mc.duke.edu

Dr Tom BÖHLING
Department of Pathology
Haartman Institute, University of Helsinki
Haartmansgatan 3, POB 21
SF-00014 Helsinki
FINLAND
Tel: +358 9 1912 6419
Fax: +358 9 1912 6700
tom.bohling@helsinki.fi

Dr Sebastian BRANDNER *
Institute of Neuropathology
University Hospital Zurich
Schmelzbergstrasse 12
CH-8091 Zurich
SWITZERLAND
Tel: +41 1 255 2849
Fax: +41 1 255 4402
seb@pathol.unizh.ch

Dr Daniel J. BRAT
Dept. of Pathology and Lab. Medicine
Emory University Hospital, H-190
1364 Clifton Rd. NE
Atlanta, GA 30322
USA
Tel: +1 404 712 7004
Fax: +1 404 712 0148
dbrat@emory.edu

Dr Garrett M. BRODEUR
Division of Oncology
Children's Hospital of Philadelphia
Abramson Research Center, Rm. 902-D
3416 Civic Center Blvd.
Philadelphia, PA 19104-4318
USA
Tel: +1 215 390 2817
Fax: +1 215 590 3770
brodeur@email.chop.edu

Dr Janet M. BRUNER
Neuropathology, Box 85
MD Anderson Cancer Center
1515 Holcombe Blvd.
Houston, TX 77030
USA
Tel: +1 713 792 6127
Fax: +1 713 794 1695
jbruner@mdanderson.org

Dr Herbert BUDKA *
Allgemeines Krankenhaus 4 J
Institute of Neurology, Univ. of Vienna
Währinger Gürtel 18-20, Postfach 48
A-1097 Vienna
AUSTRIA
Tel: +43 1 40400 5501
Fax: +43 1 40400 5511
h.budka@akh-wien.ac.at or h.budka@ac.at

Dr Peter C. BURGER *
Pathology Building, Room 706
The Johns Hopkins Hospital
600 N. Wolfe Street
Baltimore, MD 21287
USA
Tel: +1 410 955 8378
Fax: +1 410 614 9310
pburger@jhmi.edu

Dr Webster K. CAVENEE *
Ludwig Institute for Cancer Research
University of California, San Diego
9500 Gilman Drive,
La Jolla, CA 92093-0660
USA
Tel: +1 858 534 7802
Fax: +1 858 534 7750
wcavenee@ucsd.edu

Dr Georgia CHENEVIX-TRENCH
Queensland Institute of
Medical Research
Royal Brisbane Hospital
Herston, QLD 4029
AUSTRALIA
Tel: +61 7 3362 0930
Fax: +61 7 3362 0105
georgiaT@qimr.edu.au

Dr Leila CHIMELLI
Department of Pathology
University Hospital CFF - UFRJ
Ilha de Fundao - CEP 21941-590
Rio de Janeiro RJ
BRAZIL
Tel: +55 21 562 2450
Fax: +55 21 270 2193
chimelli@hucff.ufrj.br

Dr Pauline CHOU
Department of Pathology and Lab. Services
Children's Memorial Hospital
2300 Children's Plaza, #17
Chicago, IL 60614
USA
Tel: +1 773 880 4610
Fax: +1 773 880 8127
pmchou@nwu.edu

Dr V. Peter COLLINS *
Department of Histopathology, Box 235
Addenbrooke's Hospital
Hills Road
Cambridge CB2 2QQ
UNITED KINGDOM
Tel: +44 1223 336072/217164
Fax: +44 1223 216980
vpc20@cam.ac.uk

Dr Stephen W. COONS
Department of Neuropathology
Barrow Neurological Institute
350 W. Thomas Rd.
Phoenix, AZ 85013-4496
USA
Tel: +1 602 406 7088
Fax: +1 602 406 7169
scoons@mha.chw.edu

Dr Selina C. CORTEZ
Department of Pathology
Rhode Island Hospital
593 Eddy Street
Providence, RI 02903
USA
Tel: +1 401 444 4000

Dr Felix F. CRUZ-SANCHEZ
Inst. of Neurological & Gerontological
Sciences
International University of Catalonia
c/ Inmaculada 22
E-08017 Barcelona
SPAIN
Tel: +34 93 254 1816
Fax: +34 93 254 1841
fcruz@unica.edu

Dr Catherine DAUMAS-DUPORT *
Service d'Anatomie Pathologique
H™pital Sainte-Anne
1 rue Cabanis
F-75014 Paris
FRANCE
Tel: +33-1-4565-8205
Fax: +33-1-4565-8728
daumas@chsa.broca.inserm.fr or
cdaumas75@hotmail.com

Dr Richard L. DAVIS
Neuropathology Unit, HSW-501
Medical School
University of California
San Francisco, CA 94143-0506
USA
Tel: +1 415 476 5236
Fax: +1 415 476 9672
richardd@email.his.ucsf.edu

Dr Martina DECKERT-SCHLÜTER
Institute of Neuropathology
University Hospital
Sigmund-Freud-Str.
D-53127 Bonn
GERMANY
Tel: +49 228 287 6523
Fax: +49 228 287 4331
mds@uni-bonn.de

Dr Wolfgang FEIDEN
Institute of Pathology
Homburg Medical School
D-66421Homburg/Saar
GERMANY
Tel: +49 6841 163865
Fax: +49 6841 163877
pawfei@med-rz.uni-sb.de

Dr Dominique FIGARELLA-BRANGER *
Neuropathology Laboratory
Faculty of Medicine
27 boulevard Jean Moulin
F-13385 Marseille
FRANCE
Tel: +33 (0)4 91 38 55 28
Fax: +33 (0)4 91 25 42 32
dominique.figarella-branger@medecine.univ-mrs.fr or dfigarel@ap-hm.fr

Dr Sydney D. FINKELSTEIN
Department of Anatomic Pathology
University of Pittsburgh Medical Center
200 Lothrop Street, PUH A610.2
Pittsburgh, PA 15213
USA
Tel: +1 412 647 3735/6594
Fax: +1 412 647 6251
finkelsteinsd@msx.upmc.edu

Dr Rosemary FOSTER
Molecular Neurogenetics Unit
Massachussetts General Hospital
Building 149, 13th St.
Charlestown, MA 02129
USA
Tel: +1 617 724 9619
Fax: +1 617 726 5736
foster@helix.mgh.harvard.edu

Dr Frank B. FURNARI
Ludwig Institute for Cancer Research
University of California, San Diego
9500 Gilman Dr., CMM-East Rm. 3071
La Jolla, CA 92093-0660
USA
Tel: +1 858 534 7808
Fax: +1 858 534 7816
ffurnari@ucsd.edu

Dr Felice GIANGASPERO *
Institute of Anatomical Pathology
Bufalini Hospital
Via Ghirotti, 286
47023 Cesena
ITALY
Tel: +39 0547 352737
Fax: +39 0547 300066
giangi@ausl-cesena.emr.it

Dr Caterina GIANNINI *
Anatomia Patologica
Ospedale Regionale di Vincenza
Via Generale Basso 14, Bassano del Grappa
36061Vincenza
ITALY
Tel: +39 0424 514371
Fax: +39 0424 514371
ricagna@tin.it

Dr Maria Teresa GIORDANA
Second Department of Neurology
University of Torino
Via Cherasco, 15
I-10126 Torino
ITALY
Tel: +39 011 663 8135/5439
Fax: +39 011 696 3487
giordana@medfarm.unito.it or
giordana@molinette.unito.it

Dr A.J. GREEN
Department of Pathology
University of Cambridge
Addenbrooke's Hospital
Cambridge CB1 1QP
UNITED KINGDOM
Tel:
Fax: +44 1223 333346

Dr Hannu HAAPASALO
Department of Pathology
Tampere University Hospital
POB 2000
SF-33521 Tampere
FINLAND
Tel: +358 3 247 6560
Fax: +358 3 247 5503
hhaapasalo@tays.fi

Dr Pierre HAINAUT
Molecular Carcinogenesis Group
Intl. Agency for Res. on Cancer (IARC)
150 cours Albert-Thomas
69372Lyon Cedex 08
FRANCE
Tel: +33 4 72 73 85 32
Fax: +33 4 72 73 85 75
hainaut@iarc.fr

Dr Matti J. HALTIA *
Department of Pathology
University of Helsinki
Haartmaninkatu 3, POB 21
FIN-00014 Helsinki
FINLAND
Tel: +358 9 1912 6337
Fax: +358 9 1912 6700
matti.j.haltia@helsinki.fi

Dr Michael N. HART
Department of Pathology, 505 SMI
University of Wisconsin Medical School
1300 University Avenue
Madison, WI 53706-1532
USA
Tel: +1 608 262 1188
Fax: +1 608 265 3301
mnhart@facstaff.wisc.edu

Dr Jacques HASSOUN
Laboratoire de Neuropathologie
Facult+ de M+decine
27 blvd. Jean Moulin
F-13005 Marseille
FRANCE
Tel: +33 (0)4 91 83 44 43
Fax: +33 (0)4 91 25 42 32
jacques.hassoun@medecine.univ-mrs.fr

Dr Monika HEGI
Centre Hospitalier Universitaire Vaudois
Department of Neurosurgery
Laboratory of Tumour Biology and Genetics
CH-1011Lausanne
SWITZERLAND
Tel: +41 21 314 2582
Fax: +41 21 314 2587
monika.hegi@chuv.hospvd.ch

Dr Takanori HIROSE
Department of Pathology
Saitama Medical School
Morohongo 38, Moroyama
350-0495Saitama
JAPAN
Tel: +81 492 76 1158
Fax: +81 492 76 1583
thirose@saitama-med.ac.jp

Dr Huei-Jen Su HUANG
Ludwig Institute for Cancer Research
University of California, San Diego
9500 Gilman Dr., CMM-East Rm. 3071
La Jolla, CA 92093-0660
USA
Tel: +1 858 534 7814
Fax: +1 858 534 7750
hjshuang@ucsd.edu

Dr Mark A. ISRAEL *
Preuss Lab. for Molecular Neuro-Oncology
University of California, San Francisco
HSE 722, 513 Parnassus Ave.
San Francisco, CA 94143-0520
USA
Tel: +1 415 476 6662
Fax: +1 415 476 0388
israel@cgl.ucsf.edu

Dr Juha JÄÄSKELÄINEN
Department of Neurosurgery
Helsinki University Hospital
Topeliuksenkatu 5
SF-00260 Helsinki
FINLAND
Tel: +358 9 4718 7415
Fax: +358 9 4718 7560
juha.jaaskelainen@huch.fi

Dr Robert-Charles JANZER *
Division of Neuropathology
University Institute of Pathology
27 rue du Bugnon
CH-1011 Lausanne
SWITZERLAND
Tel: +41 21 314 7171
Fax: +41 21 314 7175
rjanzer@chuv.hospvd.ch

Dr Kurt JELLINGER
PKH/B Bldg.
Ludwig Boltzmann Inst. Clin. Neurobiol.
Baumgartner Hoehe 1
A-1140 Vienna
AUSTRIA
Tel: +43 1 91060 14248/14244
Fax: +43 1 91060 49862
kurt.jellinger@univie.ac.at

Dr Vijay JOSHI
Pathology and Laboratory Medicine
Hartford Hospital
80 Seymour St., POB 5037
Hartford, CT 06102-5037
USA
Tel: +1 860 545 2249
Fax: +1 860 545 5206

Dr Anne JOUVET *
Laboratory of Neuropathology
Neurology Hospital
59 boulevard Pinel
69003 Lyon
FRANCE
Tel: +33 4 72 35 76 34
Fax: +33 4 72 35 70 67
jouvet@laennec.univ-lyon1.fr

Dr Hannu KALIMO
Department of Pathology
Turku University Central Hospital
FIN-20520 Turku
FINLAND
Tel: +358 2 261 1685
Fax: +358 2 333 7459
hkalimo@utu.fi

Dr John J. KEPES
Dept. of Pathology / Lab Medicine
University of Kansas Medical Center
3901 Rainbow Blvd.
Kansas City, KS 66160-7410
USA
Tel: +1 913 588 7169
Fax: +1 913 588 7073
kulgener@kumc.edu

Dr Paul KLEIHUES *
International Agency for
Research on Cancer (IARC)
150 cours Albert Thomas
69372Lyon Cedex 08
FRANCE
Tel: +33 4 72 73 85 77
Fax: +33 4 72 73 85 64
kleihues@iarc.fr

Dr Helen P. KOUREA
Dept. of Pathology
Univ. of Patras Hospital
Markora 20
26442 Patras
GREECE
Tel: +30 61 438 985
kouma@otenet.gr

Dr Winfrid KRONE
Dept. of Human Genetics
University of Ulm
Albert-Einstein-Allee 11
D-89070 Ulm
GERMANY
Tel: +49 731 502 3420/3421
Fax: +49 731 502 3427
winfrid.krone@medizin.uni-ulm.de

Dr Johan M. KROS *
Div. of Pathology/Neuropathology
University Hospital Rotterdam-Dijkzigt
Dr. Molewaterplein 40
NL-3015 GD Rotterdam
THE NETHERLANDS
Tel: +31 10 408 7905
Fax: +31 10 408 9487
kros@path.fgg.eur.nl

Dr Peter L. LANTOS *
Department of Neuropathology
Institute of Psychiatry
De Crespigny Park
Denmark Hill
London SE5 8AF
UNITED KINGDOM
Tel: +44 171 919 3272
Fax: +44 171 708 3895
i.hart@iop.kcl.ac.uk

Dr Ching C. LAU *
Baylor College of Medicine
Texas Children's Hospital
6621 Fannin St., MC 3-3320
Houston, TX 77030-4202
USA
Tel: +1 713 770 4200
Fax: +1 713 770 4038
clau@txccc.org

Dr. Beatriz S. LOPES
Dept. of Pathology/Neuropathol.
Univ. of Virginia Health Sciences Center
Box 214
Charlottesville, VA 22908
USA
Tel: +1 804 924 9175
Fax: +1 804 924 9177
msl2e@virginia.edu

Dr David N. LOUIS *
Molecular Neuro-Oncology Laboratory, CNY6
Massachusetts General Hospital
149 Thirteenth St.
Charlestown, MA 02129
USA
Tel: +1 617 726 5510
Fax: +1 617 726 5079
louis@helix.mgh.harvard.edu

Dr Lorraine A. MARIN *
Preuss Foundation for Brain Tumor Research
2223 Avenida de la Playa, Suite 220
La Jolla, CA 92093-0660
USA
Tel: +1 858 454-0200
+1 718 470-7194
Fax: +1 718 470-9756
marin@lij.edu

Dr Masao MATSUTANI
Department of Neurosurgery
Saitama Medical School
Moroyamamachi Morohongo 38
350-04 Saitama
JAPAN
Tel: +81 492 76 1551
Fax: +81 492 76 1551
matutani@saitama-med.ac.jp

Dr Roger E. MCLENDON *
Department of Pathology
Duke University Medical Center
Box 3712
Durham, NC 27710
USA
Tel: +1 919 684 3300
Fax: +1 919 684 3324
roger.mclendon@duke.edu

Dr Hernando MENA *
Department of Neuropathology
Armed Forces Institute of Pathology
Alaska Avenue at 14th Street
Washington, DC 20306-6000
USA
Tel: +1 202 782 1620
Fax: +1 202 782 4099
mena@afip.osd.mil

Dr Susan MORGELLO
Dept. of Pathology, Neuropathology
The Mount Sinai Medical Center
1 Gustave L. Levy Place
New York, NY 10029
USA
Tel: +1 212 241 9118
Fax: +1 212 996 1343
smorgello@smtplink.mssm.edu

Dr Motoo NAGANE
Ludwig Institute for Cancer Research
University of California, San Diego
9500 Gilman Dr., CMM-East Rm. 3071
La Jolla, CA 92093-0660
USA
Tel: +1 858 534 7808
Fax: +1 858 534 7816
mnagane@ucsd.edu

Dr Yoichi NAKAZATO *
Department of Pathology
Gunma University School of Medicine
3-39-22 Showamachi
Maebashi Gunma 371
JAPAN
Tel: +81 27 220 7970
Fax: +81 27 220 7978
nakazato@akagi.sb.gunma-u.ac.jp

Dr James S. NELSON *
Department of Pathology, Box P5-1
Louisiana State University Medical Center
1901 Perdido Street
New Orleans, Louisiana 70112
USA
Tel: +1 504 568 6082
Fax: +1 504 568 6037
jsnilsson@aol.com

Dr Hartmut P.H. NEUMANN
Dpt. of Nephrology and Hypertension
Albert-Ludwigs-University
Hugstetter Strasse 55
D-79106 Freiburg
Germany
Tel: +49 761 270 3578/3401
Fax: +49 761 270 3778
neumann@mm41.ukl.uni-freiburg.de

Dr Elizabeth W. NEWCOMB
Department of Pathology, MSB 531
NYU Medical Center
550 First Avenue
New York, NY 10016
USA
Tel: +1 212 263 8757
Fax: +1 212 263 8211
newcoe01@mcrcr.med.nyu.edu

Dr Mark D. NOBLE *
Huntsman Cancer Institute
University of Utah Health Sciences Center
Biopolymers Bldg., Room 410
Salt Lake City, UT 84112
USA
Tel: +1 801 585 7167
Fax: +1 801 585 7120
mark.noble@hci.utah.edu

Dr Hiroko OHGAKI *
Unit of Molecular Pathology
Intl. Agency for Research on Cancer (IARC)
150 cours Albert-Thomas
69372 Lyon
FRANCE
Tel: +33 4 72 73 84 34
Fax: +33 4 72 73 85 64
ohgaki@iarc.fr

Dr George W. PADBERG
Department of Neurology
University Hospital
PO Box 9101
HB-6500 Nijmegen
NETHERLANDS
Tel: +31 24 361 8860
Fax: +31 24 354 1122
g.padberg@czzoneu.azn.nl

Dr Werner PAULUS *
Institute of Neuropathology
University of Münster
Domagkstr. 19
D-48129 Münster/Westf.
GERMANY
Tel: +49 251 83 56966
Fax: +49 251 83 56971
werner.paulus@uni-muenster.de

Dr Aurelia PERAUD
Department of Neurosurgery
Ludwig Maximilians University
Marchioninistrasse 15
D-81377 Munich
GERMANY
Tel: +49 89 7095 4789
Fax: +49 89 7095 5694
aurelia.peraud@nc.med.uni-muenchen.de

Dr Iver PETERSEN
Institute of Pathology
University Hospital Charité
Schumannstr. 20-21
D-10117Berlin
GERMANY
Tel: +49 30 2802 2611
Fax: +49 30 2802 3407
iver.petersen@charite.de

Dr Torsten PIETSCH
Department of Neuropathology
University of Bonn Medical Center
Sigmund-Freud Str. 25
D-53105 Bonn
Germany
Tel: +49 228 287 4332/4398
Fax: +49 228 287 4331
pietsch-t@uni-bonn.de

Dr Karl H. PLATE *
Laboratory of Neuropathology
University Erlangen-Nurnberg
Krankenhausstr. 8-10
D-91054 Erlangen
GERMANY
Tel: +49 9131 852 6031/32
Fax: +49 9131 852 6033
plate@rzmail.uni-erlangen.de

Dr Richard A. PRAYSON
Department of Anatomic Pathology
Cleveland Clinic Foundation
Cleveland, OH 44195
USA
Tel: +1 216 444 8805
Fax: +1 216 445 6967
praysor@cesmtp.ccf.org

Peter PREUSS *
President
The Preuss Foundation, Inc.
2223 Avenida de la Playa, Suite 220
La Jolla, CA 92093-0660
USA
Tel: +1 858 454 0200
Fax: +1 858 454 4449
preussp@sdsc.edu

Dr Guido REIFENBERGER *
Institute of Neuropathology
University Hospital
Sigmund-Freud Str. 25
D-53105 Bonn
GERMANY
Tel: +49 228 287 6523
Fax: +49 228 287 4331
reifenb@rz.uni-duesseldorf.de or
g.reifenberger@uni-bonn.de

Dr Rui REIS
Unit of Molecular Pathology
Intl. Agency for Res. on Cancer (IARC)
150 cours Albert-Thomas
69372 Lyon Cedex 08
FRANCE
Tel: +33 (0)4 72 73 85 78
Fax: +33 (0)4 72 73 85 64
reis@iarc.fr

Dr Lucy B. RORKE *
Dept. of Pathology & Lab. Medicine
The Children's Hospital of Philadelphia
34th Street and Civic Center Blvd.
Philadelphia, PA 19104-4399
USA
Tel: +1 215 590 1734
Fax: +1 215 590 1736
rorke@email.chop.edu

Dr Marc K. ROSENBLUM *
Department of Pathology
Memorial Sloan Kettering Cancer Center
1275 York Avenue
New York, NY 10021
USA
Tel: +1 212 639 5905
Fax: +1 212 717 3203
rosenbl1@mskcc.org

Dr Bernd W. SCHEITHAUER *
Dept. of Laboratory Medicine & Pathology
Mayo Clinic
200 First Street South West
Rochester, MN 55901
USA
Tel: +1 507 284 8350
Fax: +1 507 284 1599
scheithauer.bernd@mayo.edu

Dr Davide SCHIFFER *
Second Dept. of Neurology
University of Turin
Via Cherasco no. 15
I-10126 Turin
ITALY
Tel: +39 011 663 6327
Fax: +39 011 696 3487
schiffer@molinette.unito.it

Dr Manfred SCHWAB *
Division of Cytogenetics - 0825
German Cancer Research Centre
Im Neuenheimer Feld 280
D-69120 Heidelberg
GERMANY
Tel: +49 6221 423220
Fax: +49 6221 423277
m.schwab@dkfz-heidelberg.de

Dr M.C. SHARMA
Department of Pathology
All India Institute of Medical Sciences
Ansari Nagar
New Delhi 110029
INDIA
Tel: +91 11 659 3371
Fax: +91 11 686 2663
sarkarch@medinst.ernet.in

Dr Hiroyuki SHIMADA
Department of Pathology & Lab. Medicine
Children's Hospital Los Angeles, MS#43
4650 Sunset Blvd.
Los Angeles, CA 90027
USA
Tel: +1 323 669 2377
Fax: +1 323 667 1123
hshimada@chla.usc.edu

Dr Shanop SHUANGSHOTI
Department of Pathology
Shulalongkorn University
Bangkok 10250
THAILAND
Tel: +66 2 215 0871
Fax: +66 2 215 4804
shanshua@rph.health.wa.gov.au

Dr Leslie H. SOBIN *
Division of Gastrointestinal Pathology
Armed Forces Institute of Pathology
Alaska Avenue at 14th St
Washington, DC 20306-6000
USA
Tel: +1 202 782 2880
Fax: +1 202 782 9020
sobin@afip.osd.mil

Dr Dov SOFFER *
Department of Pathology
Hadassah University Hospital
Kiryat Hadassah, POB 12000
IL-91120 Jerusalem
ISRAEL
Tel: +972 2 675 8207
Fax: +972 2 642 6268
soffer@cc.huji.ac.il

Dr Figen SÖYLEMEZOGLU
Department of Pathology
Haceteppe University
Tip Fakultesi, Patoloji Anabilim Dali
Ankara 06100
TURKEY
Tel: +90 312 230 6728
Fax: +90 312 231 5182
soylemez@ato.org.tr

Dr Peter A. STECK
Neuro-Oncology & Tumor Biology
UT M.D. Anderson Cancer Center
1515 Holcombe Blvd.
Houston, TX 77030
USA
Tel: +1 713 792 3003
Fax: +1 713 745 1183
steckpa@utmdacc.mda.uth.tmc.edu

Dr Anat O. STEMMER-RACHAMIMOV
Molecular Neuro-Oncology Laboratory, CNY6
Massachusetts General Hospital
149 Thirteenth St.
Charlestown, MA 02129
USA
Tel: +1 617 726 5510
Fax: +1 617 726 5079
rachammimov@helix.mgh.harvard.edu

Dr Janusz SZYMAS
Department of Pathology
University of Medical Sciences
Przybyszewski Str. 49
60-355 Poznan
POLAND
Tel: +48 61 869 1498/867
Fax: +48 61 867 9913 ?
jszymas@ampat.amu.edu.pl

Dr Ana Lia TARATUTO *
Department of Neuropathology
Inst. de Invest. Neurol. "R. Carrea"
Montañeses 2325 p. 3º
1428 Buenos Aires
ARGENTINA
Tel: +54 11 4788 3444
Fax: +54 11 4784 7620
ataratuto@fleni.org.ar

Dr John Q. TROJANOWSKI
Dept. of Pathology & Laboratory Medicine
Univ. of Pennsylvania School of Medicine
HUP-Maloney, 3rd floor, 36th and Spruce St.
Philadelphia, PA 19104-4283
USA
Tel: +1 215 662 6399
Fax: +1 215 349 5909
trojanow@uphs1.uphs.upenn.edu

Dr Erwin G. VAN MEIR
Neurosurgery/Molecular Neuro-Oncology
Emory University School of Medicine
1365-B Clifton Rd., N.E,. Suite B 5103
Atlanta, GA 30322
USA
Tel: +1 404 778 5227/2267
Fax: +1 404 778 5240/4472
evanmei@emory.edu

Dr Scott R. VANDENBERG
Department of Neuropathology
Univeristy of Virginia School of Medicine
Charlottesville, VA 22908
USA
Tel: +1 804 924 9175
Fax: +1 804 924 8060
srv@unix.mail.virginia.edu

Dr Harry V. VINTERS
Pathology Department
UCLA Medical School, CHS 18-170
10833 Le Conte Avenue
Los Angeles, CA
USA
Tel: +1 310 825 6191
Fax: +1 310 206 5178
hvinters@pathology.medsch.ucla.edu

Dr Anne VITAL
Laboratory of Neuropathology
Victor Segalen University, Bordeaux 2
146, rue Leo-Saignat
33076 Bordeaux Cedex
FRANCE
Tel: +33 (0)5 57 57 16 69
Fax: +33 (0)5 57 57 16 70
anne.vital@neuropath.u-bordeaux2.fr

Dr Silke VOGELGESANG
Department of Neuropathology
University of Greifswald
17489 Greifswald
GERMANY
Tel: +49 3834 865716
Fax: +49 3834 865704
vogelgesang@mail.uni-greifswald.de

Dr Andreas VON DEIMLING *
Institute of Neuropathology
University Hospital Charité
Austenburger Platz 1
D-13353 Berlin
GERMANY
Tel: +49 30 450 56013
Fax: +49 30 450 56940
andreas.von_deimling@charite.de

Dr Rolf W. WARZOK
Department of Neuropathology
University of Greifswald
17489 Greifswald
GERMANY
Tel: +49 3834 865715
Fax: +49 3834 865704
warzok@mail.uni-greifswald.de

Dr Kunihiko WATANABE
Department of Neurosurgery
Dokkyo Medical College
880 Kita-Kobayashi Mibu-cho Shimotsugagun
321-0293Tochigi 321-02
JAPAN
Tel: +81 282 87 21 59
Fax: +81 282 86 32 76
kunihiko@dokkyomed.ac.jp

Dr Michael WELLER
Department of Neurology
University of Tübingen School of Medicine
Hoppe-Seyler-Strasse 3
D-72076 Tübingen
GERMANY
Tel: +49 7071 298 6529
Fax: +49 7071 295260
michael.weller@uni-tuebingen.de

Dr Manfred M. WESTPHAL *
Neurosurgical Clinic
University of Hamburg
Martinstrasse 52
D-20246 Hamburg
GERMANY
Tel: +49 40 4280 33751
Fax: +49 40 4280 34596
westphal@plexus.uke.uni-hamburg.de

Dr Otmar D. WIESTLER *
Institute of Neuropathology
University Hospital
Sigmund-Freud Str. 25
D-53105 Bonn
GERMANY
Tel: +49 228 287 6523
Fax: +49 228 287 4331
neuropath@uni-bonn.de

Dr James M. WOODRUFF *
Department of Pathology
Memorial Sloan Kettering Cancer Center
1275 York Avenue
New York, NY 10021
USA
Tel: +1 212 639 5905
Fax: +1 212 717 3203
woodrufj@mskcc.org

Sources of charts and photographs

1.1	E.W. Newcomb
1.2	W.K. Cavenee
1.3	W.K. Cavenee
1.4	P. Kleihues
1.5	M.E. Berens
1.6	K.H. Plate
1.7	K.H. Plate
1.8	M. Weller
1.9	P. Kleihues
1.10	M. Westphal
1.11	P. Kleihues
1.12	M. Westphal
1.13A,B	Y. Nakazato
1.13C-D	P. Kleihues
1.14A	Y. Nakazato
1.14B	H. Ohgaki
1.15A	J.M. Kros
1.15B	Y. Nakazato
1.16	H. Ohgaki
1.17	P. Kleihues
1.18	P. Kleihues
1.19A	Y. Nakazato
1.19B	P. Kleihues
1.19C	Y. Nakazato
1.19D	P. Kleihues
1.20	P. Kleihues
1.21	Dr A. Valavanis Institute of Neuroradiology, University Hospital, 8091 Zürich, Switzerland
1.22	K.H. Plate
1.23	P.C. Burger
1.24	P. Kleihues
1.25	P. Kleihues
1.26A	Y. Nakazato
1.26B	P. Kleihues
1.26C	G. Reifenberger
1.27	P. Kleihues
1.28A	J.J. Kepes
1.28B	P. Kleihues
1.28C,D	Dr Y. Iwasaki Miyagi National Hospital Watawari-gun 989-22 Miyagi, Japan
1.29	P. Kleihues
1.30A	P. Kleihues
1.30B	Y. Nakazato
1.30C	H. Ohgaki
1.31	H. Ohgaki
1.32	H. Ohgaki
1.33	H. Ohgaki
1.34	P. Kleihues
1.35	P.C. Burger
1.36	H. Ohgaki
1.37	P. Kleihues
1.38	Y. Nakazato
1.39	W. Biernat
1.40	P. Kleihues
1.41	H. Ohgaki
1.42	H. Ohgaki
1.43	P. Kleihues
1.44A	P.C. Burger
1.44B	Dr. W.J. Huk Neuroradiology, University of Erlangen Medical School, 91054 Erlangen, Germany
1.44C,D	P.C. Burger
1.45	M. Westphal
1.46A	W. Paulus
1.46B	L.B. Rorke
1.47A,B	P.C. Burger
1.47C,D	P. Kleihues
1.48	Dr. G. Perilongo, Pediatric Oncology-Hematology, University of Padua, Italy
1.49A-D	P.C. Burger
1.49E	L.B. Rorke
1.49F	P.C. Burger
1.50	J. Szymas
1.51	C. Giannini
1.52	W. Paulus
1.53	J.M. Kros
1.54A-C	W. Paulus
1.54D	J.M. Kros
1.54E,F	W. Paulus
1.55	J.J. Kepes
2.1	G. Reifenberger
2.2	M. Westphal
2.3	P. Kleihues
2.4	P. Kleihues
2.5A,B	Y. Nakazato
2.5C	V.P. Collins
2.5D	Y. Nakazato
2.6	J.M. Kros
2.7	J.M. Kros
2.8A	Y. Nakazato
2.8B	J.M. Kros
2.9	G. Reifenberger
2.10A	Dr. S. VandenBerg
2.10B	Y. Nakazato
2.11A	Y. Nakazato
2.11B,C	G. Reifenberger
2.11D	P. Kleihues
2.12	O.D. Wiestler
2.13	G. Reifenberger
2.14	G. Reifenberger
3.1	D. Schiffer
3.2	M. Westphal
3.3	P. Kleihues
3.4	M. Rosenblum
3.5A	D. Schiffer
3.5B	P. Kleihues
3.5C	D. Schiffer
3.5D	D.N. Louis
3.6A	P. Kleihues
3.6B	M. Rosenblum
3.6C	Y. Nakazato
3.6D	P. Kleihues
3.7	M. Westphal
3.8	K. Jellinger
3.9	O.D. Wiestler
3.10A	M. Rosenblum
3.10B	D. Schiffer
3.10C	M. Rosenblum
3.10D	P. Kleihues
3.11	O.D. Wiestler
3.12	Y. Nakazato
3.13	O.D. Wiestler
3.14A	P. Kleihues
3.14B	W. Paulus
3.15	P. Kleihues
4.1	W. Paulus
4.2	A. Vital
4.3A	L.B. Rorke
4.3B	M.K. Rosenblum
4.4	A. Aguzzi
4.5A	S. Brandner
4.5B	W. Paulus
4.5C	L.B. Rorke
4.5D	P. Kleihues
4.6	D.N. Louis
5.1	M.K. Rosenblum
5.2	M.K. Rosenblum
5.3A,B	D.J. Brat
5.3C	P.C. Burger
5.4	M.T. Jennings
5.5A	C. Daumas-Duport
5.5B	P. Kleihues
5.6A	P.L. Lantos
5.6B	L.B. Rorke
6.1A	O.D. Wiestler
6.1B	M.K. Rosenblum
6.2A	Y. Nakazato
6.2B	O.D. Wiestler
6.2C	J.M. Bruner
6.2D	J.S. Nelson
6.2E,F	P. Kleihues
6.3	A.L. Taratuto

6.4A	Dr R.A. Zimmerman, Neuroradiology Department, The Children's Hospital of Philadelphia, Philadelphia, PA 19104-4301, U.S.A.
6.4B	A.L. Taratuto
6.5	A.L. Taratuto
6.6A	A.L. Taratuto
6.6B	Y. Nakazato
6.6C,D	L.B. Rorke
6.7A	Y. Nakazato
6.7B	A.L. Taratuto
6.8	C. Daumas-Duport
6.9A,B	C. Daumas-Duport
6.9C	O.D. Wiestler
6.10	C. Daumas-Duport
6.11	O.D. Wiestler
6.12	C. Daumas-Duport
6.13	C. Daumas-Duport
6.14	Y. Nakazato
6.15	C. Daumas-Duport
6.16	F. Söylemezoglu
6.17	P.C. Burger
6.18	D. Soffer
6.19A	P. Kleihues
6.19B	Y. Nakazato
6.19C	P.C. Burger
6.19D	P. Kleihues
6.20	P.C. Burger
6.21	D. Figarella-Branger
6.22A	Y. Nakazato
6.22B	P. Kleihues
6.22C	D. Figarella-Branger
6.23	S. Brandner
6.24A,B	F. Giangaspero
6.24C,D	P. Kleihues
6.25	D. Soffer
6.26	D. Soffer
6.27A,B	D. Soffer
6.27C	P. Kleihues
6.27D	D. Soffer
6.28	D. Soffer
7.1	H. Mena
7.2	H. Mena
7.3A	A.L. Taratuto
7.3B	M.K. Rosenblum
7.4A	M.K. Rosenblum
7.4B	H. Mena
7.4C	J.M. Kros
7.4D	Y. Nakazato
7.5	H. Mena
7.6	H. Mena
7.7	Y. Nakazato
7.8A	Y. Nakazato
7.8B	P. Kleihues
7.8C,D	H. Mena
7.8E	Y. Nakazato
7.8F	H. Mena
7.9	B.W. Scheithauer
7.10A	H. Mena
7.10B	A. Jouvet
7.10C	Y. Nakazato
7.10D	S.R. Vandenberg
8.1A	L.E. Becker
8.1B	D. Figarella-Branger
8.2A	Y. Nakazato
8.2B,C	L.E. Becker
8.3A	F. Giangaspero
8.3B	J.M. Kros
8.4A	Y. Nakazato
8.4B	P. Kleihues
8.4C	Y. Nakazato
8.4D	P. Kleihues
8.5	F. Giangaspero
8.6A	V. Joshi
8.6B	P. Kleihues
8.7	P. Kleihues
8.8A	M. Westphal
8.8B	D. Figarella-Branger
8.8C,D	P. Kleihues
8.9A,B	P. Kleihues
8.9C	L.B. Rorke
8.9D,E	P. Kleihues
8.9F	L.B. Rorke
8.10A	F. Giangaspero
8.10B-D	P. Kleihues
8.11A-C	P.C. Burger
8.11D	F. Giangaspero
8.12	P. Kleihues
8.13	F. Giangaspero
8.14A,B	F. Giangaspero
8.14C	O.D. Wiestler
8.14D	P. Kleihues
8.14E	O.D. Wiestler
8.14F	P. Kleihues
8.15	S.H. Bigner
8.16	S.H. Bigner
8.17A	Y. Nakazato
8.17B	H. Kalimo
8.17C	O.D. Wiestler
8.18	Dr F. Garcia-Bragado, Department of Pathology, Hospital Virgen del Camino, 31008 Pamplona, Spain
8.19	M. Westphal
8.20	Y. Nakazato
8.21A,B	R.E. McLendon
8.21C,D	L.B. Rorke
8.22	R.E. McLendon
8.23A,B	R.E. McLendon
8.23C	Y. Nakazato
8.23D	P. Kleihues
8.24	L.B. Rorke
8.25	R.A. Zimmerman (see 6.4A)
8.26	L.B. Rorke
8.27	Y. Nakazato
8.28	L.B. Rorke
9.1	S.D. Finkelstein
9.2	Dr J. Martinez, Department of Pathology, University of Pittsburgh Medical Center, Pittsburgh, PA 15213, U.S.A.
9.3	Dr J. Martinez (see 9.2)
9.4A,B	Dr J. Martinez (see 9.2)
9.5	J.M. Kros
9.6	R.A. Zimmerman (see 6.4A)
9.7	H. Shimada
9.8	H. Shimada
9.9	J.M. Kros
9.10	M. Schwab
10.1	P. Kleihues
10.2A	D. Soffer
10.2B	P. Kleihues
10.3A	P. Kleihues
10.3B	D. Soffer
10.4A,B	Y. Nakazato
10.4C	P. Kleihues
10.4D	J.M. Woodruff
10.5A	J.M. Woodruff
10.5B	Y. Nakazato
10.5C,D	J.M. Woodruff
10.6	Y. Nakazato
10.7	J.M. Woodruff
10.8	H. Budka
10.9	C. Giannini
10.10	C. Giannini
10.11	C. Giannini
10.12	C. Giannini
10.13	C. Giannini
10.14	C. Giannini
10.15	J.M. Woodruff
10.16	J.M. Woodruff
11.1A	Dr P.W. Schaefer, Department of Radiology, Massachusetts General Hospital and Havard Medical School, Boston, MA 02114, U.S.A.
11.1B	D.N. Louis
11.2	P. Kleihues
11.3A-E	P. Kleihues
11.3F	H. Budka
11.4	Dr. K. Mori, Department of Neurosurgery, Juntendo University, Izunagaoka Hospital, Shizuoka 410-2295, Japan
11.5A	H. Budka
11.5B	P. Kleihues
11.6	P. Kleihues
11.7A,B	D.N. Louis
11.7C	Y. Nakazato
11.7D	D.N. Louis
11.7E,F	Y. Nakazato
11.8	H. Budka
11.9	P. Kleihues
11.10	D. Figarella-Branger
11.11	H. Budka
11.12	D.N. Louis
11.13	Y. Nakazato
11.14A	D.N. Louis
11.14B	P. Kleihues
11.14C,D	Y. Nakazato
11.15	Y. Nakazato
11.16	Dr. L.F. Bleggy-Torres and J.S. Reis Filho, Department of Pathology, Federal University of Parana, Curitiba, Brazil
11.17A	Y. Nakazato
11.17B	H. Budka
11.17C	Y. Nakazato
11.17D	J.M. Kros
11.18	W. Paulus

11.19 D.N. Louis
11.20A P. Kleihues
11.20B B.W. Scheithauer
11.20C W. Paulus
11.21A B.W. Scheithauer
11.21B W. Paulus
11.22A B.W. Scheithauer
11.22B M.J. Haltia
11.23 J. Jääskeläinen
11.24 J. Jääskeläinen
11.25 J. Jääskeläinen
11.26A,B M.J. Haltia
11.26C Y. Nakazato
11.26D,E M.J. Haltia
11.26F Y. Nakazato
11.27 K. Jellinger
11.28 Y. Nakazato
11.29 K. Jellinger
11.30A D. Soffer
11.30B J.M. Kros
11.31A D.N. Louis
11.31B,C L.B. Rorke
11.32 Y. Nakazato

12.1 W. Paulus
12.2A Dr W.J. Huk (see 1.44B)
12.2B P. Kleihues
12.3A-C P. Kleihues
12.3D K. Jellinger
12.4 Y. Nakazato
12.5 M.J. Haltia
12.6A,B Y. Nakazato
12.6C-E W. Paulus
12.6F D.N. Louis
12.7 W. Paulus
12.8 Dr C.H. Rickert, Inst. of Neuropathology, University of Münster, 48129 Münster, Germany
12.9 Y. Nakazato
12.10A Dr. J. Peiffer, Institute for Brain Research, University of Tübingen, 72076 Tübingen, Germany
12.10B-D Y. Nakazato
12.11 Dr. M. Fartasch, Department of Dermatology, University of Erlangen, 91054 Erlangen, Germany
12.12A Dr. R.V. Jones, AFIP, Dept. of Neuropathology, Washington DC 20306, USA
12.12B R.V. Jones (see 12.12A)
12.13A W. Paulus
12.13B Dr. W. Brück, Institute of Neuro- pathology, University of Göttingen, 37075 Göttingen, Germany

13.1 M.K. Rosenblum
13.2 M.K. Rosenblum
13.3 Dr J.E. Olvera-Rabiela, Department of Pathology, Memorial Sloan Kettering Cancer Center, New York, NY 10021, U.S.A
13.4 M. Westphal
13.5 M.K. Rosenblum
13.6 M.K. Rosenblum
13.7 M.K. Rosenblum

14.1 J.M. Kros
14.2 J.S. Nelson
14.3 P.C. Burger
14.4 P. Kleihues
14.5 D.N. Louis
14.6A K.H. Plate
14.6B,C Dr P.W. Schaefer (see 11.2A)
14.7 O.D. Wiestler
14.8 O.D. Wiestler
14.9A O.D. Wiestler
14.9B D.N. Louis
14.10 O.D. Wiestler
14.11A O.D. Wiestler
14.11B-D D.N. Louis
14.12 Dr. V. Ramesh, Molecular Neurogenetics Unit, Massachusetts General Hospital, Charlestown, MA 02129, USA
14.13 T. Böhling
14.14A K.H. Plate
14.14B J.M. Kros
14.15A M. Westphal
14.15B W. Paulus
14.16 P. Kleihues
14.17A Y. Nakazato
14.17B O.D. Wiestler
14.17C J.M. Kros
14.17D K.H. Plate
14.17E T. Böhling
14.17F,G K.H. Plate
14.18 Dr. S. Gläsker, Department of Nephrology and Hyperten- sion, Albert-Ludwigs Univer- sity, 71906 Freiburg, Germany
14.19 O.D. Wiestler
14.20 M. Westphal
14.21 M. Westphal
14.22 Dr. J.-P. Vonsattel, Depart- ment of Neuropathology and Neurosurgery, Massachusetts General Hospital and Havard Medical School, Boston, MA 02114, U.S.A.
14.23 W. Paulus
14.24A W. Paulus
14.24B P. Kleihues
14.24C,D B.S. Lopes
14.25 H. Ohgaki
14.26 A. Vital
14.27 H. Ohgaki
14.28 P. Hainaut
14.29 H. Ohgaki
14.30 Dr C.B. Sonier, Service de Neuroradiologie, Hospital Laennec, 44000 Nantes, France
14.31A G. Reifenberger
14.31B Y. Nakazato
14.32A,B Dr. M.M. Ruchoux, Depart- ment of Neuropathology, Hospital Roger Salengro, Centre Hospitalier Regional Universitaire de Lille, 59037 Lille Cedex, France
14.32C W. Paulus
14.32D A. Vital
14.33 O.D. Wiestler
14.34 W.E. Cavenee
14.35 G. Reifenberger

15.1 R.C. Janzer
15.2 P.C. Burger
15.3 P. Kleihues
15.4A P. Kleihues
15.4B J.M. Bruner
15.5 Dr. G.P. Pizzolato, Division of Neuropathology, Department of Pathology, University Hospital, 1211 Geneva, Switzerland
15.6A P.C. Burger
15.6B,C F. Giangaspero
15.6D P.C. Burger
15.7 W. Paulus
15.8 R.W. Warzok
15.9 R.W. Warzok
15.10A,B W. Feiden
15.10C-F R.W. Warzok

16.1 M. Westphal
16.2A-D P. Kleihues
16.2E R.C. Janzer
16.2F P. Kleihues
16.2G R.C. Janzer
16.2H-S P. Kleihues
16.3 J.S. Nelson
16.4 I. Petersen

References

1. Abe M, Tabuchi K, Tsuji A, Shiraishi T, Koga H, Takagi M (1995). Dysembryoplastic neuroepithelial tumor: report of three cases. *Surg Neurol* 43: 240-245.

2. Abeliovich D, Gelman K, Silverstein S, Lerer I, Chemke J, Merin S, Zlotogora J (1995). Familial cafe au lait spots: a variant of neurofibromatosis type. *J Med Genet* 32: 985-986.

3. Aboody-Guterman K, Hair L, Morgello S (1996). Epstein-Barr virus and AIDS-related primary central nervous system lymphoma: viral detection by immunohistochemistry, RNA in situ hybridization, and polymerase chain reaction. *Clin Neuropathol* 15: 79-86.

4. Abs R, Van Vyve M, Willems PJ, Neetens I, Van der Auwera B, Van den Ende E, Van de Kelft E, Beckers A, Van Marck E, Martin JJ (1992). The association of astrocytoma and pituitary adenoma in a patient with alcaptonuria. *J Neurol Sci* 108: 32-34.

5. Adamson TE, Wiestler OD, Kleihues P, Yasargil MG (1990). Correlation of clinical and pathological features in surgically treated craniopharyngiomas. *J Neurosurg* 73: 12-17.

6. Adesina AM, Nalbantoglu J, Cavenee WK (1994). p53 gene mutation and mdm2 gene amplification are uncommon in medulloblastoma. *Cancer Res* 54: 5649-5651.

7. Agamanolis DP, Malone JM (1995). Chromosomal abnormalities in 47 pediatric brain tumors. *Cancer Genet Cytogenet* 81: 125-134.

8. Ahlsen G, Gillberg IC, Lindblom R, Gillberg C (1994). Tuberous sclerosis in Western Sweden. A population study of cases with early childhood onset. *Arch Neurol* 51: 76-81.

9. Aho R, Haapasalo H, Alanen K, Haltia M, Paetau A, Kalimo H (1995). Proliferative activity and DNA index do not significantly predict survival in primary central nervous system lymphoma. *J Neuropathol Exp Neurol* 54: 826-832.

10. Aho R, Kalimo H, Salmi M, Smith D, Jalkanen S (1997). Binding of malignant lymphoid cells to the white matter of the human central nervous system: Role of different CD44 isoforms, beta1, beta2 and beta7 Integrins and L-selectin. *J Neuropath Exp Neurol* 56: 557-568.

11. Aida T, Abe H, Itoh T, Nagashima K, Inoue K (1993). Desmoplastic infantile ganglioglioma—case report. *Neurol Med Chir Tokyo* 33: 463-466.

12. al Ahwal M, Jha N, Nabholtz JM, Hugh J, Birchall I, Nguyen GK (1994). Olfactory neuroblastoma: report of a case associated with inappropriate antidiuretic hormone secretion. *J Otolaryngol* 23: 437-439.

13. al Sarraj S, Bridges LR (1995). p53 immunoreactivity in astrocytomas and its relationship to survival. *Br J Neurosurg* 9: 143-149.

14. Albert FK, Forsting M, Sartor K, Adams HP, Kunze S (1994). Early postoperative magnetic resonance imaging after resection of malignant glioma: objective evaluation of residual tumor and its influence on regrowth and prognosis. *Neurosurgery* 34: 45-60.

15. Albrecht S, Armstrong DL, Mahoney DH, Cheek WR, Cooley LD (1993). Cytogenetic demonstration of gene amplification in a primary intracranial germ cell tumor. *Genes Chromosomes Cancer* 6: 61-63.

16. Albrecht S, Bruner JM, Segall GK (1993). Immunoglobulin heavy chain rearrangements in primary brain lymphomas. A study using PCR to amplify CDR-III. *J Pathol* 169: 297-302.

17. Albrecht S, Connelly JH, Bruner JM (1993). Distribution of p53 protein expression in gliosarcomas: an immunohistochemical study. *Acta Neuropathol (Berl)* 85: 222-226.

18. Albrecht S, Haber RM, Goodman JC, Duvic M (1992). Cowden syndrome and Lhermitte-Duclos disease. *Cancer* 70: 869-876.

19. Albrecht S, Rouah E, Becker LE, Bruner J (1991). Transthyretin immunoreactivity in choroid plexus neoplasms and brain metastases. *Mod Pathol* 4: 610-614.

20. Albrecht S, von Deimling A, Pietsch T, Giangaspero F, Brandner S, Kleihues P, Wiestler OD (1994). Microsatellite analysis of loss of heterozygosity on chromosomes 9q, 11p and 17p in medulloblastomas. *Neuropathol Appl Neurobiol* 20: 74-81.

21. Albright AL, Wisoff JH, Zeltzer P, Boyett J, Rorke LB, Stanley P, Geyer JR, Milstein JM (1995). Prognostic factors in children with supratentorial (nonpineal) primitive neuroectodermal tumors. A neurosurgical perspective from the Children's Cancer Group. *Pediatr Neurosurg* 22: 1-7.

22. Albuquerque L, Pimentel J, Costa A, Cristina L (1992). Cerebral granular cell tumors: report of a case and a note on their nature and expected behaviour. *Acta Neuropathol (Berl)* 84: 680-685.

23. Alderson L, Fetell MR, Sisti M, Hochberg F, Cohen M, Louis DN (1996). Sentinel lesions of primary CNS lymphoma. *J Neurol Neurosurg Psychiatry* 60: 102-105.

24. Alguacil G, Pettigrew NM, Sima AA (1986). Secretory meningioma. A distinct subtype of meningioma. *Am J Surg Pathol* 10: 102-111.

25. Allcutt D, Michowiz S, Weitzman S, Becker L, Blaser S, Hoffman HJ, Humphreys RP, Drake JM, Rutka JT (1993). Primary leptomeningeal melanoma: an unusually aggressive tumor in childhood. *Neurosurgery* 32: 721-729.

26. Allegranza A, Girlando S, Arrigoni GL, Veronese S, Mauri FA, Gambacorta M, Pollo B, Dalla P, Barbareschi M (1991). Proliferating cell nuclear antigen expression in central nervous system neoplasms. *Virchows Arch A Pathol Anat Histopathol* 419: 417-423.

27. Alpers CE, Davis RL, Wilson CB (1982). Persistence and late malignant transformation of childhood cerebellar astrocytoma. Case report. *J Neurosurg* 57: 548-551.

28. Alvarez F, Roda JM, Perez R, Morales C, Sarmiento MA, Blazquez MG (1987). Malignant and atypical meningiomas: a reappraisal of clinical, histological, and computed tomographic features. *Neurosurgery* 20: 688-694.

29. Alvarez JA, Cohen ML, Hlavin ML (1996). Primary intrinsic brainstem oligodendroglioma in an adult. Case report and review of the literature. *J Neurosurg* 85: 1165-1169.

30. Ambler M, Pogacar S, Sidman R (1969). Lhermitte-Duclos disease (granule cell hypertrophy of the cerebellum) pathological analysis of the first familial cases. *J Neuropathol Exp Neurol* 28: 622-647.

31. Ambros IM, Zellner A, Roald B, Amann G, Ladenstein R, Printz D, Gadner H, Ambros PF (1996). Role of ploidy, chromosome 1p, and Schwann cells in the maturation of neuroblastoma. *N Engl J Med* 334: 1505-1511.

32. Amler LC, Corvi R, Praml C, Savelyeva L, Le Paslier D, Schwab M (1995). A reciprocal translocation (1;15) (36.2;q24) in a neuroblastoma cell line is accompanied by DNA duplication and may signal the site of a putative tumor suppressor-gene. *Oncogene* 10: 1095-1101.

33. Ammirati M, Vick N, Liao YL, Ciric I, Mikhael M (1987). Effect of the extent of surgical resection on survival and quality of life in patients with supratentorial glioblastomas and anaplastic astrocytomas. *Neurosurgery* 21: 201-206.

34. Andrews JM,Schumann GB (1992). *Neurocytopathology.* Wiliams and Wilkins: Philadelphia.

35. Antinheimo J, Haapasalo H, Seppala M, Sainio M, Carpen O, Jaaskelainen J (1995). Proliferative potential of sporadic and neurofibromatosis 2- associated schwannomas as studied by MIB-1 (Ki-67) and PCNA labeling. *J Neuropathol Exp Neurol* 54: 776-782.

36. Anzil AP (1970). Glioblastoma multiforme with extracranial metastases in the absence of previous craniotomy. Case report. *J Neurosurg* 33: 88-94.

37. Aoyama I, Makita Y, Nabeshima S, Motomochi M, Masuda A (1980). Extradural nasal and orbital extension of glioblastoma multiforme without previous surgical intervention. *Surg Neurol* 14: 343-347.

38. Aozasa K, Saeki K, Horiuchi K, Yoshimine T, Ikeda H, Nakao K, Hayakawa T (1993). Primary lymphoma of the brain developing in a boy after a 5-year history of encephalitis: polymerase chain reaction and in situ hybridization analyses for Epstein-Barr virus. *Hum Pathol* 24: 802-805.

39. Arap W, Nishikawa R, Furnari FB, Cavenee WK, Huang HJ (1995). Replacement of the p16/CDKN2 gene suppresses human glioma cell growth. *Cancer Res* 55: 1351-1354.

40. Arens R, Marcus D, Engelberg S, Findler G, Goodman RM, Passwell JH (1988). Cerebral germinomas and Klinefelter syndrome. A review. *Cancer* 61: 1228-1231.

41. Arita N, Taneda M, Hayakawa T (1994). Leptomeningeal dissemination of malignant gliomas. Incidence, diagnosis and outcome. *Acta Neurochir Wien* 126: 84-92.

42. Ariza A, Kim JH (1988). Kaposi's sarcoma of the dura mater. *Hum Pathol* 19: 1461-1463.

43. Arnesen MA, Scheithauer BW, Freeman S (1994). Cushing's syndrome secondary to olfactory neuroblastoma. *Ultrastruct Pathol* 18: 61-68.

44. Arnoldus EP, Wolters LB, Voormolen JH, van Duinen SG, Raap AK, van der Ploeg M, Peters AC (1992). Interphase cytogenetics: a new tool for the study of genetic changes in brain tumors. *J Neurosurg* 76: 997-1003.

45. Arseni C, Ciurea AV (1981). Statistical survey of 276 cases of medulloblastoma (1935—1978). *Acta Neurochir Wien* 57: 159-162.

46. Artigas J, Cervos N, Iglesias JR, Ebhardt G (1985). Gliomatosis cerebri: clinical and histological findings. *Clin Neuropathol* 4: 135-148.

47. Aso T, Lane WS, Conaway JW, Conaway RC (1995). Elongin (SIII): a multisubunit regulator of elongation by RNA polymerase II. *Science* 269: 1439-1443.

48. Auer RN, Becker LE (1983). Cerebral medulloepithelioma with bone, cartilage, and striated muscle. Light microscopic and immunohistochemical study. *J Neuropathol Exp Neurol* 42: 256-267.

49. Auperin I, Mikolt J, Oksenhendler E, Thiebaut JB, Brunet M, Dupont B, Morinet F (1994). Primary central nervous system malignant non-Hodgkin's lymphomas from HIV-infected and non-infected patients: expression of cellular surface proteins and Epstein-Barr viral markers. *Neuropathol Appl Neurobiol* 20: 243-252.

50. Aydin F, Ghatak NR, Salvant J, Muizelaar P (1993). Desmoplastic cerebral astrocytoma of infancy. A case report with immunohistochemical, ultrastructural and proliferation studies. *Acta Neuropathol (Berl)* 86: 666-670.

51. Azar CG, Scavarda NJ, Reynolds CP, Brodeur GM (1990). Multiple defects of the nerve growth factor receptor in human neuroblastomas. *Cell Growth Differ* 1: 421-428.

52. Azzarelli B, Rekate HL, Roessmann U (1977). Subependymoma: a case report with ultrastructural study. *Acta Neuropathol (Berl)* 40: 279-282.

53. Badiali M, Pession A, Basso G, Andreini L, Rigobello L, Galassi E, Giangaspero F (1991). N-myc and c-myc oncogenes amplification in medulloblastomas. Evidence of particularly aggressive behavior of a tumor with c- myc amplification. *Tumori* 77: 118-121.

54. Bagan JV, Penarrocha M, Vera S (1989). Cowden syndrome: clinical and pathologi-

cal considerations in two new cases. *J Oral Maxillofac Surg* 47: 291-294.

55. Bailey P, Bucy PC (1929). Oligodendrogliomas of the brain. *J Path Bact* 32: 735-751.

56. Bailey P, Bucy PC (1930). Astroblastomas of the brain. *Acta Psychiatr Neurol* 5: 439-461.

57. Bailey P, Cushing H (1925). Medulloblastoma cerebelli: a common type of mid-cerebellar glioma of childhood. *Arch Neurol Psychiatry* 14: 192-224.

58. Bailey P, Cushing H (1926). *A Classification of Tumors of the Glioma Group on a Histogenetic Basis with a Correlation Study of Prognosis.* Lippincott: Philadelphia.

59. Baker DL, Molenaar WM, Trojanowski JQ, Evans AE, Ross AH, Rorke LB, Packer RJ, Lee VM, Pleasure D (1991). Nerve growth factor receptor expression in peripheral and central neuroectodermal tumors, other pediatric brain tumors, and during development of the adrenal gland. *Am J Pathol* 139: 115-122.

60. Balko MG, Blisard KS, Samaha FJ (1992). Oligodendroglial gliomatosis cerebri. *Hum Pathol* 23: 706-707.

61. Balmaceda C, Heller G, Rosenblum M, Diez B, Villablanca JG, Kellie S, Maher P, Vlamis V, Walker RW, Leibel S, Finlay JL (1996). Chemotherapy without irradiation—a novel approach for newly diagnosed CNS germ cell tumors: results of an international cooperative trial. The First International Central Nervous System Germ Cell Tumor Study. *J Clin Oncol* 14: 2908-2915.

62. Balmaceda CM, Fetell MR, O'Brien JL, Housepian EH (1993). Nevus of Ota and leptomeningeal melanocytic lesions. *Neurology* 43: 381-386.

63. Banerjee AK, Sharma BS, Kak VK, Ghatak NR (1989). Gliosarcoma with cartilage formation. *Cancer* 63: 518-523.

64. Barak Y, Gottlieb E, Juven G, Oren M (1994). Regulation of mdm2 expression by p53: alternative promoters produce transcripts with nonidentical translation potential. *Genes Dev* 8: 1739-1749.

65. Barker FG, Davis RL, Chang SM, Prados MD (1996). Necrosis as a prognostic factor in glioblastoma multiforme. *Cancer* 77: 1161-1166.

66. Barkovich AJ, Frieden IJ, Williams ML (1994). MR of neurocutaneous melanosis. *AJNR Am J Neuroradiol* 15: 859-867.

67. Barnard RO, Bradford TS, Thomas DGT (1986). Gliomyosarcoma: Report of a case of rhabdomyosarcoma arising in malignant glioma. *Acta Neuropathol (Berl)* 69: 23-27.

68. Barnard RO, Geddes JF (1987). The incidence of multifocal cerebral gliomas. A histologic study of large hemisphere sections. *Cancer* 60: 1519-1531.

69. Barnes L, Kapadia SB (1994). The biology and pathology of selected skull base tumors. *J Neurooncol* 20: 213-240.

70. Bartram CR, Berthold F (1987). Amplification and expression of the N-myc gene in neuroblastoma. *Eur J Pediatr* 146: 162-165.

71. Barzilay JI, Pazianos AG (1989). Adrenocortical carcinoma. *Urologenic Clincs N America* 16: 457-468.

72. Bashir R, Chamberlain M, Ruby E, Hochberg FH (1996). T-cell infiltration of primary CNS lymphoma. *Neurology* 46: 440-444.

73. Batra SK, McLendon RE, Koo JS, Castelino P, Fuchs HE, Krischer JP, Friedman HS, Bigner DD, Bigner SH (1995). Prognostic implications of chromosome 17p deletions in human medulloblastomas. *J Neurooncol* 24: 39-45.

74. Batra SK, Rasheed BK, Bigner SH, Bigner DD (1994). Biology of disease. Oncogenes and anti-oncogenes in human central nervous system tumors. *Lab Invest* 71: 621-637.

75. Batzdorf U, Malamud U (1963). The problem of multicentric gliomas. *J Neurosurg* 20: 122-136.

76. Bauman GS, Gaspar LE, Fisher BJ, Halperin EC, Macdonald DR, Cairncross JG (1994). A prospective study of short-course radiotherapy in poor prognosis glioblastoma multiforme. *Int J Radiat Oncol Biol Phys* 29: 835-839.

77. Bauman GS, Wara WM, Ciricillo SF, Davis RL, Zoger S, Edwards MSB (1997). Primary intracerebral osteosarcoma: a case report. *J Neurooncol* 32: 209-213.

78. Baysal BE, Farr JE, Rubinstein WS, Galus RA, Johnson KA, Aston CE, Myers EN, Johnson JT, Carrau R, Kirkpatric SJ, Myssiorek D, Singh D, Saha S, Gollin SM, Evans GA, James MR, Richard C (1997). Fine mapping of an imprinted gene for familial nonchromaffin paraganliomas, on chromosome 11q23. *Am J Hum Genet* 60: 121-132.

79. Bechtel JT, Patton JM, Takei Y (1978). Mixed mesenchymal and neuroectodermal tumor of the cerebellum. *Acta Neuropathol (Berl)* 41: 261-263.

80. Becker DP, Benyo R, Roessman V (1967). Glial origin of monstrocellular tumor: Case report of prolonged survival. *J Neurosurg* 26: 72-77.

81. Beckwith JB, Martin RF (1968). Observations on the histopathology of neuroblastomas. *J Pediatr Surg* 3: 106-110.

82. Bello MJ, Leone PE, Nebreda P, de Campos JM, Kusak ME, Vaquero J, Sarasa JL, Garcia M, Queizan A, Hernandez M (1995). Allelic status of chromosome 1 in neoplasms of the nervous system. *Cancer Genet Cytogenet* 83: 160-164.

83. Bello MJ, Leone PE, Vaquero J, de Campos JM, Kusak ME, Sarasa JL, Pestana A, Rey JA (1995). Allelic loss at 1p and 19q frequently occurs in association and may represent early oncogenic events in oligodendroglial tumors. *Int J Cancer* 64: 207-210.

84. Bello MJ, Rey JA, de Campos JM, Kusak ME (1993). Chromosomal abnormalities in a pineocytoma. *Cancer Genet Cytogenet* 71: 185-186.

85. Bello MJ, Vaquero J, de Campos JM, Kusak ME, Sarasa JL, Saez Castresana J, Pestana A, Rey JA (1994). Molecular analysis of chromosome 1 abnormalities in human gliomas reveals frequent loss of 1p in oligodendroglial tumors. *Int J Cancer* 57: 172-175.

86. Belloni E, Muenke M, Roessler E, Traverso G, Siegel B, Frumkin A, Mitchell HF, Donis K, Helms C, Hing AV, Heng HH, Koop B, Martindale D, Rommens JM, Tsui LC, Scherer SW (1996). Identification of Sonic hedgehog as a candidate gene responsible for holoprosencephaly. *Nat Genet* 14: 353-356.

87. Benli K, Inci S (1995). Solitary dural plasmacytoma: case report. *Neurosurgery* 36: 1206-1209.

88. Bennett JP, Jr., Rubinstein LJ (1984). The biological behavior of primary cerebral neuroblastoma: a reappraisal of the clinical course in a series of 70 cases. *Ann Neurol* 16: 21-27.

89. Berger MS, Deliganis AV, Dobbins J, Keles GE (1994). The effect of extent of resection on recurrence in patients with low grade cerebral hemisphere gliomas. *Cancer* 74: 1784-1791.

90. Bergmann M, Blasius S, Bankfalvi A, Mellin W (1996). Primary non-Hodgkin lymphomas of the CNS-proliferation, oncoproteins and Epstein-Barr-virus. *Gen Diagn Pathol* 141: 235-242.

91. Bergmann M, Terzija W, Blasius S, Kuchelmeister K, Kryne K, Gerhard L, Beneicke U, Berlit P (1994). Intravascular lymphomatosis of the CNS: clinicopathologic study and search for expression of oncoproteins and Epstein-Barr virus. *Clin Neurol Neurosurg* 96: 236-243.

92. Bergsagel DJ, Finegold MJ, Butel JS, Kupsky WJ, Garcea RL (1992). DNA sequences similar to those of simian virus 40 in ependymomas and choroid plexus tumors of childhood. *N Engl J Med* 326: 988-993.

93. Berkman RA, Clark WC, Saxena A, Robertson JT, Oldfield EH, Ali IU (1992). Clonal composition of glioblastoma multiforme. *J Neurosurg* 77: 432-437.

94. Berkman RA, Merrill MJ, Reinhold WC, Monacci WT, Saxena A, Clark WC, Robertson JT, Ali IU, Oldfield EH (1993). Expression of the vascular permeability factor/vascular endothelial growth factor gene in central nervous system neoplasms. *J Clin Invest* 91: 153-159.

95. Bernards A (1995). Neurofibromatosis type 1 and Ras-mediated signaling: filling in the GAPs. *Biochim Biophys Acta* 1242: 43-59.

96. Bernell WR, Kepes JJ, Seitz EP (1972). Late malignant recurrence of childhood cerebellar astrocytoma. Report of two cases. *J Neurosurg* 37: 470-474.

97. Bernstein JJ, Woodard CA (1995). Glioblastoma cells do not intravasate into blood vessels. *Neurosurgery* 36: 124-132.

98. Barron KD, Hirano A, Araki S, Terry RD (1958). Experiences with neoplasms involving the spinal cord. *Neurology* 9: 91-106.

99. Berthold F (1990). Overview: biology of neuroblastoma. In: *Neuroblastoma: Tumor Biology and Therapy*, Pochedly C (eds). CRC Press: Boca Raton.

100. Bessell EM, Graus F, Punt JA, Firth JL, Hope DT, Moloney AJ, Lopez G, Villa S (1996). Primary non-Hodgkin's lymphoma of the CNS treated with BVAM or CHOD/BVAM chemotherapy before radiotherapy. *J Clin Oncol* 14: 945-954.

101. Best PV (1973). A medulloblastoma-like tumour with melanin formation. *J Pathol* 110: 109-111.

102. Best PV (1987). Malignant triton tumour in the cerebellopontine angle. Report of a case. *Acta Neuropathol (Berl)* 74: 92-96.

103. Bickerstaff ER, Connolly RC, Woolf AL (1967). Cerebellar medulloblastoma occurring in brothers. *Acta Neuropathol (Berl)* 8: 104-107.

104. Biegel JA, Allen CS, Kawasaki K, Shimizu N, Budarf ML, Bell CJ (1996). Narrowing the critical region for a rhabdoid tumor locus in 22q11. *Genes Chromosomes Cancer* 16: 94-105.

105. Biegel JA, Burk CD, Barr FG, Emanuel BS (1992). Evidence for a 17p tumor related locus distinct from p53 in pediatric primitive neuroectodermal tumors. *Cancer Res* 52: 3391-3395.

106. Biegel JA, Janss AJ, Raffel C, Sutton L, Rorke LB, Harper JM, Phillips PC (1997). Prognostic significance of chromosome 17p deletions in childhood primitive neuroectodermal tumors (medulloblastomas) of the central nervous system. *Clin Cancer Res* 3: 473-478.

107. Biegel JA, Perilongo G, Rorke LB, Parmiter AH, Emanuel BS (1992). Malignant fibrous histiocytoma of the brain in a six-year-old girl. *Genes Chromosomes Cancer* 4: 309-313.

108. Biegel JA, Rorke LB, Packer RJ, Emanuel BS (1990). Monosomy 22 in rhabdoid or atypical tumors of the brain. *J Neurosurg* 73: 710-714.

109. Biegel JA, Rorke LB, Janss AJ, Sutton LN, Parmiter AH (1995). Isochromosome 17q demonstrated by interphase fluorescence in situ hybridization in primitive neuroectodermal tumors of the central nervous system. *Genes Chromosomes Cancer* 14: 85-96.

110. Biegel JA, Wentz E (1997). No preferential parent of origin for the isochromosome 17q in childhood primitive neuroectodermal tumor (medulloblastoma). *Genes Chromosomes Cancer* 18: 143-146.

111. Biegel JA, White PS, Marshall HN, Fujimori M, Zackai EH, Scher CD, Brodeur GM, Emanuel BS (1993). Constitutional 1p36 deletion in a child with neuroblastoma. *Am J Hum Genet* 52: 176-182.

112. Biernat W, Aguzzi A, Sure U, Grant JW, Kleihues P, Hegi ME (1995). Identical mutations of the p53 tumor suppressor gene in the gliomatous and the sarcomatous components of gliosarcomas suggest a common origin from glial cells. *J Neuropathol Exp Neurol* 54: 651-656.

113. Biernat W, Kleihues P, Yonekawa Y, Ohgaki H (1997). Amplification and overexpression of MDM2 in primary (de novo) glioblastomas. *J Neuropathol Exp Neurol* 56: 180-185.

114. Biggs PJ, Garen PD, Powers JM, Garvin AJ (1987). Malignant rhabdoid tumor of the central nervous system. *Hum Pathol* 18: 332-337.

115. Bignami A, Adelman LS, Perides G, Dahl D (1989). Glial hyaluronate-binding protein in polar spongioblastoma. *J Neuropathol Exp Neurol* 48: 187-196.

116. Bigner SH (1992). Cerebrospinal fluid (CSF) cytology: current status and diagnostic applications. *J Neuropathol Exp Neurol* 51: 235-245.

117. Bigner SH, Burger PC, Wong AJ, Werner MH, Hamilton SR, Muhlbaier LH, Vogelstein B, Bigner DD (1988). Gene amplification in malignant human gliomas: clinical and histopathologic aspects. *J Neuropathol Exp Neurol* 50: 8017-8022.

118. Bigner SH, Friedman HS, Vogelstein B, Oakes WJ, Bigner DD (1990). Amplification of the c-myc gene in human medulloblastoma cell lines and xenografts. *Cancer Res* 50: 2347-2350.

119. Bigner SH, Humphrey PA, Wong AJ, Vogelstein B, Mark J, Friedman HS, Bigner DD (1990). Characterization of the epidermal growth factor receptor in human glioma cell lines and xenografts. *Cancer Res* 50: 8017-8022.

120. Bigner SH, Mark J, Friedman HS, Biegel

JA, Bigner DD (1988). Structural chromosomal abnormalities in human medulloblastoma. *Cancer Genet Cytogenet* 30: 91-101.

121. Bigner S, McLendon R, Fuchs HE, McKeever PE, Friedman HS (1997). Chromosomal characteristics of childhood brain tumors. *Cancer Genet Cytogenet* 97: 125-134.

122. Bigner SH, Vogelstein B (1990). Cytogenetics and molecular genetics of malignant gliomas and medulloblastoma. *Brain Pathol* 1: 12-18.

123. Bijlsma EK, Leenstra S, Westerveld A, Bosch DA, Hulsebos TJ (1994). Amplification of the anonymous marker D17S67 in malignant astrocytomas. *Genes Chromosomes Cancer* 9: 148-152.

124. Bijlsma EK, Merel P, Bosch DA, Westerveld A, Delattre O, Thomas G, Hulsebos TJ (1994). Analysis of mutations in the SCH gene in schwannomas. *Genes Chromosomes Cancer* 11: 7-14.

125. Bijlsma EK, Voesten AM, Bijleveld EH, Troost D, Westerveld A, Merel P, Thomas G, Hulsebos TJ (1995). Molecular analysis of genetic changes in ependymomas. *Genes Chromosomes Cancer* 13: 272-277.

126. Bindal AK, Blisard KS, Melin-Aldama H, Warnick RE (1997). Primary T-cell lymphoma of the brain in acquired immunodeficiency syndrome: case report. *J Neurooncol* 31: 267-271.

127. Birch BD, Johnson JP, Parsa A, Desai RD, Yoon JT, Lycette CA, Li YM, Bruce JN (1996). Frequent type 2 neurofibromatosis gene transcript mutations in sporadic intramedullary spinal cord ependymomas. *Neurosurgery* 39: 135-140.

128. Birch JM, Hartley AL, Blair V, Kelsey AM, Harris M, Teare MD, Jones PH (1990). Cancer in the families of children with soft tissue sarcoma. *Cancer* 66: 2239-2248.

129. Bjornsson J, Scheithauer BW, Okazaki H, Leech RW (1985). Intracranial germ cell tumors: pathobiological and immunohistochemical aspects of 70 cases. *J Neuropathol Exp Neurol* 44: 32-46.

130. Blades DA, Hardy RW, Cohen M (1991). Cervical paraganglioma with subsequent intracranial and intraspinal metastases. Case report. *J Neurosurg* 75: 320-323.

131. Blaeker H, Rasheed BK, McLendon RE, Friedman HS, Batra SK, Fuchs HE, Bigner SH (1996). Microsatellite analysis of childhood brain tumors. *Genes Chromosomes Cancer* 15: 54-63.

132. Blair V, Birch JM (1994). Patterns and temporal trends in the incidence of malignant disease in children: II. Solid tumours of childhood. *Eur J Cancer* 30A: 1498-1511.

133. Bobele GB, Sexauer C, Barnes PA, Krous HF, Bodensteiner JB (1994). Esthesioneuroblastoma presenting as an orbital mass in a young child. *Med Pediatr Oncol* 22: 269-273.

134. Bodey B, Bodey B, Jr., Siegel SE (1995). Immunophenotypic characterization of infiltrating polynuclear and mononuclear cells in childhood brain tumors. *Mod Pathol* 8: 333-338.

135. Boerman RH, Anderl K, Herath J, Borell T, Johnson N, Schaeffer-Klein J, Kirchhof A, Raap AK, Scheithauer BW, Jenkins RB (1996). The glial and mesenchymal elements of gliosarcomas share similar genetic alterations. *J Neuropathol Exp Neurol* 55: 973-981.

136. Boesel CP, Suhan JP, Sayers MP (1978). Melanotic medulloblastoma. Report of a case with ultrastructural findings. *J Neuropathol Exp Neurol* 37: 531-543.

137. Bogler O, Huang HJ, Cavenee WK (1995). Loss of wild-type p53 bestows a growth advantage on primary cortical astrocytes and facilitates their in vitro transformation. *Cancer Res* 55: 2746-2751.

138. Bogler O, Huang HJ, Kleihues P, Cavenee WK (1995). The p53 gene and its role in human brain tumors. *Glia* 15: 308-327.

139. Bohling T, Hatva E, Kujala M, Claesson Welsh L, Alitalo K, Haltia M (1996). Expression of growth factors and growth factor receptors in capillary hemangioblastoma. *J Neuropathol Exp Neurol* 55: 522-527.

140. Bohling T, Maenpaa A, Timonen T, Vantunen L, Paetau A, Haltia M (1996). Different expression of adhesion molecules in stromal cells and endothelial cells of capillary hemangioblastoma. *Acta Neuropathol* 92: 461-466.

141. Bohling T, Paetau A, Ekblom P, Haltia M (1983). Distribution of endothelial and basement membrane markers in angiogenic tumors of the nervous system. *Acta Neuropathol (Berl)* 62: 67-72.

142. Bohling T, Turunen O, Jaaskelainen J, Carpen O, Sainio M, Wahlstrom T, Vaheri A, Haltia M (1996). Ezrin expression in stromal cells of capillary hemangioblastoma. An immunohistochemical survey of brain tumors. *Am J Pathol* 148: 367-373.

143. Boker DK, Wassmann H, Solymosi L (1983). Paragangliomas of the spinal canal. *Surg Neurol* 19: 461-468.

144. Bonnin JM, Rubinstein LJ (1989). Astroblastomas: a pathological study of 23 tumors, with a postoperative follow-up in 13 patients. *Neurosurgery* 25: 6-13.

145. Bonnin JM, Rubinstein LJ, Palmer NF, Beckwith JB (1984). The association of embryonal tumors originating in the kidney and in the brain. A report of seven cases. *Cancer* 54: 2137-2146.

146. Boop FA, Chadduck WM, Sawyer J, Husain M (1991). Congenital aneurysmal hemorrhage and astrocytoma in an infant. *Pediatr Neurosurg* 17: 44-47.

147. Borberg A (1951). Clinical and genetic investigations into tuberous sclerosis and Recklinghausen's neurofibromatosis. *Acta Psychiatr Neurol Scand* 71: 1-239.

148. Borit A, Blackwood W, Mair WG (1980). The separation of pineocytoma from pineoblastoma. *Cancer* 45: 1408-1418.

149. Borovich B, Doron Y (1986). Recurrence of intracranial meningiomas: the role played by regional multicentricity. *J Neurosurg* 64: 58-63.

150. Bosch EP, Murphy MJ, Cancilla PA (1981). Peripheral neurofibromatosis and peroneal muscular atrophy. *Neurology* 31: 1408-1414.

151. Bourhis J, De Vathaire F, Wilson GD, Hartmann O, Terrier L, Boccon G, McNally NJ, Lemerle J, Riou G, Benard J (1991). Combined analysis of DNA ploidy index and N-myc genomic content in neuroblastoma. *Cancer Res* 51: 33-36.

152. Bourn D, Carter SA, Mason S, Gareth D, Evans R, Strachan T (1994). Germline mutations in the neurofibromatosis type 2 tumour suppressor gene. *Hum Mol Genet* 3: 813-816.

153. Brada M, Ford D, Ashley S, Bliss JM, Crowley S, Mason M, Rajan B, Traish D (1992). Risk of second brain tumour after conservative surgery and radiotherapy for pituitary adenoma. *Br Med J* 304: 1343-1346.

154. Brandis A, Mirzai S, Tatagiba M, Walter GF, Samii M, Ostertag H (1993). Immunohistochemical detection of female sex hormone receptors in meningiomas: correlation with clinical and histological features. *Neurosurgery* 33: 212-217.

155. Briner J, Bannwart F, Kleihues P, Odermott B, Janzer R, Willi U, Boltshauser E (1985). Malignant small cell tumor of the brain with intermediate filaments - a case of primary cerebral rhabdoid tumors. *Pediatr Pathol* 3;117-118.

156. Brinster RL, Chen HY, Messing A, Van Dyke T, Levine AJ, Palmiter RD (1984). Transgenic mice harboring SV40 T-antigen genes develop characteristic brain tumors. *Cell* 37: 367-379.

157. Britz GW, Kim DK, Loeser JD (1996). Hydrocephalus secondary to diffuse villous hyperplasia of the choroid plexus. Case report and review of the literature. *J Neurosurg* 85: 689-691.

158. Brodeur GM, Castleberry RP (1993). Neuroblastoma. In: *Principles and Practice of Pediatric Oncology*, Pizzo PA, Poplack DG (eds), 2nd ed. J.B. Lippincott: Philadelphia. pp. 739-767.

159. Brodeur GM, Pritchard J, Berthold F, Carlsen NL, Castel V, Castleberry RP, DeBarnardi B, Evans AE, Favrot M, Hedborg F, Kaneko M, Kemshead J, Lampert F, Lee REJ, Look AT, Pearson ADJ, Philip T, Roald B, Sawada T, Seeger RC, Tsuchida Y, Voute PA (1993). Revisions of the international criteria for neuroblastoma diagnosis, staging, and response to treatment. *J Clin Oncol* 17: 1466-1477.

160. Broggi G, Franzini A, Cajola L, Pluchino F (1994). Cell kinetic investigations in craniopharyngioma: preliminary results and considerations. *Pediatr Neurosurg* 21 Suppl 1: 21-23.

161. Brooks JS, Freeman M, Enterline HT (1985). Malignant "Triton" tumors. Natural history and immunohistochemistry of nine new cases with literature review. *Cancer* 55: 2543-2549.

162. Brooks WH, Markesbery WR, Gupta GD, Roszman TL (1978). Relationship of lymphocyte invasion and survival of brain tumor patients. *Ann Neurol* 4: 219-224.

163. Brown MT, McClendon RE, Gockerman JP (1995). Primary central nervous system lymphoma with systemic metastasis: case report and review. *J Neurooncol* 23: 207-221.

164. Brownstein MH, Mehregan AH, Bikowski JB, Lupulescu A, Patterson JC (1979). The dermatopathology of Cowden's syndrome. *Br J Dermatol* 100: 667-673.

165. Bruce JN, Stein BM (1990). Pineal tumors. *Neurosurg Clin N Am* 1: 123-138.

166. Brunner HG, Hulsebos T, Steijlen PM, der K, Steen A, Hamel BC (1993). Exclusion of the neurofibromatosis 1 locus in a family with inherited cafe-au-lait spots. *Am J Med Genet* 46: 472-474.

167. Brustle O, Ohgaki H, Schmitt HP, Walter GF, Ostertag H, Kleihues P (1992). Primitive neuroectodermal tumors after prophylactic central nervous system irradiation in children. Association with an activated K-ras gene. *Cancer* 69: 2385-2392.

168. Budka H (1974). Intracranial lipomatous hamartomas (intracranial "lipomas"). A study of 13 cases including combinations with medulloblastoma, colloid and epidermoid cysts, angiomatosis and other malformations. *Acta Neuropathol (Berl)* 28: 205-222.

169. Budka H, Chimelli L (1994). Lipomatous medulloblastoma in adults: a new tumor type with possible favorable prognosis. *Hum Pathol* 25: 730-731.

170. Bullard DE, Rawlings CE, Phillips B, Cox EB, Schold SC, Jr., Burger P, Halperin EC (1987). Oligodendroglioma. An analysis of the value of radiation therapy. *Cancer* 60: 2179-2188.

171. Burger PC (1996). Pathology of brain stem astrocytomas. *Pediatr Neurosurg* 24: 35-40.

172. Burger PC, Breiter SN, Fisher PG (1996). Pilocytic and fibrillary astrocytomas of the brain stem - a comparative clinical, radiological and pathological study. *J Neuropathol Exp Neurol* 55;640.

173. Burger PC, Dubois PJ, Schold SC, Jr., Smith KR, Jr., Odom GL, Crafts DC, Giangaspero F (1983). Computerized tomographic and pathologic studies of the untreated, quiescent, and recurrent glioblastoma multiforme. *J Neurosurg* 58: 159-169.

174. Burger PC, Grahmann FC, Bliestle A, Kleihues P (1987). Differentiation in the medulloblastoma. A histological and immunohistochemical study. *Acta Neuropathol (Berl)* 73: 115-123.

175. Burger PC, Green SB (1987). Patient age, histologic features, and length of survival in patients with glioblastoma multiforme. *Cancer* 59: 1617-1625.

176. Burger PC, Heinz ER, Shibata T, Kleihues P (1988). Topographic anatomy and CT correlations in the untreated glioblastoma multiforme. *J Neurosurg* 68: 698-704.

177. Burger PC, Kleihues P (1989). Cytologic composition of the untreated glioblastoma with implications for evaluation of needle biopsies. *Cancer* 63: 2014-2023.

178. Burger PC, Rawlings CE, Cox EB, McLendon RE, Schold SC, Jr., Bullard DE (1987). Clinicopathologic correlations in the oligodendroglioma. *Cancer* 59: 1345-1352.

179. Burger PC, Scheithauer BW (1994). Tumors of paraganglionic tissue. In: *Tumors of the Central Nervous System. Atlas of Tumor Pathology*, Armed Forces Institute of Pathology: Washington D.C. pp. 317-320.

180. Burger PC, Scheithauer BW (1994). *Tumors of the Central Nervous System.* Armed Forces Institute of Pathology: Washington.

181. Burger PC, Scheithauer BW, Vogel FS (1991). *Surgical Pathology of the Nervous System and its Coverings.* 3rd ed, Churchill Livingstone: London.

182. Burger PC, Shibata T, Kleihues P (1986). The use of the monoclonal antibody Ki-67 in the identification of proliferating cells: application to surgical neuropathology. *Am J Surg Pathol* 10: 611-617.

183. Burger PC, Vogel FS, Green SB, Strike TA (1985). Glioblastoma multiforme and anaplastic astrocytoma. Pathologic criteria and prognostic implications. *Cancer* 56: 1106-1111.

184. Burger PC, Vollmer RT (1980). Histologic factors of prognostic significance in the glioblastoma multiforme. *Cancer* 46: 1179-1186.

185. Bussey HJR (1975). *Familial Polyposis Coli*. John Hopkins University: Baltimore.

186. Byravan S, Foster LM, Phan T, Verity AN, Campagnoni AT (1994). Murine oligodendroglial cells express nerve growth factor. *Proc Natl Acad Sci USA* 91: 8812-8816.

187. Cabello A, Madero S, Castresana A, Diaz L (1991). Astroblastoma: electron microscopy and immunohistochemical findings: case report. *Surg Neurol* 35: 116-121.

188. Caccamo DV, Herman MM, Rubinstein LJ (1989). An immunohistochemical study of the primitive and maturing elements of human cerebral medulloepitheliomas. *Acta Neuropathol (Berl)* 79: 248-254.

189. Caccamo DV, Ho KL, Garcia JH (1992). Cauda equina tumor with ependymal and paraganglionic differentiation. *Hum Pathol* 23: 835-838.

190. Camilleri-Broet S, Davi F, Feuillard J, Seilhean D, Michiels JF, Brousset P, Epardeau B, Navratil E, Mokhtari K, Bourgeois C, Marelle L, Raphael M, Hauw JJ (1997). AIDS-related primary brain lymphomas: histopathologic and immunohisochemical study of 51 cases. The French study group for HIV-associated tumors. *Hum Pathol* 28: 367-374.

191. Campbell AN, Chan HS, Becker LE, Daneman A, Park TS, Hoffman HJ (1984). Extracranial metastases in childhood primary intracranial tumors. A report of 21 cases and review of the literature. *Cancer* 53: 974-981.

192. Carbonara C, Longa L, Grosso E, Mazzucco G, Borrone C, Garre ML, Brisigotti M, Filippi G, Scabar A, Giannotti A, Falzoni P, Monga G, Garini G, Gabrielli M, Riegler P, Danesino C, Ruggieri M, Magro G, Migone N (1996). Apparent preferential loss of heterozygosity at TSC2 over TSC1 chromosomal region in tuberous sclerosis hamartomas. *Genes Chromosomes Cancer* 15: 18-25.

193. Carbone M, Pass HI, Rizzo P, Marinetti M, Di Muzio M, Mew DJ, Levine AS, Procopio A (1994). Simian virus 40-like DNA sequences in human pleural mesothelioma. *Oncogene* 9: 1781-1790.

194. Carbone M, Rizzo P, Procopio A, Giuliano M, Pass HI, Gebhardt MC, Mangham C, Hansen M, Malkin DF, Bushart G, Pompetti F, Picci P, Levine AS, Bergsagel JD, Garcea RL (1996). SV40-like sequences in human bone tumors. *Oncogene* 13: 527-535.

195. Carlson SS,Hockfield S (1996). Central nervous system. In: *Extracellular Matrix*, Comper WD (eds). Overseas Publishers: Amsterdam. pp. 1-23.

196. Carneiro SS, Scheithauer BW, Nascimento AG, Hirose T, Davis DH (1996). Solitary fibrous tumor of the meninges: a lesion distinct from fibrous meningioma. A clinicopathologic and immunohistochemical study. *Am J Clin Pathol* 106: 217-224.

197. Carney JA (1990). Psammomatous melanotic schwannoma. A distinctive, heritable tumor with special associations, including cardiac myxoma and the Cushing syndrome. *Am J Surg Pathol* 14: 206-222.

198. Carney JA, Gordon H, Carpenter PC, Shenoy BV, Go VL (1985). The complex of myxomas, spotty pigmentation, and endocrine overactivity. *Medicine Baltimore* 64: 270-283.

199. Carney ME, O'Reilly RC, Sholevar B, Buiakova OI, Lowry LD, Keane WM, Margolis FL, Rothstein JL (1995). Expression of the human Achaete-scute 1 gene in olfactory neuroblastoma (esthesioneuroblastoma). *J Neurooncol* 26: 35-43.

200. Caron H, van Sluis P, de Kraker J, Bokkerink J, Egeler M, Laureys G, Slater R, Westerveld A, Voute PA, Versteeg R (1996). Allelic loss of chromosome 1p as a predictor of unfavorable outcome in patients with neuroblastoma. *N Engl J Med* 334: 225-230.

201. Caron H, van Sluis P, van Roy N, de Kraker J, Speleman F, Voute PA, Westerveld A, Slater R, Versteeg R (1994). Recurrent 1;17 translocations in human neuroblastoma reveal nonhomologous mitotic recombination during the S/G2 phase as a novel mechanism for loss of heterozygosity. *Am J Hum Genet* 55: 341-347.

202. Carrie C, Lasset C, Alapetite C, Haie M, Hoffstetter S, Demaille MC, Kerr C, Wagner JP, Lagrange JL, Maire JP (1994). Multivariate analysis of prognostic factors in adult patients with medulloblastoma. Retrospective study of 156 patients. *Cancer* 74: 2352-2360.

203. Carrol RS, Glowacka D, Dashner K, Black PM (1993). Progesterone receptor expression in meningiomas. *Cancer Res* 53: 1312-1316.

204. Casadei GP, Komori T, Scheithauer BW, Miller GM, Parisi JE, Kelly PJ (1993). Intracranial parenchymal schwannoma. A clinicopathological and neuroimaging study of nine cases. *J Neurosurg* 79: 217-222.

205. Casadei GP, Scheithauer BW, Hirose T, Manfrini M, Van Houton C, Wood MB (1995). Cellular schwannoma. A clinicopathologic, DNA flow cytometric, and proliferation marker study of 70 patients. *Cancer* 75: 1109-1119.

206. Casalone R, Righi R, Granata P, Portentoso P, Minelli E, Meroni, Solero CL, Allegranza A (1994). Cerebral germ cell tumor and XXY karyotype. *Cancer Genet Cytogenet* 74: 25-29.

207. Castaneda VL, Cheah MS, Saldivar VA, Richmond CM, Parmley RT (1991). Cytogenetic and molecular evaluation of clinically aggressive esthesioneuroblastoma. *Am J Pediatr Hematol Oncol* 13: 62-70.

208. Cavender JF, Conn A, Epler M, Lacko H, Tevethia MJ (1995). Simian virus 40 large T antigen contains two independent activities that cooperate with a ras oncogene to transform rat embryo fibroblasts. *J Virol* 69: 923-934.

209. Cavin LW, Dalrymple GV, McGuire EL, Maners AW, Broadwater JR (1990). CNS tumor induction by radiotherapy: a report of four new cases and estimate of dose required. *Int J Radiat Oncol Biol Phys* 18: 399-406.

210. Celli P, Cervoni L, Cantore G (1993). Ependymoma of the filum terminale: treatment and prognostic factors in a series of 28 cases. *Acta Neurochir Wien* 124: 99-103.

211. Celli P, Nofrone I, Palma L, Cantore G, Fortuna A (1994). Cerebral oligodendroglioma: prognostic factors and life history. *Neurosurgery* 35: 1018-1034.

212. Cenacchi G, Giangaspero A, Cerasoli S, Manetto V, Martinelli GN (1996). Ultrastructural characterization of oligodendroglial-like cells in central nervous system tumors. *Ultrastruct Pathol* 20: 537-547.

213. Centeno BA, Louis DN, Kupsky WJ, Preffer FI, Sobel RA (1993). The AgNOR technique, PCNA immunohistochemistry, and DNA ploidy in the evaluation of choroid plexus biopsy specimens. *Am J Clin Pathol* 100: 690-696.

214. Central Brain Tumor Registry of the United States (1995). *First Annual Report*.

215. Cerda-Nicolas M, Kepes JJ (1993). Gliofibromas (including malignant forms), and gliosarcomas: a comparative study and review of the literature. *Acta Neuropathol (Berl)* 85: 349-361.

216. Cerda-Nicolas M, Lopez-Gines C, Peydro O, Llombart-Bosch A (1993). Central neurocytoma: a cytogenetic case study. *Cancer Genet Cytogenet* 65: 173-174.

217. Cervera-Pierot P, Varlet P, Chodkiewicz JP, Daumas D (1997). Dysembryoplastic neuroepithelial tumors in the caudate nucleus area. *Neurosurg* 40: 1065-1069.

218. Chaganti RS, Rodriguez E, Bosl GJ (1993). Cytogenetics of male germ-cell tumors. *Urol Clin North Am* 20: 55-66.

219. Challa VR, Goodman HO, Davis CH, Jr. (1983). Familial brain tumors: studies of two families and review of recent literature. *Neurosurgery* 12: 18-23.

220. Chamberlain MC (1994). Long survival in patients with acquired immune deficiency syndrome-related primary central nervous system lymphoma. *Cancer* 73: 1728-1730.

221. Chan GL, Little JB (1983). Cultured diploid fibroblasts from patients with the nevoid basal cell carcinoma syndrome are hypersensitive to ionizing radiation. *Am J Pathol* 111: 50-55.

222. Chang CH, Housepian EM, Herbert C, Jr. (1969). An operative staging system and a megavoltage radiotherapeutic technique for cerebellar medulloblastomas. *Radiology* 93: 1351-1359.

223. Chang SM, Lillis H, Larson DA, Wara WM, Bollen AW, Prados MD (1995). Pineoblastoma in adults. *Neurosurgery* 37: 383-390.

224. Chapin JE, Davis LE, Kornfeld M, Mandler RN (1995). Neurologic manifestations of intravascular lymphomatosis. *Acta Neurol Scand* 91: 494-499.

225. Chaubal A, Paetau A, Zoltick P, Miettinen M (1994). CD34 immunoreactivity in nervous system tumors. *Acta Neuropathol (Berl)* 88: 454-458.

226. Chen F, Slife L, Kishida T, Mulvihill J, Tisherman SE, Zbar B (1996). Genotype-phenotype correlation in von Hippel-Lindau disease: identification of a mutation associated with VHL type 2A. *J Med Genet* 33: 716-717.

227. Chen R, Macdonald DR, Ramsay DA (1995). Primary diffuse leptomeningeal oligodendroglioma. Case report. *J Neurosurg* 83: 724-728.

228. Chen WY, Liu HC (1990). Atypical (anaplastic) meningioma: relationship between histologic features and recurrence—a clinicopathologic study. *Clin Neuropathol* 9: 74-81.

229. Cheng SY, Huang HJ, Nagane M, Ji XD, Wang D, Shih CC, Arap W, Huang CM, Cavenee WK (1996). Suppression of glioblastoma angiogenicity and tumorigenicity by inhibition of endogenous expression of vascular endothelial growth factor. *Proc Natl Acad Sci USA* 93: 8502-8507.

230. Chidambaram A, Goldstein AM, Gailani MR, Gerrard B, Bale SJ, DiGiovanna JJ, Bale AE, Dean M (1996). Mutations in the human homologue of the Drosophila patched gene in Caucasian and African-American nevoid basal cell carcinoma syndrome patients. *Cancer Res* 56: 4599-4601.

231. Chiechi MV, Smirniotopoulos JG, Mena H (1995). Pineal parenchymal tumors: CT and MR features. *J Comput Assist Tomogr* 19: 509-517.

232. Chimelli L, Hahn MD, Budka H (1991). Lipomatous differentiation in a medulloblastoma. *Acta Neuropathol (Berl)* 81: 471-473.

233. Chin HW, Hazel JJ, Kim TH, Webster JH (1980). Oligodendrogliomas. I. A clinical study of cerebral oligodendrogliomas. *Cancer* 45: 1458-1466.

234. Cho KG, Hoshino T, Nagashima T, Murovic JA, Wilson CB (1986). Prediction of tumor doubling time in recurrent meningiomas. Cell kinetics studies with bromodeoxyuridine labeling. *J Neurosurg* 65: 790-794.

235. Cho KG, Hoshino T, Pitts LH, Nomura K, Shimosato Y (1988). Proliferative potential of brain metastases. *Cancer* 62: 512-515.

236. Cho Y, Gorina S, Jeffrey PD, Pavletich NP (1994). Crystal structure of a p53 tumor suppressor-DNA complex: understanding tumorigenic mutations. *Science* 265: 346-355.

237. Choi BH, Kim RC (1984). Expression of glial fibrillary acidic protein in immature oligodendroglia. *Science* 223: 407-409.

238. Choi BH, Matthias SC (1987). Cortical dysplasia associated with massive ectopia of neurons and glial cells within the subarachnoid space. *Acta Neuropathol (Berl)* 73: 105-109.

239. Chou SM, Anderson JS (1991). Primary CNS malignant rhabdoid tumor (MRT): report of two cases and review of literature. *Clin Neuropathol* 10: 1-10.

240. Chou TM, Chou SM (1989). Tuberous sclerosis in the premature infant: a report of a case with immunohistochemistry on the CNS. *Clin Neuropathol* 8: 45-52.

241. Chowdhury C, Roy S, Mahapatra AK, Bhatia R (1985). Medullomyoblastoma. A teratoma. *Cancer* 55: 1495-1500.

242. Chow CW, Brittingham J (1987). Perivascular pseudorosettes in childhood brain tumours: an ultrastructural and immunohistochemical study. *Pathology* 19: 12-16.

244. Chozick BS, Benzil DL, Stopa EG, Pezzullo JC, Knuckey NW, Epstein MH, Finkelstein SD, Finch PW (1996). Immunohistochemical evaluation of erbB-2 and p53 protein expression in benign and atypical human meningiomas. *J Neurooncol* 27: 117-126.

245. Chozick BS, Pezzullo JC, Epstein MH, Finch PW (1994). Prognostic implications of p53 overexpression in supratentorial astrocytic tumors. *Neurosurgery* 35: 831-837.

246. Christensen WN, Strong EW, Bains MS, Woodruff JM (1988). Neuroendocrine differentiation in the glandular peripheral nerve sheath tumor. Pathologic distinction from the biphasic synovial sarcoma with glands. *Am J Surg Pathol* 12: 417-426.

247. Christiansen H, Lampert F (1988). Tumour karyotype discriminates between good and bad prognostic outcome in neuroblastoma. *Br J Cancer* 57: 121-126.

248. Christiansen H, Sahin K, Berthold F, Hero B, Terpe HJ, Lampert F (1995). Comparison of DNA aneuploidy, chromosome 1 abnor-

malities, MYCN amplification and CD44 expression as prognostic factors in neuroblastoma. *Eur J Cancer* 31A: 541-544.

249. Chu CT, Everiss KD, Wikstrand CJ, Batra SK, Kung HJ, Bigner DD (1997). Receptor dimerization is not a factor in the signalling activity of a transforming variant epidermal growth factor receptor (EGFRvIII). *Biochem J* 324: 855-861.

250. Chun HC, Schmidt U, Wolfson A, Tercilla OF, Sagerman RH, King GA (1990). External beam radiotherapy for primary spinal cord tumors. *J Neurooncol* 9: 211-217.

251. Cinalli G, Zerah M, Carteret M, Doz F, Vinikoff L, Lellouch T, Husson B, Pierre K (1997). Subdural sarcoma associated with chronic subdural hematoma. Report of two cases and review of the literature. *J Neurosurg* 86: 553-557.

252. Cinque P, Brytting M, Vago L, Castagna A, Parravicini C, Zanchetta N, D'Arminio M, Wahren B, Lazzarin A, Linde A (1993). Epstein-Barr virus DNA in cerebrospinal fluid from patients with AIDS-related primary lymphoma of the central nervous system. *Lancet* 342: 398-401.

253. Claassen U, Kuntz G, Schmitt HP (1990). Malignant intracerebral granular cell tumor reacts positively with anti-alpha-1-antichymotripsin and the MB2 antibody: a clue to the histogenesis of the brain granular cell? *Clin Neuropathol* 9: 82-88.

254. Claesson W (1994). Platelet-derived growth factor receptor signals. *J Biol Chem* 269: 32023-32026.

255. Clarenbach P, Kleihues P, Metzel E, Dichgans J (1979). Simultaneous clinical manifestation of subependymoma of the fourth ventricle in identical twins. Case report. *J Neurosurg* 50: 655-659.

256. Clark GB, Henry JM, McKeever PE (1985). Cerebral pilocytic astrocytoma. *Cancer* 56: 1128-1133.

257. Clark WC, Callihan T, Schwartzberg L, Fontanesi J (1992). Primary intracranial Hodgkin's lymphoma without dural attachment. Case report. *J Neurosurg* 76: 692-695.

258. Coca S, Moreno M, Martos JA, Rodriguez J, Barcena A, Vaquero J (1994). Neurocytoma of spinal cord. *Acta Neuropathol (Berl)* 87: 537-540.

259. Coca S, Vaquero J, Escandon J, Moreno M, Peralba J, Rodriguez J (1992). Immunohistochemical characterization of pineocytomas. *Clin Neuropathol* 11: 298-303.

260. Coffin CM, Braun JT, Wick MR, Dehner LP (1990). A clinicopathologic and immunohistochemical analysis of 53 cases of medulloblastoma with emphasis on synaptophysin expression. *Mod Pathol* 3: 164-170.

261. Coffin CM, Wick MR, Braun JT, Dehner LP (1986). Choroid plexus neoplasms. Clinicopathologic and immunohistochemical studies. *Am J Surg Pathol* 10: 394-404.

262. Cogen PH (1991). Prognostic significance of molecular genetic markers in childhood brain tumors. *Pediatr Neurosurg* 17: 245-250.

263. Cogen PH, Daneshvar L, Metzger AK, Duyk G, Edwards MS, Sheffield VC (1992). Involvement of multiple chromosome 17p loci in medulloblastoma tumorigenesis. *Am J Hum Genet* 50: 584-589.

264. Cogen PH, McDonald JD (1996). Tumor suppressor genes and medulloblastoma. *J Neurooncol* 29: 103-112.

265. Cohn SL, Look AT, Joshi VV, Holbrook T, Salwen H, Chagnovich D, Chesler L, Rowe ST, Valentine MB, Komuro H (1995). Lack of correlation of N-myc gene amplification with prognosis in localized neuroblastoma: a Pediatric Oncology Group study. *Cancer Res* 55: 721-726.

266. Collins VP, James CD (1993). Gene and chromosomal alterations associated with the development of human gliomas. *FASEB J* 7: 926-930.

267. Colman SD, Williams CA, Wallace MR (1995). Benign neurofibromas in type 1 neurofibromatosis (NF1) show somatic deletions of the NF1 gene. *Nat Genet* 11: 90-92.

268. Combaret V, Gross N, Lasset C, Frappaz D, Peruisseau G, Philip T, Beck D, Favrot MC (1996). Clinical relevance of CD44 cell-surface expression and N-myc gene amplification in a multicentric analysis of 121 pediatric neuroblastomas. *J Clin Oncol* 14: 25-34.

269. Combaret V, Ladenstein R, Coze C (1993). Analysis of the prognostic value of N-*myc* amplification and expression on the progression-free survival of children with neuroblastoma. In: *Human Neuroblastoma. Recent Advances in Clinical and Genetic Analysis*, Schwab M, Tonini GP, Bernard J (eds). Harwood Academic Publishers: Philadelphia. pp. 147-161.

270. Connor JM, Pirrit LA, Yates JR, Fryer AE, Ferguson Smith MA (1987). Linkage of the tuberous sclerosis locus to a DNA polymorphism detected by v-abl. *J Med Genet* 24: 544-546.

271. Constantini S, Soffer D, Siegel T, Shalit MN (1989). Paraganglioma of the thoracic spinal cord with cerebrospinal fluid metastasis. *Spine* 14: 643-645.

272. Coons SW, Johnson PC (1993). Regional heterogeneity in the proliferative activity of human gliomas as measured by the Ki-67 labeling index. *J Neuropathol Exp Neurol* 52: 609-618.

273. Coons SW, Johnson PC, Pearl DK, Olafsen AG (1994). Prognostic significance of flow cytometry deoxyribonucleic acid analysis of human oligodendrogliomas. *Neurosurgery* 34: 680-687.

274. Coons SW, Johnson PC, Scheithauer BW, Yates AJ, Pearl DK (1997). Improving diagnostic accuracy and interobserver concordance in the classification and grading of primary gliomas. *Cancer* 79: 1381-1393.

275. Cooper ERA (1935). The relation of oligodendrocytes and astrocytes in cerebral tumours. *J Path Bact* 41: 259-266.

276. Cooper PR, Epstein F (1985). Radical resection of intramedullary spinal cord tumors in adults. Recent experience in 29 patients. *J Neurosurg* 63: 492-499.

277. Corn B, Curtis MT, Lynch D, Gomori JM (1994). Malignant oligodendroglioma arising after radiation therapy for lymphoma [clinical conference]. *Med Pediatr Oncol* 22: 45-52.

278. Corvi R, Amler LC, Savelyeva L, Gehring M, Schwab M (1994). *MYCN* is retained in single copy at chromosome 2 band p23-24 during amplification in human neuroblastoma cells. *Proc Natl Acad Sci USA* 91: 5523-5527.

279. Corvi R, Savelyeva L, Breit S, Wenzel A, Handgretinger R, Barak J, Oren M, Amler LC, Schwab M (1995). Non-syntenic amplification of MDM2 and MYCN in human neuroblastoma. *Oncogene* 10: 1081-1086.

280. Corvi R, Savelyeva L, Schwab M (1995). Duplication of *N-MYC* at its resident site 2p24 may be a mechanism of activation alternative to amplification in human neuroblastoma cells. *Cancer Res* 55: 3471-3474.

281. Costello JF, Berger MS, Huang HJS, Cavenee WK (1996). Silencing of p16/CDKN2 expression in human gliomas by methylation and chromatin condensation. *Cancer Res* 56: 2405-2410.

282. Costello JF, Plass C, Arap W, Chapman VM, Held WA, Berger MS, Huang HJS, Cavenee WK (1997). Cyclin-dependent kinase 6 (CDK6) amplification in human gliomas identified using two-dimensional separation of genomic DNA. *Cancer Res* 57: 1250-1254.

283. Cote TR, Manns A, Hardy CR, Yellin FJ, Hartge P (1996). Epidemiology of brain lymphoma among people with or without acquired immunodeficiency syndrome. AIDS/Cancer Study Group. *J Natl Cancer Inst* 88: 675-679.

284. Cottingham SL, Boesel CP, Yates AJ (1996). Pilocytic astrocytoma in infants: a distinctive histologic pattern. *J Neuropathol Exp Neurol* 55: 654.

285. Coulon RA, Till K (1977). Intracranial ependymomas in children: a review of 43 cases. *Childs Brain* 3: 154-168.

286. Crail HW (1949). Multiple primary malignancies arising in the rectum, brain and thyroid. *US Nav Bull* 49: 123-128.

287. Crino PB, Trojanowski JQ, Dichter MA, Eberwine J (1996). Embryonic neuronal markers in tuberous sclerosis: single-cell molecular pathology. *Proc Natl Acad Sci USA* 93: 14152-14157.

288. Crotty TB, Scheithauer BW, Young WF, Jr., Davis DH, Shaw EG, Miller GM, Burger PC (1995). Papillary craniopharyngioma: a clinicopathological study of 48 cases. *J Neurosurg* 83: 206-214.

289. Cruz S, Haustein J, Rossie ML, Cervos N, Hughs JT (1988). Ependymoblastoma: a histological, immunohistological and ultrastructural study of five cases. *Histopathology* 12: 17-27.

290. Cruz S, Miquel R, Rossi ML, Figols J, Palacin A, Cardesa A (1993). Clinico-pathological correlations in meningiomas: a DNA and immunohistochemical study. *Histol Histopathol* 8: 1-8.

291. Cruz S, Rossi ML, Buller JR, Carboni P, Jr., Fineron PW, Coakham HB (1991). Oligodendrogliomas: a clinical, histological, immunocytochemical and lectin-binding study. *Histopathology* 19: 361-367.

292. Cushing H (1930). Experiences with the cerebellar medulloblastoma: a critical review. *Acta Pathol Microbiol Scand* 7: 1-86.

293. Cushing H (1931). Experiences with the cerebellar astrocytomas. A critical review of seventy-six cases. *Surg Gynecol Obstet* 52: 1129-1204.

294. Cushing H, Eisenhardt L (1938). *Meningiomas, their Classification, Regional Behaviour, Life History, and End Surgical Results.* Charles C. Thomas: Springfield.

295. Cybulski GR, Nijensohn E, Brody BA, Meyer PR, Jr., Cohen B (1991). Spinal cord compression from a thoracic paraganglioma: case report. *Neurosurgery* 28: 306-309.

296. Czarnecki EJ, Silbergleit, Guttierez JA (1997). MR of spinal meningeal melanocytoma. *Am J Neuroradiol* 18: 180-182.

297. Czerwionka M, Korf HW, Hoffmann O, Busch H, Schachenmayr W (1989). Differentiation in medulloblastomas: correlation between the immunocytochemical demonstration of photoreceptor markers (S- antigen, rod-opsin) and the survival rate in 66 patients. *Acta Neuropathol (Berl)* 78: 629-636.

298. D'Andrea AD, Packer RJ, Rorke LB, Bilaniuk LT, Sutton LN, Bruce DA, Schut L (1987). Pineocytomas of childhood. A reappraisal of natural history and response to therapy. *Cancer* 59: 1353-1357.

299. Dameron KM, Volpert OV, Tainsky MA, Bouck N (1994). Control of angiogenesis in fibroblasts by p53 regulation of thrombospondin-1. *Science* 265: 1582-1584.

300. Dardick I, Hammar SP, Scheithauer BW (1989). Ultrastructural spectrum of hemangiopericytoma: a comparative study of fetal, adult, and neoplastic pericytes. *Ultrastruct Pathol* 13: 111-154.

301. Daumas-Duport C (1993). Dysembryoplastic neuroepithelial tumours. *Brain Pathol* 3: 283-295.

302. Daumas-Duport C (1995). Dysembryoplastic neuroepithelial tumours in epilepsy surgery. In: *Dysplasia of Cerebral Cortex and Epilepsy*, Guerrini R (eds). Raven Press: New York. pp. 125-147.

303. Daumas Duport C (1995). Patterns of tumor growth and problems associated with histological typing of low-grade gliomas. In: *Benign Cerebral Gliomas*, Apuzzo LJ (eds). AANS: Park Ridge. pp. 125-147.

304. Daumas-Duport C, Scheithauer B, O'Fallon J, Kelly P (1988). Grading of astrocytomas. A simple and reproducible method. *Cancer* 62: 2152-2165.

305. Daumas-Duport C, Scheithauer BW, Chodkiewicz JP, Laws ER, Jr., Vedrenne C (1988). Dysembryoplastic neuroepithelial tumor: a surgically curable tumor of young patients with intractable partial seizures. Report of thirty-nine cases. *Neurosurgery* 23: 545-556.

306. Daumas-Duport C, Scheithauer BW, Kelly PJ (1987). A histologic and cytologic method for the spatial definition of gliomas. *Mayo Clin Proc* 62: 435-449.

307. Daumas-Duport C, Tucker ML, Kolles H, Cervera P, Beuvon F, Varlet P, Udo N, Koziak M, Chodkiewicz JP (1997). Oligodendrogliomas. Part II: A new grading system based on morphological and imaging criteria. *J Neurooncol* 34: 61-78.

308. David KM, Casey ATH, Hayward RD, Harkness WFJ, Phipps K, Wade AM (1997). Medulloblastoma: is the 5-year survival rate improving? *J Neurosurg* 86: 13-21.

309. Davis DG, Wilson D, Schmitz M, Markesbery WR (1993). Lipidized medulloblastoma in adults. *Hum Pathol* 24: 990-995.

310. Davis RL, Onda K, Shubuya M, Lamborn K, Hoshino T (1995). Proliferation markers in gliomas: a comparison of BUDR, KI-67, and MIB-1. *J Neurooncol* 24: 9-12.

311. Dayal Y, Tallberg KA, Nunnemacher G, DeLellis RA, Wolfe HJ (1986). Duodenal carcinoids in patients with and without neurofibromatosis. A comparative study. *Am J Surg Pathol* 10: 348-357.

312. de Bruin TW, Slater RM, Defferrari R, Geurts vK, Suijkerbuijk RF, Jansen G, de

Jong B, Oosterhuis JW (1994). Isochromosome 12p-positive pineal germ cell tumor. *Cancer Res* 54: 1542-1544.

313. de Chadarevian JP, Guyda HJ, Hollenberg RD (1984). Hypothalamic polar spongioblastoma associated with the diencephalic syndrome. Ultrastructural demonstration of a neuro- endocrine organization. *Virchows Arch A Pathol Anat Histopathol* 402: 465-474.

314. de Chadarevian JP, Montes JL, O'Gorman AM, Freeman CR (1987). Maturation of cerebellar neuroblastoma into ganglioneuroma with melanosis. A histologic, immunocytochemical, and ultrastructural study. *Cancer* 59: 69-76.

315. de Chadarevian JP, Pattisapu JV, Faerber EN (1990). Desmoplastic cerebral astrocytoma of infancy. Light microscopy, immunocytochemistry, and ultrastructure. *Cancer* 66: 173-179.

316. De Jesus O, Rifkinson N (1995). Pleomorphic xanthoastrocytoma with invasion of the tentorium and falx. *Surg Neurol* 43: 77-79.

317. de la Monte SM (1989). Uniform lineage of oligodendrogliomas. *Am J Pathol* 135: 529-540.

318. de la Monte SM, Flickinger J, Linggood RM (1986). Histopathologic features predicting recurrence of meningiomas following subtotal resection. *Am J Surg Pathol* 10: 836-843.

319. De Potter P, Shields CL, Shields JA (1994). Clinical variations of trilateral retinoblastoma: a report of 13 cases. *J Pediatr Ophthalmol Strabismus* 31: 26-31.

320. De Vitis LR, Tedde A, Vitelli F, Ammannati F, Mennonna P, Bigozzi U, Montali E, Papi L (1996). Screening for mutations in the neurofibromatosis type 2 (NF2) gene in sporadic meningiomas. *Hum Genet* 97: 632-637.

321. de Vries J, Scheremet R, Altmannsberger M, Michilli R, Lindemann A, Hinkelbein W (1993). Primary leiomyosarcoma of the spinal leptomeninges. *J Neurooncol* 18: 25-31.

322. DeCaprio JA, Ludlow JW, Figge J, Shew JY, Huang CM, Lee WH, Marsilio E, Paucha E, Livingston DM (1988). SV40 large tumor antigen forms a specific complex with the product of the retinoblastoma susceptibility gene. *Cell* 54: 275-283.

323. Deck JH (1969). Cerebral medulloepithelioma with maturation into ependymal cells and ganglion cells. *J Neuropathol Exp Neurol* 28: 442-454.

324. Deckert M, Reifenberger G, Wechsler W (1989). Determination of the proliferative potential of human brain tumors using the monoclonal antibody Ki-67. *J Cancer Res Clin Oncol* 115: 179-188.

325. DeDavid M, Orlow SJ, Provost N, Marghoob AA, Rao BK, Wasti Q, Huang CL, Kopf AW, Bart RS (1996). Neurocutaneous melanosis: clinical features of large congenital melanocytic nevi in patients with manifest central nervous system melanosis. *J Am Acad Dermatol* 35: 529-538.

326. DeGirolami U, Schmidek H (1973). Clinicopathological study of 53 tumors of the pineal region. *J Neurosurg* 39: 455-462.

327. Del Bigio MR, Deck JH (1993). Rosenthal fibers producing a granular cell appearance in a glioblastoma. *Acta Neuropathol (Berl)* 86: 100-104.

328. del Carpio-O'Donovan R, Korah I, Salazar A, Melancon D (1996). Gliomatosis cerebri. *Radiology* 198: 831-835.

329. Delattre JY, Krol G, Thaler HT, Posner JB (1988). Distribution of brain metastases. *Arch Neurol* 45: 741-744.

330. Demirci A, Kawamura Y, Sze G, Duncan C (1995). MR of parenchymal neurocutaneous melanosis. *AJNR Am J Neuroradiol* 16: 603-606.

331. Devaney K, Wenig BM, Abbondanzo SL (1996). Olfactory neuroblastoma and other round cell lesions of the sinonasal region. *Mod Pathol* 9: 658-663.

332. Devaux BC, O'Fallon JR, Kelly PJ (1993). Resection, biopsy, and survival in malignant glial neoplasms. A retrospective study of clinical parameters, therapy, and outcome. *J Neurosurg* 78: 767-775.

333. Di Fiore PP, Pierce JH, Fleming TP, Hazan R, Ullrich A, King CR, Schlessinger J, Aaronson SA (1987). Overexpression of the human EGF receptor confers an EGF- dependent transformed phenotype to NIH 3T3 cells. *Cell* 51: 1063-1070.

334. DiCarlo EF, Woodruff JM, Bansal M, Erlandson RA (1986). The purely epithelioid malignant peripheral nerve sheath tumor. *Am J Surg Pathol* 10: 478-490.

335. Dickson DW, Hart MN, Menezes A, Cancilla PA (1983). Medulloblastoma with glial and rhabdomyoblastic differentiation. A myoglobin and glial fibrillary acidic protein immunohistochemical and ultrastructural study. *J Neuropathol Exp Neurol* 42: 639-647.

336. Diengdoh JV, Shaw MD (1993). Oncocytic variant of choroid plexus papilloma. Evolution from benign to malignant "oncocytoma". *Cancer* 71: 855-858.

337. Dinda AK, Kharbanda K, Sarkar C, Roy S, Mathur M, Banerji AK (1993). In-vivo proliferative potential of primary human brain tumors; its correlation with histological classification and morphological features: II. Nonglial tumors. *Pathology* 25: 10-14.

338. Dinda AK, Sarkar C, Roy S (1990). Rosenthal fibres: an immunohistochemical, ultrastructural and immunoelectron microscopic study. *Acta Neuropathol (Berl)* 79: 456-460.

339. Dirks PB, Jay V, Becker LE, Drake JM, Humphreys RP, Hoffman HJ, Rutka JT (1994). Development of anaplastic changes in low-grade astrocytomas of childhood. *Neurosurgery* 34: 68-78.

340. Disclafani A, Hudgins RJ, Edwards MS, Wara W, Wilson CB, Levin VA (1989). Pineocytomas. *Cancer* 63: 302-304.

341. Dohrmann GJ, Farwell JR, Flannery JT (1976). Glioblastoma multiforme in children. *J Neurosurg* 44: 442-448.

342. Dohrmann GJ, Farwell JR, Flannery JT (1976). Ependymomas and ependymoblastomas in children. *J Neurosurg* 273-283.

343. Dolman CL (1988). Melanotic medulloblastoma. A case report with immunohistochemical and ultrastructural examination. *Acta Neuropathol (Berl)* 76: 528-531.

344. Donat JF, Okazaki H, Gomez MR, Reagan TJ, Baker HL, Jr., Laws ER, Jr. (1978). Pineal tumors. A 53-year experience. *Arch Neurol* 35: 736-740.

345. Doran SE, Blaivas M, Dauser RC (1995). Bone formation within a choroid plexus papilloma. *Pediatr Neurosurg* 23: 216-218.

346. Dou QP, An B, Antoku K, Johnson DE (1997). Fas stimulation induces RB dephosphorilation and proteolysis that is blocked by inhibitors of the ICE protease family. *J Cell Biochem* 64: 586-594.

347. Dou QP, Lui VW (1995). Failure to dephosphorylate retinoblastoma protein in drug- resistant cells. *Cancer Res* 55: 5222-5225.

348. Drago G, Pasquiev B, Pasquev D, Pinel N, Rouault-Plantaz V, Dyon JF, Durand C, Armari-Alla C, Plantaz D (1997). Malignant peripheral sheath tumor arising in a "DeNovo" ganglioneuroma: a case report and review of literature. *Med Pediatr Oncol* 28: 216-222.

349. Duan DR, Pause A, Burgess WH, Aso T, Chen DY, Garrett KP, Conaway RC, Conaway JW, Linehan WM, Klausner RD (1995). Inhibition of transcription elongation by the VHL tumor suppressor protein. *Science* 269: 1402-1406.

350. Ducatman BS, Scheithauer BW (1983). Postirradiation neurofibrosarcoma. *Cancer* 51: 1028-1033.

351. Ducatman BS, Scheithauer BW (1984). Malignant peripheral nerve sheath tumors with divergent differentiation. *Cancer* 54: 1049-1057.

352. Ducatman BS, Scheithauer BW, Piepgras DG, Reiman HM (1984). Malignant peripheral nerve sheath tumors in childhood. *J Neurooncol* 2: 241-248.

353. Ducatman BS, Scheithauer BW, Piepgras DG, Reiman HM, Ilstrup DM (1986). Malignant peripheral nerve sheath tumors. A clinicopathologic study of 120 cases. *Cancer* 57: 2006-2021.

354. Duffell D, Farber L, Chou S, Hartmann JF, Nelson E (1963). Electron microscopic observations on astrocytomas. *Am J Pathol* 43: 539-554.

355. Duffner PK, Burger PC, Cohen ME, Sanford RA, Krischer JP, Elterman R, Aronin PA, Pullen J, Horowitz ME, Parent A (1994). Desmoplastic infantile gangliogliomas: an approach to therapy. *Neurosurgery* 34: 583-589.

356. Duffner PK, Cohen ME, Sanford RA, Horowitz ME, Krischer JP, Burger PC, Friedman HS, Kun LE (1995). Lack of efficacy of postoperative chemotherapy and delayed radiation in very young children with pineoblastoma. Pediatric Oncology Group. *Med Pediatr Oncol* 25: 38-44.

357. Dumanski JP, Carlbom E, Collins VP, Nordenskjold M (1987). Deletion mapping of a locus on human chromosome 22 involved in the oncogenesis of meningioma. *Proc Natl Acad Sci USA* 84: 9275-9279.

358. Dumanski JP, Rouleau GA, Nordenskjold M, Collins VP (1990). Molecular genetic analysis of chromosome 22 in 81 cases of meningioma. *Cancer Res* 50: 5863-5867.

359. Duncan JA,Hoffman HJ (1995). Intracranial ependymomas. In: *Brain Tumors*, Kaye AH, Lows ER, Jr. (eds). Churchill Livingstone: Edinburgh. pp. 493-504.

360. Easton DF, Ponder MA, Huson SM, Ponder BA (1993). An analysis of variation in expression of neurofibromatosis (NF) type 1 (NF1): evidence for modifying genes. *Am J Hum Genet* 53: 305-313.

361. Edvardsen K, Pedersen PH, Bjerkvig R, Hermann GG, Zeuthen J, Laerum OD, Walsh FS, Bock E (1994). Transfection of glioma cells with the neural-cell adhesion molecule NCAM: effect on glioma-cell invasion and growth in vivo. *Int J Cancer* 58: 116-122.

362. Edwards MK, Terry JG, Montebello JF, Hornback NB, Kuharik MA (1986). Gliomas in children following radiation therapy for lymphoblastic leukemia. *Acta Radiol Suppl Stockh* 369: 651-653.

363. Edwards MS, Hudgins RJ, Wilson CB, Levin VA, Wara WM (1988). Pineal region tumors in children. *J Neurosurg* 68: 689-697.

364. Ehret M, Jacobi G, Hey A, Segerer S (1987). Embryonal brain neoplasms in the neonatal period and early infancy. *Clin Neuropathol* 6: 218-223.

365. Eibl RH, Kleihues P, Jat PS, Wiestler OD (1994). A model for primitive neuroectodermal tumors in transgenic neural transplants harboring the SV40 large T antigen. *Am J Pathol* 144: 556-564.

366. Ekstrand AJ, James CD, Cavenee WK, Seliger B, Pettersson RF, Collins VP (1991). Genes for epidermal growth factor receptor, transforming growth factor alpha, and epidermal growth factor and their expression in human gliomas in vivo. *Cancer Res* 51: 2164-2172.

367. Ekstrand AJ, Sugawa N, James CD, Collins VP (1992). Amplified and rearranged epidermal growth factor receptor genes in human glioblastomas reveal deletions of sequences encoding portions of the N- and/ or C-terminal tails. *Proc Natl Acad Sci USA* 89: 4309-4313.

368. El Deiry WS, Harper JW, O'Connor PM, Velculescu VE, Canman CE, Jackman J, Pietenpol JA, Burrell M, Hill DE, Wang Y (1994). WAF1/CIP1 is induced in p53-mediated G1 arrest and apoptosis. *Cancer Res* 54: 1169-1174.

369. El Deiry WS, Tokino T, Velculescu VE, Levy DB, Parsons R, Trent JM, Lin D, Mercer WE, Kinzler KW, Vogelstein B (1993). WAF1, a potential mediator of p53 tumor suppression. *Cell* 75: 817-825.

370. El Rouby S, Thomas A, Costin D, Rosenberg CR, Potmesil M, Silber R, Newcomb EW (1993). p53 gene mutation in B-cell chronic lymphocytic leukemia is associated with drug resistance and is independent of MDR1/MDR3 gene expression. *Blood* 82: 3452-3459.

371. Ellison DW, Steart PV, Gatter KC, Weller RO (1995). Apoptosis in cerebral astrocytic tumours and its relationship to expression of the bcl-2 and p53 proteins. *Neuropathol Appl Neurobiol* 21: 352-361.

372. Ellison DW, Zygmunt SC, Weller RO (1993). Neurocytoma/lipoma (neurolipocytoma) of the cerebellum. *Neuropathol Appl Neurobiol* 19: 95-98.

373. Emadian SM, McDonald JD, Gerken SC, Fults D (1997). Correlation of chromosome 17p loss with clinical outcome in medulloblastoma. *Clin Cancer Res* 2: 1559-1564.

374. Eng C, Murday V, Seal S, Mohammed S, Hodgson SV, Chaudary MA, Fentiman IS, Ponder BA, Eeles RA (1994). Cowden syndrome and Lhermitte-Duclos disease in a family: a single genetic syndrome with pleiotropy? *J Med Genet* 31: 458-461.

375. Eng DY, DeMonte F, Ginsberg L, Fuller GN, Jaeckle K (1997). Craniospinal dissemination of central neurocytoma - report of two cases. *J Neurosurg* 86: 547-552.

376. Engebraaten O, Bjerkvig R, Pedersen

PH, Laerum OD (1993). Effects of EGF, bFGF, NGF and PDGF(bb) on cell proliferative, migratory and invasive capacities of human brain-tumour biopsies in vitro. *Int J Cancer* 53: 209-214.

377. Enzinger FM, Smith BH (1976). Hemangiopericytoma. An analysis of 106 cases. *Hum Pathol* 7: 61-82.

378. Enzinger FM,Weiss SW (1995). *Soft Tissue Tumors.* 3rd ed, Mosby: St Louis.

379. Enzinger FM,Weiss SW (1995). Paraganglioma. In: *Soft Tissue Tumors*, Enzinger FM, Weiss SW (eds), 3rd ed. Mosby: St. Louis. pp. 965-990.

380. Eppenberger U, Mueller H (1994). Growth factor receptors and their ligands. *J Neurooncol* 22: 249-254.

381. Erlandson RA (1994). Paragangliomas. In: *Diagnostic Transmission Electron Microscopy of Tumors*, Raven Press: New York. pp. 615-622.

382. Erlandson RA, Woodruff JM (1982). Peripheral nerve sheath tumors: an electron microscopic study of 43 cases. *Cancer* 49: 273-287.

383. Evans AE, Gerson J, Schnaufer L (1976). Spontaneous regression of neuroblastoma. *NCI Monogr* 44: 49-54.

384. Evans DG, Farndon PA, Burnell LD, Gattamaneni HR, Birch JM (1991). The incidence of Gorlin syndrome in 173 consecutive cases of medulloblastoma. *Br J Cancer* 64: 959-961.

385. Evans DG, Huson SM, Donnai D, Neary W, Blair V, Newton V, Harris R (1992). A clinical study of type 2 neurofibromatosis. *Q J Med* 84: 603-618.

386. Evans DG, Ladusans EJ, Rimmer S, Burnell LD, Thakker N, Farndon PA (1993). Complications of the naevoid basal cell carcinoma syndrome: results of a population based study. *J Med Genet* 30: 460-464.

387. Fabiani A, Trebini F, Favero M, Peres B, Palmucci L (1977). The significance of atypical mitoses in malignant meningiomas. *Acta Neuropathol (Berl)* 38: 229-231.

388. Fairburn B, Urich H (1971). Malignant gliomas occurring in identical twins. *J Neurol Neurosurg Psychiatry* 34: 718-722.

389. Fanning E, Knippers R (1992). Structure and function of simian virus 40 large tumor antigen. *Annu Rev Biochem* 61: 55-85.

390. Farndon PA, Del Mastro RG, Evans DG, Kilpatrick MW (1992). Location of gene for Gorlin syndrome. *Lancet* 339: 581-582.

391. Farwell J, Flannery JT (1984). Cancer in relatives of children with central-nervous-system neoplasms. *N Engl J Med* 311: 749-753.

392. Farwell JR, Dohrmann GJ, Flannery JT (1984). Medulloblastoma in childhood: an epidemiological study. *J Neurosurg* 61: 657-664.

393. Favrot MC, Combaret V, Lasset C (1993). CD44-a new prognostic marker for neuroblastoma. *N Engl J Med* 329: 1965-1965.

394. Fazeli A, Dickinson SL, Hermiston ML, Tighe RV, Steen RG, Small CG, Stoeckli ET, KeinoMasu K, Masu M, Rayburn H, Simons J, Bronson RT, Gordon JI, Tessier L, Weinberg RA (1997). Phenotype of mice lacking functional Deleted in colorectal cancer (Dcc) gene. *Nature* 386: 796-804.

395. Fearon ER, Cho KR, Nigro JM, Kern SE, Simons JW, Ruppert JM, Hamilton SR, Preisinger AC, Thomas G, Kinzler KW, Vogelstein B (1990). Identification of a chromosome 18q gene that is altered in colorectal cancers. *Science* 247: 49-56.

396. Feigin I, Epstein F, Mangiardi J (1983). Extensive advanced maturation of medulloblastoma to astrocytoma and ependymoma. *J Neurooncol* 1: 95-108.

397. Feigin IM, Ransohoff J, Lieberman A (1976). Sarcoma arising in oligodendroglioma of the brain. *J Neuropath Exp Neurol* 35: 679-684.

398. Feigin IM, Allen LB, Lipkin L, Gross SW (1958). The endothelial hyperplasia of the cerebral blood vessels, and its sarcomatous transformation. *Cancer* 11: 264-277.

399. Feigin I, Gross SW (1955). Sarcoma arising in glioblastoma of the brain. *Am J Pathol* 31: 633-653.

400. Felix I, Becker LE (1990). Intracranial germ cell tumors in children: an immunohistochemical and electron microscopic study. *Pediatr Neurosurg* 16: 156-162.

401. Feng X, Zhang S, Ichikawa T, Koga H, Washiyama K, Motoyama T, Kumanishi T (1995). Intracranial germ cell tumors: detection of p53 gene mutations by single-strand conformation polymorphism analysis. *Jpn J Cancer Res* 86: 555-561.

402. Ferracini R, Pileri S, Bergmann M, Sabattini E, Rigobello L, Gambacorta M, Galli C, Manetto V, Frank G, Godano U (1993). Non-Hodgkin lymphomas of the central nervous system. Clinico- pathologic and immunohistochemical study of 147 cases. *Pathol Res Pract* 189: 249-260.

403. Ferraresi S, Servello D, De Lorenzi L, Allegranza A (1989). Familial frontal lobe oligodendroglioma. Case report. *J Neurosurg Sci* 33: 317-318.

404. Ferrer I, Fabregues I, Coll J, Ribalta T, Rives A (1984). Tuberous sclerosis: a Golgi study of cortical tuber. *Clin Neuropathol* 3: 47-51.

405. Ferreri AJ, Reni M, Zoldan MC, Terreni MR, Villa E (1996). Importance of complete staging in non-Hodgkin's lymphoma presenting as a cerebral mass lesion. *Cancer* 77: 827-833.

406. Figarella B, Durbec PL, Rougon GN (1990). Differential spectrum of expression of neural cell adhesion molecule isoforms and L1 adhesion molecules on human neuroectodermal tumors. *Cancer Res* 50: 6364-6370.

407. Figarella B, Pellissier JF, Daumas D, Delisle MB, Pasquier B, Parent M, Gambarelli D, Rougon G, Hassoun J (1992). Central neurocytomas. Critical evaluation of a small-cell neuronal tumor. *Am J Surg Pathol* 16: 97-109.

408. Fine H, Mayer R (1993). Primary central nervous system lymphoma. *Ann Intern Med* 119: 1093-1104.

409. Fink KL, Rushing EJ, Schold SC, Jr., Nisen PD (1996). Infrequency of p53 gene mutations in ependymomas. *J Neurooncol* 27: 111-115.

410. Finkelstein SD, Przygodzki R, Pricolo VE, Sakallah SA, Swalsky PA, Bakker A, Lanning R, Bland KI, Cooper DL (1996). Prediction of biologic aggressiveness in colorectal cancer by p53/K-ras-2 topographic genotyping. *Molec Diag* 1: 5-28.

411. Firsching R, Tieben R, Schroder R, Stutzer R (1994). Long-term prognosis of low grade astrocytoma. *Zentralbl Neurochir* 55: 10-15.

412. Fischer BJN, Siddiqui J, Macdonald D, Cairney AE, Ramsey D, Munoz D, DelMaestro R (1996). Malignant rhabdoid tumor of brain: an aggressive clinical entity. *Can J Neurol Sci* 23: 257-263.

413. Fix SE, Nelson J, Schochet SS, Jr. (1989). Focal leptomeningeal rhabdomyomatosis of the posterior fossa. *Arch Pathol Lab Med* 113: 872-873.

414. Fletcher CD, Davies SE (1986). Benign plexiform (multinodular) schwannoma: a rare tumour unassociated with neurofibromatosis. *Histopathology* 10: 971-980.

415. Flint EW, Claassen D, Pang D, Hirsch WL (1993). Intrasellar and suprasellar paraganglioma: CT and MR findings. *AJNR Am J Neuroradiol* 14: 1191-1193.

416. Fogelholm R, Uutela T, Murros K (1984). Epidemiology of central nervous system neoplasms. A regional survey in central Finland. *Acta Neurol Scand* 69: 129-136.

417. Fokes EC, Jr., Earle KM (1969). Ependymomas: clinical and pathological aspects. *J Neurosurg* 30: 585-594.

418. Foley KM, Woodruff JM, Ellis FT, Posner JB (1980). Radiation-induced malignant and atypical peripheral nerve sheath tumors. *Ann Neurol* 7: 311-318.

419. Fong CT, Dracopoli NC, White PS, Merrill PT, Griffith RC, Housman DE, Brodeur GM (1989). Loss of heterozygosity for the short arm of chromosome 1 in human neuroblastomas: correlation with N-myc amplification. *Proc Natl Acad Sci USA* 86: 3753-3757.

420. Font RL, Truong LD (1984). Melanotic schwannoma of soft tissues. Electron-microscopic observations and review of literature. *Am J Surg Pathol* 8: 129-138.

421. Foote RL, Morita A, Ebersold MJ, Olsen KD, Lewis JE, Quast LM, Ferguson JA, O'Fallon WM (1993). Esthesioneuroblastoma: the role of adjuvant radiation therapy. *Int J Radiat Oncol Biol Phys* 27: 835-842.

422. Forrester K, Lupold SE, Ott VL, Chay CH, Band V, Wang XW, Harris CC (1995). Effects of p53 mutants on wild-type p53-mediated transactivation are cell type dependent. *Oncogene* 10: 2103-2111.

423. Forsyth PA, Shaw EG, Scheithauer BW, O'Fallon JR, Layton DD, Jr., Katzmann JA (1993). Supratentorial pilocytic astrocytomas. A clinicopathologic, prognostic, and flow cytometric study of 51 patients. *Cancer* 72: 1335-1342.

424. Fort DW, Tonk VS, Tomlinson GE, Timmons CF, Schneider NR (1994). Rhabdoid tumor of the kidney with primitive neuroectodermal tumor of the central nervous system: associated tumors with different histologic, cytogenetic, and molecular findings. *Genes Chromosomes Cancer* 11: 146-152.

425. Fortuna A, Celli P, Palma L (1980). Oligodendrogliomas of the spinal cord. *Acta Neurochir Wien* 52: 305-329.

426. Fowler M, Simpson DA (1962). Malignant melanin-forming tumour of the cerebellum. *J Pathol Bacteriol* 84: 307-311.

427. Frankel RH, Bayona W, Koslow M, Newcomb EW (1992). p53 mutations in human malignant gliomas: comparison of loss of heterozygosity with mutation frequency. *Cancer Res* 52: 1427-1433.

428. Franks AJ (1985). Epithelioid neurilemmoma of the trigeminal nerve: an immunohistochemical and ultrastructural study. *Histopathology* 9: 1339-1350.

429. Freilich RJ, Thompson SJ, Walker RW, Rosenblum MK (1995). Adenocarcinomatous transformation of intracranial germ cell tumors. *Am J Surg Pathol* 19: 537-544.

430. Frenk E, Marazzi A (1984). Neurofibromatosis of von Recklinghausen: a quantitative study of the epidermal keratinocyte and melanocyte populations. *J Invest Dermatol* 83: 23-25.

431. Friedlander DR, Zagzag D, Shiff B, Cohen H, Allen JC, Kelly PJ, Grumet M (1996). Migration of brain tumor cells on extracellular matrix proteins in vitro correlates with tumor type and grade and involves alphaV and beta1 integrins. *Cancer Res* 56: 1939-1947.

432. Friesen C, Herr I, Krammer PH, Debatin KM (1996). Involvement of the CD95 (APO-1/FAS) receptor/ligand system in drug-induced apoptosis in leukemia cells. *Nat Med* 2: 574-577.

433. Frost G, Patel K, Bourne S, Coakham HB, Kemshead JT (1991). Expression of alternative isoforms of the neural cell adhesion molecule (NCAM) on normal brain and a variety of brain tumours. *Neuropathol Appl Neurobiol* 17: 207-217.

434. Fu YS, Chen AT, Kay S, Young H (1974). Is subependymoma (subependymal glomerate astrocytoma) an astrocytoma or ependymoma? A comparative ultrastructural and tissue culture study. *Cancer* 34: 1992-2008.

435. Fulham MJ, Melisi JW, Nishimiya J, Dwyer AJ, Di Chiro G (1993). Neuroimaging of juvenile pilocytic astrocytomas: an enigma. *Radiology* 189: 221-225.

436. Fuller GN, Bigner SH (1992). Amplified cellular oncogenes in neoplasms of the human central nervous system. *Mutat Res* 276: 299-306.

437. Fults D, Brockmeyer D, Tullous MW, Pedone CA, Cawthon RM (1992). p53 mutation and loss of heterozygosity on chromosomes 17 and 10 during human astrocytoma progression. *Cancer Res* 52: 674-679.

438. Fults D, Pedone CA, Thomas GA, White R (1990). Allelotype of human malignant astrocytoma. *Cancer Res* 50: 5784-5789.

439. Fung KM, Trojanowski JQ (1995). Animal models of medulloblastomas and related primitive neuroectodermal tumors. A review. *J Neuropath Exp Neurol* 54: 285-296.

440. Furnari FB, Huang HJ, Cavenee WK (1996). Molecular biology of malignant degeneration of astrocytoma. *Pediatr Neurosurg* 24: 41-49.

441. Furness PN, Lowe J, Tarrant GS (1990). Subepithelial basement membrane deposition and intermediate filament expression in choroid plexus neoplasms and ependymomas. *Histopathology* 16: 251-255.

442. Furuta A, Takahashi H, Ikuta F, Onda K, Takeda N, Tanaka R (1992). Temporal lobe tumor demonstrating ganglioglioma and pleomorphic xanthoastrocytoma components. Case report. *J Neurosurg* 77: 143-147.

443. Gabos S, Berkel J (1992). Meta-analysis of progestin and estrogen receptors in human meningiomas. *Neuroepidemiology* 11: 255-260.

444. Gailani MR, Bale SJ, Leffell DJ, DiGiovanna JJ, Peck GL, Poliak S, Drum MA, Pastakia B, McBride OW, Kase R (1992). Developmental defects in Gorlin syndrome

related to a putative tumor suppressor gene on chromosome 9. *Cell* 69: 111-117.

445. Gailani MR, Stahle B, Leffell DJ, Glynn M, Zaphiropoulos PG, Pressman C, Unden AB, Dean M, Brash DE, Bale AE, Toftgard R (1996). The role of the human homologue of Drosophila patched in sporadic basal cell carcinomas. *Nat Genet* 14: 78-81.

446. Gajjar A, Bhargava R, Jenkins JJ, Heideman R, Sanford RA, Langston JW, Walter AW, Kuttesch JF, Muhlbauer M, Kun LE (1995). Low-grade astrocytoma with neuraxis dissemination at diagnosis. *J Neurosurg* 83: 67-71.

447. Gajjar AJ, Heideman RL, Douglass EC, Kun LE, Kovnar EH, Sanford RA, Fairclough DL, Ayers D, Look AT (1993). Relation of tumor-cell ploidy to survival in children with medulloblastoma. *J Clin Oncol* 11: 2211-2217.

448. Galatioto S, Gaddoni G (1971). [Primary myosarcomas of the CNS]. *Acta Neurol Napoli* 26: 297-302.

449. Galatioto S, Marafioti T, Cavallari V, Batolo D (1993). Gliomatosis cerebri. Clinical, neuropathological, immunohistochemical and morphometric studies. *Zentralbl Pathol* 139: 261-267.

450. Gambarelli D, Hassoun J, Choux M, Toga M (1982). Complex cerebral tumor with evidence of neuronal, glial and Schwann cell differentiation: a histologic, immunocytochemical and ultrastructural study. *Cancer* 49: 1420-1428.

451. Ganju V, Jenkins RB, O'Fallon JR, Scheithauer BW, Ransom DT, Katzmann JA, Kimmel DW (1994). Prognostic factors in gliomas. A multivariate analysis of clinical, pathologic, flow cytometric, cytogenetic, and molecular markers. *Cancer* 74: 920-927.

452. Gannett DE, Wisbeck WM, Silbergeld DL, Berger MS (1994). The role of postoperative irradiation in the treatment of oligodendroglioma. *Int J Radiat Oncol Biol Phys* 30: 567-573.

453. Garber JE, Goldstein AM, Kantor AF, Dreyfus MG, Fraumeni JF, Jr., Li FP (1991). Follow-up study of twenty-four families with Li-Fraumeni syndrome. *Cancer Res* 51: 6094-6097.

454. Garcia B, Cabello A, Guarch R, Ruiz dA, Ezpeleta I (1990). [Melanotic medulloblastoma. Ultrastructural and histochemical study of a case]. *Arch Neurobiol Madr* 53: 8-12.

455. Garner A,Klinworth GK (1982). Tumors of the orbit, optic nerve and lacrimal sac. In: *Pathobiology of Ocular Disease*, Marcel Dekker: New York. pp. 741.

456. Garty BZ, Laor A, Danon YL (1994). Neurofibromatosis type 1 in Israel: survey of young adults. *J Med Genet* 31: 853-857.

457. Garvin JH, Jr., Lack EE, Berenberg W, Frantz CN (1984). Ganglioneuroma presenting with differentiated skeletal metastases. Report of a case. *Cancer* 54: 357-360.

458. Gaspar LE, Mackenzie IR, Gilbert JJ, Kaufmann JC, Fisher BF, Macdonald DR, Cairncross JG (1993). Primary cerebral fibrosarcomas. Clinicopathologic study and review of the literature. *Cancer* 72: 3277-3281.

459. Geddes JF, Thom M, Robinson SFD, Revesz T (1996). Granular cell change in astrocytic tumors. *Am J Surg Pathol* 20: 55-63.

460. Gehring M, Berthold F, Edler L, Schwab M, Amler LC (1995). The 1p deletion is not a reliable marker for the prognosis of patients with neuroblastoma. *Cancer Res* 55: 5366-5369.

461. Gentry WC, Jr., Eskritt NR, Gorlin RJ (1974). Multiple hamartoma syndrome (Cowden disease). *Arch Dermatol* 109: 521-525.

462. Geyer JR, Zeltzer PM, Boyett JM, Rorke LB, Stanley P, Albright AL, Wisoff JH, Milstein JM, Allen JC, Finlay JL, Ayers GD, Shurin SB, Stevens KR, Bleyer WA (1994). Survival of infants with primitive neuroectodermal tumors or malignant ependymomas of the CNS treated with eight drugs in 1 day: a report from the Childrens Cancer Group. *J Clin Oncol* 12: 1607-1615.

463. Gherardi R, Baudrimont M, Nguyen JP, Gaston A, Cesaro P, Degos JD, Caron JP, Poirier J (1986). Monstrocellular heavily lipidized malignant glioma. *Acta Neuropathol (Berl)* 69: 28-32.

464. Giangaspero F, Burger PC, Osborne DR, Stein RB (1984). Suprasellar papillary squamous epithelioma ("papillary craniopharyngioma"). *Am J Surg Pathol* 8: 57-64.

465. Giangaspero F, Cenacchi G, Losi L, Cerasoli S, Bisceglia M, Burger PC (1997). Extraventricular neoplasms with neurocytoma features: A clinicopathological study of 11 cases. *Am J Surg Pathol* 21: 206-212.

466. Giangaspero F, Cenacchi G, Roncaroli F, Rigobello L, Gambacorta M,Allegranza A (1995). Medullocytoma (lipidized medulloblastoma). a cerebellar neoplasm of adults with favorable prognosis. *J Neuropathol Exp Neurol* 54;423.

467. Giangaspero F, Cenacchi G, Roncaroli F, Rigobello L, Manetto V, Gambacorta M, Allegranza A (1996). Medullocytoma (lipidized medulloblastoma): a cerebellar neoplasm of adults with favorable prognosis. *Am J Surg Pathol* 20: 656-664.

468. Giangaspero F, Chieco P, Ceccarelli C, Lisignoli G, Pozuolli R, Gambacorta M, Rossi G, Burger PC (1991). "Desmoplastic" versus "classic" medulloblastoma: comparison of DNA content, histopathology and differentiation. *Virchows Arch A Pathol Anat Histopathol* 418: 207-214.

469. Giangaspero F, Doglioni C, Rivano MT, Pileri S, Gerdes J, Stein H (1987). Growth fraction in human brain tumors defined by the monoclonal antibody Ki-67. *Acta Neuropathol (Berl)* 74: 179-182.

470. Giangaspero F, Rigobello L, Badiali M, Loda M, Andreini L, Basso G, Zorzi F, Montaldi A (1992). Large cell medulloblastomas. A distinct variant with highly aggressive behavior. *Am J Surg Pathol* 16: 687-693.

471. Giannini C, Scheithauer BW (1997). Classification and grading of low-grade astrocytic tumors in children. *Brain Pathol* 7: 785-798.

472. Giese A, Loo MA, Rief MD, Tran N, Berens ME (1995). Substrates for astrocytoma invasion. *Neurosurgery* 37: 294-301.

473. Giordana MT, Bradac GB, Pagni CA, Marino S, Attanasio A (1995). Primary diffuse leptomeningeal gliomatosis with anaplastic features. *Acta Neurochir (Wien)* 132: 154-159.

474. Giordana MT, Cavalla P, Chio A, Marino S, Soffietti R, Vigliani MC, Schiffer D (1995). Prognostic factors in human medulloblastoma. A clinicopathologic study. *Tumori* 81: 338-346.

475. Giordana MT, Cavalla P, Dutto A, Borsotti L, Chio A, Schiffer D (1997). Is medulloblastoma the same tumor in children and adults? *J Neurooncol* 35: 169-176.

476. Giordano MJ, Mahadeo DK, He YY, Geist RT, Hsu C, Gutmann DH (1996). Increased expression of the neurofibromatosis 1 (*NF1*) gene product, neurofibromin, in astrocytes in response to cerebral ischemia. *J Neurosci Res* 43: 246-253.

477. Gjerris F, Klinken L (1978). Long-term prognosis in children with benign cerebellar astrocytoma. *J Neurosurg* 49: 179-184.

478. Gladson CL, Wilcox JN, Sanders L, Gillespie GY, Cheresh DA (1995). Cerebral microenvironment influences expression of the vitronectin gene in astrocytic tumors. *J Cell Sci* 108: 947-956.

479. Glass J, Hochberg FH, Gruber ML, Louis DN, Smith D, Rattner B (1992). The treatment of oligodendrogliomas and mixed oligodendroglioma- astrocytomas with PCV chemotherapy. *J Neurosurg* 76: 741-745.

480. Glavac D, Neumann HP, Wittke C, Jaenig H, Masek O, Streicher T, Pausch F, Engelhardt D, Plate KH, Hofler H, Chen F, Zbar B, Brauch H (1996). Mutations in the VHL tumor suppressor gene and associated lesions in families with von Hippel-Lindau disease from central Europe. *Hum Genet* 98: 271-280.

481. Globus JH, Strauss I (1925). Spongioblastoma multiforme. *Arch Neurol Psychiatry* 14: 139-151.

482. Gnarra JR, Zhou S, Merrill MJ, Wagner JR, Krumm A, Papavassiliou E, Oldfield EH, Klausner RD, Linehan WM (1996). Post-transcriptional regulation of vascular endothelial growth factor mRNA by the product of the VHL tumor suppressor gene. *Proc Natl Acad Sci USA* 93: 10589-10594.

483. Goebel HH, Cravioto H (1972). Ultrastructure of human and experimental ependymomas. A comparative study. *J Neuropathol Exp Neurol* 31: 54-71.

484. Goellner JR, Laws ER, Jr., Soule EH, Okazaki H (1978). Hemangiopericytoma of the meninges. Mayo Clinic experience. *Am J Clin Pathol* 70: 375-380.

485. Goldberg S, Gadoth N, Stern S, Cohen IJ, Zaizov R, Sandbank U (1991). The prognostic significance of glial fibrillary acidic protein staining in medulloblastoma. *Cancer* 68: 568-573.

486. Goldman JE, Corbin E (1991). Rosenthal fibers contain ubiquitinated alpha B-crystallin. *Am J Pathol* 139: 933-938.

487. Goldwein JW, Leahy JM, Packer RJ, Sutton LN, Curran WJ, Rorke LB, Schut L, Littman PS,D'Angio GJ (1988). Intracranial ependymomas in children. *Pediatr Neurosci* 14;149.

488. Gomez M, Fueyo J, Kyritsis AP, Steck PA, Roth JA, McDonnell TJ, Steck KD, Levin VA, Yung WK (1996). Adenovirus-mediated transfer of the p53 gene produces rapid and generalized death of human glioma cells via apoptosis. *Cancer Res* 56: 694-699.

489. Gomez MR (1991). Phenotypes of the tuberous sclerosis complex with a revision of diagnostic criteria. *Ann N Y Acad Sci* 615: 1-7.

490. Gonzalez C, Goldschmidt RA, Hsueh W, Trujillo YP (1982). Infantile sarcoma with intracytoplasmic filamentous inclusions: distinctive tumor of possible histiocytic origin. *Cancer* 49: 2365-2375.

491. Gonzalez Gomez I, Rowland JM (1997). Immunohistochemical panel for differential diagnosis of small blue cell tumors in childhood. *Lab Invest* 76: 3p-

492. Gorlin RJ, Goltz RW (1960). Multiple nevoid basal-cell epithelioma, jaw cysts and bifid rib: a syndrome. *N Engl J Med* 262: 908-912.

493. Gorski GK, McMorrow LE, Donaldson MH, Freed M (1992). Multiple chromosomal abnormalities in a case of craniopharyngioma. *Cancer Genet Cytogenet* 60: 212-213.

494. Goto S, Nagahiro S, Ushio Y, Kitaoka M, Nishio S, Fukui M (1993). Immunocytochemical detection of calcineurin and microtubule- associated protein 2 in central neurocytoma. *J Neurooncol* 16: 19-24.

495. Gottschalk J, Jautzke G, Paulus W, Goebel S, Cervos N (1993). The use of immunomorphology to differentiate choroid plexus tumors from metastatic carcinomas. *Cancer* 72: 1343-1349.

496. Gould VE, Jansson DS, Molenaar WM, Rorke LB, Trojanowski JQ, Lee VM, Packer RJ, Franke WW (1990). Primitive neuroectodermal tumors of the central nervous system. Patterns of expression of neuroendocrine markers, and all classes of intermediate filament proteins. *Lab Invest* 62: 498-509.

497. Gould VE, Rorke LB, Jansson DS, Molenaar WM, Trojanowski JQ, Lee VM, Packer RJ, Franke WW (1990). Primitive neuroectodermal tumors of the central nervous system express neuroendocrine markers and may express all classes of intermediate filaments. *Hum Pathol* 21: 245-252.

498. Goutelle A, Fischer G (1977). Les ependymomes, intracraniens et intrarachidiens. *Neurochirurgie* 23: 5-6.

499. Grady EF, Schwab M, Rosenau W (1987). Expression of N-myc and c-src during the development of fetal human brain. *Cancer Res* 47: 2931-2936.

500. Grant JW (1983). Histiocytic origin of the sarcomatous elements in gliosarcomas. *Neuropathol Appl Neurobiol* 9: 335.

501. Grant JW, Steart PV, Aguzzi A, Jones DB, Gallagher PJ (1989). Gliosarcoma: an immunohistochemical study. *Acta Neuropathol (Berl)* 79: 305-309.

502. Gratas C, Tohma Y, Van Meir EG, Klein M, Tenan M, Ishii N, Tachibana O, Kleihues P, Ohgaki H (1997). Fas ligand expression in glioblastoma cell lines and primary astrocytic brain tumors. *Brain Pathol* 7: 863-869.

503. Green AJ, Smith M, Yates JR (1994). Loss of heterozygosity on chromosome 16p13.3 in hamartomas from tuberous sclerosis patients. *Nat Genet* 6: 193-196.

504. Greenblatt MS, Bennett WP, Hollstein M, Harris CC (1994). Mutations in the *p53* tumor suppressor gene: clues to cancer etiology and molecular pathogenesis. *Cancer Res* 54: 4855-4878.

505. Griepentrog F, Pauly H (1957). Intra- und extracranielle, fruhmanifeste Medulloblastome bei erbgleichen Zwillingen. *Zentralbl Neurochir* 17: 129-140.

506. Griesser H (1993). Applied molecular genetics in the diagnosis of malignant non-Hodgkin's lymphoma. *Diagn Mol Pathol* 2: 177-191.

507. Griffin CA, Hawkins AL, Packer RJ, Rorke LB, Emanuel BS (1988). Chromosome abnormalities in pediatric brain tumors. *Cancer Res* 48: 175-180.

508. Griffin CA, Long PP, Carson BS, Brem H (1992). Chromosome abnormalities in low-grade central nervous system tumors. *Cancer Genet Cytogenet* 60: 67-73.

509. Griffiths DF, Williams GT, Williams ED (1987). Duodenal carcinoid tumours, phaeochromocytoma and neurofibromatosis: islet cell tumour, phaeochromocytoma and the von Hippel-Lindau complex: two distinctive neuroendocrine syndromes. *Q J Med* 64: 769-782.

510. Grinspan JB, Stern JL, Franceschini B, Pleasure D (1993). Trophic effects of basic fibroblast growth factor (bFGF) on differentiated oligodendroglia: a mechanism for regeneration of the oligodendroglial lineage. *J Neurosci Res* 36: 672-680.

511. Grossman RI,Yousem DM (1994). *Neuroradiology. The Requisites.* Mosby-Yearbook: St. Louis.

512. Grove A, Vyberg M (1993). Primary leptomeningeal T-cell lymphoma: a case and a review of primary T-cell lymphoma of the central nervous system. *Clin Neuropathol* 12: 7-12.

513. Gunthert U, Stauder R, Mayer B, Terpe HJ, Finke L, Friedrichs K (1995). Are CD44 variant isoforms involved in human tumour progression? *Cancer Surveys* 24: 19-42.

514. Gusella JF, Ramesh V, MacCollin M, Jacoby LB (1996). Neurofibromatosis 2: loss of merlin's protective spell. *Curr Opin Genet Dev* 6: 87-92.

515. Guthrie BL, Ebersold MJ, Scheithauer BW, Shaw EG (1989). Meningeal hemangiopericytoma: histopathological features, treatment, and long-term follow-up of 44 cases. *Neurosurgery* 25: 514-522.

516. Gutmann DH, Giordano MJ, Mahadeo DK, Lau N, Silbergeld D, Guha A (1996). Increased neurofibromatosis 1 gene expression in astrocytic tumors: positive regulation by p21-ras. *Oncogene* 12: 2121-2127.

517. Gyure KA, Prayson RA (1997). Subependymal giant cell astrocytoma: a clinicopathologic study with HMB-45 and MIB1 immunohistochemistry. *Mod Pathol* 10: 313-317.

518. Haapasalo HK, Sallinen PK, Helen PT, Rantala IS, Helin HJ, Isola JJ (1993). Comparison of three quantitation methods for PCNA immunostaining: applicability and relation to survival in 83 astrocytic neoplasms. *J Pathol* 171: 207-214.

519. Haataja L, Raffel C, Ledbetter DH, Tanigami A, Petersen D, Heisterkamp N, Groffen J (1997). Deletion within the D17S34 locus in a primitive neuroectodermal tumor. *Cancer Res* 57: 32-34.

520. Hachitanda Y, Hata J (1996). Stage IVS neuroblastoma: a clinical, histological, and biological analysis of 45 cases. *Hum Pathol* 27: 1135-1138.

521. Haddad SF, Hitchon PW, Godersky JC (1991). Idiopathic and glucocorticoid-induced spinal epidural lipomatosis. *J Neurosurg* 74: 38-42.

522. Haddad SF, Moore SA, Schelper RL, Goeken JA (1992). Vascular smooth muscle hyperplasia underlies the formation of glomeruloid vascular structures of glioblastoma multiforme. *J Neuropathol Exp Neurol* 51: 488-492.

523. Haddad SF, Moore SA, Schelper RL, Goeken JA (1992). Smooth muscle can comprise the sarcomatous component of gliosarcomas. *J Neuropathol Exp Neurol* 51: 493-498.

524. Hahn H, Wicking C, Zaphiropoulos PG, Gailani MR, Shanley S, Chidambaram A, Vorechovsky I, Holmberg E, Unden AB, Gillies S, Negus K, Smyth I, Pressman C, Leffell DJ, Gerrard B, Goldstein AM, Dean M, Toftgard R, Chenevix T, Wainwright B, Bale AE (1996). Mutations of the human homolog of Drosophila patched in the nevoid basal cell carcinoma syndrome. *Cell* 85: 841-851.

525. Hahn JF, Sperber EE, Netsky MG (1976). Melanotic neuroectodermal tumors of the brain and skull. *J Neuropathol Exp Neurol* 35: 508-519.

526. Hainaut P, Soussi T, Shomer B, Hollstein M, Greenblatt M, Hovig E, Harris CC, Montesano R (1997). Database of p53 gene somatic mutations in human tumors and cell lines: updated compilation and future prospects. *Nucleic Acids Res* 25: 151-157.

527. Haines DS, Landers JE, Engle LJ, George DL (1994). Physical and functional interaction between wild-type p53 and mdm2 proteins. *Mol Cell Biol* 14: 1171-1178.

528. Hair LS, Symmans F, Powers JM, Carmel P (1992). Immunohistochemistry and proliferative activity in Lhermitte- Duclos disease. *Acta Neuropathol (Berl)* 84: 570-573.

529. Hall PA, Meek D, Lane DP (1996). p53—integrating the complexity. *J Pathol* 180: 1-5.

530. Halling KC, Scheithauer BW, Halling AC, Nascimento AG, Ziesmer SC, Roche PC, Wollan PC (1996). p53 expression in neurofibroma and malignant peripheral nerve sheath tumor. An immunohistochemical study of sporadic and NF1- associated tumors. *Am J Clin Pathol* 106: 282-288.

531. Hamilton MG, Demetrick DJ, Tranmer BI, Curry B (1994). Isolated cerebellar lymphomatoid granulomatosis progressing to malignant lymphoma. Case report. *J Neurosurg* 80: 314-320.

532. Hamilton RL, Pollack IF (1997). The molecular biology of ependymomas. *Brain Pathol* 7: 807-822.

533. Hamilton SR, Liu B, Parsons RE, Papadopoulos N, Jen J, Powell SM, Krush AJ, Berk T, Cohen Z, Tetu B, Burger PC, Wood PA, Tagi F, Booker SV, Peterson GM, Offerhaus GJA, Tersmette AC, Giardiello FM, Vogelstein B, Kinzler RW (1995). The molecular basis of Turcot's syndrome. *N Engl J Med* 332: 839-847.

534. Han DH, Kim DG, Chi JG, Park SH, Jung HW, Kim YG (1992). Malignant triton tumor of the acoustic nerve. Case report. *J Neurosurg* 76: 874-877.

535. Hanssen AM, Fryns JP (1995). Cowden syndrome. *J Med Genet* 32: 117-119.

536. Hanssen AM, Werquin H, Suys E, Fryns JP (1993). Cowden syndrome: report of a large family with macrocephaly and increased severity of signs in subsequent generations. *Clin Genet* 44: 281-286.

537. Hara A, Araki Y, Shinoda J, Hirayama H, Niikawa S, Sakai N, Yamada H (1993). Central neurocytoma: proliferative assessment by nucleolar organizer region staining. *Surg Neurol* 39: 343-347.

538. Hara A, Sakai N, Yamada H, Tanaka T, Mori H (1991). Assessment of proliferative potential in gliomatosis cerebri. *J Neurol* 238: 80-82.

539. Hardwidge C, Diengdoh J, Husband D, Nash J (1990). Primary cerebral lymphoma: a clinico-pathological study. *Clin Neuropathol* 9: 217-223.

540. Harper JW, Adami GR, Wei N, Keyomarsi K, Elledge SJ (1993). The p21 Cdk-interacting protein Cip1 is a potent inhibitor of G1 cyclin-dependent kinases. *Cell* 75: 805-816.

541. Harris CP, Townsend JJ, Brockmeyer DL, Heilbrun MP (1991). Cerebral granular cell tumor occurring with glioblastoma multiforme: case report. *Surg Neurol* 36: 202-206.

542. Harris NL, Jaffe ES, Stein H, Banks PM, Chan JK, Cleary ML, Delsol G, De Wolf P, Falini B, Gatter KC (1994). A revised European-American classification of lymphoid neoplasms: a proposal from the International Lymphoma Study Group. *Blood* 84: 1361-1392.

543. Harrison MJ, Wolfe DE, Lau TS, Mitnick RJ, Sachdev VP (1991). Radiation-induced meningiomas: experience at the Mount Sinai Hospital and review of the literature. *J Neurosurg* 75: 564-574.

544. Hart MN, Earle KM (1973). Primitive neuroectodermal tumors of the brain in children. *Cancer* 32: 890-897.

545. Hart MN, Petito CK, Earle KM (1974). Mixed gliomas. *Cancer* 33: 134-140.

546. Hartwell L (1992). Defects in a cell cycle checkpoint may be responsible for the genomic instability of cancer cells. *Cell* 71: 543-546.

547. Harwood-Nash DC (1994). Neuroimaging of childhood craniopharyngioma. *Pediatr Neurosurg* 21 Suppl 1: 2-10.

548. Hashimoto T, Sasagawa I, Ishigooka M, Kubota Y, Nakada T, Fujita T, Nakai O (1995). Down's syndrome associated with intracranial germinoma and testicular embryonal carcinoma. *Urol Int* 55: 120-122.

549. Hassin GB, Munch-Petersen CJ (1951). Central neurogenic tumors (neuroblastoma and ganglioneuroma). A pathologic study of two cases. *J Neuropathol Clin Neurol* 1: 63-80.

550. Hassoun J, Gambarelli D, Grisoli F, Pellet W, Salamon G, Pellisier JF, Toga M (1982). Central neurocytoma. An electron-microscopic study of two cases. *Acta Neuropathol (Berl)* 56: 151-156.

551. Hassoun J, Soylemezoglu F, Gambarelli D, Figarella B, von Ammon K, Kleihues P (1993). Central neurocytoma: a synopsis of clinical and histological features. *Brain Pathol* 3: 297-306.

552. Hatva E, Bohling T, Jaaskelainen J, Persico MG, Haltia M, Alitalo K (1996). Vascular growth factors and receptors in capillary hemangioblastomas and hemangiopericytomas. *Am J Pathol* 148: 763-775.

553. Hatva E, Kaipainen A, Mentula P, Jaaskelainen J, Paetau A, Haltia M, Alitalo K (1995). Expression of endothelial cell-specific receptor tyrosine kinases and growth factors in human brain tumors. *Am J Pathol* 146: 368-378.

554. Haupt Y, Maya R, Kazaz A, Oren M (1997). Mdm2 promotes the rapid degradation of p53. *Nature* 387: 296-299.

555. Hayakawa T, Takakura K, Abe H, Yoshimoto T, Tanaka R, Sugita K, Kikuchi H, Uozumi T, Hori T, Fukui H (1994). Primary central nervous system lymphoma in Japan—a retrospective, co-operative study by CNS-Lymphoma Study Group in Japan. *J Neurooncol* 19: 197-215.

556. Hayashi K, Ohara N, Jeon HJ, Akagi S, Takahashi K, Akagi T, Namba S (1993). Gliosarcoma with features of chondroblastic osteosarcoma. *Cancer* 72: 850-855.

557. Hayashi Y, Kanda N, Inaba T, Hanada R, Nagahara N, Muchi H, Yamamoto K (1989). Cytogenetic findings and prognosis in neuroblastoma with emphasis on marker chromosome 1. *Cancer* 63: 126-132.

558. Hayashi Y, Ueki K, Waha A, Wiestler OD, Louis DN, von Deimling A (1997). Association of *EGFR* gene amplification and *CDKN2* (*p16/MTS1*) gene deletion in glioblastoma multiforme. *Brain Pathol* 7: 871-875.

559. Hayostek CJ, Shaw EG, Scheithauer B, O'Fallon JR, Weiland TL, Schomberg PJ, Kelly PJ, Hu TC (1993). Astrocytomas of the cerebellum. A comparative clinicopathologic study of pilocytic and diffuse astrocytomas. *Cancer* 72: 856-869.

560. Hazuka MB, DeBiose DA, Henderson RH, Kinzie JJ (1992). Survival results in adult patients treated for medulloblastoma. *Cancer* 69: 2143-2148.

561. Hecht BK, Turc C, Chatel M, Lonjon M, Roche JL, Gioanni J, Hecht F, Gaudray P (1995). Chromosomes in gliomatosis cerebri. *Genes Chromosomes Cancer* 14: 149-153.

562. Hecht F, Grix A, Jr., Hecht BK, Berger C, Bixenman H, Szucs S, O'Keeffe D, Finberg HJ (1984). Direct prenatal chromosome diagnosis of a malignancy. *Cancer Genet Cytogenet* 11: 107-111.

563. Heegaard S, Sommer HM, Broholm H, Broendstrup O (1995). Proliferating cell nuclear antigen and Ki-67 immunohistochemistry of oligodendrogliomas with special reference to prognosis. *Cancer* 76: 1809-1813.

564. Heimdal K, Evensen SA, Fossa SD, Hirscberg H, Langholm R, Brogger A, Moller P (1991). Karyotyping of a hematologic neoplasia developing shortly after treatment for cerebral extragonadal germ cell tumor. *Cancer Genet Cytogenet* 57: 41-46.

565. Heiss JD, Papavassiliou E, Merrill MJ, Nieman L, Knightly JJ, Walbridge S, Edwards NA, Oldfield EH (1996). Mechanism of dexamethasone suppression of brain tumor-associated vascular permeability in rats. Involvement of the glucocorticoid receptor and vascular permeability factor. *J Clin Invest* 98: 1400-1408.

566. Heldin CH, Westermark B (1990). Platelet-derived growth factor: mechanism of action and possible in vivo function. *Cell Regul* 1: 555-566.

567. Helle T, Britt R, Colby T (1984). Primary lymphoma of the central nervous system: clinicopathologic study of experience at Stanford. *J Neurosurg* 60: 94-103.

568. Helseth A, Mork SJ (1989). Neoplasms of the central nervous system in Norway. III. Epidemiological characteristics of intracranial gliomas according to histology. *APMIS* 97: 547-555.

569. Hendrick EB,Raffel C (1989). Tumors of the fourth ventricle: ependymomas, choroid plexus papillomas and dermoid cysts. In: *Pediatric Neurosurgery*, Saunders: Philadelphia. pp. 366-371.

570. Henn W, Wullich B, Thonnes M, Steudel WI, Feiden W, Zang KD (1993). Recurrent t(12;19)(q13;q13.3) in intracranial and extrac-

ranial hemangiopericytoma. *Cancer Genet Cytogenet* 71: 151-154.

571. Henske EP, Scheithauer BW, Short MP, Wollmann R, Nahmias J, Hornigold N, van Slegtenhorst M, Welsh CT, Kwiatkowski DJ (1996). Allelic loss is frequent in tuberous sclerosis kidney lesions but rare in brain lesions. *Am J Hum Genet* 59: 400-406.

572. Henson JW, Schnitker BL, Correa KM, von Deimling A, Fassbender F, Xu HJ, Benedict WF, Yandell DW, Louis DN (1994). The retinoblastoma gene is involved in malignant progression of astrocytomas. *Ann Neurol* 36: 714-721.

573. Herath SE, Stalboerger PG, Dahl RJ, Parisi JE, Jenkins RB (1994). Cytogenetic studies of four hemangiopericytomas. *Cancer Genet Cytogenet* 72: 137-140.

574. Herholz K, Pietrzyk U, Voges J, Schroder R, Halber M, Treuer H, Sturm V, Heiss WD (1993). Correlation of glucose consumption and tumor cell density in astrocytomas. A stereotactic PET study. *J Neurosurg* 79: 853-858.

575. Herman JG, Jen J, Merlo A, Baylin SB (1996). Hypermethylation-associated inactivation indicates a tumor suppressor role for p15INK4B. *Cancer Res* 56: 722-727.

576. Hermanson M, Funa K, Hartman M, Claesson W, Heldin CH, Westermark B, Nister M (1992). Platelet-derived growth factor and its receptors in human glioma tissue: expression of messenger RNA and protein suggests the presence of autocrine and paracrine loops. *Cancer Res* 52: 3213-3219.

577. Hermanson M, Funa K, Koopmann J, Maintz D, Waha A, Westermark B, Heldin CH, Wiestler OD, Louis DN, von Deimling A, Nister M (1996). Association of loss of heterozygosity on chromosome 17p with high platelet-derived growth factor alpha receptor expression in human malignant gliomas. *Cancer Res* 56: 164-171.

578. Herpers MJHM, Budka H (1984). Glial fibrillary acidic protein (GFAP) in oligodendroglial tumors: gliofibrillary oligodendroglioma and transitional oligoastrocytoma as subtypes of oligodendroglioma. *Acta Neuropathol (Berl)* 64: 265-272.

579. Herpers MJ, Ramaekers FC, Aldeweireldt J, Moesker O, Slooff J (1986). Co-expression of glial fibrillary acidic protein- and vimentin- type intermediate filaments in human astrocytomas. *Acta Neuropathol (Berl)* 70: 333-339.

580. Herpers MJHM, Freling G, Beuls EAM (1994). Pleomorphic xanthoastrocytoma in the spinal cord. Case report. *J Neurosurg* 80: 564-569.

581. Herregodts P, Vloeberghs M, Schmedding E, Goossens A, Stadnik T, D'Haens J (1991). Solitary dorsal intramedullary schwannoma. Case report. *J Neurosurg* 74: 816-820.

582. Herrick MK, Rubinstein LJ (1979). The cytological differentiating potential of pineal parenchymal neoplasms (true pinealomas). A clinicopathological study of 28 tumours. *Brain* 102: 289-320.

583. Herva R, Serlo W, Laitinen J, Becker LE (1996). Intraventricular rhabdomyosarcoma after resection of hyperplastic choroid plexus. *Acta Neuropathol (Berl)* 92: 213-216.

584. Hessler RB, Lopes MB, Frankfurter A, Reidy J, VandenBerg SR (1992). Cytoskeletal immunohistochemistry of central neurocytomas. *Am J Surg Pathol* 16: 1031-1038.

585. Hetelekidis S, Barnes PD, Tao ML, Fischer EG, Schneider L, Scott RM, Tarbell NJ (1993). 20-year experience in childhood craniopharyngioma. *Int J Radiat Oncol Biol Phys* 27: 189-195.

586. Heutink P, van Schothorst EM, van der Mey AG, Bardoel A, Breedveld G, Pertijs J, Sandkuijl LA, van Ommen GJ, Cornelisse CJ, Oostra BA (1994). Further localization of the gene for hereditary paragangliomas and evidence for linkage in unrelated families. *Eur J Hum Genet* 2: 148-158.

587. Hiesiger EM, Hayes RL, Pierz DM, Budzilovich GN (1993). Prognostic relevance of epidermal growth factor receptor (EGF-R) and c-neu/erbB2 expression in glioblastomas (GBMs). *J Neurooncol* 16: 93-104.

588. Hirano A (1978). Some contributions of electron microscopy to the diagnosis of brain tumors. *Acta Neuropathol (Berl)* 43: 119-128.

589. Hirato J, Nakazato Y, Ogawa A (1994). Expression of non-glial intermediate filament proteins in gliomas. *Clin Neuropathol* 13: 1-11.

590. Hirose T, Kannuki S, Nishida K, Matsumoto K, Sano T, Hizawa K (1992). Anaplastic ganglioglioma of the brain stem demonstrating active neurosecretory features of neoplastic neuronal cells. *Acta Neuropathol (Berl)* 83: 365-370.

591. Hirose T, Scheithauer BW, Lopes MB, Gerber HA, Altermatt HJ, Harner SG, VandenBerg SR (1995). Olfactory neuroblastoma. An immunohistochemical, ultrastructural, and flow cytometric study. *Cancer* 76: 4-19.

592. Hirose T, Scheithauer BW, Lopes MB, Gerber HA, Altermatt HJ, Hukee MJ, VandenBerg SR, Charlesworth JC (1995). Tuber and subependymal giant cell astrocytoma associated with tuberous sclerosis: an immunohistochemical, ultrastructural, and immunoelectron and microscopic study. *Acta Neuropathol (Berl)* 90: 387-399.

593. Hirose T, Scheithauer BW, Lopes MB, VandenBerg SR (1994). Dysembryoplastic neuroeptiehelial tumor (DNT): an immunohistochemical and ultrastructural study. *J Neuropathol Exp Neurol* 53: 184-195.

594. Hirose T, Scheithauer BW, Lopes MBS, Gerber HA, Altermatt HJ, VandenBerg SR (1997). Ganglioglioma: An ultrastructural and immunohistochemical study. *Cancer* 79: 989-1003.

595. Hirsch JF, Pierre K (1988). Lumbosacral lipomas with spina bifida. *Childs Nerv Syst* 4: 354-360.

596. Hitotsumatsu T, Iwaki T, Kitamati T, Mizoguchi M, Suzuki SO, Hamada Y, Fukui M, Tateishi J (1997). Expression of neurofibromatosis 2 protein in human brain tumors: an immunohistochemical study. *Acta Neuropathol* 93: 225-232.

597. Ho DM, Liu HC (1992). Primary intracranial germ cell tumor. Pathologic study of 51 patients. *Cancer* 70: 1577-1584.

598. Ho KL, Wolfe DE (1981). Concurrence of multiple sclerosis and primary intracranial neoplasms. *Cancer* 47: 2913-2919.

599. Ho YS, Wei CH, Tsai MD, Wai YY (1992). Intracerebral malignant fibrous histiocytoma: case report and review of the literature. *Neurosurgery* 31: 567-571.

600. Hochstrasser H, Boltshauser E, Valavanis A (1988). Brain tumors in children with von Recklinghausen neurofibromatosis. *Skeletal Radiol* 1: 25-28.

601. Hodges LC, Smith JL, Garrett A, Tate S (1992). Prevalence of glioblastoma multiforme in subjects with prior therapeutic radiation. *J Neurosci Nurs* 24: 79-83.

602. Hoffman HJ, Duffner PK (1985). Extraneural metastases of central nervous system tumors. *Cancer* 59: 1778-1782.

603. Hoffman HJ, Otsubo H, Hendrick EB, Humphreys RP, Drake JM, Becker LE, Greenberg M, Jenkin D (1991). Intracranial germ-cell tumors in children. *J Neurosurg* 74: 545-551.

604. Hoffman HJ, Yoshida M, Becker LE, Hendrick EB, Humphreys RP (1983). Pineal region tumors in childhood. Experience at the Hospital for Sick Children. *Pediatr Neurosurg* 21: 91-103.

605. Hoffman JM, Waskin HA, Schifter T, Hanson MW, Gray L, Rosenfeld S, Coleman RE (1993). FDG-PET in differentiating lymphoma from nonmalignant central nervous system lesions in patients with AIDS. *J Nucl Med* 34: 567-575.

606. Hoffman S, Rorke L (1971). On finding striated muscle in the brain. *J Neurol Neurosurg Psychiatry* 34: 761-764.

607. Hoffmeyer S, Assum G, Griesser J, Kaufmann D, Nurnberg P, Krone W (1995). On unequal allelic expression of the neurofibromin gene in neurofibromatosis type 1. *Hum Mol Genet* 4: 1267-1272.

608. Holl T, Kleihues P, Yasargil MG, Wiestler OD (1991). Cerebellar medullomyoblastoma with advanced neuronal differentiation and hamartomatous component. *Acta Neuropathol (Berl)* 82: 408-413.

609. Hollstein MC, Rice K, Greenblatt MS, Soussi T, Fuchs R, Sorlie T, Hovig E, Smith-Sorensen B, Montesano R, Harris CC (1994). Database of *p53* gene somatic mutations in human tumors and cell lines. *Nucleic Acids Res* 22: 3551-3555.

610. Honan WP, Anderson M, Carey MP, Williams B (1987). Familial subependymomas. *Br J Neurosurg* 1: 317-321.

611. Honavar M, Janota I (1994). 73 cases of dysembryoplastic neuroepithelial tumour: the range of histological appearances. *Brain Pathol* 4: 428.

612. Hopewell JW (1975). The subependymal plate and genesis of gliomas. *J Pathol* 117: 101-103.

613. Horn M, Schlote W, Lerch KD, Steudel WI, Harms D, Thomas E (1992). Malignant rhabdoid tumor: primary intracranial manifestation in an adult. *Acta Neuropathol (Berl)* 83: 445-448.

614. Horoupian DS, Kerson LA, Sainotz H, Valsamis M (1974). Paraganglioma of cauda equina. Clinicopathologic and ultrastructural studies of an unusual case. *Cancer* 33: 1337-1348.

615. Horten BC, Rubinstein LJ (1976). Primary cerebral neuroblastoma. A clinicopathological study of 35 cases. *Brain* 99: 735-756.

616. Horten BC, Urich H, Rubinstein LJ, Montague SR (1977). The angioblastic meningioma: a reappraisal of a nosological problem. Light-, electron-microscopic, tissue, and organ culture observations. *J Neurol Sci* 31: 387-410.

617. Hoshino T (1991). Cell kinetics in brain tumors. In: *Neurobiology of Brain Tumors*, Salcman M (eds). Williams & Wilkins: Baltimore. pp. 145-159.

618. Hoshino T, Ahn D, Prados MD, Lamborn K, Wilson CB (1993). Prognostic significance of the proliferative potential of intracranial gliomas measured by bromodeoxyuridine labeling. *Int J Cancer* 53: 550-555.

619. Hoshino T, Kobayashi S, Townsend JJ, Wilson CB (1985). A cell kinetic study on medulloblastomas. *Cancer* 55: 1711-1713.

620. Hoshino T, Rodriguez LA, Cho KG, Lee KS, Wilson CB, Edwards MS, Levin VA, Davis RL (1988). Prognostic implications of the proliferative potential of low- grade astrocytomas. *J Neurosurg* 69: 839-842.

621. Hoshino T, Wilson BC, Ellis WG (1975). Gemistocytic astrocytes in gliomas. An autoradiographic study. *J Neuropathol Exp Neurol* 263-281.

622. Hosokawa Y, Tsuchihashi Y, Okabe H, Toyama M, Namura K, Kuga M, Yonezawa T, Fujita S, Ashihara T (1991). Pleomorphic xanthoastrocytoma. Ultrastructural, immunohistochemical and DNA cytofluorometric study of a case. *Cancer* 68: 853-859.

623. Howley PM, Levine AJ, Li FP, Livingston DM, Rabson AS (1991). Lack of SV40 DNA in tumors from scientists working with SV40 virus. *N Engl J Med* 324: 494-494.

624. Hoyt WF, Baghdassarian SA (1969). Optic glioma of childhood. Natural history and rationale for conservative management. *Br J Ophthalmol* 53: 793-798.

625. Hruban RH, Shiu MH, Senie RT, Woodruff JM (1990). Malignant peripheral nerve sheath tumors of the buttock and lower extremity. A study of 43 cases. *Cancer* 66: 1253-1265.

626. Hsiang J, Ng H, Poon W (1996). Atypical monoclonal plasma cell hyperplasia: its identity and treatment. *J Neurosurg* 85: 697-700.

627. Hsu DW, Efird JT, Hedley Whyte ET (1997). Progesterone and estrogen receptors in meningiomas: prognostic considerations. *J Neurosurg* 86: 113-120.

628. Hsu DW, Pardo FS, Efird JT, Linggood RM, Hedley W (1994). Prognostic significance of proliferative indices in meningiomas. *J Neuropathol Exp Neurol* 53: 247-255.

629. Hsu SC, Volpert OV, Steck PA, Mikkelsen T, Polverini PJ, Rao S, Chou P, Bouck NP (1996). Inhibition of angiogenesis in human glioblastomas by chromosome 10 induction of thrombospondin-1. *Cancer Res* 56: 5684-5691.

630. Huang CI, Chiou WH, Ho DM (1987). Oligodendroglioma occurring after radiation therapy for pituitary adenoma. *J Neurol Neurosurg Psychiatry* 50: 1619-1624.

631. Huang HJS, Nagane M, Klingbeil CK, Lin H, Nishikawa R, Ji XD, Huang CM, Gill GN, Wiley HS, Cavenee WK (1997). The enhanced tumorigenic activity of a mutant epidermal growth factor receptor common in human cancers is mediated by threshold levels of constitutive tyrosine phosphorylation and unattenuated signalling. *J Biol Chem* 272: 2927-2935.

632. Hubbard JL, Scheithauer BW, Kispert DB, Carpenter SM, Wick MR, Laws ER, Jr. (1989). Adult cerebellar medulloblastomas: the pathological, radiographic, and clinical disease spectrum. *J Neurosurg* 70: 536-544.

633. Huddart SN, Muir KR, Parkes SE, Mann JR, Stevens MC, Raafat F, Smith K (1993). Retrospective study of prognostic value of DNA ploidy and proliferative activity in neuroblastoma. *J Clin Pathol* 46: 1101-1104.

634. Hulbanni S, Goodman PA (1976). Glioblastoma multiforme with extraneural metastases in the absence of previous surgery. *Cancer* 37: 1577-1583.

635. Humphrey PA, Gangarosa LM, Wong AJ, Archer GE, Lund Johansen M, Bjerkvig R, Laerum OD, Friedman HS, Bigner DD (1991). Deletion-mutant epidermal growth factor receptor in human gliomas: effects of type II mutation on receptor function. *Biochem Biophys Res Commun* 178: 1413-1420.

636. Humphrey PA, Wong AJ, Vogelstein B, Zalutsky MR, Fuller GN, Archer GE, Friedman HS, Kwatra MM, Bigner SH, Bigner DD (1990). Anti-synthetic peptide antibody reacting at the fusion junction of deletion-mutant epidermal growth factor receptors in human glioblastoma. *Proc Natl Acad Sci USA* 87: 4207-4211.

637. Hung KL, Wu CM, Huang JS, How SW (1990). Familial medulloblastoma in siblings: report in one family and review of the literature. *Surg Neurol* 33: 341-346.

638. Hurtt MR, Moossy J, Donovan-Peluso M, Locker J (1992). Amplification of epidermal growth factor receptor gene in gliomas: histopathology and prognosis. *J Neuropathol Exp Neurol* 51: 84-90.

639. Husain AN, Leestma JE (1986). Cerebral astroblastoma: immunohistochemical and ultrastructural features. Case report. *J Neurosurg* 64: 657-661.

640. Huson SM (1994). Neurofibromatosis 1: a clinical and genetic overview. In: *The Neurofibromatoses. A Pathogenetic and Clinical Overview*, Huson SM, Hughes RAC (eds). Chapman & Hall Medical: London. pp. 160-179.

641. Huson SM, Harper PS, Compston DA (1988). Von Recklinghausen neurofibromatosis. A clinical and population study in south-east Wales. *Brain* 111: 1355-1381.

642. Huttenlocher PR, Heydemann PT (1984). Fine structure of cortical tubers in tuberous sclerosis: a Golgi study. *Ann Neurol* 16: 595-602.

643. Huynh DP, Maunter V, Baser ME, Stavrou D, Pulst S (1997). Immunohistochemical detection of schwannomin and neurofibromin in vestibular schwannomas, ependymomas and meningiomas. *J Neuropath Exp Neurol* 56: 382-390.

644. Ichimura K, Schmidt EE, Goike HM, Collins VP (1996). Human glioblastomas with no alterations of the *CDK2A* (*p16^INK4A^*, *MTS1*) and *CDK4* genes have frequent mutations of the retinoblastoma gene. *Oncogene* 13: 1065-1072.

645. Ikeda E, Achen MG, Breier G, Risau W (1995). Hypoxia-induced transcriptional activation and increased mRNA stability of vascular endothelial growth factor in C6 glioma cells. *J Biol Chem* 270: 19761-19766.

646. Ilgren EB, Stiller CA, Hughes JT, Silberman D, Steckel N, Kaye A (1984). Ependymomas: a clinical and pathologic study. Part II. Survival features. *Clin Neuropathol* 3: 122-127.

647. Illum N, Korf HW, Julian K, Rasmussen T, Herning M, Krabbe S (1992). Concurrent uveoretinitis and pineocytoma in a child suggests a causal relationship. *Br J Ophthalmol* 76: 574-576.

648. Inoue H, Tamura M, Koizumi H, Nakamura M, Naganuma H, Ohye C (1984). Clinical pathology of malignant meningiomas. *Acta Neurochir Wien* 73: 179-191.

649. Ito S, Chandler KL, Prados MD, Lamborn K, Wynne J, Malec MK, Wilson CB, Davis RL, Hoshino T (1994). Proliferative potential and prognostic evaluation of low-grade astrocytomas. *J Neurooncol* 19: 1-9.

650. Ito S, Hoshino T, Prados MD, Edwards MS (1992). Cell kinetics of medulloblastomas. *Cancer* 70: 671-678.

651. Ito S, Hoshino T, Shibuya M, Prados MD, Edwards MS, Davis RL (1992). Proliferative characteristics of juvenile pilocytic astrocytomas determined by bromodeoxyuridine labeling. *Neurosurgery* 31: 413-418.

652. Ito T, Takahashi H, Ikuta F, Sato H (1994). Metastatic pineocytoma of the spinal cord after long-term dormancy. *Pathol Int* 44: 860-864.

653. Itoh H, Ohsato K (1985). Turcot syndrome and its characteristic colonic manifestations. *Dis Colon Rectum* 28: 399-402.

654. Itoyama T, Sadamori N, Tsutsumi K, Tokunaga Y, Soda H, Tomonaga M, Yamamori S, Masuda Y, Oshima K, Kikuchi M (1994). Primary central nervous system lymphomas. Immunophenotypic, virologic, and cytogenetic findings of three patients without immune defects. *Cancer* 73: 455-463.

655. Iuzzolino P, Ghimenton C, Nicolato A, Giorgiutti F, Fina P, Doglioni C, Barbareschi M (1994). p53 protein in low-grade astrocytomas: a study with long-term follow-up. *Br J Cancer* 69: 586-591.

656. Iwadate Y, Fujimoto S, Tagawa M, Namba H, Sueyoshi K, Hirose M, Sakiyama S (1996). Association of p53 gene mutation with decreased chemosensitivity in human malignant gliomas. *Int J Cancer* 69: 236-240.

657. Iwaki T, Fukui M, Kondo A, Matsushima T, Takeshita I (1987). Epithelial properties of pleomorphic xanthoastrocytomas determined in ultrastructural and immunohistochemical studies. *Acta Neuropathol (Berl)* 74: 142-150.

658. Iwashita T, Enjoji M (1987). Plexiform neurilemmoma: a clinicopathological and immunohistochemical analysis of 23 tumours from 20 patients. *Virchows Arch A Pathol Anat Histopathol* 411: 305-309.

659. Jaaskelainen J (1986). Seemingly complete removal of histologically benign intracranial meningioma: late recurrence rate and factors predicting recurrence in 657 patients. A multivariate analysis. *Surg Neurol* 26: 461-469.

660. Jaaskelainen J, Haltia M, Laasonen E, Wahlstrom T, Valtonen S (1985). The growth rate of intracranial meningiomas and its relation to histology. An analysis of 43 patients. *Surg Neurol* 24: 165-172.

661. Jaaskelainen J, Haltia M, Servo A (1986). Atypical and anaplastic meningiomas: radiology, surgery, radiotherapy, and outcome. *Surg Neurol* 25: 233-242.

662. Jaaskelainen J, Paetau A, Pyykko I, Blomstedt G, Palva T, Troupp H (1994). Interface between the facial nerve and large acoustic neurinomas. Immunohistochemical study of the cleavage plane in NF2 and non-NF2 cases. *J Neurosurg* 80: 541-547.

663. Jaaskelainen J, Servo A, Haltia M, Kallio M, Troupp H (1991). Meningeal hemangiopericytoma. In: *Meningiomas and Their Surgical Treatment*, Schmidek H (eds). Saunders Company: Orlando. pp. 73-82.

664. Jaaskelainen J, Servo A, Haltia M, Wahlstrom T, Valtonen S (1985). Intracranial hemangiopericytoma: radiology, surgery, radiotherapy, and outcome in 21 patients. *Surg Neurol* 23: 227-236.

665. Jack CR, Jr., Bhansali DT, Chason JL, Boulos RS, Mehta BA, Patel SC, Sanders WP (1987). Angiographic features of gliosarcoma. *AJNR Am J Neuroradiol* 8: 117-122.

666. Jacoby LB, MacCollin M, Barone R, Ramesh V, Gusella JF (1996). Frequency and distribution of NF2 mutations in schwannomas. *Genes Chromosomes Cancer* 17: 45-55.

667. Jacoby LB, MacCollin M, Louis DN, Mohney T, Rubio MP, Pulaski K, Trofatter JA, Kley N, Seizinger B, Ramesh V, et al (1994). Exon scanning for mutation of the NF2 gene in schwannomas. *Hum Mol Genet* 3: 413-419.

668. Jacoby LB, Pulaski K, Rouleau GA, Martuza RL (1990). Clonal analysis of human meningiomas and schwannomas. *Cancer Res* 50: 6783-6786.

669. Jaenisch W, Schreiber D,Guthert H (1988). Primare melanome der ZNS. In: *Neuropathologie. Tumoren des Nervensystems*, Gustav Fischer: Stuttgart. pp. 347-353.

670. Jagadha V, Halliday WC, Becker LE (1986). Glial fibrillary acidic protein (GFAP) in oligodendrogliomas: a reflection of transient GFAP expression by immature oligodendroglia. *Can J Neurol Sci* 13: 307-311.

671. Jakacki RI, Zeltzer PM, Boyett JM, Albright AL, Allen JC, Geyer JR, Rorke LB, Stanley P, Stevens KR, Wisoff J, McGuire C, Milstein JM, Packer F, Finlay JL (1995). Survival and prognostic factors following radiation and/or chemotherapy for primitive neuroectodermal tumors of the pineal region in infants and children: a report of the Childrens Cancer Group. *J Clin Oncol* 13: 1377-1383.

672. Jalkanen S, Aho R, Kallajoki M, Ekfors T, Nortamo P, Gahmberg C, Duijvestijn A, Kalimo H (1989). Lymphocyte homing receptors and adhesion molecules in intravascular malignant lymphomatosis. *Int J Cancer* 44: 777-782.

673. Jallo GI, Zagzag D, Epstein F (1996). Intramedullary subependymoma of the spinal cord. *Neurosurgery* 38: 251-257.

674. James CD, Carlbom E, Dumanski JP, Hausen M, Nordenskjold MD, Collins VP, Cavenee WK (1988). Clonal genomic alterations in glioma malignancy stages. *Cancer Res* 48: 5546-5551.

675. James CD, He J, Carlbom E, Mikkelsen T, Ridderheim PA, Cavenee WK, Collins VP (1990). Loss of genetic information in central nervous system tumors common to children and young adults. *Genes Chromosomes Cancer* 2: 94-102.

676. James CD, He J, Carlbom E, Nordenskjold M, Cavenee WK, Collins VP (1991). Chromosome 9 deletion mapping reveals interferon alpha and interferon beta-1 gene deletions in human glial tumors. *Cancer Res* 51: 1684-1688.

677. Jamjoom ZA, Sadiq S, Naim UR, Malabary T (1991). Cerebello-pontine angle paraganglioma simulating an acoustic neurinoma. *Br J Neurosurg* 5: 307-312.

678. Janisch W, Janda J, Link I (1994). [Primary diffuse leptomeningeal leiomyomatosis]. *Zentralbl Pathol* 140: 195-200.

679. Janisch W, Staneczek W (1989). [Primary tumors of the choroid plexus. Frequency, localization and age]. *Zentralbl Allg Pathol* 135: 235-240.

680. Jansen GH, Troost D, Dingemans KP (1990). Polar spongioblastoma: an immunohistochemical and electron microscopical study. *Acta Neuropathol (Berl)* 81: 228-232.

681. Janss AJ, Yachnis AT, Silber JH, Trojanowski JQ, Lee VM, Sutton LN, Perilongo G, Rorke LB, Phillips PC (1996). Glial differentiation predicts poor clinical outcome in primitive neuroectodermal brain tumors. *Ann Neurol* 39: 481-489.

682. Jaque CM, Kujas M, Poreau A, Raoul M, Collier P, Racadot J, Baumann NA (1979). GFA and S 100 protein levels as an index for malignancy in human gliomas and neurinomas. *J Natl Cancer Inst* 62: 479-483.

683. Jaros E, Perry RH, Adam L, Kelly PJ, Crawford PJ, Kalbag RM, Mendelow AD, Sengupta RP, Pearson ADJ (1992). Prognostic implications of p53 protein, epidermal growth factor receptor, and Ki-67 labelling in brain tumours. *Br J Cancer* 66: 373-385.

684. Jaskolsky D, Zawirski M, Papierz W, Kotwica Z (1987). Mixed gliomas. Their clinical course and results of surgery. *Zentralbl Neurochir* 48: 120-123.

685. Jay V, Edwards V, Squire J, Rutka J (1993). Astroblastoma: report of a case with ultrastructural, cell kinetic, and cytogenetic analysis. *Pediatr Pathol* 13: 323-332.

686. Jay V, Squire J, Becker LE, Humphreys R (1994). Malignant transformation in a ganglioglioma with anaplastic neuronal and astrocytic components. Report of a case with flow cytometric and cytogenetic analysis. *Cancer* 73: 2862-2868.

687. Jayawickreme DP, Hayward RD, Harkness WF (1995). Intracranial ependymomas in childhood: a report of 24 cases followed for 5 years. *Childs Nerv Syst* 11: 409-413.

688. Jellinger K (1986). Vascular malformations of the central nervous system: a morphological overview. *Neurosurg Rev* 9: 177-216.

689. Jellinger K, Boeck F, Brenner H (1988). Meningeal melanocytoma. Report of a case and review of the literature. *Acta Neurochir Wien* 94: 78-87.

690. Jellinger K, Paulus W (1991). Mesenchymal, non-meningothelial tumors of the central nervous system. *Brain Pathol* 1: 79-87.

691. Jellinger K, Paulus W, Slowik F (1991). The enigma of meningeal hemangiopericytoma. *Brain Tumor Pathol* 8: 33-43.

692. Jellinger K, Radaskiewicz TH, Slowik F (1975). Primary malignant lymphomas of the central nervous system in man. *Acta Neuropathol Suppl Berl* Suppl 6: 95-102.

693. Jellinger K, Seitelberger F (1975). Malignant Lymphomas of the Nervous System. International Symposium Wien 1974. *Acta Neuropathol* Suppl 6: 1-301.

694. Jellinger K, Slowik F (1975). Histological subtypes and prognostic problems in meningiomas. *J Neurol* 208: 279-298.

695. Jellinger KA, Paulus W (1992). Primary central nervous system lymphomas—an update. *J Cancer Res Clin Oncol* 119: 7-27.

696. Jen J, Harper JW, Bigner SH, Bigner DD, Papadopoulos N, Markowitz S, Willson JK, Kinzler KW, Vogelstein B (1994). Dele-

tion of p16 and p15 genes in brain tumors. *Cancer Res* 54: 6353-6358.

697. Jenkins RB, Kimmel DW, Moertel CA, Schultz CG, Scheithauer BW, Kelly PJ, Dewald GW (1989). A cytogenetic study of 53 human gliomas. *Cancer Genet Cytogenet* 39: 253-279.

698. Jennings MT, Frenchman M, Shehab T, Johnson MD, Creasy J, LaPorte K, Dettbarn WD (1995). Gliomatosis cerebri presenting as intractable epilepsy during early childhood. *J Child Neurol* 10: 37-45.

699. Jennings MT, Gelman R, Hochberg F (1985). Intracranial germ-cell tumors: natural history and pathogenesis. *J Neurosurg* 63: 155-167.

700. Jennings RW, LaQuaglia MP, Leong K, Hendren WH, Adzick NS (1993). Fetal neuroblastoma: prenatal diagnosis and natural history. *J Pediatr Surg* 28: 1168-1174.

701. Jhanwar SC, Chen Q, Li FP, Brennan MF, Woodruff JM (1994). Cytogenetic analysis of soft tissue sarcomas. Recurrent chromosome abnormalities in malignant peripheral nerve sheath tumors (MPNST). *Cancer Genet Cytogenet* 78: 138-144.

702. Jimenez CL, Carpenter BF, Robb IA (1987). Melanotic cerebellar tumor. *Ultrastruct Pathol* 11: 751-759.

703. Jin Y, Mertens F, Arheden K, Mandahl N, Wennerberg J, Dictor M, Heim S, Mitelman F (1995). Karyotypic features of malignant tumors of the nasal cavity and paranasal sinuses. *Int J Cancer* 60: 637-641.

704. Johannsson O, Ostermeyer EA, Hakansson S, Friedman LS, Johansson U, Sellberg G, Brondum N, Sele V, Olsson H, King MC, Borg A (1996). Founding BRCA1 mutations in hereditary breast and ovarian cancer in southern Sweden. *Am J Hum Genet* 58: 441-450.

705. Johnson RL, Rothman AL, Xie J, Goodrich LV, Bare JW, Bonifas JM, Quinn AG, Myers RM, Cox DR, Epstein EH, Jr., Scott MP (1996). Human homolog of patched, a candidate gene for the basal cell nevus syndrome. *Science* 272: 1668-1671.

706. Jones H, Steart PV, Weller RO (1991). Spindle-cell glioblastoma or gliosarcoma? *Neuropathol Appl Neurobiol* 17: 177-187.

707. Joseph JT, Lisle DK, Jacoby LB, Paulus W, Barone R, Cohen ML, Roggendorf WH, Bruner JM, Gusella JF, Louis DN (1995). *NF2* gene analysis distinguishes hemangiopericytoma from meningioma. *Am J Pathol* 147: 1450-1455.

708. Joshi VV, Cantor AB, Altshuler G, Larkin EW, Neill JS, Shuster JJ, Holbrook CT, Hayes FA, Nitschke R, Duncan MH (1992). Age-linked prognostic categorization based on a new histologic grading system of neuroblastomas. A clinicopathologic study of 211 cases from the Pediatric Oncology Group. *Cancer* 69: 2197-2211.

709. Joshi VV, Cantor AB, Altshuler G, Larkin EW, Neill JS, Shuster JJ, Holbrook CT, Hayes FA, Castleberry RP (1992). Recommendations for modification of terminology of neuroblastic tumors and prognostic significance of Shimada classification. A clinicopathologic study of 213 cases from the Pediatric Oncology Group. *Cancer* 69: 2183-2196.

710. Joshi VV, Cantor AB, Brodeur GM, Look AT, Shuster JJ, Altshuler G, Larkin EW, Holbrook CT, Silverman JF, Norris HT, Hayes FA, Smith EI, Castleberry RP (1993). Correlation between morphologic and other prognostic markers of neuroblastoma. A study of histologic grade, DNA index, N-myc gene copy number, and lactic dehydrogenase in patients in the Pediatric Oncology Group. *Cancer* 71: 3173-3181.

711. Joshi VV, Chatten J, Sather HN, Shimada H (1991). Evaluation of the Shimada classification in advanced neuroblastoma with a special reference to the mitosis- karyorrhexis index: a report from the Childrens Cancer Study Group. *Mod Pathol* 4: 139-147.

712. Joshi VV, Kelly DR, Cantor AB, Smith EI, Brodeur GM, Look AT, Catrou P, Larkin EW, Silverman JF, Norris HT, Shuster JJ, Castleberry RP (1994). Prognostic significance (PS) of histopathologic features (HFs) of neuroblastomas (NBs) resected at second look surgery. A report from the Pediatric Oncology Group. *Pediatr Pathol Lab Med* 14: 540.

713. Joshi VV, Rao PV, Cantor AB, Altshuler G, Shuster JJ, Castleberry RP (1996). Modified histologic grading of neuroblastomas by replacement of mitotic rate with mitosis karyorrhexis index. A clinicopathologic study of 223 cases from the Pediatric Oncology Group. *Cancer* 77: 1582-1588.

714. Joshi VV, Silverman JF (1994). Pathology of neuroblastic tumors. *Semin Diagn Pathol* 11: 107-117.

715. Joshi VV, Silverman JF, Altshuler G, Cantor AB, Larkin EW, Neill JS, Norris HT, Shuster JJ, Holbrook CT, Hayes FA (1993). Systematization of primary histopathologic and fine-needle aspiration cytologic features and description of unusual histopathologic features of neuroblastic tumors: a report from the Pediatric Oncology Group. *Hum Pathol* 24: 493-504.

716. Joshi VV, Tsongalis GA (1997). Correlation between morphologic and non-morphologic prognostic markers in neuroblastoma. *Ann N Y Acad Sci* 824: 71-83.

717. Jouvet A, Fevre M, Besancon R, Derrington E, Saint P, Belin MF, Pialat J, Lapras C (1994). Structural and ultrastructural characteristics of human pineal gland, and pineal parenchymal tumors. *Acta Neuropathol (Berl)* 88: 334-348.

718. Jung JM, Bruner JM, Ruan S, Langford LA, Kyritsis AP, Kobayashi T, Levin VA, Zhang W (1995). Increased levels of p21WAF1/Cip1 in human brain tumors. *Oncogene* 11: 2021-2028.

719. Kadish S, Goodman M, Wang CC (1976). Olfactory neuroblastoma. A clinical analysis of 17 cases. *Cancer* 37: 1571-1576.

720. Kalimo H, Paljarvi L, Ekfors T, Pelliniemi LJ (1987). Pigmented primitive neuroectodermal tumor with multipotential differentiation in cerebellum (pigmented medullomyoblastoma). A case with light- and electron-microscopic, and immunohistochemical analysis. *Pediatr Neurosci* 13: 188-195.

721. Kallio M, Sankila R, Hakulinen T, Jaaskelainen J (1992). Factors affecting operative and excess long-term mortality in 935 patients with intracranial meningioma. *Neurosurgery* 31: 2-12.

722. Kalyan R, Olivero WC (1987). Ganglioglioma: a correlative clinicopathological and radiological study of ten surgically treated cases with follow-up. *Neurosurgery* 20: 428-433.

723. Kandt RS, Haines JL, Smith M, Northrup H, Gardner RJ, Short MP, Dumars K, Roach ES, Steingold S, Wall S (1992). Linkage of an important gene locus for tuberous sclerosis to a chromosome 16 marker for polycystic kidney disease. *Nat Genet* 2: 37-41.

724. Kanno H, Kondo K, Ito S, Yamamoto I, Fujii S, Torigoe S, Sakai N, Hosaka M, Shuin T, Yao M (1994). Somatic mutations of the von Hippel-Lindau tumor suppressor gene in sporadic central nervous system hemangioblastomas. *Cancer Res* 54: 4845-4847.

725. Kanzawa T, Takahashi H, Hayano M, Mori S, Shimbo Y, Kitazana T (1997). Melanotic cerebral astrocytoma - case report and literature review. *Acta Neuropathol* 93: 200-204.

726. Kapadia SB, Frisman DM, Hitchcock CL, Ellis GL, Popek EJ (1993). Melanotic neuroectodermal tumor of infancy. Clinicopathological, immunohistochemical, and flow cytometric study. *Am J Surg Pathol* 17: 566-573.

727. Kapadia SB, Popek EJ, Barnes L (1994). Pediatric otorhinolaryngic pathology: diagnosis of selected lesions. *Pathol Annu* 29 Pt 1: 159-209.

728. Karamitopoulou E, Perentes E, Diamantis I, Maraziotis T (1994). Ki-67 immunoreactivity in human central nervous system tumors: a study with MIB 1 monoclonal antibody on archival material. *Acta Neuropathol (Berl)* 87: 47-54.

729. Karch SB, Urich H (1972). Medulloepithelioma: definition of an entity. *J Neuropathol Exp Neurol* 31: 27-53.

730. Karlbom AE, James CD, Boethius J, Cavenee WK, Collins VP, Nordenskjöld M, Larsson C (1993). Loss of heterozygosity in malignant gliomas involves at least three distinct regions on chromosome 10. *Hum Genet* 92: 169-174.

731. Karnes PS, Tran TN, Cui MY, Raffel C, Gilles FH, Barranger JA, Ying KL (1992). Cytogenetic analysis of 39 pediatric central nervous system tumors. *Cancer Genet Cytogenet* 59: 12-19.

732. Karsdorp N, Elderson A, Wittebol P, Hene RJ, Vos J, Feldberg MA, van Gils AP, Jansen Sv, V, Vroom TM, Hoppener JW (1994). Von Hippel-Lindau disease: new strategies in early detection and treatment. *Am J Med* 97: 158-168.

733. Kaschten B, Flandroy P, Reznik M, Hainaut H, Stevenaert A (1995). Radiation-induced gliosarcoma. Case report and review of the literature. *J Neurosurg* 83: 154-162.

734. Kato H, Uchimura I, Morohoshi M, Fujisawa K, Kobayashi Y, Numano F, Goseki N, Endo M, Tamura A, Nagashima C (1996). Multiple endocrine neoplasia type 1 associated with spinal ependymoma. *Intern Med* 35: 285-289.

735. Kato S, Hirano A, Kato M, Herz F, Ohama E (1993). Comparative study on the expression of stress-response protein (srp) 72, srp 27, alpha B-crystallin and ubiquitin in brain tumours. An immunohistochemical investigation. *Neuropathol Appl Neurobiol* 19: 436-442.

736. Katsetos CD, Burger PC (1994). Medulloblastoma. *Semin Diagn Pathol* 11: 85-97.

737. Katsetos CD, Frankfurter A, Christakos S, Mancall EL, Vlachos IN, Urich H (1993). Differential localization of class III, beta-tubulin isotype and calbindin-D28k defines distinct neuronal types in the developing human cerebellar cortex. *J Neuropathol Exp Neurol* 52: 655-666.

738. Katsetos CD, Herman MM, Frankfurter A, Gass P, Collins VP, Walker CC, Rosemberg S, Barnard RO, Rubinstein LJ (1989). Cerebellar desmoplastic medulloblastomas. A further immunohistochemical characterization of the reticulin-free pale islands. *Arch Pathol Lab Med* 113: 1019-1029.

739. Katsetos CD, Herman MM, Krishna L, Vender JR, Vinores SA, Agamanolis DP, Schiffer D, Burger PC, Urich H (1995). Calbindin-D28k in subsets of medulloblastomas and in the human medulloblastoma cell line D283 Med. *Arch Pathol Lab Med* 119: 734-743.

740. Katsetos CD, Krishna L, Friedberg E, Reidy J, Karkavelas G, Savory J (1994). Lobar pilocytic astrocytomas of the cerebral hemispheres: II. Pathobiology- Morphogenesis of the eosinophilic granular bodies. *Clin Neuropathol* 13: 306-314.

741. Katsetos CD, Krishna L (1994). Lobar pilocytic astrocytomas of the cerebral hemispheres: I. Diagnosis and nosology. *Clin Neuropathol* 13: 295-305.

742. Katsetos CD, Liu HM, Zacks SI (1988). Immunohistochemical and ultrastructural observations on Homer Wright (neuroblastic) rosettes and the "pale islands" of human cerebellar medulloblastomas. *Hum Pathol* 19: 1219-1227.

743. Kaufmann T, Nisce LZ, Coleman M (1996). A comparison of survival of patients treated for AIDS-related central nervous system lymphoma with and without tissue diagnosis. *Int J Radiat Oncol Biol Phys* 36: 429-432.

744. Kawano H, Hayashi M, Sato K, Hosotani K, Kubota T, Hirano A (1989). [Histological study of malignant cerebral granular cell tumor]. *No To Shinkei* 41: 955-960.

745. Kawano N, Yada K, Aihara M, Yagishita S (1983). Oligodendroglioma-like cells (clear cells) in ependymoma. *Acta Neuropathol (Berl)* 62: 141-144.

746. Keles GE, Berger MS, Schofield D, Bothwell M (1993). Nerve growth factor receptor expression in medulloblastomas and the potential role of nerve growth factor as a differentiating agent in medulloblastoma cell lines. *Neurosurgery* 32: 274-280.

747. Kelly DR,Joshi VV (1996). Neuroblastoma and Related Tumors. In: *Pediatric Neoplasia: Morphology and Biology*, Parham DM (eds). Lippincott-Review Publishers: Philadelphia. pp. 105-152.

748. Kennedy PG, Watkins BA, Thomas DG, Noble MD (1987). Antigenic expression by cells derived from human gliomas does not correlate with morphological classification. *Neuropathol Appl Neurobiol* 13: 327-347.

749. Kepes JJ (1971). Differential diagnosis problems of brain tumors. In: *Pathology of the Nervous System*, Minckler J (eds). McGraw-Hill: New York. pp. 2219-2237.

750. Kepes JJ (1978). Transitional cell tumor of the pituitary gland developing from a Rathke's cleft cyst. *Cancer* 41: 337-343.

751. Kepes JJ (1979). 'Xanthomatous' lesions of the central nervous system: definition, classification and some recent observations. *Prog Neuropathol* 4: 179-213.

752. Kepes JJ (1987). Astrocytomas: old and newly recognized variants, their spectrum of morphology and antigen expression. *Can J Neurol Sci* 14: 109-121.

753. Kepes JJ (1993). Pleomorphic xanthoastrocytoma: the birth of a diagnosis and a concept. *Brain Pathol* 3: 269-274.

754. Kepes JJ, Belton K, Roessmann U, Ketcherside WJ (1985). Primitive neuroectodermal tumors of the cauda equina in adults with no detectable primary intracranial neoplasm—three case studies. *Clin Neuropathol* 4: 1-11.

755. Kepes JJ, Chen WY, Connors MH, Vogel FS (1988). "Chordoid" meningeal tumors in young individuals with peritumoral lymphoplasmacellular infiltrates causing systemic manifestations of the Castleman syndrome. A report of seven cases. *Cancer* 62: 391-406.

756. Kepes JJ, Fulling KH, Garcia JH (1982). The clinical significance of "adenoid" formations of neoplastic astrocytes, imitating metastatic carcinoma, in gliosarcomas. A review of five cases. *Clin Neuropathol* 1: 139-150.

757. Kepes JJ, Kepes M, Slowik F (1973). Fibrous xanthomas and xanthosarcomas of the meninges and the brain. *Acta Neuropathol (Berl)* 23: 187-199.

758. Kepes JJ, Rubinstein LJ (1981). Malignant gliomas with heavily lipidized (foamy) tumor cells: a report of three cases with immunoperoxidase study. *Cancer* 47: 2451-2459.

759. Kepes JJ, Rubinstein LJ, Ansbacher L, Schreiber DJ (1989). Histopathological features of recurrent pleomorphic xanthoastrocytomas: further corroboration of the glial nature of this neoplasm. A study of three cases. *Acta Neuropathol* 78: 585-593.

760. Kepes JJ, Rubinstein LJ, Chiang H (1984). The role of astrocytes in the formation of cartilage in gliomas. An immunohistochemical study of four cases. *Am J Pathol* 117: 471-483.

761. Kepes JJ, Rubinstein LJ, Eng LF (1979). Pleomorphic xanthoastrocytoma: a distinctive meningocerebral glioma of young subjects with relatively favorable prognosis; a study of 12 cases. *Cancer* 44: 1839-1852.

762. Kerfoot C, Wienecke R, Menchine M, Emelin J, Maize JCJ, Welsh CT, Norman MG, DeClue JE, Vinters HV (1996). Localization of tuberous sclerosis 2 mRNA and its protein product tuberin in normal human brain and in cerebral lesions of patients with tuberous sclerosis. *Brain Pathol* 6: 367-377.

763. Kernohan JW, Mabon RF, Svien HJ, Adson AW (1949). A simplified classification of gliomas. *Proc Staff Meet Mayo Clin* 24: 71-75.

764. Khatib Z, Heidemann R, Kovnar E (1992). Pilocytic dorsally exophytic brainstem gliomas: a distinct clinicopathological entity. *Ann Neurol* 32: 458-459.

765. Khoddami M, Becker LE (1997). Immunohistochemistry of medulloepithelioma and neural tube. *J Ped Pathol Lab Med* 17: 913-925.

766. Kibel A, Iliopoulos O, DeCaprio JA, Kaelin WG, Jr. (1995). Binding of the von Hippel-Lindau tumor suppressor protein to Elongin B and C. *Science* 269: 1444-1446.

767. Kida S, Ellison DW, Steart PV, Weller RO (1995). Characterisation of perivascular cells in astrocytic tumours and peritumoral oedematous brain. *Neuropathol Appl Neurobiol* 21: 121-129.

768. Kikuchi T, Rempel SA, Rutz HP, de Tribolet N, Mulligan L, Cavenee WK, Jothy S, Leduy L, Van Meir EG (1993). Turcot's syndrome of glioma and polyposis occurs in the absence of germ line mutations of exons 5 to 9 of the p53 gene. *Cancer Res* 53: 957-961.

769. Kim DG, Kim JS, Chi JG, Park SH, Jung HW, Choi KS, Han DH (1996). Central neurocytoma: proliferative potential and biological behavior. *J Neurosurg* 84: 742-747.

770. Kim KJ, Li B, Winer J, Armanini M, Gillett N, Phillips HS, Ferrara N (1993). Inhibition of vascular endothelial growth factor-induced angiogenesis suppresses tumour growth in vivo. *Nature* 362: 841-844.

771. Kim L, Hochberg FH, Thornton AF, Harsh GR, Patel H, Finkelstein D, Louis DN (1996). Procarbazine, lomustine, and vincristine (PCV) chemotherapy for grade III and grade IV oligoastrocytomas. *J Neurosurg* 85: 602-607.

772. Kim TS, Halliday AL, Hedley W, Convery K (1991). Correlates of survival and the Daumas-Duport grading system for astrocytomas. *J Neurosurg* 74: 27-37.

773. Kimura M, Takayasu M, Suzuki Y, Negoro M, Nagasaka T, Nakashima N, Sugita K (1992). Primary choroid plexus papilloma located in the suprasellar region: case report. *Neurosurgery* 31: 563-566.

774. Kimura T, Budka H, Soler F (1986). An immunocytochemical comparison of the glia-associated proteins glial fibrillary acidic protein (GFAP) and S-100 protein (S100P) in human brain tumors. *Clin Neuropathol* 5: 21-27.

775. Kindblom LG, Ahlden M, Meis K, Stenman G (1995). Immunohistochemical and molecular analysis of p53, MDM2, proliferating cell nuclear antigen and Ki67 in benign and malignant peripheral nerve sheath tumours. *Virchows Arch* 427: 19-26.

776. Kirkpatrick PJ, Honavar M, Janota I, Polkey CE (1993). Control of temporal lobe epilepsy following en bloc resection of low-grade tumors. *J Neurosurg* 78: 19-25.

777. Kirschstein RL, Gerber P (1962). Ependymomas produced after intracerebral inoculation of SV40 into newborn hamsters. *Nature* 195: 299-300.

778. Kitanaka C, Shitara N, Nakagomi T, Nakamura H, Genka S, Nakagawa K, Akanuma A, Aoyama H, Takakura K (1989). Postradiation astrocytoma. Report of two cases. *J Neurosurg* 70: 469-474.

779. Kleihues P, Burger PC, Scheithauer BW (1993). *Histological Typing of Tumours of the Central Nervous System. World Health Organization International Histological Classification of Tumours.* 2nd ed, Springer Verlag: Berlin Heidelberg.

780. Kleihues P, Burger PC, Scheithauer BW (1993). The new WHO classification of brain tumours. *Brain Pathol* 3: 255-268.

781. Kleihues P, Kiessling M, Janzer RC (1987). Morphological markers in neuro-oncology. *Curr Top Pathol* 77: 307-338.

782. Kleihues P, Ohgaki H, Aguzzi A (1995). Gliomas. In: *Neuroglia*, Kettenmann H, Ransom BR (eds). Oxford University Press: Oxford. pp. 1044-1063.

783. Kleihues P, Ohgaki H (1997). Genetics of glioma progression and the definition of primary and secondary glioblastoma. *Brain Pathol* 7: 1131-1136.

784. Kleihues P, zur Hausen A, Schauble B, Ohgaki H (1997). Tumours associated with p53 germline mutations. A synopsis of 91 families. *Am J Pathol* 150: 1-13.

785. Klein R, Jing SQ, Nanduri V, O'Rourke E, Barbacid M (1991). The trk proto-oncogene encodes a receptor for nerve growth factor. *Cell* 65: 189-197.

786. Kleinschmidt D, Lillehei KO (1995). Radiation-induced meningioma with a 63-year latency period. Case report. *J Neurosurg* 82: 487-488.

787. Kliewer KE, Cochran AJ (1989). A review of the histology, ultrastructure, immunohistology, and molecular biology of extra-adrenal paragangliomas. *Arch Pathol Lab Med* 113: 1209-1218.

788. Kliewer KE, Wen DR, Cancilla PA, Cochran AJ (1989). Paragangliomas: assessment of prognosis by histologic, immunohistochemical, and ultrastructural techniques. *Hum Pathol* 20: 29-39.

789. Ko LJ, Prives C (1996). p53: puzzle and paradigm. *Genes Dev* 10: 1054-1072.

790. Kobayashi T, Yoshida J, Kida Y (1989). Bilateral germ cell tumors involving the basal ganglia and thalamus. *Neurosurgery* 24: 579-583.

791. Kochi N, Budka H (1987). Contribution of histiocytic cells to sarcomatous development of the gliosarcoma. An immunohistochemical study. *Acta Neuropathol (Berl)* 73: 124-130.

792. Koeller KK, Dillon WP (1992). Dysembryoplastic neuroepithelial tumors: MR appearance. *AJNR Am J Neuroradiol* 13: 1319-1325.

793. Koga H, Zhang S, Ichikawa T, Washiyama K, Kuroiwa T, Tanaka R, Kumanishi T (1994). Primary malignant lymphoma of the brain: demonstration of the p53 gene mutations by PCR-SSCP analysis and immunohistochemistry. *Noshuyo Byori* 11: 151-155.

794. Kogner P, Barbany G, Dominici C, Castello MA, Raschella G, Persson H (1993). Coexpression of messenger RNA for TRK protooncogene and low affinity nerve growth factor receptor in neuroblastoma with favorable prognosis. *Cancer Res* 53: 2044-2050.

795. Kolles H, Niedermayer I, Schmitt C, Henn W, Feld R, Steudel WI, Zang KD, Feiden W (1995). Triple approach for diagnosis and grading of meningiomas: histology, morphometry of Ki-67/Feulgen stainings, and cytogenetics. *Acta Neurochir Wien* 137: 174-181.

796. Kondziolka D, Bilbao JM (1988). Mixed ependymoma-astrocytoma (subependymoma?) of the cerebral cortex. *Acta Neuropathol (Berl)* 76: 633-637.

797. Koopmann J, Maintz D, Schild S, Schramm J, Louis DN, Wiestler OD, von Deimling A (1995). Multiple polymorphisms, but no mutations, in the WAF1/CIP1 gene in human brain tumours. *Br J Cancer* 72: 1230-1233.

798. Kordek R, Biernat W, Sapieja W, Alwasiak J, Liberski P (1995). Pleomorphic xanthoastrocytoma with a gangliomatous component, an immunohistochemical and ultrastructural study. *Acta Neuropathol* 89: 194-197.

799. Kordek R, Klimek A, Karpinska A, Alwasiak J, Debiec R, Liberski P (1996). The immunohistochemistry and ultrastructure of ganglioglioma with chromosomal alterations: a case report. *Pol J Pathol* 47: 37-39.

800. Korf BR, Prasad C, Schneider G, Anthony D (1996). A family with multiple neurofibromas and non-linkage to NF1 and NF2. *FASEB Summer Research Conference On Neurofibromatosis, Snowmass, Co, USA*

801. Korf HW, Schachenmayr W, Chader GJ, Wiggert B (1992). Immunocytochemical demonstration of interphotoreceptor retinoid-binding protein in cerebellar medulloblastomas. *Acta Neuropathol (Berl)* 83: 482-487.

802. Kovalic JJ, Flaris N, Grigsby PW, Pirkowski M, Simpson JR, Roth KA (1993). Intracranial ependymoma long term outcome, patterns of failure. *J Neurooncol* 15: 125-131.

803. Kozmik Z, Sure U, Ruedi D, Busslinger M, Aguzzi A (1995). Deregulated expression of *PAX5* in medulloblastoma. *Proc Natl Acad Sci USA* 92: 5709-5713.

804. Kraichoke S, Cosgrove M, Chandrasoma PT (1988). Granulomatous inflammation in pineal germinoma. A cause of diagnostic failure at stereotaxic brain biopsy. *Am J Surg Pathol* 12: 655-660.

805. Kramer S, Ward E, Meadows AT, Malone KE (1987). Medical and drug risk factors associated with neuroblastoma: a case-control study. *J Natl Cancer Inst* 78: 797-804.

806. Krammer PH, Behrmann I, Daniel P, Dhein J, Debatin KM (1994). Regulation of apoptosis in the immune system. *Curr Opin Immunol* 6: 279-289.

807. Kraus JA, Bolln C, Wolf HK, Neumann J, Kindermann D, Fimmers R, Forster F, Baumann A, Schlegel U (1994). TP53 alterations and clinical outcome in low grade astrocytomas. *Genes Chromosomes Cancer* 10: 143-149.

808. Kraus JA, Koopmann J, Kaskel P, Maintz D, Brandner S, Schramm J, Louis DN, Wiestler OD, von Deimling A (1995). Shared allelic losses on chromosomes 1p and 19q suggest a common origin of oligodendroglioma and oligoastrocytoma. *J Neuropathol Exp Neurol* 54: 91-95.

809. Kreth FW, Warnke PC, Scheremet R, Ostertag CB (1993). Surgical resection and radiation therapy versus biopsy and radiation therapy in the treatment of glioblastoma multiforme. *J Neurosurg* 78: 762-766.

810. Kricheff II, Becker M, Schenk SA, Taveras JM (1964). Intracranial ependymomas; factors influencing prognosis. *J Neurosurg* 21: 7-14.

811. Krieg P, Amtmann E, Jonas D, Fischer H, Zang K, Sauer G (1981). Episomal simian virus 40 genomes in human brain tumors. *Proc Natl Acad Sci USA* 78: 6446-6450.

812. Krieg P, Scherer G (1984). Cloning of SV40 genomes from human brain tumors. *Virology* 138: 336-340.

813. Kriho VK, Zang H, Moskal JR, Skalli O (1997). Keratin expression in astrocytomas: an immunofluorescent and biochemical reassessment. *Virchows Arch* 431: 139-147.

814. Kristof RA, Van Roost D, Wolf HK, Schramm J (1997). Intravascular papillary endothelial hyperplasia of the sellar region. Report of three cases and review of the literature. *J Neurosurg* 86: 558-563.

815. Kroemer G, Zamzani N, Susin SA (1997). Mitochondrial control of apoptosis. *Immunol Today* 18: 44-51.

816. Kros JM, Stefanko SZ, de Jong AA, van Vroonhoven CC, van der Heul RO, van der

Kwast TH (1991). Ultrastructural and immunohistochemical segregation of gemistocytic subsets. *Hum Pathol* 22: 33-40.

817. Kros JM, Godschalk JJ, Krishnadath KK, Van Eden CG (1993). Expression of p53 in oligodendrogliomas. *J Pathol* 171: 285-290.

818. Kros JM, Hop WC, Godschalk JJ, Krishnadath KK (1996). Prognostic value of the proliferation-related antigen Ki-67 in oligodendrogliomas. *Cancer* 78: 1107-1113.

819. Kros JM, Lie ST, Stefanko SZ (1994). Familial occurrence of polymorphous oligodendroglioma. *Neurosurgery* 34: 732-736.

820. Kros JM, Pieterman H, Van Eden CG, Avezaat CJ (1994). Oligodendroglioma: the Rotterdam-Dijkzigt experience. *Neurosurgery* 34: 959-966.

821. Kros JM, Troost D, Van Eden CG, van der Werf AJ, Uylings HB (1988). Oligodendroglioma. A comparison of two grading systems. *Cancer* 61: 2251-2259.

822. Kros JM, van den Brink WA, van Loon-van Luyt JJM, Stefanko SZ (1997). Signet-ring cell oligodendroglioma - report of two cases and discussion of the differential diagnosis. *Acta Neuropathol* 93: 638-643.

823. Kros JM, Van Eden CG, Stefanko SZ, Waayer-Van Batenburg M, van der Kwast TH (1990). Prognostic implications of glial fibrillary acidic protein containing cell types in oligodendrogliomas. *Cancer* 66: 1204-1212.

824. Kros JM, Van Eden CG, Vissers CJ, Mulder AH, van der Kwast TH (1992). Prognostic relevance of DNA flow cytometry in oligodendroglioma. *Cancer* 69: 1791-1798.

825. Kros JM, Vecht CJ, Stefanko SZ (1991). The pleomorphic xanthoastrocytoma and its differential diagnosis: a study of five cases. *Hum Pathol* 22: 1128-1135.

826. Krouwer HG, Davis RL, Silver P, Prados M (1991). Gemistocytic astrocytomas: a reappraisal. *J Neurosurg* 74: 399-406.

827. Kubbutat MHG, Jones SN, Vousden KH (1997). Regulation of p53 stability by Mdm2. *Nature* 387: 289-303.

828. Kubo O, Sasahara A, Tajika Y, Kawamura H, Kawabatake H, Takakura K (1996). Pleomorphic xanthoastrocytoma with neurofibromatosis type 1: case report. *Noshuyo Byori* 13: 79-83.

829. Kubota T, Hayashi M, Kawano H, Kabuto M, Sato K, Ishise J, Kawamoto K, Shirataki K, Iizuka H, Tsunoda S (1991). Central neurocytoma: immunohistochemical and ultrastructural study. *Acta Neuropathol (Berl)* 81: 418-427.

830. Kuchelmeister K, Demirel T, Schlorer E, Bergmann M, Gullotta F (1995). Dysembryoplastic neuroepithelial tumour of the cerebellum. *Acta Neuropathol (Berl)* 89: 385-390.

831. Kuchelmeister K, von Borcke IM, Klein H, Bergmann M, Gullotta F (1994). Pleomorphic pineocytoma with extensive neuronal differentiation: report of two cases. *Acta Neuropathol (Berl)* 88: 448-453.

832. Kudo H, Oi S, Tamaki N, Nishida Y, Matsumoto S (1990). Ependymoma diagnosed in the first year of life in Japan in collaboration with the International Society for Pediatric Neurosurgery. *Childs Nerv Syst* 6: 375-378.

833. Kudo M, Matsumoto M, Terao H (1983). Malignant nerve sheath tumor of acoustic nerve. *Arch Pathol Lab Med* 107: 293-297.

834. Kuijten RR, Strom SS, Rorke LB, Boesel CP, Buckley JD, Meadows AT, Bunin GR (1993). Family history of cancer and seizures in young children with brain tumors: a report from the Childrens Cancer Group (United States and Canada). *Cancer Causes Control* 4: 455-464.

835. Kultursay N, Gelal F, Mutluer S, Senrecper S, Oziz E, Oral R (1995). Antenatally diagnosed neonatal craniopharyngioma. *J Perinatol* 15: 426-428.

836. Kumanishi T, Washiyama K, Nishiyama A, Abe S, Saito T, Ichikawa T (1989). Primary malignant lymphoma of the brain: demonstration of immunoglobulin gene rearrangements in four cases by the Southern blot hybridization technique. *Acta Neuropathol (Berl)* 79: 23-26.

837. Kumanishi T, Zhang S, Ichikawa T, Endo S, Washiyama K (1996). Primary malignant lymphoma of the brain: demonstration of frequent p16 and p15 gene deletions. *Jpn J Cancer Res* 87: 691-695.

838. Kuppner MC, Hamou MF, de Tribolet N (1990). Activation and adhesion molecule expression on lymphoid infiltrates in human glioblastomas. *J Neuroimmunol* 29: 229-238.

839. Kuppner MC, Van Meir E, Gauthier T, Hamou MF, de Tribolet N (1992). Differential expression of the CD44 molecule in human brain tumours. *Int J Cancer* 50: 572-577.

840. Kuroiwa T, Bergey GK, Rothman MI, Zoarski GH, Wolf A, Zagardo MT, Kristt DA, Hudson LP, Krumholz A, Barry E (1995). Radiologic appearance of the dysembryoplastic neuroepithelial tumor. *Radiology* 197: 233-238.

841. Kurt E, Beute GN, Sluzewski M, van Rooij WJ, Teepen JL (1996). Giant chondroma of the falx. Case report and review of the literature. *J Neurosurg* 85: 1161-1164.

842. Kusaka H, Hirano A, Bornstein MB, Raine CS (1985). Basal lamina formation by astrocytes in organotypic cultures of mouse spinal cord tissue. *J Neuropathol Exp Neurol* 44: 295-303.

843. Kushner BH, Gilbert F, Helson L (1986). Familial neuroblastoma. Case reports, literature review, and etiologic considerations. *Cancer* 57: 1887-1893.

844. Kyritsis AP, Bondy ML, Xiao M, Berman EL, Cunningham JE, Lee PS, Levin VA, Saya H (1994). Germline p53 gene mutations in subsets of glioma patients. *J Natl Cancer Inst* 86: 344-349.

845. Kyritsis AP, Yung WK, Bruner J, Gleason MJ, Levin VA (1993). The treatment of anaplastic oligodendrogliomas and mixed gliomas. *Neurosurg* 32: 365-370.

846. Lach B, Duggal N, DaSilva VF, Benoit BG (1996). Association of pleomorphic xanthoastrocytoma with cortical dysplasia and neuronal tumors. A report of three cases. *Cancer* 78: 2551-2563.

847. Lach B, Duncan E, Rippstein P, Benoit BG (1994). Primary intracranial pleomorphic angioleiomyoma—a new morphologic variant. An immunohistochemical and electron microscopic study. *Cancer* 74: 1915-1920.

848. Lach B, Sikorska M, Rippstein P, Gregor A, Staines W, Davie TR (1991). Immunoelectron microscopy of Rosenthal fibers. *Acta Neuropathol (Berl)* 81: 503-509.

849. Lack EE (1994). Paragangliomas. In: *Diagnostic Surgical Pathology*, Sternberg SS (eds), 2nd ed. Raven Press: New York. pp. 559-621.

850. Lack EE, Cubilla AL, Woodruff JM (1979). Paragangliomas of the head and neck region. A pathologic study of tumors from 71 patients. *Hum Pathol* 10: 191-218.

851. Lacombe D, Chateil JF, Fontan D, Battin J (1990). Medulloblastoma in the nevoid basal-cell carcinoma syndrome: case reports and review of the literature. *Genet Couns* 1: 273-277.

852. Lampl Y, Eshel Y, Gilad R, Sarova-Pinchas I (1990). Glioblastoma multiforme with bone metastase and cauda equina syndrome. *J Neurooncol* 8: 167-172.

853. Lane DP (1992). Cancer. p53, guardian of the genome. *Nature* 358: 15-16.

854. Lang FF, Epstein FJ, Ransohoff J, Allen JC, Wisoff J, Abbott IR, Miller DC (1993). Central nervous system gangliogliomas. Part 2: Clinical outcome. *J Neurosurg* 79: 867-873.

855. Lang FF, Miller DC, Koslow M, Newcomb EW (1994). Pathways leading to glioblastoma multiforme: a molecular analysis of genetic alterations in 65 astrocytic tumors. *J Neurosurg* 81: 427-436.

856. Lang FF, Miller DC, Pisharody S, Koslow M, Newcomb EW (1994). High frequency of p53 protein accumulation without p53 gene mutation in human juvenile pilocytic, low grade and anaplastic astrocytomas. *Oncogene* 9: 949-954.

857. Langford LA (1986). The ultrastructure of the ependymoblastoma. *Acta Neuropathol (Berl)* 71: 136-141.

858. Langford LA, Camel MH (1987). Palisading pattern in cerebral neuroblastoma mimicking the primitive polar spongioblastoma. An ultrastructural study. *Acta Neuropathol (Berl)* 73: 153-159.

859. Lantos PL, VandenBerg SR, Kleihues P (1996). Tumours of the Nervous System. In: *Greenfield's Neuropathology*, Graham DI, Lantos PL (eds), 6th ed. Arnold: London. pp. 583-879.

860. Larson JJ, Tew JM, Jr., Simon M, Menon AG (1995). Evidence for clonal spread in the development of multiple meningiomas. *J Neurosurg* 83: 705-709.

861. Laskin WB, Weiss SW, Bratthauer GL (1991). Epithelioid variant of malignant peripheral nerve sheath tumor (malignant epithelioid schwannoma). *Am J Surg Pathol* 15: 1136-1145.

862. Lasser DM, DeVivo DC, Garvin J, Wilhelmsen KC (1994). Turcot's syndrome: evidence for linkage to the adenomatous polyposis coli (APC) locus. *Neurology* 44: 1083-1086.

863. Latif F, Tory K, Gnarra J, Yao M, Duh FM, Orcutt ML, Stackhouse T, Kuzmin I, Modi W, Geil L (1993). Identification of the von Hippel-Lindau disease tumor suppressor gene. *Science* 260: 1317-1320.

864. Lauer DH, Enzinger FM (1980). Cranial fasciitis of childhood. *Cancer* 45: 401-406.

865. Laureys G, Speleman F, Opdenakker G, Benoit Y, Leroy J (1990). Constitutional translocation t(1;17)(p36;q12-21) in a patient with neuroblastoma. *Genes Chromosomes Cancer* 2: 252-254.

866. Lednicky JA, Garcea RL, Bergsagel DJ, Butel JS (1995). Natural simian virus 40 strains are present in human choroid plexus and ependymoma tumors. *Virology* 212: 710-717.

867. Lee JH, Sundaram V, Stein J, Kinney SE, Stacey DW, Golubic M (1997). Reduced expression of schwannomin/merlin in human sporadic meningiomas. *Neurosurgery* 40: 578-587.

868. Lee YY, Van Tassel P (1989). Intracranial oligodendrogliomas: imaging findings in 35 untreated cases. *AJR Am J Roentgenol* 152: 361-369.

869. Lee YY, Van Tassel P, Bruner JM, Moser RP, Share JC (1989). Juvenile pilocytic astrocytomas: CT and MR characteristics. *AJR Am J Roentgenol* 152: 1263-1270.

870. Leestma JE, Earle KM (1973). Neoplasms of the central nervous system in infants 2 years of age and under. Analysis of 163 cases. *J Neuropathol Exp Neurol* 32;155-156.

871. Legius E, Dierick H, Wu R, Hall BK, Marynen P, Cassiman JJ, Glover TW (1994). TP53 mutations are frequent in malignant NF1 tumors. *Genes Chromosomes Cancer* 10: 250-255.

872. Legius E, Marchuk DA, Collins FS, Glover TW (1993). Somatic deletion of the neurofibromatosis type 1 gene in a neurofibrosarcoma supports a tumour suppressor gene hypothesis. *Nat Genet* 3: 122-126.

873. Leibel SA, Scott CB, Loeffler JS (1994). Contemporary approaches to the treatment of malignant gliomas with radiation therapy. *Semin Oncol* 21: 198-219.

874. Leisti EL, Pyhtinen J, Poyhonen M (1996). Spontaneous decrease of a pilocytic astrocytoma in neurofibromatosis type I. *AJNR Am J Neuroradiol* 17: 363-370.

875. Lekanne D, Bianchi AB, Groen NA, Seizinger BR, Hagemeijer A, van Drunen E, Bootsma D, Koper JW, Avezaat CJ, Kley N (1994). Frequent NF2 gene transcript mutations in sporadic meningiomas and vestibular schwannomas. *Am J Hum Genet* 54: 1022-1029.

876. Lekanne D, Riegman PH, Groen NA, Warringa UL, van Biezen NA, Molijn AC, Bootsma D, de Jong PJ, Menon AG, Kley NA (1995). Cloning and characterization of MN1, a gene from chromosome 22q11, which is disrupted by a balanced translocation in a meningioma. *Oncogene* 10: 1521-1528.

877. Lellouch T, Bourgeois M, Vekemans M, Robain O (1995). Dysembryoplastic neuroepithelial tumors in two children with neurofibromatosis type 1. *Acta Neuropathol (Berl)* 90: 319-322.

878. Lennert K, Feller AC (1992). *Histopathology of Non-Hodgkin's Lymphomas (Based on the Updated Kiel Classification)*. 2nd ed, Springer: Berlin.

879. Leone A, Seeger RC, Hong CM, Hu YY, Arboleda MJ, Brodeur GM, Stram D, Slamon DJ, Steeg PS (1993). Evidence for nm23 RNA overexpression, DNA amplification and mutation in aggressive childhood neuroblastomas. *Oncogene* 8: 855-865.

880. Lerman RI, Kaplan ES, Daman L (1972). Ganglioneuroma-paraganglioma of the intradural filum terminale. Case report. *J Neurosurg* 36: 652-658.

881. Lesser GJ, Grossman S (1994). The chemotherapy of high-grade astrocytomas. *Semin Oncol* 21: 220-223.

882. Leung SY, Gwi E, Ng HK, Fung CF, Yam KY (1994). Dysembryoplastic neuroepithelial tumor. A tumor with small neuronal cells resembling oligodendroglioma. *Am J Surg Pathol* 18: 604-614.

883. Levine A (1997). p53: the cellular

gatekeeper for growth and division. *Cell* 89: 323-331.

884. Levy AP, Levy NS, Goldberg MA (1996). Hypoxia-inducible protein binding to vascular endothelial growth factor mRNA and its modulation by the von Hippel-Lindau protein. *J Biol Chem* 271: 25492-25497.

885. Lewis JH, Ginsberg AL, Toomey KE (1983). Turcot's syndrome. Evidence for autosomal dominant inheritance. *Cancer* 51: 524-528.

886. Lewis JJ, Brennan MF (1996). Soft tissue sarcomas. *Curr Probl Surg* 33: 817-872.

887. Lewis RA, Gerson LP, Axelson KA, Riccardi VM, Whitford RP (1984). von Recklinghausen neurofibromatosis. II. Incidence of optic gliomata. *Ophthalmology* 91: 929-935.

888. Lhermitte J, Duclos P (1920). Sur un ganglioneurome diffus du coertex du cervelet. *Bull Assoc Fran Etude Cancer* 9: 99-107.

889. Li FP, Fraumeni JF, Jr. (1969). Soft-tissue sarcomas, breast cancer, and other neoplasms. A familial syndrome? *Ann Intern Med* 71: 747-752.

890. Li FP, Fraumeni JF, Jr., Mulvihill JJ, Blattner WA, Dreyfus MG, Tucker MA, Miller RW (1988). A cancer family syndrome in twenty-four kindreds. *Cancer Res* 48: 5358-5362.

891. Li FP, Little JB, Bech H, Paterson MC, Arlett C, Garnick MB, Mayer RJ (1983). Acute leukemia after radiotherapy in a patient with Turcot's syndrome. Impaired colony formation in skin fibroblast cultures after irradiation. *Am J Med* 74: 343-348.

892. Li H, Hamou MF, de Tribolet N, Jaufeerally R, Hofmann M, Diserens AC, Van Meir EG (1993). Variant CD44 adhesion molecules are expressed in human brain metastases but not in glioblastomas. *Cancer Res* 53: 5345-5349.

893. Li J, Yen C, Liaw D, Podsypanina K, Bose S, Wang SI, Puc J, Miliaresis C, Rodgers L, McCombie R, Bigner SH, Giovanella BC, Ittmann M, Tycko B, Hibshoosh H, Wigler MH, Parsons R (1997). *PTEN*, a putative protein tyrosine phosphatase gene mutated in human brain, breast, and prostate cancer. *Science* 275: 1943-1947.

894. Li YS, Ramsay DA, Fan YS, Armstrong RF, Del Maestro RF (1995). Cytogenetic evidence that a tumor suppressor gene in the long arm of chromosome 1 contributes to glioma growth. *Cancer Genet Cytogenet* 84: 46-50.

895. Liaw D, Marsh DJ, Li J, Dahia PLM, Wang SI, Zheng Z, Bose S, Call KM, Tsou HC, Peacocke M, Eng C, Parsons R (1997). Germline mutations of the *PTEN* gene in Cowden disease, an inherited breast and thyroid cancer syndrome. *Nat Genet* 16: 64-67.

896. Libermann TA, Nusbaum HR, Razon N, Kris R, Lax I, Soreq H, Whittle N, Waterfield MD, Ullrich A, Schlessinger J (1985). Amplification, enhanced expression and possible rearrangement of EGF receptor gene in primary human brain tumours of glial origin. *Nature* 313: 144-147.

897. Lin SL, Wang JS, Huang CS, Tseng HH (1996). Primary intracerebral leiomyoma: a case with eosinophilic inclusions of actin filaments. *Histopathology* 28: 365-369.

898. Lindau A (1926). Studien uber Kleinhirncysten. Bau, Pathogenese und Beziehungen zur Angiomatosis Retinae. *Acta Pathol Microbiol Scand* Suppl 1.

899. Lindblom A, Ruttledge M, Collins VP, Nordenskjold M, Dumanski JP (1994). Chromosomal deletions in anaplastic meningiomas suggest multiple regions outside chromosome 22 as important in tumor progression. *Int J Cancer* 56: 354-357.

900. Lindboe C, Cappelen J, Kepes J (1992). Pleomorphic xanthoastrocytoma as a component of a cerebellar ganglioglioma: case report. *Neurosurgery* 31: 353-355.

901. Lipper S, Decker RE (1984). Paraganglioma of the cauda equina. A histologic, immunohistochemical, and ultrastructural study and review of the literature. *Surg Neurol* 22: 415-420.

902. Listernick R, Charrow J, Greenwald M, Mets M (1994). Natural history of optic pathway tumors in children with neurofibromatosis type 1: a longitudinal study. *J Pediatr* 125: 63-66.

903. Liszka U, Drlicek M, Hitzenberger P, Machacek E, Mayer H, Stockhammer G, Grisold W (1994). Intravascular lymphomatosis: a clinicopathological study of three cases. *J Cancer Res Clin Oncol* 120: 164-168.

904. Litofsky NS, Zee CS, Breeze RE, Chandrasoma PT (1992). Meningeal melanocytoma: diagnostic criteria for a rare lesion. *Neurosurgery* 31: 945-948.

905. Liu HM, Boogs J, Kidd J (1976). Ependymomas of childhood. I. Histological survey and clinicopathological correlation. *Childs Brain* 2: 92-110.

906. Lloyd KM, Dennis M (1963). Cowden's disease: a possible new symptom complex with multiple system involvement. *Ann Intern Med* 58: 136-142.

907. Lodding P, Kindblom LG, Angervall L (1986). Epithelioid malignant schwannoma. A study of 14 cases. *Virchows Arch A Pathol Anat Histopathol* 409: 433-451.

908. Lodding P, Kindblom LG, Angervall L, Stenman G (1990). Cellular schwannoma. A clinicopathologic study of 29 cases. *Virchows Arch A Pathol Anat Histopathol* 416: 237-248.

909. Look AT, Hayes FA, Nitschke R, McWilliams NB, Green AA (1984). Cellular DNA content as a predictor of response to chemotherapy in infants with unresectable neuroblastoma. *N Engl J Med* 311: 231-235.

910. Look AT, Hayes FA, Shuster JJ, Douglass EC, Castleberry RP, Bowman LC, Smith EI, Brodeur GM (1991). Clinical relevance of tumor cell ploidy and N-myc gene amplification in childhood neuroblastoma: a Pediatric Oncology Group study. *J Clin Oncol* 9: 581-591.

911. Lopes MB, Gonzalez F, Scheithauer BW, VandenBerg SR (1993). Differential expression of retinal proteins in a pineal parenchymal tumor. *J Neuropathol Exp Neurol* 52: 516-524.

912. Lorberboym M, Estok L, Machac J, Germano I, Sacher M, Feldman R, Wallach F, Dorfman D (1996). Rapid differential diagnosis of cerebral toxoplasmosis and primary central nervous system lymphoma by thallium-201 SPECT. *J Nucl Med* 37: 1150-1154.

913. Los M, Jansen GH, Kaelin WG, Lips CJ, Blijham GH, Voest EE (1996). Expression pattern of the von Hippel-Lindau protein in human tissues. *Lab Invest* 75: 231-238.

914. Lothe RA, Slettan A, Saeter G, Brogger A, Borresen AL, Nesland JM (1995). Alterations at chromosome 17 loci in peripheral nerve sheath tumors. *J Neuropathol Exp Neurol* 54: 65-73.

915. Louis DN (1994). The p53 gene and protein in human brain tumors. *J Neuropathol Exp Neurol* 53: 11-21.

916. Louis DN, Cavenee WK (1997). Molecular biology of central nervous system neoplasms. In: *Cancer: Principles and Practice of Oncology*, DeVita VT, Hellman S, Rosenberg SA (eds), 5th ed. Lippincott-Raven Publishers: Philadelphia. pp. 2013-2022.

917. Louis DN, Edgerton S, Thor AD, Hedley Whyte ET (1991). Proliferating cell nuclear antigen and Ki-67 immunohistochemistry in brain tumors: a comparative study. *Acta Neuropathol (Berl)* 81: 675-679.

918. Louis DN, Hamilton AJ, Sobel RA, Ojemann RG (1991). Pseudopsammomatous meningioma with elevated serum carcinoembryonic antigen: a true secretory meningioma. Case report. *J Neurosurg* 74: 129-132.

919. Louis DN, Ramesh V, Gusella JF (1995). Neuropathology and molecular genetics of neurofibromatosis 2 and related tumors. *Brain Pathol* 5: 163-172.

920. Louis DN, Rubio MP, Correa KM, Gusella JF, von Deimling A (1993). Molecular genetics of pediatric brain stem gliomas. Application of PCR techniques to small and archival brain tumor specimens. *J Neuropathol Exp Neurol* 52: 507-515.

921. Louis DN, Swearingen B, Linggood RM, Dickersin GR, Kretschmar C, Bhan AK, Hedley Whyte ET (1990). Central nervous system neurocytoma and neuroblastoma in adults— report of eight cases. *J Neurooncol* 9: 231-238.

922. Louis DN, von Deimling A (1995). Hereditary tumor syndromes of the nervous system: overview and rare syndromes. *Brain Pathol* 5: 145-151.

923. Louis DN, von Deimling A, Dickersin GR, Dooling EC, Seizinger BR (1992). Desmoplastic cerebral astrocytomas of infancy: a histopathologic, immunohistochemical, ultrastructural, and molecular genetic study. *Hum Pathol* 23: 1402-1409.

924. Lowe SW, Ruley HE, Jacks T, Housman DE (1993). p53-dependent apoptosis modulates the cytotoxicity of anticancer agents. *Cell* 74: 957-967.

925. Lubbe J, von Ammon K, Watanabe K, Hegi ME, Kleihues P (1995). Familial brain tumor syndrome associated with a *p53* germline deletion of codon 236. *Brain Pathol* 5: 15-23.

926. Ludwig CL, Smith MT, Godfrey AD, Armbrustmacher VW (1986). A clinicopathological study of 323 patients with oligodendrogliomas. *Ann Neurol* 19: 15-21.

927. Ludwin SK, Rubinstein LJ, Russell DS (1975). Papillary meningioma: a malignant variant of meningioma. *Cancer* 36: 1363-1373.

928. Lueder GT, Judisch GF, Wen BC (1991). Heritable retinoblastoma and pinealoma. *Arch Ophthalmol* 109: 1707-1709.

929. Lyons CJ, Wilson CB, Horton JC (1993). Association between meningioma and Cowden's disease. *Neurology* 43: 1436-1437.

930. Macaulay R, Jay V, Hoffman H, Becker L (1993). Increase mitotic activity as a negative prognostic indicator in pleomorphic xanthoastrocytoma. *J Neurosurg* 79: 761-768.

931. MacCollin M, Braverman N, Viskochil D, Ruttledge M, Davis K, Ojemann R, Gusella J, Parry DM (1996). A point mutation associated with a severe phenotype of neurofibromatosis 2. *Ann Neurol* 40: 440-445.

932. MacCollin M, Ramesh V, Jacoby LB, Louis DN, Rubio MP, Pulaski K, Trofatter JA, Short MP, Bove C, Eldridge R, Parry D, Gusella JF (1994). Mutational analysis of patients with neurofibromatosis 2. *Am J Hum Genet* 55: 314-320.

933. MacCollin M, Woodfin W, Kronn D, Short MP (1996). Schwannomatosis: a clinical and pathologic study. *Neurology* 46: 1072-1079.

934. Macdonald DR, O'Brien RA, Gilbert JJ, Cairncross JG (1989). Metastatic anaplastic oligodendroglioma. *Neurology* 39: 1593-1596.

935. Mack EE, Wilson CB (1993). Meningiomas induced by high-dose cranial irradiation. *J Neurosurg* 79: 28-31.

936. Mackenzie IR, Girvin JP, Lee D (1996). Symptomatic osteolipoma of the tuber cinereum. *Clin Neuropathol* 15: 60-62.

937. Maddock JR, Moran A, Maher EA, Teare MD, Norman A, Payne SJ, Whitehouse R, Dodd C, Lavin M, Hartely N, Super M, Evans DGR (1996). A genetic register for von Hippel-Lindau disease. *J Med Genet* 33: 120-127.

938. Magnani I, Guerneri S, Pollo B, Cirenei N, Colombo BM, Broggi G, Galli C, Bugiani O, DiDonato S, Finocchiaro G (1994). Increasing complexity of the karyotype in 50 human gliomas. Progressive evolution and de novo occurrence of cytogenetic alterations. *Cancer Genet Cytogenet* 75: 77-89.

939. Maguire JA, Bilbao JM, Kovacs K, Resch L (1992). Hypothalamic neurocytoma with vasopressin immunoreactivity: immunohistochemical and ultrastructural observations. *Endocr Pathol* 3: 99-104.

940. Maher ER, Iselius L, Yates JR, Littler M, Benjamin C, Harris R, Sampson J, Williams A, Ferguson Smith MA, Morton N (1991). Von Hippel-Lindau disease: a genetic study. *J Med Genet* 28: 443-447.

941. Maher ER, Yates JR, Ferguson S (1990). Statistical analysis of the two stage mutation model in von Hippel-Lindau disease, and in sporadic cerebellar haemangioblastoma and renal cell carcinoma. *J Med Genet* 27: 311-314.

942. Mahmood A, Caccamo DV, Tomecek FJ, Malik GM (1993). Atypical and malignant meningiomas: a clinicopathological review. *Neurosurgery* 33: 955-963.

943. Maier H, Ofner D, Hittmair A, Kitz K, Budka H (1992). Classic, atypical, and anaplastic meningioma: three histopathological subtypes of clinical relevance. *J Neurosurg* 77: 616-623.

944. Maier H, Wanschitz J, Sedivy R, Rossler K, Ofner D, Budka H (1997). Proliferation and DNA fragmentation in meningioma subtypes. *Neuropathol Appl Neurobiol* 23: 496-506.

945. Maintz D, Fiedler K, Koopmann J, Rollbrocker B, Nechev S, Lenartz D, Stangl AP, Louis DN, Schramm J, Wiestler OD, von Deimling A (1997). Molecular genetic evidence for subtypes of oligoastrocytomas. *J Neuropathol Exp Neurol* 56: 1098-1104.

946. Maire JP, Guerin J, Rivel J, San Galli F,

Bernard C, Dautheribes M, Caudry M (1992). [Medulloblastoma in children. Prognostic incidence of vascular hyperplasia, coagulation necrosis and postoperative clinical state on survival]. *Neurochirurgie* 38: 80-88.

947. Maiuri F, Stella L, Benvenuti D, Giamundo A, Pettinato G (1990). Cerebral gliosarcomas: correlation of computed tomographic findings, surgical aspect, pathological features, and prognosis. *Neurosurgery* 26: 261-267.

948. Major EO, Di Mayorca G (1973). Malignant transformation of BHK21 clone 13 cells by BK virus—a human papovavirus. *Proc Natl Acad Sci USA* 70: 3210-3212.

949. Malkin D (1994). p53 and the Li-Fraumeni syndrome. *Biochim Biophys Acta* 1198: 197-213.

950. Malkin D, Li FP, Strong LC, Fraumeni JF, Nelson CE, Kim DH, Kassel J, Gryka MA, Bishoff FZ, Tainsky MA (1990). Germ line *p53* mutations in a familial syndrome of breast cancer, sarcomas, and other neoplasms. *Science* 250: 1233-1238.

951. Mallory FB (1914). *Principles of Pathologic Histology.* Saunders: Philadelphia.

952. Mamelak AN, Prados MD, Obana WG, Cogen PH, Edwards MS (1994). Treatment options and prognosis for multicentric juvenile pilocytic astrocytoma. *J Neurosurg* 81: 24-30.

953. Mandahl N, Orndal C, Heim S, Willen H, Rydholm A, Bauer HC, Mitelman F (1993). Aberrations of chromosome segment 12q13-15 characterize a subgroup of hemangiopericytomas. *Cancer* 71: 3009-3013.

954. Mandel M, Toren A, Hadani M, Engelberg I, Martinowitz U, Rechavi G (1994). Ependymoblastoma in an HIV-positive hemophilic girl. *Med Pediatr Oncol* 23: 441-443.

955. Mannoji H, Becker LE (1988). Ependymal and choroid plexus tumors. Cytokeratin and GFAP expression. *Cancer* 61: 1377-1385.

956. Marano SR, Johnson PC, Spetzler RF (1988). Recurrent Lhermitte-Duclos disease in a child. Case report. *J Neurosurg* 69: 599-603.

957. Maraziotis T, Perentes E, Karamitopoulou E, Nakagawa Y, Gessaga EC, Probst A, Frankfurter A (1992). Neuron-associated class III beta-tubulin isotype, retinal S- antigen, synaptophysin, and glial fibrillary acidic protein in human medulloblastomas: a clinicopathological analysis of 36 cases. *Acta Neuropathol (Berl)* 84: 355-363.

958. Marcus DM, Lasudry JG, Carpenter JL, Windle J, Howes KA, al Ubaidi MR, Baehr W, Overbeek PA, Font RL, Albert DM (1996). Trilateral tumors in four different lines of transgenic mice expressing SV40 T-antigen. *Invest Ophthalmol Vis Sci* 37: 392-396.

959. Margetts JC, Kalyan R (1989). Giant-celled glioblastoma of brain. A clinico-pathological and radiological study of ten cases (including immunohistochemistry and ultrastructure). *Cancer* 63: 524-531.

960. Marigo V, Davey RA, Zuo Y, Cunningham JM, Tabin CJ (1996). Biochemical evidence that patched is the Hedgehog receptor. *Nature* 384: 176-179.

961. Mariman EC, van Beersum SE, Cremers CW, Struycken PM, Ropers HH (1995). Fine mapping of a putatively imprinted gene for familial non- chromaffin paragangliomas to chromosome 11q13.1: evidence for genetic heterogeneity. *Hum Genet* 95: 56-62.

962. Marinesco G, Goldstein M (1933). Sur une forme anatomique, non encore decrite, de medulloblastome: medullo-myoblastome. *Ann Anat Pathol* 10: 513-525.

963. Maris JM, White PS, Beltinger CP, Sulman EP, Castleberry RP, Shuster JJ, Look AT, Brodeur GM (1995). Significance of chromosome 1p loss of heterozygosity in neuroblastoma. *Cancer Res* 55: 4664-4669.

964. Mark RJ, Lutge WR, Shimizu KT, Tran LM, Selch MT, Parker RG (1995). Craniopharyngioma: treatment in the CT and MR imaging era. *Radiology* 197: 195-198.

965. Markesbery WR, Haugh RM, Young AB (1981). Ultrastructure of pineal parenchymal neoplasms. *Acta Neuropathol (Berl)* 55: 143-149.

966. Martin DS, Levy B, Awwad EE, Pittman T (1991). Desmoplastic infantile ganglioglioma: CT and MR features. *AJNR Am J Neuroradiol* 12: 1195-1197.

967. Martinez-Salazar A, Supler M, Rojiani AM (1997). Primary intracerebral malignant fibrous histiocytoma: immunohistochemical findings and etiopathogenetic considerations. *Mod Pathol* 10: 149-154.

968. Martuza RL, Eldridge R (1988). Neurofibromatosis 2 (bilateral acoustic neurofibromatosis). *N Engl J Med* 318: 684-688.

969. Mathews T, Moossy J (1974). Gliomas containing bone and cartilage. *J Neuropathol Exp Neurol* 33: 456-471.

970. Matsuda M, Yasui K, Nagashima K, Mori W (1987). Origin of the medulloblastoma experimentally induced by human polyomavirus JC. *J Natl Cancer Inst* 79: 585-591.

971. Matsuno A, Fujimaki T, Sasaki T, Nagashima T, Ide T, Asai A, Matsuura R, Utsunomiya H, Kirino T (1996). Clinical and histopathological analysis of proliferative potentials of recurrent and non-recurrent meningiomas. *Acta Neuropathol (Berl)* 91: 504-510.

972. Matsutani M, Sano K, Takakura K, Fujimaki T, Nakamura O, Funata N, Seto T (1997). Primary intracranial germ cell tumors: a clinical analysis of 153 histologically verified cases. *J Neurosurg* 86: 446-455.

973. Maxwell M, Galanopoulos T, Antoniades HN (1996). Expression of cyclin D1 proto-oncogene mRNA in primary meningiomas may contribute to tumorigenesis. *Int J Oncol* 9: 1213-1217.

974. McDonald JD, Daneshvar L, Willert JR, Matsumura K, Waldman F, Cogen PH (1994). Physical mapping of chromosome 17p13.3 in the region of a putative tumor suppressor gene important in medulloblastoma. *Genomics* 23: 229-232.

975. McGirr SJ, Kelly PJ, Scheithauer BW (1987). Stereotactic resection of juvenile pilocytic astrocytomas of the thalamus and basal ganglia. *Neurosurgery* 20: 447-452.

976. McGrogan G, Rivel J, Vital C, Guerin J (1992). A pineal tumour with features of "pineal anlage tumour". *Acta Neurochir Wien* 117: 73-77.

977. McKinnon RD, Piras G, Ida JA, Jr., Dubois D (1993). A role for TGF-beta in oligodendrocyte differentiation. *J Cell Biol* 121: 1397-1407.

978. McKusick VA (1994). *Mendelian Inheritance in Man: a Catalogue of Human Genes and Genetic Disorders.* 11th ed, The John Hopkins University Press: Baltimore & London. See also: http://www.ncbi.nlm.nih.gov/omim

979. McLean CA, Jolley D, Cukier E, Giles G, Gonzales MF (1993). Atypical and malignant meningiomas: importance of micronecrosis as a prognostic indicator. *Histopathology* 23: 349-353.

980. McLean CA, Laidlaw JD, Brownbill DS, Gonzales MF (1990). Recurrence of acoustic neurilemoma as a malignant spindle-cell neoplasm. Case report. *J Neurosurg* 73: 946-950.

981. McLean IW, Burnier MN, Zimmerman LE,Jakobiec FA (1994). *Tumors of the Eye and the Ocular Adnexa.* Armed Forces Institute of Pathology: Washington, DC.

982. Meeker TC, Shiramizu B, Kaplan L, Herndier B, Sanchez H, Grimaldi JC, Baumgartner J, Rachlin J, Feigal E, Rosenblum M (1991). Evidence for molecular subtypes of HIV-associated lymphoma: division into peripheral monoclonal, polyclonal and central nervous system lymphoma. *AIDS* 5: 669-674.

983. Meese E, Blin N, Zang KD (1987). Loss of heterozygosity and the origin of meningioma. *Hum Genet* 77: 349-351.

984. Meinke W, Goldstein DA, Smith RA (1979). Simian virus 40-related DNA sequences in a human brain tumor. *Neurology* 29: 1590-1594.

985. Meis-Kindblom JM, Stenman G, Kindblom LG (1996). Differential diagnosis of small round cell tumors. *Semin Diagn Pathol* 13: 213-241.

986. Meis JM, Enzinger FM, Martz KL, Neal JA (1992). Malignant peripheral nerve sheath tumors (malignant schwannomas) in children. *Am J Surg Pathol* 16: 694-707.

987. Meis JM, Ho KL, Nelson JS (1990). Gliosarcoma: a histologic and immunohistochemical reaffirmation. *Mod Pathol* 3: 19-24.

988. Meis JM, Martz KL, Nelson JS (1991). Mixed glioblastoma multiforme and sarcoma. A clinicopathologic study of 26 radiation therapy oncology group cases. *Cancer* 67: 2342-2349.

989. Meitar D, Crawford SE, Rademaker AW, Cohn SL (1996). Tumor angiogenesis correlates with metastatic disease, N-myc amplification, and poor outcome in human neuroblastoma. *J Clin Oncol* 14: 405-414.

990. Mena H, Ribas JL, Enzinger FM, Parisi JE (1991). Primary angiosarcoma of the central nervous system. Study of eight cases and review of the literature. *J Neurosurg* 75: 73-76.

991. Mena H, Ribas JL, Pezeshkpour GH, Cowan DN, Parisi JE (1991). Hemangiopericytoma of the central nervous system: a review of 94 cases. *Hum Pathol* 22: 84-91.

992. Mena H, Rushing EJ, Ribas JL, Delahunt B, McCarthy WF (1995). Tumors of pineal parenchymal cells: a correlation of histological features, including nucleolar organizer regions, with survival in 35 cases. *Hum Pathol* 26: 20-30.

993. Menon AG, Anderson KM, Riccardi VM, Chung RY, Whaley JM, Yandell DW, Farmer GE, Freiman RN, Lee JK, Li FP, Barker DF, Ledbetter DH, Kleider A, Martuza RL, Gusella JF, Seizinger BR (1990). Chromosome 17p deletions and p53 gene mutations associated with the formation of malignant neurofibrosarcomas in von Recklinghausen neurofibromatosis. *Proc Natl Acad Sci USA* 87: 5435-5439.

994. Menon AG, Rutter JL, von Sattel JP, Synder H, Murdoch C, Blumenfeld A, Martuza RL, von Deimling A, Gusella JF, Houseal TW (1997). Frequent loss of chromosome 14 in atypical and malignant meningioma: Identification a putative'tumor progression' locus. *Oncogene* 14: 611-616.

995. Mercer WE, Shields MT, Amin M, Sauve GJ, Appella E, Romano JW, Ullrich SJ (1990). Negative growth regulation in a glioblastoma tumor cell line that conditionally expresses human wild-type p53. *Proc Natl Acad Sci USA* 87: 6166-6170.

996. Merel P, Khe HX, Sanson M, Bijlsma E, Rouleau G, Laurent P, Pulst S, Baser M, Lenoir G, Sterkers JM (1995). Screening for germ-line mutations in the NF2 gene. *Genes Chromosomes Cancer* 12: 117-127.

997. Merlo A, Rochlitz C, Scott R (1996). Survival of patients with Turcot's syndrome and glioblastoma. *N Engl J Med* 334: 736-737.

998. Mertens F, Rydholm A, Bauer HF, Limon J, Nedoszytko B, Szadowska A, Willen H, Heim S, Mitelman F, Mandahl N (1995). Cytogenetic findings in malignant peripheral nerve sheath tumors. *Int J Cancer* 61: 793-798.

999. Metzger AK, Sheffield VC, Duyk G, Daneshvar L, Edwards MS, Cogen PH (1991). Identification of a germ-line mutation in the *p53* gene in a patient with an intracranial ependymoma. *Proc Natl Acad Sci USA* 88: 7825-7829.

1000. Meyer-Puttlitz B, Hayashi Y, Waha A, Rollbrocker B, Bostrom J, Wiestler OD, Louis DN, Reifenberger G, von Deimling A (1997). Molecular genetic analysis of giant cell glioblastomas. *Am J Pathol* 151: 853-857.

1001. Michieli P, Chedid M, Lin D, Pierce JH, Mercer WE, Givol D (1994). Induction of WAF1/CIP1 by a p53-independent pathway. *Cancer Res* 54: 3391-3395.

1002. Milbouw G, Born JD, Martin D, Collignon J, Hans P, Reznik M, Bonnal J (1988). Clinical and radiological aspects of dysplastic gangliocytoma (Lhermitte-Duclos disease): a report of two cases with review of the literature. *Neurosurgery* 22: 124-128.

1003. Millauer B, Shawver LK, Plate KH, Risau W, Ullrich A (1994). Glioblastoma growth inhibited in vivo by a dominant-negative Flk- 1 mutant. *Nature* 367: 576-579.

1004. Millen SJ, Campbell BH, Meyer GA, Ho KC (1985). Mixed glioma of the cerebellopontine angle. *Am J Otol* 6: 503-507.

1005. Miller CA, Torack RM (1970). Secretory ependymoma of the filum terminale. *Acta Neuropathol (Berl)* 15: 240-250.

1006. Miller DC, Goodman ML, Pilch BZ, Shi SR, Dickersin GR, Halpern H, Norris CM, Jr. (1984). Mixed olfactory neuroblastoma and carcinoma. A report of two cases. *Cancer* 54: 2019-2028.

1007. Miller DC, Hochberg FH, Harris NL, Gruber ML, Louis DN, Cohen H (1994). Pathology with clinical correlations of primary central nervous system non-Hodgkin's lymphoma. The Massachusetts General Hospital experience 1958-1989. *Cancer* 74: 1383-1397.

1008. Miller DC, Kim R,Zagzag D (1992). Neurocytomas: non-classical sites and mixed elements. *J Neuropath Exp Neurol* 51;364A.

1009. Miller DC, Lang FF, Epstein FJ (1993). Central nervous system gangliogliomas. Part 1: Pathology. *J Neurosurg* 79: 859-866.

1010. Min KW (1995). Usefulness of electron microscopy in the diagnosis of "small" round cell tumors of the sinonasal region. *Ultrastruct Pathol* 19: 347-363.

1011. Min KW, Cashman RE, Brumback RA (1995). Glioneurocytoma: tumor with glial and neuronal differentiation. *J Child Neurol* 10: 219-226.

1012. Min KW, Scheithauer BW (1990). Pineal germinomas and testicular seminoma: a comparative ultrastructural study with special references to early carcinomatous transformation. *Ultrastruct Pathol* 14: 483-496.

1013. Min KW, Scheithauer BW, Bauserman SC (1994). Pineal parenchymal tumors: an ultrastructural study with prognostic implications. *Ultrastruct Pathol* 18: 69-85.

1014. Min KW, Seo IS, Song J (1987). Postnatal evolution of the human pineal gland. An immunohistochemical study. *Lab Invest* 57: 724-728.

1015. Minehan KJ, Shaw EG, Scheithauer BW, Davis DL, Onofrio BM (1995). Spinal cord astrocytoma: pathological and treatment considerations. *J Neurosurg* 83: 590-595.

1016. Miranda RN, Glantz LK, Myint MA, Levy N, Jackson CL, Rhodes CH, Glantz MJ, Medeiros LJ (1996). Stage IE non-Hodgkin's lymphoma involving the dura: A clinicopathologic study of five cases. *Arch Pathol Lab Med* 120: 254-260.

1017. Mishima K, Nakamura M, Nakamura H, Nakamura O, Funata N, Shitara N (1992). Leptomeningeal dissemination of cerebellar pilocytic astrocytoma. Case report. *J Neurosurg* 77: 788-791.

1018. Mitchell A, Scheithauer BW, Ebersold MJ, Forbes GS (1991). Intracranial fibromatosis. *Neurosurgery* 29: 123-126.

1019. Mitchell A, Scheithauer BW, Unni KK, Forsyth PJ, Wold LE, McGivney DJ (1993). Chordoma and chondroid neoplasms of the spheno-occiput. An immunohistochemical study of 41 cases with prognostic and nosologic implications. *Cancer* 72: 2943-2949.

1020. Miyamori T, Mizukoshi H, Yamano K, Takayanagi N, Sugino M, Hayase H, Ito H (1990). Intracranial chondrosarcoma—case report. *Neurol Med Chir Tokyo* 30: 263-267.

1021. Molenaar WM, de Leij L, Trojanowski JQ (1991). Neuroectodermal tumors of the peripheral and the central nervous system share neuroendocrine N-CAM-related antigens with small cell lung carcinomas. *Acta Neuropathol (Berl)* 83: 46-54.

1022. Molenaar WM, Rorke LB,Trojanowski JQ (1993). Neural tumors. In: *Diagnostic Immunopathology*, Calvin RB, Bhan AK, McCluskey RT (eds), 2nd ed. Raven Press: New York. pp. 651-668.

1023. Molenaar WM, Trojanowski JQ (1994). Primitive neuroectodermal tumors of the central nervous system in childhood: tumor biological aspects. *Crit Rev Oncol Hematol* 17: 1-25.

1024. Molloy PT, Yachnis AT, Rorke LB, Dattilo JJ, Needle MN, Millar WS, Goldwein JW, Sutton LN, Phillips PC (1996). Central nervous system medulloepithelioma: a series of eight cases including two arising in the pons. *J Neurosurg* 84: 430-436.

1025. Momand J, Zambetti GP, Olson DC, George D, Levine AJ (1992). The mdm-2 oncogene product forms a complex with the p53 protein and inhibits p53-mediated transactivation. *Cell* 69: 1237-1245.

1026. Momozaki N, Ikezaki K, Abe M, Fukui M, Fujii K, Kishikawa T (1992). Cystic pineocytoma—case report. *Neurol Med Chir Tokyo* 32: 169-171.

1027. Montine TJ, Vandersteenhoven JJ, Aguzzi A, Boyko OB, Dodge RK, Kerns BJ, Burger PC (1994). Prognostic significance of Ki-67 proliferation index in supratentorial fibrillary astrocytic neoplasms. *Neurosurgery* 34: 674-678.

1028. Morantz RA, Kepes JJ, Batnitzky S, Masterson BJ (1979). Extraspinal ependymomas. Report of three cases. *J Neurosurg* 51: 383-391.

1029. Morgello S (1995). Pathogenesis and classification of primary central nervous system lymphoma: an update. *Brain Pathol* 5: 383-393.

1030. Morgello S, Maiese K, Petito CK (1989). T-cell lymphoma in the CNS: clinical and pathologic features. *Neurology* 39: 1190-1196.

1031. Morgello S, Petito CK, Mouradian JA (1990). Central nervous system lymphoma in the acquired immunodeficiency syndrome. *Clin Neuropathol* 9: 205-215.

1032. Morgello S, Tagliati M, Ewart MR (1997). HHV-8 and AIDS-related CNS lymphoma. *Neurology* 48: 1333-1335.

1033. Mori T, Nagase H, Horii A, Miyoshi Y, Shimano T, Nakatsuru S, Aoki T, Arakawa H, Yanagisawa A, Ushio Y, Takano S, Ogaura M, Karamura M, Shibuya M, Nishikawa R, Matsutani M, Hayashi Y, Jakahashi H, Ikuta F, Nishihara T, Mori S, Nakamura Y (1994). Germ-line and somatic mutations of the APC gene in patients with Turcot syndrome and analysis of APC mutations in brain tumors. *Genes Chromosomes Cancer* 9: 168-172.

1034. Morier P, Merot Y, Paccaud D, Beck D, Frenk E (1990). Juvenile chronic granulocytic leukemia, juvenile xanthogranulomas, and neurofibromatosis. Case report and review of the literature. *J Am Acad Dermatol* 22: 962-965.

1035. Morimura T, Maier H, Budka H (1996). Intermediate filament protein expression in gliomas: Correlation with proliferation rate. *Virchows Arch*

1036. Mork SJ, Halvorsen TB, Lindegaard KF, Eide GE (1986). Oligodendroglioma. Histologic evaluation and prognosis. *J Neuropathol Exp Neurol* 45: 65-78.

1037. Mork SJ, Lindegaard KF, Halvorsen TB, Lehmann EH, Solgaard T, Hatlevoll R, Harvei S, Ganz J (1985). Oligodendroglioma: incidence and biological behavior in a defined population. *J Neurosurg* 63: 881-889.

1038. Mork SJ, Rubinstein LJ (1985). Ependymoblastoma. A reappraisal of a rare embryonal tumor. *Cancer* 55: 1536-1542.

1039. Mork SJ, Rubinstein LJ, Kepes JJ, Perentes E, Uphoff DF (1988). Patterns of epithelial metaplasia in malignant gliomas II. Squamous differentiation of epithelial-like formations in gliosarcomas and glioblastomas. *J Neuropath Exp Neurol* 47: 101-118.

1040. Morris HH, Estes ML, Gilmore R, Van Ness PC, Barnett GH, Turnbull J (1993). Chronic intractable epilepsy as the only symptom of primary brain tumor. *Epilepsia* 34: 1038-1043.

1041. Mortimer EA, Jr., Lepow ML, Gold E, Robbins FC, Burton GJ, Fraumeni JF, Jr. (1981). Long-term follow-up of persons inadvertently inoculated with SV40 as neonates. *N Engl J Med* 305: 1517-1518.

1042. Moss TH (1984). Observations on the nature of subependymoma: an electron microscopic study. *Neuropathol Appl Neurobiol* 10: 63-75.

1043. Motoi M, Yoshino T, Hayashi K, Nose S, Horie Y, Ogawa K (1985). Immunohistochemical studies on human brain tumors using anti-Leu 7 monoclonal antibody in paraffin-embedded specimens. *Acta Neuropathol (Berl)* 66: 75-77.

1044. Mrak RE, Flanigan S, Collins CL (1994). Malignant acoustic schwannoma. *Arch Pathol Lab Med* 118: 557-561.

1045. Muller W, Bramisch R, Afra D, Schwenzfeger A (1977). [Cytophotometric investigations of the nuclear DNA content in ependymomas and plexuspapillomas]. *Acta Neuropathol (Berl)* 39: 255-259.

1046. Mullins JD (1980). A pigmented differentiating neuroblastoma. A light and ultrastructural study. *Cancer* 46: 522-528.

1047. Munoz EL, Eberhard DA, Lopes MBS, Schneider BF, Gonzalez F,VandenBerg SR (1996). Proliferative activity and *p53* mutation as prognostic indicators in pleomorphic xanthoastrocytoma. *J Neuropathol Exp Neurol* 55;606.

1048. Muragaki Y, Chou T, Kaplan D, Trojanowski JQ, Lee VMY (1997). Nerve growth factor (NGF) induces apoptosis in a human medulloblastoma cell lines that express TrkA receptors. *J Neurosci* 17: 530-542.

1049. Musa BS, Pople IK, Cummins BH (1995). Intracranial meningiomas following irradiation—a growing problem? *Br J Neurosurg* 9: 629-637.

1050. Myers SL, Hardy DA, Wiebe CB, Shiffman J (1994). Olfactory neuroblastoma invading the oral cavity in a patient with inappropriate antidiuretic hormone secretion. *Oral Surg Oral Med Oral Pathol* 77: 645-650.

1051. Nagashima T, Hoshino T, Cho KG (1987). Proliferative potential of vascular components in human glioblastoma multiforme. *Acta Neuropathol (Berl)* 73: 301-305.

1052. Nagashima T, Hoshino T, Cho KG, Senegor M, Waldman F, Nomura K (1988). Comparison of bromodeoxyuridine labeling indices obtained from tissue sections and flow cytometry of brain tumors. *J Neurosurg* 68: 388-392.

1053. Nakagawa Y, Perentes E, Rubinstein LJ (1986). Immunohistochemical characterization of oligodendrogliomas: an analysis of multiple markers. *Acta Neuropathol (Berl)* 72: 15-22.

1054. Nakagawa Y, Perentes E, Rubinstein LJ (1987). Non-specificity of anti-carbonic anhydrase C antibody as a marker in human neurooncology. *J Neuropathol Exp Neurol* 46: 451-460.

1055. Nakagawara A, Arima N, Scavarda NJ, Azar CG, Cantor AB, Brodeur GM (1993). Association between high levels of expression of the TRK gene and favorable outcome in human neuroblastoma. *N Engl J Med* 328: 847-854.

1056. Nakamura Y, Becker LE, Mancer K, Gillespie R (1982). Peripheral medulloepithelioma. *Acta Neuropathol (Berl)* 57: 137-142.

1057. Nakasu S, Nakasu Y, Nioka H, Nakajima M, Handa J (1994). bcl-2 protein expression in tumors of the central nervous system. *Acta Neuropathol* 88: 520-526.

1058. Nakazato Y (1993). Central nervous system. In: *Melanocytic Tumors*, Nakajima T, Ishikara K (eds). Bunkodo: Tokyo. pp. 140-144.

1059. Narod SA, Parry DM, Parboosingh J, Lenoir GM, Ruttledge M, Fischer G, Eldridge R, Martuza RL, Frontali M, Haines J (1992). Neurofibromatosis type 2 appears to be a genetically homogeneous disease. *Am J Hum Genet* 51: 486-496.

1060. Naudin tC, Vermeij K, Smit DA, Cohen O, Gerssen S, Dijkhuizen T (1995). Intracranial teratoma with multiple fetuses: pre- and post-natal appearance. *Hum Pathol* 26: 804-807.

1061. Nazar GB, Hoffman HJ, Becker LE, Jenkin D, Humphreys RP, Hendrick EB (1990). Infratentorial ependymomas in childhood: prognostic factors and treatment. *J Neurosurg* 72: 408-417.

1062. Nazzaro JM, Neuwelt EA (1990). The role of surgery in the management of supratentorial intermediate and high-grade astrocytomas in adults. *J Neurosurg* 73: 331-344.

1063. Neglia JP, Meadows AT, Robison LL, Kim TH, Newton WA, Ruymann FB, Sather HN, Hammond JD (1991). Second neoplasms after acute lymphoblastic leukemia in childhood. *New Engl J Med* 325: 1330-1336.

1064. Nelen MR, Padberg GW, Peeters EAJ, Lin AY, van den Helm B, Frants RR, Coulon V, Goldstein AM, van Reen MMM, Easton DF, Eeles RA, Hodgson S, Mulvihill JJ, Murday VA, Tucker MA, Mariman ECM, Starink TM, Ponder BAJ, Ropers HH, Kremer H, Longy M, Eng C (1996). Localization of the gene for Cowden disease to chromosome 10q22-23. *Nat Genet* 13: 114-116.

1065. Nelson JS, Tsukada Y, Schoenfeld D, Fulling K, Lamarche J, Peress N (1983). Necrosis as a prognostic criterion in malignant supratentorial, astrocytic gliomas. *Cancer* 52: 550-554.

1066. Nelson RS, Perlman EJ, Askin FB (1995). Is esthesioneuroblastoma a peripheral neuroectodermal tumor? *Hum Pathol* 26: 639-641.

1067. Neumann E, Kalousek DK, Norman MG, Steinbok P, Cochrane DD, Goddard K (1993). Cytogenetic analysis of 109 pediatric central nervous system tumors. *Cancer Genet Cytogenet* 71: 40-49.

1068. Neumann HP, Wiestler OD (1994). Von Hippel-Lindau disease: a syndrome providing insights into growth control and tumorigenesis. *Nephrol Dial Transplant* 9: 1832-1833.

1069. Nevin S (1938). Gliomatosis cerebri. *Brain* 61: 170-191.

1070. Newcomb EW (1995). P53 gene mutations in lymphoid diseases and their possible relevance to drug resistance. *Leuk Lymphoma* 17: 211-221.

1071. Newcomb EW, Bhalla SK, Parrish CL, Hayes RL, Cohen H, Miller DC (1997). bcl-2 expression in astrocytomas in relation to patient survival and p53 gene status. *Acta Neuropathol* 94: 369-375.

1072. Newcomb EW, Madonia WJ, Pisharody S, Lang FF, Koslow M, Miller DC (1993). A correlative study of p53 protein alteration and p53 gene mutation in glioblastoma multiforme. *Brain Pathol* 3: 229-235.

1073. Newham P, Humphries MJ (1996). Integrin adhesion receptors: structure, function and implications for biomedicine. *Mol Med Today* 2: 304-313.

1074. Ng HK (1995). Cytologic diagnosis of intracranial germinomas in smear preparations. *Acta Cytol* 39: 693-697.

1075. Ng HK, Poon WS (1990). Gliosarcoma of the posterior fossa with features of a malignant fibrous histiocytoma. *Cancer* 65: 1161-1166.

1076. Ng HK, Tang NL, Poon WS (1994). Polar spongioblastoma with cerebrospinal fluid metastases. *Surg Neurol* 41: 137-142.

1077. Ng TH, Fung CF, Ma LT (1990). The pathological spectrum of desmoplastic infantile gangliogliomas. *Histopathology* 16: 235-241.

1078. Niikawa S, Hara A, Ando T, Sakai N, Yamada H, Shimokawa K (1992). Dolichos biflorus agglutinin binding to intracranial germ-cell tumors: detection of embryonal components in germinomas. *Acta Neuropathol (Berl)* 83: 347-351.

1079. Nijjar TS, Simpson WJ, Gadalla T, McCartney M (1993). Oligodendroglioma. The Princess Margaret Hospital experience (1958-1984). *Cancer* 71: 4002-4006.

1080. Nishikawa R, Furnari FB, Lin H, Arap W, Berger MS, Cavenee WK, Su H (1995). Loss of P16INK4 expression is frequent in high grade gliomas. *Cancer Res* 55: 1941-1945.

1081. Nishio S, Takeshita I, Fukui M (1990). Primary cerebral ganglioneurocytoma in an adult. *Cancer* 66: 358-362.

1082. Nishio S, Takeshita I, Fukui M, Yamashita M, Tateishi J (1988). Anaplastic evolution of childhood optico-hypothalamic pilocytic astrocytoma: report of an autopsy case. *Clin Neuropathol* 7: 254-258.

1083. Nishio S, Takeshita I, Kaneko Y, Fukui M (1992). Cerebral neurocytoma. A new subset of benign neuronal tumors of the cerebrum. *Cancer* 70: 529-537.

1084. Nishioka H, Ito H, Miki T (1996). Difficulties in the antemortem diagnosis of gliomatosis cerebri: report of a case with diffuse increase of gemistocyte-like cells, mimicking reactive gliosis. *Br J Neurosurg* 10: 103-107.

1085. Nitta T, Uda K, Ebato M, Ikezaki K, Fukui M, Sato K (1995). Primary peripheral-postthymic T-cell lymphoma in the central nervous system: immunological and molecular approaches to diagnosis. *J Neurosurg* 82: 77-82.

1086. NNFF INGAC (1999). Index to Mutation Types. http://www.nf.org/nf1gene/secure_data/nf1gene_mutdata.index.html

1087. Noble M, Gutowski N, Bevan K, Engel U, Linskey M, Urenjak J, Bhakoo K, Williams S (1995). From rodent glial precursor cell to human glial neoplasia in the oligodendrocyte-type-2 astrocyte lineage. *Glia* 15: 222-230.

1088. Nora FE, Scheithauer BW (1996). Primary epithelioid hemangioendothelioma of the brain. *Am J Surg Pathol* 20: 707-714.

1089. Numoto RT (1994). Pineal parenchymal tumors: cell differentiation and prognosis. *J Cancer Res Clin Oncol* 120: 683-690.

1090. O'Brien PC, Roos DE, Liew KH, Trotter GE, Barton MB, Walker QJ, Poulsen MG, Olver IN (1996). Preliminary results of combined chemotherapy and radiotherapy for non-AIDS primary central nervous system lymphoma. Trans- Tasman Radiation Oncology Group (TROG). *Med J Aust* 165: 424-427.

1091. O'Brien TF, Moran M, Miller JH, Hensley SD (1995). Meningeal melanocytoma. An uncommon diagnostic pitfall in surgical neuropathology. *Arch Pathol Lab Med* 119: 542-546.

1092. O'Marcaigh AS, Ledger GA, Roche PC, Parisi JE, Zimmerman D (1995). Aromatase expression in human germinomas with possible biological effects. *J Clin Endocrinol Metab* 80: 3763-3766.

1093. O'Neill B, Illig J (1989). Primary central nervous system lymphoma. *Mayo Clin Proc* 64: 1005-1020.

1094. Oberstrass J, Reifenberger G, Reifenberger J, Wechsler W, Collins VP (1996). Mutation of the Von Hippel-Lindau tumour suppressor gene in capillary haemangioblastomas of the central nervous system. *J Pathol* 179: 151-156.

1095. Ogasawara H, Inagawa T, Yamamoto M, Kamiya K, Yano T, Utsunomiya H (1988). Medulloblastoma in infancy associated with omphalocele, malrotation of the intestine, and extrophy of the bladder. *Childs Nerv Syst* 4: 108-111.

1096. Ohgaki H, Eibl RH, Schwab M, Reichel MB, Mariani L, Gehring M, Petersen I, Holl T, Wiestler OD, Kleihues P (1993). Mutations of the p53 tumor suppressor gene in neoplasms of the human nervous system. *Mol Carcinog* 8: 74-80.

1097. Ohgaki H, Eibl RH, Wiestler OD, Yasargil MG, Newcomb EW, Kleihues P (1991). p53 mutations in nonastrocytic human brain tumors. *Cancer Res* 51: 6202-6205.

1098. Ohgaki H, Schauble B, zur H, von Ammon K, Kleihues P (1995). Genetic alterations associated with the evolution and progression of astrocytic brain tumours. *Virchows Arch* 427: 113-118.

1099. Ohnishi T, Arita N, Hayakawa T, Kawahara K, Kato K, Kakinuma A (1993). Purification of motility factor (GMF) from human malignant glioma cells and its biological significance in tumor invasion. *Biochem Biophys Res Commun* 193: 518-525.

1100. Oikawa S, Sakamoto K, Kobayashi N (1994). A neonatal huge subependymal giant cell astrocytoma: case report. *Neurosurgery* 35: 748-750.

1101. Okada H, Yoshida J, Sokabe M, Wakabayashi T, Hagiwara M (1996). Suppression of CD44 expression decreases migration and invasion of human glioma cells. *Int J Cancer* 66: 255-260.

1102. Oliner JD, Kinzler KW, Meltzer PS, George DL, Vogelstein B (1992). Amplification of a gene encoding a p53-associated protein in human sarcomas. *Nature* 358: 80-83.

1103. Olopade OI, Jenkins RB, Ransom DT, Malik K, Pomykala H, Nobori T, Cowan JM, Rowley JD, Diaz MO (1992). Molecular analysis of deletions of the short arm of chromosome 9 in human gliomas. *Cancer Res* 52: 2523-2529.

1104. Olson DC, Marechal V, Momand J, Chen J, Romocki C, Levine AJ (1993). Identification and characterization of multiple mdm-2 proteins and mdm-2-p53 protein complexes. *Oncogene* 8: 2353-2360.

1105. Olson JM, Breslow NE, Barce J (1993). Cancer in twins of Wilms tumor patients. *Am J Med Genet* 47: 91-94.

1106. Onda K, Davis RL, Shibuya M, Wilson CB, Hoshino T (1994). Correlation between the bromodeoxyuridine labeling index and the MIB-1 and Ki-67 proliferating cell indices in cerebral gliomas. *Cancer* 74: 1921-1926.

1107. Onda K, Davis RL, Wilson CB, Hoshino T (1994). Regional differences in bromodeoxyuridine uptake, expression of Ki-67 protein, and nucleolar organizer region counts in glioblastoma multiforme. *Acta Neuropathol (Berl)* 87: 586-593.

1108. Ono Y, Ueki K, Joseph JT, Louis DN (1996). Homozygous deletions of the CDKN2/p16 gene in dural hemangiopericytomas. *Acta Neuropathol (Berl)* 91: 221-225.

1109. Oro AE, Higgins KM, Hu Z, Bonifas JM, Epstein EH, Jr., Scott MP (1997). Basal cell carcinomas in mice overexpressing Sonic hedgehog. *Science* 276: 817-821.

1110. Ory K, Legros Y, Auguin C, Soussi T (1994). Analysis of the most representative tumour-derived p53 mutants reveals that changes in protein conformation are not correlated with loss of transactivation or inhibition of cell proliferation. *EMBO J* 13: 3496-3504.

1111. Osborne AG (1994). *Diagnostic Neuroradiology.* Mosby: St. Louis.

1112. Ota S, Crabbe DC, Tran TN, Triche TJ, Shimada H (1993). Malignant rhabdoid tumor. A study with two established cell lines. *Cancer* 71: 2862-2872.

1113. Owen S, Zhang W, Cusack JC, Angelo LS, Santee SM, Fujiwara T, Roth JA, Deisseroth AB, Zhang WW, Kruzel E (1995). Wild-type human p53 and a temperature-sensitive mutant induce Fas/APO-1 expression. *Mol Cell Biol* 15: 3032-3040.

1114. Ozek MM, Sav A, Pamir MN, Ozer AF, Ozek E, Erzen C (1993). Pleomorphic xanthoastrocytoma associated with von Recklinghausen neurofibromatosis. *Childs Nerv Syst* 9: 39-42.

1115. Packer RJ, Perilongo G, Johnson D, Sutton LN, Vezina G, Zimmerman RA, Ryan J, Reaman G, Schut L (1992). Choroid plexus carcinoma of childhood. *Cancer* 69: 580-585.

1116. Packer RJ, Sutton LN, Elterman R, Lange B, Goldwein J, Nicholson HS, Mulne L, Boyett J, D'Angio G, Wechsler Jentzsch K, et al (1994). Outcome for children with medulloblastoma treated with radiation and cisplatin, CCNU, and vincristine chemotherapy. *J Neurosurg* 81: 690-698.

1117. Packer RJ, Sutton LN, Rorke LB, Littman PA, Sposto R, Rosenstock JG, Bruce DA, Schut L (1984). Prognostic importance of cellular differentiation in medulloblastoma of childhood. *J Neurosurg* 61: 296-301.

1118. Packer RJ, Sutton LN, Rorke LB, Zimmerman RA, Littman P, Bruce DA, Schut L (1985). Oligodendroglioma of the posterior fossa in childhood. *Cancer* 56: 195-199.

1119. Packer RJ, Sutton LN, Rosenstock JG, Rorke LB, Bilaniuk LT, Zimmerman RA, Littman PA, Bruce DA, Schut L (1984). Pineal region tumors of childhood. *Pediatrics* 74: 97-102.

1120. Padberg GW, Schot JD, Vielvoye GJ, Bots GT, de Beer FC (1991). Lhermitte-Duclos disease and Cowden disease: a single phakomatosis. *Ann Neurol* 29: 517-523.

1121. Pagni CA, Giordana MT, Canavero S (1991). Benign recurrence of a pilocytic cerebellar astrocytoma 36 years after radical removal: case report. *Neurosurgery* 28: 606-609.

1122. Pahapill PA, Ramsay DA, Del Maestro RF (1996). Pleomorphic xanthoastrocytoma: case report and analysis of the literature concerning the efficacy of resection and the significance of necrosis. *Neurosurgery* 38: 822-828.

1123. Palma L, Celli P, Cantore G (1993). Supratentorial ependymomas of the first two decades of life. Long-term follow-up of 20 cases (including two subependymomas). *Neurosurgery* 32: 169-175.

1124. Palma L, Celli P, Maleci A, Di Lorenzo N, Cantore G (1989). Malignant monstrocellular brain tumours. A study of 42 surgically treated cases. *Acta Neurochir Wien* 97: 17-25.

1125. Palma L, Di Lorenzo N, Guidetti B (1978). Lymphocytic infiltrates in primary glioblastomas and recidivous gliomas: Incidence, fate, and relevance to prognosis in 228 operated cases. *J Neurosurg* 49: 854-861.

1126. Palma L, Russo A, Mercuri S (1983). Cystic cerebral astrocytomas in infancy and childhood: long-term results. *Childs Brain* 10: 79-91.

1127. Palma L, Russo A, Celli P (1984). Prognosis of the so-called "diffuse" cerebellar astrocytoma. *Neurosurgery* 15: 315-317.

1128. Papadaki H, Kounelis S, Kapadia SB, Bakker A, Swalsky PA, Finkelstein SD (1996). Relationship of p53 gene alterations with tumor progression and recurrence in olfactory neuroblastoma. *Am J Surg Pathol* 20: 715-721.

1129. Papi L, De Vitis LR, Vitelli F, Ammannati F, Mennonna P, Montali E, Bigozzi U (1995). Somatic mutations in the neurofibromatosis type 2 gene in sporadic meningiomas. *Hum Genet* 95: 347-351.

1130. Paraf F, Jothy S, Van Meir EG (1997). Brain tumor-polyposis syndrome: two genetic diseases? *J Clin Oncol* 15: 2744-2758.

1131. Parisi JE,Scheithauer BW (1993). Glial tumors. In: *Principles and Practice of Neuropathology,* Nelson JS, Parisi JE, Schochet SS, Jr. (eds). Mosby: St. Louis. pp. 123-183.

1132. Parisi JE, Scheithauer BW, Priest JR, Okazaki H,Komori T (1992). Desmoplastic infantile ganglioglioma (DIG): a form of gangliogliomatosis? *J Neuropath Exp Neurol* 51;365.

1133. Park JP, Chaffee S, Noll WW, Rhodes CH (1996). Constitutional de novo t(1;22)(p22;q11.2) and ependymoma. *Cancer Genet Cytogenet* 86: 150-152.

1134. Parkinson D, Hall CW (1962). Case Reports. Oligodendrogliomas. Simultaneous appearance in frontal lobes of siblings. *J Neurosurg* 19: 424-426.

1135. Pasquier B, Couderc P, Pasquier D, Panh MH, N'Golet A (1978). Sarcoma arising in oligodendroglioma of the brain: a case with intramedullary and subarachnoid spinal metastases. *Cancer* 42: 2753-2758.

1136. Pasquier B, Gasnier F, Pasquier D, Keddari E, Morens A, Couderc P (1986). Papillary meningioma. Clinicopathologic study of seven cases and review of the literature. *Cancer* 58: 299-305.

1137. Pasquier B, Pasquier D, Golet AN, Panh MH, Couderc P (1980). Extraneural metastases of astrocytomas and glioblastomas: clinicopathological study of two cases and review of the literature. *Cancer* 45: 112-125.

1138. Pasquier B, Pasquier D, N'Golet A, Panh MH, Couderc P (1979). [The metastatic potential of primary central nervous tumours]. *Rev Neurol Paris* 135: 263-278.

1139. Patil A, McComb RD, Gelber B, McConnell J, Sasse S (1990). Intraventricular neurocytoma: a report of two cases. *Neurosurg* 26: 140-144.

1140. Patronas NJ, Di Chiro G, Kufta C, Bairamian D, Kornblith PL, Simon R, Larson SM (1985). Prediction of survival in glioma patients by means of positron emission tomography. *J Neurosurg* 62: 816-822.

1141. Patt S, Gries H, Giraldo M, Cervos N, Martin H, Janisch W, Brockmoller J (1996). p53 gene mutations in human astrocytic brain tumors including pilocytic astrocytomas. *Hum Pathol* 27: 586-589.

1142. Patt S, Schmidt H, Labrakakis C, Weydt P, Fritsch M, Cervos N, Kettenmann H (1996). Human central neurocytoma cells show neuronal physiological properties in vitro. *Acta Neuropathol (Berl)* 91: 209-214.

1143. Paulus W, Baur I, Beutler AS, Reeves SA (1996). Diffuse brain invasion of glioma cells requires beta 1 integrins. *Lab Invest* 75: 819-826.

1144. Paulus W, Baur I, Huettner C, Schmausser B, Roggendorf W, Schlingensiepen KH, Brysch W (1995). Effects of transforming growth factor-beta1 on collagen synthesis, integrin expression, adhesion and invasion of glioma cells. *J Neuropathol Exp Neurol* 52: 236-244.

1145. Paulus W, Baur I, Schuppan D, Roggendorf W (1993). Characterization of integrin receptors in normal and neoplastic human brain. *Am J Pathol* 143: 154-163.

1146. Paulus W, Bayas A, Ott G, Roggendorf W (1994). Interphase cytogenetics of glioblastoma and gliosarcoma. *Acta Neuropathol* 88: 420-425.

1147. Paulus W, Grothe C, Sensenbrenner M, Janet T, Baur I, Graf M, Roggendorf W (1990). Localization of basic fibroblast growth factor, a mitogen and angiogenic factor, in human brain tumors. *Acta Neuropathol (Berl)* 79: 418-423.

1148. Paulus W, Janisch W (1990). Clinicopathologic correlations in epithelial choroid plexus neoplasms: a study of 52 cases. *Acta Neuropathol (Berl)* 80: 635-641.

1149. Paulus W, Jellinger K (1993). Comparison of integrin adhesion molecules expressed by primary brain lymphomas and nodal lymphomas. *Acta Neuropathol (Berl)* 86: 360-364.

1150. Paulus W, Jellinger K, Hallas C, Ott G, Muller Hermelink HK (1993). Human herpesvirus-6 and Epstein-Barr virus genome in primary cerebral lymphomas. *Neurology* 43: 1591-1593.

1151. Paulus W, Lisle DK, Tonn JC, Wolf HK, Roggendorf W, Reeves SA, Louis DN (1996). Molecular genetic alterations in pleomorphic xanthoastrocytoma. *Acta Neuropathol* 91: 293-297.

1152. Paulus W, Ott MM, Strik H, Keil V, Muller Hermelink HK (1994). Large cell anaplastic (KI-1) brain lymphoma of T-cell genotype. *Hum Pathol* 25: 1253-1256.

1153. Paulus W, Peiffer J (1988). Does the pleomorphic xanthoastrocytoma exist? Problems in the application of immunological techniques to the classification of brain tumors. *Acta Neuropathol (Berl)* 76: 245-252.

1154. Paulus W, Schlote W, Perentes E, Jacobi G, Warmuth Metz M, Roggendorf W (1992). Desmoplastic supratentorial neuroepithelial tumours of infancy. *Histopathology* 21: 43-49.

1155. Paulus W, Slowik F, Jellinger K (1991). Primary intracranial sarcomas: histopathological features of 19 cases. *Histopathology* 18: 395-402.

1156. Paulus W, Tonn JC (1994). Basement membrane invasion of glioma cells mediated by integrin receptors. *J Neurosurg* 80: 515-519.

1157. Pause A, Lee S, Worrel RA, Chen DYT, Burgess WH, Linehan WM, Klausner RD (1997). The von Hippel-Lindau tumor-suppressor gene product forms a stable complex with human CUL-2, a member of the Cdc53 family of proteins. *Proc Natl Acad Sci USA* 94: 2156-2161.

1158. Pavelic J, Hlavka V, Poljak M, Gale N, Pavelic K (1994). p53 immunoreactivity in oligodendrogliomas. *J Neurooncol* 22: 1-6.

1159. Pearl GS, Takei Y (1981). Cerebellar "neuroblastoma": nosology as it relates to medulloblastoma. *Cancer* 47: 772-779.

1160. Pearl GS, Takei Y, Bakay RA, Davis P (1985). Intraventricular primary cerebral neuroblastoma in adults: report of three cases. *Neurosurgery* 16: 847-849.

1161. Pech IV, Shuer LM, Peterson K (1997). Indolent course of disseminated juvenile pilocytic astrocytoma. *Neurology* 48: A35.

1162. Pedersen PH, Ness GO, Engebraaten O, Bjerkvig R, Lillehaug JR, Laerum OD (1994). Heterogeneous response to the growth factors [EGF, PDGF (bb), TGF-alpha, bFGF, IL-2] on glioma spheroid growth, migration and invasion. *Int J Cancer* 56: 255-261.

1163. Pedersen PH, Rucklidge GJ, Mork SJ, Terzis AJ, Engebraaten O, Lund J, Backlund EO, Laerum OD, Bjerkvig R (1994). Leptomeningeal tissue: a barrier against brain tumor cell invasion. *J Natl Cancer Inst* 86: 1593-1599.

1164. Penn I, Porat G (1995). Central nervous system lymphomas in organ allograft recipients. *Transplantation* 59: 240-244.

1165. Peraud A, Watanabe K, Plate KH, Yonekawa Y, Kleihues P, Ohgaki H (1997). *p53* Mutations versus EGF receptor expression in giant cell glioblastomas. *J Neuropath Exp Neurol* 56: 1235-1241.

1166. Percy AK, Elveback LR, Okazaki H, Kurland LT (1972). Neoplasms of the central nervous system. Epidemiologic considerations. *Neurology* 22: 40-48.

1167. Perentes E, Rubinstein LJ, Herman MM, Donoso LA (1986). S-antigen immunoreactivity in human pineal glands and pineal parenchymal tumors. A monoclonal antibody study. *Acta Neuropathol (Berl)* 71: 224-227.

1168. Perry A, Jenkins RB, Dahl RJ, Moertel CA, Scheithauer BW (1996). Cytogenetic analysis of aggressive meningiomas: possible diagnostic and prognostic implications. *Cancer* 77: 2567-2573.

1169. Peyrard M, Fransson I, Xie YG, Han FY, Ruttledge MH, Swahn S, Collins JE, Dunham I, Collins VP, Dumanski JP (1994). Characterization of a new member of the human beta-adaptin gene family from chromosome 22q12, a candidate meningioma gene. *Hum Mol Genet* 3: 1393-1399.

1170. Philips PC, Carson BS, Wharam MD, Eggleston JC, Robb PA, Strauss LC (1989). Pineal parenchymal tumors in children and adults: treatment results. *International Symposium on Pediatric Neuro-Oncology Seattle, WA* A-29.

1171. Picksley SM, Lane DP (1993). The p53-mdm2 autoregulatory feedback loop: a paradigm for the regulation of growth control by p53? *Bioessays* 15: 689-690.

1172. Pierce GB (1983). The cancer cell and its control by the embryo. Rous-Whipple Award lecture. *Am J Pathol* 113: 117-124.

1173. Pierre K, Hirsch JF, Roux FX, Renier D, Sainte R (1983). Intracranial ependymomas in childhood. Survival and functional results of 47 cases. *Childs Brain* 10: 145-156.

1174. Pietsch T, Waha A, Koch A, Kraus J, Albrecht S, Tonn J, Sorensen N, Berthold F, Henk B, Schmandt N, Wolf HK, von Deimling A, Wainwright B, Chenevix-Trench G, Wiestler OD, Wicking C (1997). Medulloblastomas of the desmoplastic variant carry mutations of the human homologue of Drosophila patched. *Cancer Res* 57: 2085-2088.

1175. Pigott TJ, Lowe JS, Palmer J (1991). Statistical modelling in analysis of prognosis in glioblastoma multiforme: a study of clinical variables and Ki-67 index. *Br J Neurosurg* 5: 61-66.

1176. Pilkington GJ (1994). Tumour cell migration in the central nervous system. *Brain Pathol* 4: 157-166.

1177. Pimentel J, Tavora L, Cristina ML, Antunes JA (1988). Intraventricular schwannoma. *Childs Nerv Syst* 4: 373-375.

1178. Pirotte B, Levivier M, Goldman S, Brucher JM, Brotchi J, Hildebrand J (1997). Glucocorticoid-induced long-term remission in primary cerebral lymphoma: case report and review of the literature. *J Neurooncol* 32: 63-69.

1179. Pitkethly DT, Major MC, Hardman JM, Kempe LG, Earle KM (1970). Angioblastic meningiomas. Clinicopathologic study of 81 cases. *J Neurosurg* 32: 539-544.

1180. Pitt MA, Jones AW, Reeve RS, Cowie RA (1992). Oligodendroglioma of the fourth ventricle with intracranial and spinal oligodendrogliomatosis: a case report. *Br J Neurosurg* 6: 371-374.

1181. Pizer BL, Moss T, Oakhill A, Webb D, Coakham HB (1995). Congenital astroblastoma: an immunohistochemical study. Case report. *J Neurosurg* 83: 550-555.

1182. Plate KH, Breier G, Farrell CL, Risau W (1992). Platelet-derived growth factor receptor-beta is induced during tumor development and upregulated during tumor progression in endothelial cells in human gliomas. *Lab Invest* 67: 529-534.

1183. Plate KH, Breier G, Risau W (1994). Molecular mechanisms of developmental and tumor angiogenesis. *Brain Pathol* 4: 207-218.

1184. Plate KH, Breier G, Weich HA, Mennel HD, Risau W (1994). Vascular endothelial growth factor and glioma angiogenesis: coordinate induction of VEGF receptors, distribution of VEGF protein and possible *in vivo* regulatory mechanisms. *Int J Cancer* 59: 520-529.

1185. Plate KH, Breier G, Weich HA, Risau W (1992). Vascular endothelial growth factor is a potential tumour angiogenesis factor in human gliomas in vivo. *Nature* 359: 845-848.

1186. Plate KH, Risau W (1995). Angiogenesis in malignant gliomas. *Glia* 15: 339-347.

1187. Platten M, Giordano MJ, Dirven CM, Gutmann DH, Louis DN (1996). Up-regulation of specific NF 1 gene transcripts in sporadic pilocytic astrocytomas. *Am J Pathol* 149: 621-627.

1188. Platten M, Meyer-Puttlitz B, Waha A, Wolf HK, Nothen MM, Louis DN, Sampson JR, von Deimling A (1997). A novel splice site-associated polymorphism in the tuberous sclerosis gene may predispose to the development of sporadic gangliogliomas. *Neuropathology* 56: 806-810.

1189. Plukker JT, Koops HS, Molenaar I, Vermey A, ten Kate LP, Oldhoff J (1988). Malignant hemangiopericytoma in three kindred members of one family. *Cancer* 61: 841-844.

1190. Pollack IF, Claassen D, al Shboul Q, Janosky JE, Deutsch M (1995). Low-grade gliomas of the cerebral hemispheres in children: an analysis of 71 cases. *J Neurosurg* 82: 536-547.

1191. Pollack IF, Gerszten PC, Martinez AJ, Lo KH, Shultz B, Albright AL, Janosky J, Deutsch M (1995). Intracranial ependymomas of childhood: long-term outcome and prognostic factors. *Neurosurgery* 37: 655-666.

1192. Pollack IF, Hoffman HJ, Humphreys RP, Becker L (1993). The long-term outcome after surgical treatment of dorsally exophytic brain-stem gliomas. *J Neurosurg* 78: 859-863.

1193. Pollack IF, Hurtt M, Pang D, Albright AL (1994). Dissemination of low grade intracranial astrocytomas in children. *Cancer* 73: 2869-2878.

1194. Pollak A, Friede RL (1977). Fine structure of medulloepithelioma. *J Neuropathol Exp Neurol* 36: 712-725.

1195. Pompili A, Calvosa F, Caroli F, Mastrostefano R, Occhipinti E, Raus L, Sciaretta F (1993). The transdural extension of gliomas. *J Neurooncol* 15: 67-74.

1196. Ponta H, Sleeman J, Herrlich P (1994). Tumor metastasis formation: cell-surface proteins confer metastasis-promoting or -suppressing properties. *Biochim Biophys Acta* 1198: 1-10.

1197. Posner JB (1995). *Neurologic Complications of Cancer.* FA Davis: Philadelphia.

1198. Posner JB, Chernik NL (1978). Intracranial metastases from systemic cancer. *Adv Neurol* 19: 579-592.

1199. Powell SZ, Yachnis AT, Rorke LB, Rojiani AM, Eskin TA (1996). Divergent differentiation in pleomorphic xanthoastrocytoma. Evidence for a neuronal element and possible relationship to ganglion cell tumors. *Am J Surg Pathol* 20: 80-85.

1200. Prados MD, Krouwer HG, Edwards MS, Cogen PH, Davis RL, Hoshino T (1992). Proliferative potential and outcome in pediatric astrocytic tumors. *J Neurooncol* 13: 277-282.

1201. Prayson RA (1996). Malignant meningioma: a clinicopathologic study of 23 patients including MIB1 and p53 immunohistochemistry. *Am J Clin Pathol* 105: 719-726.

1202. Prayson RA, Estes ML (1992). Dysembryoplastic neuroepithelial tumor. *Am J Clin Pathol* 97: 398-401.

1203. Prayson RA, Estes ML (1995). Protoplasmic astrocytoma. A clinicopathologic study of 16 tumors. *Am J Clin Pathol* 103: 705-709.

1204. Prayson RA, Estes ML, Morris HH (1993). Coexistence of neoplasia and cortical dysplasia in patients presenting with seizures. *Epilepsia* 34: 609-615.

1205. Prayson RA, Khajavi K, Comair YG (1995). Cortical architectural abnormalities and MIB1 immunoreactivity in gangliogliomas: a study of 60 patients with intracranial tumors. *J Neuropathol Exp Neurol* 54: 513-520.

1206. Preissig SH, Smith MT, Huntington HW (1979). Rhabdomyosarcoma arising in a pineal teratoma. *Cancer* 44: 281-284.

1207. Preston M, Lewis S, Winkelmann R, Borman B, Auld J, Pearce N (1993). Descriptive epidemiology of primary cancer of the brain, cranial nerves, and cranial meninges in New Zealand, 1948-88. *Cancer Causes Control* 4: 529-538.

1208. Preul MC, Leblanc R, Tampieri D, Robitaille Y, Pokrupa R (1993). Spinal angiolipomas. Report of three cases. *J Neurosurg* 78: 280-286.

1209. Pruchon E, Chauveinc L, Sabatier L, Dutrillaux AM, Ricoul M, Delattre JY, Vega F, Poisson M, Hor F, Dutrillaux B (1994). A cytogenetic study of 19 recurrent gliomas. *Cancer Genet Cytogenet* 76: 85-92.

1210. Przygodzki RM, Finkelstein SD, Langer JC, Swalsky PA, Fishback N, Bakker A, Guinee DG, Koss M, Travis WD (1996). Analysis of p53, K-ras-2, and C-raf-1 in pulmonary neuroendocrine tumors. Correlation with histological subtype and clinical outcome. *Am J Pathol* 148: 1531-1541.

1211. Przygodzki RM, Moran CA, Suster S, Khan MA, Swalsky PA, Bakker A, Koss MN, Finkelstein SD (1996). Primary mediastinal and testicular seminomas: a comparison of K- ras-2 gene sequence and p53 immunoperoxidase analysis of 26 cases. *Hum Pathol* 27: 975-979.

1212. Pulst SM, Rouleau GA, Marineau C, Fain P, Sieb JP (1993). Familial meningioma is not allelic to neurofibromatosis 2. *Neurology* 43: 2096-2098.

1213. Pyhtinen J, Paakko E (1996). A difficult diagnosis of gliomatosis cerebri. *Neuroradiology* 38: 444-448.

1214. Pykett MJ, Murphy M, Harnish PR, George DL (1994). Identification of a microsatellite instability phenotype in meningiomas. *Cancer Res* 54: 6340-6343.

1215. Rabinowicz AL, Abrey LE, Hinton DR, Couldwell WT (1995). Cerebral neurocytoma: an unusual cause of refractory epilepsy. Case report and review of the literature. *Epilepsia* 36: 1237-1240.

1216. Radotra B, McCormick D (1997). Glioma invasion in vitro is mediated by CD44-hyaluronan interactions. *J Pathol* 181: 434-438.

1217. Raff MC, Miller RH, Noble M (1983). A glial progenitor cell that develops in vitro into an astrocyte or an oligodendrocyte depending on culture medium. *Nature* 303: 390-396.

1218. Raffel C, Jenkins RB, Frederick L, Hebrink D, Alderete BE, Fults DW, James CD (1997). Sporadic medulloblastomas contain *PTCH* mutations. *Cancer Res* 57: 842-845.

1219. Raffel C, Thomas GA, Tishler DM, Lassoff S, Allen JC (1993). Absence of p53 mutations in childhood central nervous system primitive neuroectodermal tumors. *Neurosurgery* 33: 301-305.

1220. Raghavan R, Steart PV, Weller RO (1990). Cell proliferation patterns in the diagnosis of astrocytomas, anaplastic astrocytomas and glioblastoma multiforme: a Ki-67 study. *Neuropathol Appl Neurobiol* 16: 123-133.

1221. Rainho CA, Rogatto SR, de Moraes LC, Barbieri-Neto J (1992). Cytogenetic study of a pineocytoma. *Cancer Genet Cytogenet* 64: 127-132.

1222. Rainov NG, Lubbe J, Renshaw J, Pritchard J, Luthy AR, Aguzzi A (1995). Association of Wilms' tumor with primary brain tumor in siblings. *J Neuropathol Exp Neurol* 54: 214-223.

1223. Raisanen J (1993). 34th Annual Diagnostic Slide Session. *Am Ass of Neurop Meeting*

1224. Rajan B, Ashley S, Gorman C, Jose CC, Horwich A, Bloom HJ, Marsh H, Brada M (1993). Craniopharyngioma—a long-term results following limited surgery and radiotherapy. *Radiother Oncol* 26: 1-10.

1225. Ramsey H (1965). Fine structure of the surface of the cerebral cortex in the human brain. *J Cell Biol* 26: 323-333.

1226. Ramsey RG (1994). *Neuroradiology.* 3rd ed, WB Saunders: Philadelphia.

1227. Raney RB, Ater JL, Herman L, Leeds NE, Cleary KR, Womer RB, Rorke LM (1994). Primary intraspinal soft-tissue sarcoma in childhood: report of two cases with a review of the literature. *Med Pediatr Oncol* 23: 359-364.

1228. Ransom DT, Ritland SR, Kimmel DW, Moertel CA, Dahl RJ, Scheithauer BW, Kelly PJ, Jenkins RB (1992). Cytogenetic and loss of heterozygosity studies in ependymomas, pilocytic astrocytomas, and oligodendrogliomas. *Genes Chromosomes Cancer* 5: 348-356.

1230. Ransom DT, Ritland SR, Moertel CA, Dahl RJ, O'Fallon JR, Scheithauer BW, Kimmel DW, Kelly PJ, Olopade OI, Diaz MO (1992). Correlation of cytogenetic analysis and loss of heterozygosity studies in human diffuse astrocytomas and mixed oligo-astrocytomas. *Genes Chromosomes Cancer* 5: 357-374.

1231. Rao C, Friedlander ME, Klein E, Anzil AP, Sher JH (1990). Medullomyoblastoma in an adult. *Cancer* 65: 157-163.

1232. Rasheed BK, Bigner SH (1991). Genetic alterations in glioma and medulloblastoma. *Cancer Metastasis Rev* 10: 289-299.

1233. Rasheed BK, McLendon RE, Herndon JE, Friedman HS, Friedman AH, Bigner DD, Bigner SH (1994). Alterations of the *TP53* gene in human gliomas. *Cancer Res* 54: 1324-1330.

1234. Rauhut F, Reinhardt V, Budach V, Wiedemayer H, Nau HE (1989). Intramedullary pilocytic astrocytomas—a clinical and morphological study after combined surgical and photon or neutron therapy. *Neurosurg Rev* 12: 309-313.

1235. Rausing A, Ybo W, Stenflo J (1970). Intracranial meningioma - a population study of ten years. *Acta Neurol Scand* 46: 102-110.

1236. Raymond AA, Halpin SF, Alsanjari N, Cook MJ, Kitchen ND, Fish DR, Stevens JM, Harding BN, Scaravilli F, Kendall B (1994). Dysembryoplastic neuroepithelial tumor. Features in 16 patients. *Brain* 117: 461-475.

1237. Regis J, Bouillot P, Rouby V, Figarella B, Dufour H, Peragut JC (1996). Pineal region tumors and the role of stereotactic biopsy: review of the mortality, morbidity, and diagnostic rates in 370 cases. *Neurosurgery* 39: 907-912.

1238. Reifenberger G (1991). *Immunhistochemie der Tumoren des Zentralnervensystems.* Springer-Verlag: Berlin.

1239. Reifenberger G, Liu L, Ichimura K, Schmidt EE, Collins VP (1993). Amplification and overexpression of the MDM2 gene in a subset of human malignant gliomas without p53 mutations. *Cancer Res* 53: 2736-2739.

1240. Reifenberger G, Reifenberger J, Bilzer T, Wechsler W, Collins VP (1995). Coexpression of transforming growth factor-alpha and epidermal growth factor receptor in capillary hemangioblastomas of the central nervous system. *Am J Pathol* 147: 245-250.

1241. Reifenberger G, Reifenberger J, Ichimura K, Meltzer PS, Collins VP (1994). Amplification of multiple genes from chromosomal region 12q13-14 in human malignant gliomas: preliminary mapping of the amplicons shows preferential involvement of CDK4, SAS, and MDM2. *Cancer Res* 54: 4299-4303.

1242. Reifenberger G, Reifenberger J, Liu L, James CD, Wechsler W, Collins VP (1996). Molecular genetics of oligodendroglial tumors. In: *Brain Tumor Research and Therapy,* Nagai M (eds). Springer-Verlag: Tokyo. pp. 187-209.

1243. Reifenberger G, Szymas J, Wechsler W (1987). Differential expression of glial- and neuronal-associated antigens in human tumors of the central and peripheral nervous system. *Acta Neuropathol (Berl)* 74: 105-123.

1244. Reifenberger J, Reifenberger G, Liu L, James CD, Wechsler W, Collins VP (1994). Molecular genetic analysis of oligodendroglial tumors shows preferential allelic deletions on 19q and 1p. *Am J Pathol* 145: 1175-1190.

1245. Reifenberger J, Ring GU, Gies U, Cobbers L, Oberstrass J, An HX, Niederacher D, Wechsler W, Reifenberger G (1996). Analysis of p53 mutation and epidermal growth factor receptor amplification in recurrent gliomas with malignant progression. *J Neuropathol Exp Neurol* 55: 822-831.

1246. Reis A, Kuster W, Linss G, Gebel E, Hamm H, Fuhrmann W, Wolff G, Groth W, Gustafson G, Kuklik M (1992). Localisation of gene for the naevoid basal-cell carcinoma syndrome. *Lancet* 339: 617-617.

1247. Rempel SA, Schwechheimer K, Davis RL, Cavenee WK, Rosenblum ML (1993). Loss of heterozygosity for loci on chromosome 10 is associated with morphologically malignant meningioma progression. *Cancer Res* 53: 2386-2392.

1248. Rencic A, Gordon J, Otte J, Curtis M, Kovatich A, Zoltick P, Khalili K, Andrews D (1996). Detection of JC virus DNA sequence and expression of the viral oncoprotein, tumor antigen, in brain of immunocompetent patient with oligoastrocytoma. *Proc Natl Acad Sci USA* 93: 7352-7357.

1249. Reni M, Ferreri AJ, Zoldan MC, Villa E (1997). Primary brain lymphomas in patients with a prior or concomitant malignancy. *J Neurooncol* 32: 135-142.

1250. Renshaw AA, Paulus W, Joseph JT (1995). CD34 and epithelial membrane antigen distinguish dural hemangiopericytoma and meningioma. *Appl Immunohistochem* 3: 108-114.

1251. Rey JA, Bello MJ, de Campos JM, Kusak ME, Moreno S (1987). Chromosomal composition of a series of 22 human low-grade gliomas. *Cancer Genet Cytogenet* 29: 223-237.

1252. Reyes-Mugica M, Chou P, Byrd S, Ray V, Castelli M, Gattuso P, Gonzalez Crussi F (1993). Nevomelanocytic proliferations in the central nervous system of children. *Cancer* 72: 2277-2285.

1253. Reyes-Mugica M, Chou P, Gonzalez C, Tomita T (1992). Fibroma of the meninges in a child: immunohistological and ultrastructural study. Case report. *J Neurosurg* 76: 143-147.

1254. Reyes-Mugica M, Rieger-Christ K, Ohgaki H, Ekstrand BC, Helie M, Kleinman G, Yahanda A, Fearon ER, Kleihues P, Reale MA (1997). Loss of *DCC* expression and glioma progression. *Cancer Res* 57: 382-386.

1255. Rhodes CH, Glantz MJ, Glantz L, Lekos A, Sorenson GD, Honsinger C, Levy NB (1996). A comparison of polymerase chain reaction examination of cerebrospinal fluid and conventional cytology in the diagnosis of lymphomatous meningitis. *Cancer* 77: 543-548.

1256. Rhodes RH, Cole M, Takaoka Y, Roessmann U, Cotes EE, Simon J (1994). Intraventricular cerebral neuroblastoma. Analysis of subtypes and comparison with hemispheric neuroblastoma. *Arch Pathol Lab Med* 118: 897-911.

1257. Riccardi VM (1981). Von Recklinghausen neurofibromatosis. *N Engl J Med* 305: 1617-1627.

1258. Riccardi VM (1992). *Neurofibromatosis: Phenotype, Natural History and Pathogenesis.* 2nd ed, Johns Hopkins University Press: Baltimore.

1259. Ricci A, Jr., Parham DM, Woodruff JM, Callihan T, Green A, Erlandson RA (1984). Malignant peripheral nerve sheath tumors arising from ganglioneuromas. *Am J Surg Pathol* 8: 19-29.

1260. Ringertz J (1950). Grading of gliomas. *Acta Pathol Microbiol Scand* 27: 51-64.

1261. Ringertz J, Reymond A (1949). Ependymomas and choroid plexus papillomas. *J Neuropath Exp Neurol* 8: 355-380.

1262. Ritter JH, Mills SE, Nappi O, Wick MR (1995). Angiosarcoma-like neoplasms of epithelial organs: true endothelial tumors or variants of carcinoma? *Semin Diagn Pathol* 12: 270-282.

1263. Roach ES, Smith M, Huttenlocher P, Bhat M, Alcorn D, Hawley L (1992). Diagnostic criteria: tuberous sclerosis complex. Report of the Diagnostic Criteria Committee of the National Tuberous Sclerosis Association. *J Child Neurol* 7: 221-224.

1264. Robbins P, Segal A, Narula S, Stokes B, Lee M, Thomas W, Caterina P, Sinclair I, Spagnolo D (1995). Central neurocytoma. A clinicopathological, immunohistochemical and ultrastructural study of 7 cases. *Pathol Res Pract* 191: 100-111.

1265. Roberts RO, Lynch CF, Jones MP, Hart MN (1991). Medulloblastoma: a population-based study of 532 cases. *J Neuropathol Exp Neurol* 50: 134-144.

1266. Robinson JC, Challa VR, Jones DS,

Kelly DL, Jr. (1996). Pericytosis and edema generation: a unique clinicopathological variant of meningioma. *Neurosurgery* 39: 700-706.

1267. Roche PH, Figarella B, Regis J, Peragut JC (1996). Cauda equina paraganglioma with subsequent intracranial and intraspinal metastases. *Acta Neurochir (Wien)* 138: 475-479.

1268. Rodriguez HA, Berthrong M (1966). Multiple primary intracranial tumors in von Recklinghausen's neurofibromatosis. *Arch Neurol* 14: 467-475.

1269. Rodriguez LA, Edwards MS, Levin VA (1990). Management of hypothalamic gliomas in children: an analysis of 33 cases. *Neurosurgery* 26: 242-246.

1270. Roelvink NC, Kamphorst W, Lindhout D, Ponssen H (1986). Concordant cerebral oligodendroglioma in identical twins. *J Neurol Neurosurg Psychiatry* 49: 706-708.

1271. Roessler E, Belloni E, Gaudenz K, Jay P, Berta P, Scherer SW, Tsui LC, Muenke M (1996). Mutations in the human Sonic Hedgehog gene cause holoprosencephaly. *Nat Genet* 14: 357-360.

1272. Roessmann U, Velasco ME, Gambetti P, Autilio G (1983). Neuronal and astrocytic differentiation in human neuroepithelial neoplasms. An immunohistochemical study. *J Neuropathol Exp Neurol* 42: 113-121.

1273. Rogatto SR, Casartelli C, Rainho CA, Barbieri-Neto J (1993). Chromosomes in the genesis and progression of ependymomas. *Cancer Genet Cytogenet* 69: 146-152.

1274. Rogers L, Pattisapu J, Smith RR, Parker P (1988). Medulloblastoma in association with the Coffin-Siris syndrome. *Childs Nerv Syst* 4: 41-44.

1275. Rogers LR, Estes ML, Rosenbloom SA, Harrold L (1995). Primary leptomeningeal oligodendroglioma: case report. *Neurosurgery* 36: 166-168.

1276. Rohringer M, Sutherland GR, Louw DF, Sima AA (1989). Incidence and clinicopathological features of meningioma. *J Neurosurg* 71: 665-672.

1277. Rooney CM, Smith CA, Heslop HE (1997). Control of virus-induced lymphoproliferation: Epstein-Barr virus-induced lymphoproliferation and host immunity. *Mol Med Today* 3: 24-30.

1278. Roosen N, De La Porte C, Van Vyve M, Solheid C, Selosse P (1984). Familial oligodendroglioma. Case report. *J Neurosurg* 60: 848-849.

1279. Rorke LB (1983). The cerebellar medulloblastoma and its relationship to primitive neuroectodermal tumors. *J Neuropathol Exp Neurol* 42: 1-15.

1280. Rorke LB, Packer RJ, Biegel JA (1996). Central nervous system atypical teratoid/rhabdoid tumors of infancy and childhood: definition of an entity. *J Neurosurg* 85: 56-65.

1281. Rorke LB, Trojanowski JQ, Lee VMY, Zimmerman RA, Sutton LN, Biegel JA, Goldwein JW, Packer RJ (1997). Primitive neuroectodermal tumors of the central nervous system. *Brain Pathol* 7: 765-784.

1282. Rosai J, Parkash V, Reuter VE (1994). The origin of mediastinal germ cell tumors in men. *Int J Surg Pathol* 2: 73-78.

1283. Rosenberg JE, Lisle DK, Burwick JA, Ueki K, von Deimling A, Mohrenweiser HW, Louis DN (1996). Refined deletion mapping of the chromosome 19q glioma tumor suppressor gene to the D19S412-STD interval. *Oncogene* 13: 2483-2485.

1284. Rosenblum MK, Erlandson RA, Budzilovich GN (1991). The lipid-rich epithelioid glioblastoma. *Am J Surg Pathol* 15: 925-934.

1285. Ross JA, Severson RK, Pollock BH, Robison LL (1996). Childhood cancer in the United States. A geographical analysis of cases from the Pediatric Cooperative Clinical Trials groups. *Cancer* 77: 201-207.

1286. Rossi ML, Jones NR, Candy E, Nicoll JA, Compton JS, Hughes JT, Esiri MM, Moss TH, Cruz S, Coakham HB (1989). The mononuclear cell infiltrate compared with survival in high- grade astrocytomas. *Acta Neuropathol (Berl)* 78: 189-193.

1287. Rossitch E, Jr., Zeidman SM, Burger PC, Curnes JT, Harsh C, Anscher M, Oakes WJ (1990). Clinical and pathological analysis of spinal cord astrocytomas in children. *Neurosurgery* 27: 193-196.

1288. Rostad S, Kleinschmidt D, Manchester DK (1985). Two massive congenital intracranial immature teratomas with neck extension. *Teratology* 32: 163-169.

1289. Rouleau GA, Merel P, Lutchman M, Sanson M, Zucman J, Marineau C, Hoang X, Demczuk S, Desmaze C, Plougastel B (1993). Alteration in a new gene encoding a putative membrane-organizing protein causes neuro-fibromatosis type 2. *Nature* 363: 515-521.

1290. Rubie H, Hartman O, Michon J, Frappaz D, Coze C, Chastagner P, Baranzelli MC, Plantaz D, Avet-Loiseau H, Bénard J, Delattre O, Favrot M, Peyroulet MC, Thyss A, Perel Y, Bergeron C, Courbon-Collet B, Vannier JP, Lemerle J (1997). *N-MYC* gene amplification is a major prognostic factor in localized neuroblastoma: results of the French NBL 90 Study. *J Clin Pathol* 15: 1171-1182.

1291. Rubinstein LJ (1970). The definition of the ependymoblastoma. *Arch Pathol* 90: 35-45.

1292. Rubinstein LJ (1972). Cytogenesis and differentiation of primitive central neuroepithelial tumors. *J Neuropathol Exp Neurol* 31: 7-26.

1293. Rubinstein LJ (1981). Cytogenesis and differentiation of pineal neoplasms. *Hum Pathol* 12: 441-448.

1294. Rubinstein LJ (1986). The malformative central nervous system lesions in the central and peripheral forms of neurofibromatosis. A neuropathological study of 22 cases. *Ann N Y Acad Sci* 486: 14-29.

1295. Rubinstein LJ, Herman MM (1989). The astroblastoma and its possible cytogenic relationship to the tanycyte. An electron microscopic, immunohistochemical, tissue- and organ-culture study. *Acta Neuropathol (Berl)* 78: 472-483.

1296. Rubinstein LJ, Northfield DWC (1964). The medulloblastoma and the so-called "arachnoidal cerebellar sarcoma". A critical re-examination of a nosological problem. *Brain* 87: 379-412.

1297. Rubio MP, Correa KM, Ramesh V, MacCollin MM, Jacoby LB, von Deimling A, Gusella JF, Louis DN (1994). Analysis of the neurofibromatosis 2 gene in human ependymomas and astrocytomas. *Cancer Res* 54: 45-47.

1298. Ruchuox MM, Gray F, Gherardi R, Schaeffer A, Comoy J, Poirier J (1986). Orthostatic hypotension from a cerebellar gangliocytoma (Lhermitte-Duclos disease). *J Neurosurg* 65: 245-252.

1299. Rudolph P, Lappe T, Hero B, Berthold F, Parwaresch R, Harms D, Schmidt D (1997). Prognostic significance of the proliferative activity in neuroblastoma. *Am J Pathol* 150: 133-145.

1300. Rueda P, Heifetz SA, Sesterhenn IA, Clark GB (1987). Primary intracranial germ cell tumors in the first two decades of life. A clinical, light-microscopic, and immunohistochemical analysis of 54 cases. *Perspect Pediatr Pathol* 10: 160-207.

1301. Ruelle A, Tunesi G, Andrioli G (1996). Spinal meningeal melanocytoma. Case report and analysis of diagnostic criteria. *Neurosurg Rev* 19: 39-42.

1302. Rushing EJ, Armonda RA, Ansari Q, Mena H (1996). Mesenchymal chondrosarcoma: a clinicopathologic and flow cytometric study of 13 cases presenting in the central nervous system. *Cancer* 77: 1884-1891.

1303. Rushing EJ, Rorke LB, Sutton L (1993). Problems in the nosology of desmoplastic tumors of childhood. *Pediatr Neurosurg* 19: 57-62.

1304. Russell DS, Cairns H (1947). Polar spongioblastomas. *Arch Histol Norm Pathol* 3: 423-441.

1305. Russell DS,Rubinstein LJ (1977). *Pathology of Tumors of the Nervous System.* 4th ed, Arnold: London.

1306. Russell DS,Rubinstein LJ (1989). *Pathology of Tumours of the Nervous System.* 5th ed, Edward Arnold: London.

1307. Rutka JT, Giblin JR, Apodaca G, DeArmond SJ, Stern R, Rosenblum ML (1987). Inhibition of growth and induction of differentiation in a malignant human glioma cell line by normal leptomeningeal extracellular matrix proteins. *Cancer Res* 47: 3515-3522.

1308. Ruttledge MH, Xie YG, Han FY, Peyrard M, Collins VP, Nordenskjold M, Dumanski JP (1994). Deletions on chromosome 22 in sporadic meningioma. *Genes Chromosomes Cancer* 10: 122-130.

1309. Ryken TC, Robinson RA, VanGilder JC (1994). Familial occurrence of subependymoma. Report of two cases. *J Neurosurg* 80: 1108-1111.

1310. Sainz J, Figueroa K, Baser ME, Mautner VF, Pulst SM (1995). High frequency of nonsense mutations in the NF2 gene caused by C to T transitions in five CGA codons. *Hum Mol Genet* 4: 137-139.

1311. Sainz J, Huynh DP, Figueroa K, Ragge NK, Baser ME, Pulst SM (1994). Mutations of the neurofibromatosis type 2 gene and lack of the gene product in vestibular schwannomas. *Hum Mol Genet* 3: 885-891.

1312. Saito T, Tanaka R, Kouno M, Washiyama K, Abe S, Kumanishi T (1989). Tumor-infiltrating lymphocytes and histocompatibility antigens in primary intracranial germinomas. *J Neurosurg* 70: 81-85.

1313. Saitoh Y, Kuratsu J, Takeshima H, Yamamoto S, Ushio Y (1995). Expression of osteopontin in human glioma. Its correlation with the malignancy. *Lab Invest* 72: 55-63.

1314. Sakuda K, Kohda Y, Matsumoto T, Park C, Seto A, Tohma Y, Hasegawa M, Kida S, Nitta H, Yamashima T, Yamashita J (1996). Expression of NF2 gene product merlin in arachnoid villi and meningiomas. *Noshuyo Byori* 13: 145-148.

1315. Salazar OM (1983). A better understanding of CNS seeding and a brighter outlook for postoperatively irradiated patients with ependymomas. *Int J Radiat Oncol Biol Phys* 9: 1231-1234.

1316. Salcman M, Scholtz H, Kaplan RS, Kulik S (1994). Long-term survival in patients with malignant astrocytoma. *Neurosurgery* 34: 213-219.

1317. Saleh M, Stacker SA, Wilks AF (1996). Inhibition of growth of C6 glioma cells in vivo by expression of antisense vascular endothelial growth factor sequence. *Cancer Res* 56: 393-401.

1318. Salmon I, Dewitte O, Pasteels JL, Flament D, Brotchi J, Vereerstraeten P, Kiss R (1994). Prognostic scoring in adult astrocytic tumors using patient age, histopathological grade, and DNA histogram type. *J Neurosurg* 80: 877-883.

1319. Salvati M, Artico M, Caruso R, Rocchi G, Orlando ER, Nucci F (1991). A report on radiation-induced gliomas. *Cancer* 67: 392-397.

1320. Salvati M, Ciappetta P, Raco A (1993). Osteosarcomas of the skull. Clinical remarks on 19 cases. *Cancer* 71: 2210-2216.

1321. Sandberg N, Stahlbom PA, Reinecke M, Collins VP, von Holst H, Sara V (1993). Characterization of insulin-like growth factor 1 in human primary brain tumors. *Cancer Res* 53: 2475-2478.

1322. Sanford RA (1994). Craniopharyngioma: results of survey of the American Society of Pediatric Neurosurgery. *Pediatr Neurosurg* 21 Suppl 1: 39-43.

1323. Sapoznik M, Kaplan H (1983). Intracranial Hodgkin's disease. A report of 12 cases and review of the literature. *Cancer* 52: 1301-1307.

1324. Sarkar C, Roy S, Tandon PN (1988). Oligodendroglial tumors. An immunohistochemical and electron microscopic study. *Cancer* 61: 1862-1866.

1325. Sato H, Ohmura K, Mizushima M, Ito J, Kuyama H (1983). Myxopapillary ependymoma of the lateral ventricle. A study on the mechanism of its stromal myxoid change. *Acta Pathol Jpn* 33: 1017-1025.

1326. Sato K, Kubota T, Yoshida K, Murata H (1993). Intracranial extraskeletal myxoid chondrosarcoma with special reference to lamellar inclusions in the rough endoplasmic reticulum. *Acta Neuropathol (Berl)* 86: 525-528.

1327. Sato K, Schauble B, Kleihues P, Ohgaki H (1996). Infrequent alterations of the *p15, p16, CDK4* and *cyclin D1* genes in non-astrocytic human brain tumours. *Int J Cancer* 66: 305-308.

1328. Saunders JE, Kwartler JA, Wolf HK, Brackmann DE, McElveen JT, Jr. (1991). Lipomas of the internal auditory canal. *Laryngoscope* 101: 1031-1037.

1329. Savelyeva L, Corvi R, Schwab M (1994). Translocation involving 1p and 17q is a recurrent genetic alteration of human neuroblastoma cells. *Am J Hum Genet* 55: 334-340.

1330. Sawada S, Florell S, Purandare SM, Ota M, Stephens K, Viskochil D (1996). Identification of NF1 mutations in both alleles of a dermal neurofibroma. *Nat Genet* 14: 110-112.

1331. Sawyer JR, Roloson GJ, Chadduck WM, Boop FA (1991). Cytogenetic findings in a pleomorphic xanthoastrocytoma. *Cancer Genet Cytogenet* 55: 225-230.

1332. Sawyer JR, Sammartino G, Husain M, Boop FA, Chadduck WM (1994). Chromosome aberrations in four ependymomas. *Cancer Genet Cytogenet* 74: 132-138.

1333. Sawyer JR, Thomas EL, Roloson GJ, Chadduck WM, Boop FA (1992). Telomeric associations evolving to ring chromosomes in a recurrent pleomorphic xanthoastrocytoma. *Cancer Genet Cytogenet* 60: 152-157.

1334. Scheithauer BW (1978). Symptomatic subependymoma. Report of 21 cases with review of the literature. *J Neurosurg* 49: 689-696.

1335. Scheithauer BW, Halling KC, Nascimento AG, Hill EM, Sin FH,Katzmann JA (1995). Neurofibroma and malignant peripheral nerve sheath tumor: a proliferation index and DNA ploidy study. *Pathol Res Pract* 19;177-177.

1336. Scheithauer BW, Parameswaran A, Burdick B (1996). Intrasellar paraganglioma: report of a case in a sibship of von Hippel-Lindau disease. *Neurosurgery* 38: 395-399.

1337. Scheithauer BW, Rubinstein LJ (1978). Meningeal mesenchymal chondrosarcoma: report of 8 cases with review of the literature. *Cancer* 42: 2744-2752.

1338. Scheithauer BW, Woodruff JM,Erlandson RE (1997). *Tumors of the Peripheral Nerves.* Armed Forces Institute of Pathology: Washington.

1339. Scherer HJ (1938). Structural development in gliomas. *Am J Cancer* 34: 333-351.

1340. Scherer HJ (1940). Cerebral astrocytomas and their derivatives. *Am J Cancer* 40: 159-198.

1341. Scherer HJ (1940). The forms of growth in gliomas and their practical significance. *Brain* 63: 1-35.

1342. Scherneck S, Rudolph M, Geissler E, Vogel F, Lubbe L, Wahlte H, Nisch G, Weickmann F, Zimmermann W (1979). Isolation of a SV40-like Papovavirus from a human glioblastoma. *Int J Cancer* 24: 523-531.

1343. Scherrer HJ (1935). Gliomstudien. III. Angioplastische Gliome. *Virchows Arch* 294: 823-861.

1344. Scheurlen WG, Krauss J, Kuhl J (1995). No preferential loss of one parental allele of chromosome 17p13.3 in childhood medulloblastoma. *Int J Cancer* 63: 372-374.

1345. Scheurlen WG, Seranski P, Minchera A, Kuhl J, Sorensen N, Krauss J, Lichter P, Poustka A, Wilgenbus KK (1997). High-resolution deletion mapping of chromosome arm 17p in childhood primitive neuroectodermal tumors reveals a common chromosomal disruption within the Smith-Magenis Region, an unstable region in chromosome band 17p11.2. *Genes Chromosomes Cancer* 18: 50-58.

1346. Schiffer D (1993). *Brain Tumors. Pathology and its Biological Correlates.* Springer-Verlag: Berlin.

1347. Schiffer D (1997). *Brain Tumors. Biology, Pathology, and Clinical References.* 2nd ed, Springer: Berlin.

1348. Schiffer D, Cavalla P, Chio A, Giordana MT, Marino S, Mauro A, Migheli A (1994). Tumor cell proliferation and apoptosis in medulloblastoma. *Acta Neuropathol (Berl)* 87: 362-370.

1349. Schiffer D, Cavalla P, Migheli A, Chio A, Giordana MT, Marino S, Attanasio A (1995). Apoptosis and cell proliferation in human neuroepithelial tumors. *Neurosci Lett* 195: 81-84.

1350. Schiffer D, Cavalla P, Migheli A, Giordana MT, Chiado-Piat L (1996). Bcl-2 distribution in neuroepithelial tumors: an immunohistochemical study. *J Neurooncol* 27: 101-109.

1351. Schiffer D, Cavalla P,Pilkington GJ (1997). Proliferative properties of malignant brain tumors. In: *Brain Tumor Invasion. Biological, Clinical and Therapeutic Considerations,* Mikkelsen T, Bjerkvig R, Laerum O, Rosenblum ML (eds). Wiley and Soons: Chichester.

1352. Schiffer D, Chio A, Cravioto H, Giordana MT, Migheli A, Soffietti R, Vigliani MC (1991). Ependymoma: internal correlations among pathological signs: the anaplastic variant. *Neurosurgery* 29: 206-210.

1353. Schiffer D, Chio A, Giordana MT, Leone M, Soffietti R (1988). Prognostic value of histologic factors in adult cerebral astrocytoma. *Cancer* 61: 1386-1393.

1354. Schiffer D, Chio A, Giordana MT, Migheli A, Palma L, Pollo B, Soffietti R, Tribolo A (1991). Histologic prognostic factors in ependymoma. *Childs Nerv Syst* 7: 177-182.

1355. Schiffer D, Cravioto H, Giordana MT, Migheli A, Pezzulo T, Vigliani MC (1993). Is polar spongioblastoma a tumor entity? *J Neurosurg* 78: 587-591.

1356. Schiffer D, Dutto A, Cavalla P, Bosone I, Chio A, Villani R, Bellotti C (1997). Prognostic factors in oligodendroglioma. *Can J Neurol Sci* 24: 313-319.

1357. Schiffer D, Giordana MT, Mauro A, Migheli A (1984). GFAP, F VIII/RAg, laminin, and fibronectin in gliosarcomas: an immunohistochemical study. *Acta Neuropathol (Berl)* 63: 108-116.

1358. Schiffer D, Giordana MT, Pezzotta S, Pezzulo T, Vigliani MC (1992). Medullomyoblastoma: report of two cases. *Childs Nerv Syst* 8: 268-272.

1359. Schiffer J, Avidan D, Rapp A (1985). Posttraumatic meningioma. *Neurosurgery* 17: 84-87.

1360. Schifter T, Hoffman JM, Hanson MW, Boyko OB, Beam C, Paine S, Schold SC, Burger PC, Coleman RE (1993). Serial FDG-PET studies in the prediction of survival in patients with primary brain tumors. *J Comput Assist Tomogr* 17: 509-561.

1361. Schild SE, Scheithauer BW, Schomberg PJ, Hook CC, Kelly PJ, Frick L, Robinow JS, Buskirk SJ (1993). Pineal parenchymal tumors. Clinical, pathologic, and therapeutic aspects. *Cancer* 72: 870-880.

1362. Schlegel U (1994). [p53: an important or most overvalued tumor gene?]. *Laryngol Rhinol Otol* 73: 651-653.

1363. Schleiermacher G, Peter M, Michon J, Hugot JP, Vielh P, Zucker JM, Magdelenat H, Thomas G, Delattre O (1994). Two distinct deleted regions on the short arm of chromosome 1 in neuroblastoma. *Genes Chromosomes Cancer* 10: 275-281.

1364. Schlessinger J (1993). How receptor tyrosine kinase activate Ras. *Trends Biochem Sci* 18: 273-275.

1365. Schmidt EE, Ichimura K, Messerle KR, Goike HM, Collins VP (1997). Infrequent methylation of *CDKN2A(MTS1/p16)* and rare mutation of both *CDKN2A* and *CDKN2B(MTS2/p15)* in primary astrocytic tumours. *Br J Cancer* 75: 2-8.

1366. Schmidt EE, Ichimura K, Reifenberger G, Collins VP (1994). CDKN2 (p16/MTS1) gene deletion or CDK4 amplification occurs in the majority of glioblastomas. *Cancer Res* 54: 6321-6324.

1367. Schmitt HP (1983). Rapid anaplastic transformation in gliomas of adulthood. "Selection" in neuro-oncogenesis. *Pathol Res Pract* 176: 313-323.

1368. Schmitt HP (1983). Rapid anaplastic transformation of gliomas in childhood. *Neuropediatrics* 14: 137-143.

1369. Schneider BF, Shashi V, von Kap h, Golden WL (1995). Loss of chromosomes 22 and 14 in the malignant progression of meningiomas. A comparative study of fluorescence in situ hybridization (FISH) and standard cytogenetic analysis. *Cancer Genet Cytogenet* 85: 101-104.

1370. Schneider JH, Jr., Raffel C, McComb JG (1992). Benign cerebellar astrocytomas of childhood. *Neurosurgery* 30: 58-62.

1371. Schochet SS, Jr., Violett TW, Nelson J, Pelofsky S, Barnes PA (1984). Polar spongioblastoma of the cervical spinal cord: case report. *Clin Neuropathol* 3: 225-227.

1372. Schofield D, West DC, Anthony DC, Marshal R, Sklar J (1995). Correlation of loss of heterozygosity at chromosome 9q with histological subtype in medulloblastomas. *Am J Pathol* 146: 472-480.

1373. Schofield DE, Yunis EJ, Geyer JR, Albright AL, Berger MS, Taylor SR (1992). DNA content and other prognostic features in childhood medulloblastoma. Proposal of a scoring system. *Cancer* 69: 1307-1314.

1374. Schroder R, Bien K, Kott R, Meyers I, Vossing R (1991). The relationship between Ki-67 labeling and mitotic index in gliomas and meningiomas: demonstration of the variability of the intermitotic cycle time. *Acta Neuropathol (Berl)* 82: 389-394.

1375. Schroder R, Firsching R, Kochanek S (1986). Hemangiopericytoma of meninges. II. General and clinical data. *Zentralbl Neurochir* 47: 191-199.

1376. Schutz BR, Scheurlen W, Krauss J, du M, Joos S, Bentz M, Lichter P (1996). Mapping of chromosomal gains and losses in primitive neuroectodermal tumors by comparative genomic hybridization. *Genes Chromosomes Cancer* 16: 196-203.

1377. Schwab M, Alitalo K, Klempnauer KH, Varmus HE, Bishop JM, Gilbert F, Brodeur G, Goldstein M, Trent J (1983). Amplified DNA with limited homology to myc cellular oncogene is shared by human neuroblastoma cell lines and a neuroblastoma tumour. *Nature* 305: 245-248.

1378. Schwab M, Amler LC (1990). Amplification of cellular oncogenes: a predictor of clinical outcome in human cancer. *Genes Chromosomes Cancer* 1: 181-193.

1379. Schwab M, Corvi R, Amler LC (1995). N-*MYC* oncogene amplification: a consequence of genomic instability in human neuroblastoma. *The Neuroscientist* 1: 277-285.

1380. Schwab M, Praml C, Amler LC (1996). Genomic instability in 1p and human malignancies. *Genes Chromosomes Cancer* 16: 211-229.

1381. Schwab M, Varmus HE, Bishop JM, Grzeschik KH, Naylor SL, Sakaguchi AY, Brodeur G, Trent J (1984). Chromosome localization in normal human cells and neuroblastomas of a gene related to c-myc. *Nature* 308: 288-291.

1382. Segal RA, Goumnerova LC, Kwon YK, Stiles CD, Pomeroy SL (1994). Co-expression of neurotropin-3 and trk C linked to a more favorable outcome in medulloblastoma. *Proc Natl Acad Sci USA* 91: 12867-12871.

1383. Seizinger BR, Martuza RL, Gusella JF (1986). Loss of genes on chromosome 22 in tumorigenesis of human acoustic neuroma. *Nature* 322: 644-647.

1384. Seizinger BR, Rouleau GA, Ozelius LJ, Lane AH, Faryniarz AG, Chao MV, Huson S, Korf BR, Parry DM, Pericak V, Collins FS, Hobbs WJ, Falcone BG, Ianazzi JA, Roy JC, St, Tanzi RE, Bothwell MA, Upadhyaya M, Harper P, Goldstein AE, Hoover DL, Bader JL, Spence MA, Mulvihill JJ, Aylsworth AS, Vance JM, Rossenwasser GOD, Gaskell PC, Roses AD, Martuza RL, Breakefield XO, Gusella JF (1987). Genetic linkage of von Recklinghausen neurofibromatosis to the nerve growth factor receptor gene. *Cell* 49: 589-594.

1385. Selassie L, Rigotti R, Kepes JJ, Towfighi J (1994). Adipose tissue and smooth muscle in a primitive neuroectodermal tumor of cerebrum. *Acta Neuropathol (Berl)* 87: 217-222.

1386. Seppala MT, Haltia MJ, Sankila RJ, Jaaskelainen JE, Heiskanen O (1995). Long-term outcome after removal of spinal neurofibroma. *J Neurosurg* 82: 572-577.

1387. Serra A, Strain J, Ruyle S (1996). Desmoplastic cerebral astrocytoma of infancy: report and review of the imaging characteristics. *AJR Am J Roentgenol* 166: 1459-1461.

1388. Serrano M, Hannon GJ, Beach D (1993). A new regulatory motif in cell-cycle control causing specific inhibition of cyclin D/CDK4. *Nature* 336: 704-707.

1389. Serrano M, Lee HW, Chin L, Cordon-Cardo C, Beach D, De Phino RA (1996). Role of the INK4a locus in tumor suppression and cell mortality. *Cell* 85: 27-37.

1390. Shaffrey ME, Lanzino G, Lopes BS, Hessler RB, Kassel NF, VandenBerg SR (1996). Maturation of intracranial teratomas. Report of two cases. *J Neurosurg* 85: 672-676.

1391. Shah JP, Feghali J (1981). Esthesioneuroblastoma. *Am J Surg* 142: 456-458.

1392. Shah K, Nathanson N (1976). Human exposure to SV40: review and comment. *Am J Epidemiol* 103: 1-12.

1393. Shah KV (1995). Polyomaviruses. In: *Field's Virology,* Fields BN, Knipe DM, Howley PM (eds). Lippincott-Raven: Philadelphia. pp. 2027-2043.

1394. Shanley S, Ratcliffe J, Hockey A, Haan E, Oley C, Ravine D, Martin N, Wicking C, Chenevix T (1994). Nevoid basal cell carcinoma syndrome: review of 118 affected individuals. *Am J Med Genet* 50: 282-290.

1395. Shapiro S, Mealey J, Jr., Sartorius C (1989). Radiation-induced intracranial malignant gliomas. *J Neurosurg* 71: 77-82.

1396. Shaw EG, Evans RG, Scheithauer BW, Ilstrup DM, Earle JD (1986). Radiotherapeutic management of adult intraspinal ependymomas. *Int J Radiat Oncol Biol Phys* 12: 323-327.

1397. Shaw EG, Scheithauer BW, O'Fallon JR, Davis DH (1994). Mixed oligoastrocytomas: a survival and prognostic factor analysis. *Neurosurg* 34: 577-582.

1398. Shaw EG, Scheithauer BW, O'Fallon JR, Tazelaar HD, Davis DH (1992). Oligodendrogliomas: the Mayo Clinic experience. *J Neurosurg* 76: 428-434.

1399. Shein HM, Enders JF (1962). Transformation induced by simian virus 40 in human renal cell cultures. *Proc Natl Acad Sci USA* 48: 1164-1172.

1400. Shen MH, Harper PS, Upadhyaya M (1996). Molecular genetics of neurofibromatosis type 1 (NF1). *J Med Genet* 33: 2-17.

1401. Shen V, Chaparro M, Choi BH, Young R, Bernstein R (1990). Absence of isochromosome 12p in a pineal region malignant germ cell tumor. *Cancer Genet Cytogenet* 50: 153-160.

1402. Shepherd CW, Houser OW, Gomez MR (1995). MR findings in tuberous sclerosis complex and correlation with seizure development and mental impairment. *AJNR Am J Neuroradiol* 16: 149-155.

1403. Shepherd CW, Scheithauer BW, Gomez MR, Altermatt HJ, Katzmann JA (1991). Subependymal giant cell astrocytoma: a clinical, pathological, and flow cytometric study. *Neurosurgery* 28: 864-868.

1404. Shibuya M, Hoshino T, Ito S, Wacker MR, Prados MD, Davis RL, Wilson CB (1992). Meningiomas: clinical implications of a high proliferative potential determined by bromodeoxyuridine labeling. *Neurosurgery* 30: 494-497.

1405. Shimada H, Chatten J, Newton WA, Jr., Sachs N, Hamoudi AB, Chiba T, Marsden HB, Misugi K (1984). Histopathologic prognostic factors in neuroblastic tumors: definition of subtypes of ganglioneuroblastoma and an age-linked classification of neuroblastomas. *J Natl Cancer Inst* 73: 405-416.

1406. Shimada H, Stram DO, Chatten J, Joshi VV, Hachitanda Y, Brodeur GM, Lukens JN, Matthay KK, Seeger RC (1995). Identification of subsets of neuroblastomas by combined histopathologic and N-myc analysis. *J Natl Cancer Inst* 87: 1470-1476.

1407. Shimada Y, Kubo O, Tajika Y, Hiyama H, Atuji S,Takakura K (1997). Clinicopathological study of mixed oligoastrocytoma. In: *Brain Tumor Research and Therapy*, Nagai M (eds). Springer-Verlag: Tokyo. pp. 51-60.

1408. Shimizu KT, Tran LM, Mark RJ, Selch MT (1993). Management of oligodendrogliomas. *Radiology* 186: 569-572.

1409. Shin YM, Chang KH, Han MH, Myung NH, Chi JG, Cha SH, Han MC (1993). Gliomatosis cerebri: comparison of MR and CT features. *AJR Am J Roentgenol* 161: 859-862.

1410. Shinar Y, McMorris FA (1995). Developing oligodendroglia express mRNA for insulin-like growth factor-I, a regulator of oligodendrocyte development. *J Neurosci Res* 42: 516-527.

1411. Shiurba RA, Buffinger NS, Spencer EM, Urich H (1991). Basic fibroblast growth factor and somatomedin C in human medulloepithelioma. *Cancer* 68: 798-808.

1412. Short MP, Martuza RL,Huson SM (1994). Neurofibromatosis 2: clinical features, genetic counselling and management issues. In: *The Neurofibromatoses: a Pathogenetic and Clinical Overview*, Huson SM, Hughes RAC (eds). Chapman & Hall Medical: London. pp. 414-444.

1413. Short MP, Richardson EP, Jr., Haines JL, Kwiatkowski DJ (1995). Clinical, neuropathological and genetic aspects of the tuberous sclerosis complex. *Brain Pathol* 5: 173-179.

1414. Shuangshoti S, Kasantikul V, Suwanwela N (1987). Spontaneous penetretion of dura mater and bone by glioblastoma multiforme. *J Surg Oncol* 36: 36-44.

1415. Shuster D, Herrick M,Horoupian D (1994). Two unusual cases of central neurocytoma: a- concomitatntly occurring with fourth ventricular PNET, b- mixed with lipoma. *Brain Pathol* 4;433.

1416. Shweiki D, Itin A, Soffer D, Keshet E (1992). Vascular endothelial growth factor induced by hypoxia may mediate hypoxia-initiated angiogenesis. *Nature* 359: 843-845.

1417. Sidransky D, Mikkelsen T, Schwechheimer K, Rosenblum ML, Cavenee WK, Vogelstein B (1992). Clonal expansion of p53 mutant cells is associated with brain tumour progression. *Nature* 355: 846-847.

1418. Silver SA, Wiley JM, Perlman EJ (1994). DNA ploidy analysis of pediatric germ cell tumors. *Mod Pathol* 7: 951-956.

1419. Silverberg SG,Kurman RJ (1992). *Tumors of the Uterine Corpus and Gestational Trophoblastic Disease, Atlas of Tumor Pathology.* Armed Forces Institute of Pathology: Washington, DC.

1420. Silverman JF, Joshi VV (1994). FNA biopsy of small round cell tumors of childhood: cytomorphologic features and the role of ancillary studies. *Diagn Cytopathol* 10: 245-255.

1421. Simon M, Kokkino AJ, Warnick RE, Tew JM, Jr., von Deimling A, Menon AG (1996). Role of genomic instability in meningioma progression. *Genes Chromosomes Cancer* 16: 265-269.

1422. Simon M, von Deimling A, Larson JJ, Wellenreuther R, Kaskel P, Waha A, Warnick RW, Tew JM, Menon AG (1995). Allelic losses on chromosomes 14, 10, and 1 in atypical and malignant meningiomas: a genetic model of meningioma progression. *Cancer Res* 55: 4696-4701.

1423. Sklar CA (1994). Craniopharyngioma: endocrine abnormalities at presentation. *Pediatr Neurosurg* 21 Suppl 1: 18-20.

1424. Skullerud K, Stenwig AE, Brandtzaeg P, Nesland JM, Kerty E, Langmoen I, Saeter G (1995). Intracranial primary leiomyosarcoma arising in a teratoma of the pineal area. *Clin Neuropathol* 14: 245-248.

1425. Skuse GR, Kosciolek BA, Rowley PT (1989). Molecular genetic analysis of tumors in von Recklinghausen neurofibromatosis: loss of heterozygosity for chromosome 17. *Genes Chromosomes Cancer* 1: 36-41.

1426. Skuse GR, Kosciolek BA, Rowley PT (1991). The neurofibroma in von Recklinghausen neurofibromatosis has a unicellular origin. *Am J Hum Genet* 49: 600-607.

1427. Slavc I, MacCollin MM, Dunn M, Jones S, Sutton L, Gusella JF, Biegel JA (1995). Exon scanning for mutations of the NF2 gene in pediatric ependymomas, rhabdoid tumors and meningiomas. *Int J Cancer* 64: 243-247.

1428. Slowik F, Jellinger K (1990). Association of primary cerebral lymphoma with meningioma: report of two cases. *Clin Neuropathol* 9: 69-73.

1429. Slowik F, Jellinger K, Gaszo L, Fischer J (1985). Gliosarcomas: histological, immunohistochemical, ultrastructural, and tissue culture studies. *Acta Neuropathol (Berl)* 201-210.

1430. Smirniotopoulos JG, Rushing EJ, Mena H (1992). Pineal region masses: differential diagnosis. *Radiographics* 12: 577-596.

1431. Smith MT, Ludwig CL, Godfrey AD, Armbrustmacher VW (1983). Grading of oligodendrogliomas. *Cancer* 52: 2107-2114.

1432. Smith T, Davidson R (1984). Medullomyoblastoma. A histologic, immunohistochemical, and ultrastructural study. *Cancer* 54: 323-332.

1433. Smith WT, Hughes B, Ermocilla R (1966). Chemodectoma of the pineal region, with observations on the pineal body and chemoreceptor tissue. *J Pathol Bacteriol* 92: 69-76.

1434. Sneed PK, Prados MD, McDermott MW, Larson DA, Malec MK, Lamborn KR, Davis RL, Weaver KA, Wara WM, Phillips TL, Gutin PH (1995). Large effect of age on the survival of patients with glioblastoma treated with radiotherapy and brachytherapy boost. *Neurosurgery* 36: 898-904.

1435. Soffer D, Gomori JM, Pomeranz S, Siegal T (1990). Gliomas following low-dose irradiation to the head report of three cases. *J Neurooncol* 8: 67-72.

1436. Soffer D, Pittaluga S, Caine Y, Feinsod M (1983). Paraganglioma of cauda equina. A report of a case and review of the literature. *Cancer* 51: 1907-1910.

1437. Sonier CB, Feve JR, de Kersaint-Gilly A, Ruchuox MM, Rymer R, Auffray E (1992). Lhermitte-Duclos disease: a rare cause of intercranial hypertension in adults. *J Neuroradiol* 19: 133-138.

1438. Sonneland PR, Scheithauer BW, LeChago J, Crawford BG, Onofrio BM (1986). Paraganglioma of the cauda equina region. Clinicopathologic study of 31 cases with special reference to immunocytology and ultrastructure. *Cancer* 58: 1720-1735.

1439. Sonneland PR, Scheithauer BW, Onofrio BM (1985). Myxopapillary ependymoma. A clinicopathologic and immunocytochemical study of 77 cases. *Cancer* 56: 883-893.

1440. Sorensen PH, Wu JK, Berean KW, Lim JF, Donn W, Frierson HF, Reynolds CP, Lopez T, Triche TJ (1996). Olfactory neuroblastoma is a peripheral primitive neuroectodermal tumor related to Ewing sarcoma. *Proc Natl Acad Sci USA* 93: 1038-1043.

1441. Soylemezoglu F, Kleihues P, Esteve J, Scheithauer BW (1997). Atypical central neurocytoma. *J Neuropath Exp Neurol* 56: 551-556.

1442. Soylemezoglu F, Soffer D, Onol B, Schwechheimer K, Kleihues P (1996). Lipomatous medulloblastoma in adults: a distinct clinicopathological entity. *Am J Surg Pathol* 20: 413-418.

1443. Spaar FW, Blech M, Ahyai A (1986). DNA-flow fluorescence—cytometry of ependymomas. Report on ten surgically removed tumours. *Acta Neuropathol (Berl)* 69: 153-160.

1444. Sperner J, Gottschalk J, Neumann K, Schorner W, Lanksch WR, Scheffner D (1994). Clinical, radiological and histological findings in desmoplastic infantile ganglioglioma. *Childs Nerv Syst* 10: 458-462.

1445. Spiegel E (1920). Hyperplasie des Kleinhirns. *Beitr Path Anat* 67: 539-548.

1446. Srivastava S, Zou ZQ, Pirollo K, Blattner WA, Chang EH (1990). Germ-line transmission of a mutated p53 gene in a cancer-prone family with Li-Fraumeni syndrome. *Nature* 348: 747-749.

1447. Stanger BZ (1996). Looking beneath the surface: the cell death pathway of Fas/APO-1 (CD95). *Mol Med* 2: 7-20.

1448. Stangl AP, Wellenreuther R, Lenartz D, Kraus JA, Menon AG, Schramm J, Wiestler OD, von Deimling A (1997). Clonality of multiple meningioma. *J Neurosurg* 86: 853-858.

1449. Starink TM (1984). Cowden's disease: analysis of fourteen new cases. *J Am Acad Dermatol* 11: 1127-1141.

1450. Staufenbiel M, Deppert W (1983). Different structural systems of the nucleus are targets for SV40 large T antigen. *Cell* 33: 173-181.

1451. Steck PA, Pershouse MA, Jasser SA, Yung WKA, Lin H, Ligon AH, Langford LA, Baumgard ML, Hattier T, Davis T, Frye C, Hu R, Swedlund B, Teng DHF, Tavtigian SV (1997). Identification of a candidate tumour suppressor gene, *MMAC1*, at chromosome 10q23.3 that is mutated in multiple advanced cancers. *Nature Genet* 15: 356-362.

1452. Steeg PS, Bevilacqua G, Kopper L, Thorgeirsson UP, Talmadge JE, Liotta LA, Sobel ME (1988). Evidence for a novel gene associated with low tumor metastatic potential. *J Natl Cancer Inst* 80: 200-204.

1453. Steel TR, Dailey AT, Born D, Berger MS, Mayberg MR (1993). Paragangliomas of the sellar region: report of two cases. *Neurosurgery* 32: 844-847.

1454. Stefanko SZ, Vuzevski VD, Maas AI, van Vroonhoven CC (1986). Intracerebral malignant schwannoma. *Acta Neuropathol (Berl)* 71: 321-325.

1455. Steinberg GK, Shuer LM, Conley FK, Hanbery JW (1985). Evolution and outcome in malignant astroglial neoplasms of the cerebellum. *J Neurosurg* 62: 9-17.

1456. Steinbok P, Dolman CL, Kaan K (1977). Pineocytomas presenting as subarachnoid hemorrhage. Report of two cases. *J Neurosurg* 47: 776-780.

1457. Steinhoff H, Lanksch W, Kazner E (1977). Computed tomography in the diagnosis and differential diagnosis of glioblastomas. *Neuroradiology* 14: 193-200.

1458. Stemmer-Rachamimov AO, Horgan MA, Taratuto AL, Munoz DG, Smith TW, Frosch MP, Louis DN (1997). Meningioangiomatosis is associated with Neurofibromatosis 2 but not with somatic alterations of the *NF2* gene. *J Neuropathol Exp Neurol* 56: 485-489.

1459. Stern J, Jakobiec FA, Housepian EM (1980). The architecture of optic nerve gliomas with and without neurofibromatosis. *Arch Ophthalmol* 98: 505-511.

1460. Stone DM, Hynes M, Armanini M, Swanson TA, Gu Q, Johnson RL, Scott MP, Pennica D, Goddard A, Phillips H, Noll M, Hooper JE, de Sauvage F, Rosenthal A (1996). The tumour-suppressor gene patched encodes a candidate receptor for Sonic hedgehog. *Nature* 384: 129-134.

1461. Stout AP, Murray MR (1942). Hemangiopericytoma. A vascular tumor featuring Zimmermann's pericytes. *Ann Surg* 116: 26-33.

1462. Stratton MR, Darling J, Lantos PL, Cooper CS, Reeves BR (1989). Cytogenetic abnormalities in human ependymomas. *Int J Cancer* 44: 579-581.

1463. Stroebe H (1895). Uber Entstehung und Bau der Hirngliome. *Beitr Pathol Anat Allg Pathol* 18: 405-486.

1464. Stromblad LG, Anderson H, Malmstrom P, Salford LG (1993). Reoperation for malignant astrocytomas: personal experience and a review of the literature. *Br J Neurosurg* 7: 623-633.

1465. Strommer KN, Brandner S, Sarioglu AC, Sure U, Yonekawa Y (1995). Symptomatic cerebellar metastasis and late local recurrence of a cauda equina paraganglioma. Case report. *J Neurosurg* 83: 166-169.

1466. Stumpf DA, Alksne JF, Annegers JF (1988). Neurofibromatosis. NIH consensus development conference statement. *Arch Neurol* 45: 575-578.

1467. Sugawa N, Ekstrand AJ, James CD, Collins VP (1990). Identical splicing of aberrant epidermal growth factor receptor transcripts from amplified rearranged genes in human glioblastomas. *Proc Natl Acad Sci USA* 87: 8602-8606.

1468. Sugita Y, Kepes JJ, Shigemori M, Kuramoto S, Reifenberger G, Kiwit JC, Wechsler W (1990). Pleomorphic xanthoastrocytoma with desmoplastic reaction: angiomatous variant. Report of two cases. *Clin Neuropathol* 9: 271-278.

1469. Sun ZM, Genka S, Shitara N, Akanuma A, Takakura K (1988). Factors possibly influencing the prognosis of oligodendroglioma. *Neurosurgery* 22: 886-891.

1470. Sung CC, Collins R, Li J, Pearl DK, Coons SW, Scheithauer BW, Johnson PC, Yates AJ (1996). Glycolipids and myelin proteins in human oligodendrogliomas. *Glycoconj J* 13: 433-443.

1471. Sung JH, Mastri AR, Segal EL (1973). Melanotic medulloblastoma of the cerebellum. *J Neuropathol Exp Neurol* 32: 437-445.

1472. Suri C, Jones PF, Patan S, Bartunkova S, Maisonpierre PC, Davis S, Sato TN, Yancopoulos GD (1996). Requisite role of angiopoietin-1, a ligand for the TIE2 receptor, during embryonic angiogenesis. *Cell* 87: 1171-1180.

1473. Swanson PE, Lillemoe TJ, Manivel JC, Wick MR (1990). Mesenchymal chondrosarcoma. An immunohistochemical study. *Arch Pathol Lab Med* 114: 943-948.

1474. Swarz JR, Del Cerro M (1977). Lack of evidence for glial cells originating from the external granular layer in mouse cerebellum. *J Neurocytol* 6: 241-250.

1475. Szeifert GT, Pasztor E (1993). Could craniopharyngiomas produce pituitary hormones? *Neurol Res* 15: 68-69.

1476. Tabuchi K, Moriya Y, Furuta T, Ohnishi R, Nishimoto A (1982). S-100 protein in human glial tumours. Qualitative and quantitative studies. *Acta Neurochir Wien* 65: 239-251.

1477. Tachibana O, Lampe K, Kleihues P, Ohgaki H (1996). Preferential expression of Fas/APO1 (CD95) and apoptotic cell death in perinecrotic cells of the glioblastoma multiforme. *Acta Neuropathol* 92: 431-434.

1478. Tachibana O, Yamashima T, Yamashita J, Takabatake Y (1994). Immunohistochemical expression of human chorionic gonadotropin and P-glycoprotein in human pituitary glands and craniopharyngiomas. *J Neurosurg* 80: 79-84.

1479. Tada T, Katsuyama T, Aoki T (1987). Mixed glioblastoma and sarcoma with osteoid-chondral tissue. *Clin Neuropathol* 6: 160-163.

1480. Taguchi Y, Sakurai T, Takamori I, Sekino H, Tadokoro M (1993). Desmoplastic infantile ganglioglioma with extraparenchymatous cyst—case report. *Neurol Med Chir Tokyo* 33: 177-180.

1481. Takeda O, Homma C, Maseki N, Sakurai M, Kanda N, Schwab M, Nakamura Y, Kaneko Y (1994). There may be two tumor suppressor genes on chromosome arm 1p closely associated with biologically distinct subtypes of neuroblastoma. *Genes Chromosomes Cancer* 10: 30-39.

1482. Takei Y, Mirra SS, Miles ML (1976). Eosinophilic granular cells in oligodendrogliomas. An ultrastructural study. *Cancer* 38: 1968-1976.

1483. Tanaka K, Waga S, Itho H, Shimizu DM, Namiki H (1989). Superficial location of malignant glioma with heavily lipidized (foamy) tumor cells: a case report. *J Neurooncol* 7: 293-297.

1484. Tanaka M, Suda M, Ishikawa Y, Fujitake J, Fuji H, Tatsuoka Y (1996). Idiopathic hypertrophic cranial pachymeningitis associated with hydrocephalus and myocarditis: remarkable steroid-induced remission of hypertrophic dura mater. *Neurology* 46: 554-556.

1485. Tanaka T, Hiyama E, Sugimoto T, Sawada T, Tanabe M, Ida N (1995). trk A gene expression in neuroblastoma. The clinical significance of an immunohistochemical study. *Cancer* 76: 1086-1095.

1486. Taratuto AL, Molina HA, Diez B, Zuccaro G, Monges J (1985). Primary rhabdomyosarcoma of brain and cerebellum. Report of four cases in infants: an immunohistochemical study. *Acta Neuropathol (Berl)* 66: 98-104.

1487. Taratuto AL, Monges J, Lylyk P,Leiguarda R (1982). Meningocerebral astrocytoma attached to dura with "desmoplastic" reaction. *Proceedings of the IX International Congress of Neuropathology (Viena)* 5-10.

1488. Taratuto AL, Monges J, Lylyk P, Leiguarda R (1984). Superficial cerebral astrocytoma attached to dura. Report of six cases in infants. *Cancer* 54: 2505-2512.

1489. Taratuto AL, Pomata H, Sevlever G, Gallo G, Monges J (1995). Dysembryoplastic neuroepithelial tumor: morphological, immunocytochemical, and deoxyribonucleic acid analyses in a pediatric series. *Neurosurgery* 36: 474-481.

1490. Taratuto AL, Sevlever G,Schultz M (1987). Monoclonal antibodies in superficial desmoplastic cerebral astrocytoma attached to dura in infants. *J Neuropathol Exp Neurol* 46;395-395.

1491. Taratuto AL, Sevlever G, Schultz M, Gutierrez M, Monges J,Sanchez M (1994). Desmoplastic cerebral astrocytoma of infancy (DCAI). Survival data of the original series and report of two additional cases, DNA, kinetic and molecular genetic studies. *Brain Pathol* 4;423.

1492. Taruscio D, Danesi R, Montaldi A, Cerasoli S, Cenacchi G, Giangaspero F (1997). Nonrandom gain of chromosome 7 in central neurocytoma: a chromosomal analysis and fluorescence in situ hybridization study. *Virchows Arch* 430: 47-51.

1493. Tatagiba M, Samii M, Dankoweit T, Aguiar PH, Osterwald L, Babu R, Ostertag H (1995). Esthesioneuroblastomas with intracranial extension. Proliferative potential and management. *Arq Neuropsiquiatr* 53: 577-586.

1494. Tatter SB, Borges LF, Louis DN (1994). Central neurocytomas of the cervical spinal cord. Report of two cases. *J Neurosurg* 81: 288-293.

1495. Tenreiro P, Kamath SV, Knorr JR, Ragland RL, Smith TW, Lau KY (1995). Desmoplastic infantile ganglioglioma: CT and MRI features. *Pediatr Radiol* 25: 540-543.

1496. Thapar K, Stefaneanu L, Kovacs K, Scheithauer BW, Lloyd RV, Muller PJ, Laws ER, Jr. (1994). Estrogen receptor gene expression in craniopharyngiomas: an in situ hybridization study. *Neurosurgery* 35: 1012-1017.

1497. Lymphoma TN-H (1982). National Cancer Institute sponsored study of classifications of non-Hodgkin's lymphomas: summary and description of a working formulation for clinical usage. *Cancer* 49: 2112-2135.

1498. The I, Murthy AE, Hannigan GE, Jacoby LB, Menon AG, Gusella JF, Bernards A (1993). Neurofibromatosis type 1 gene mutations in neuroblastoma. *Nat Genet* 3: 62-66.

1499. Thiel G, Losanowa T, Kintzel D, Nisch G, Martin H, Vorpahl K, Witkowski R (1992). Karyotypes in 90 human gliomas. *Cancer Genet Cytogenet* 58: 109-120.

1500. Thomas A, El Rouby S, Reed JC, Krajewski S, Silber R, Potmesil M, Newcomb EW (1996). Drug-induced apoptosis in B-cell chronic lymphocytic leukemia: relationship between p53 gene mutation and bcl-2/bax proteins in drug resistance. *Oncogene* 12: 1055-1062.

1501. Thomas PK, King RH, Chiang TR, Scaravilli F, Sharma AK, Downie AW (1990). Neurofibromatous neuropathy. *Muscle Nerve* 13: 93-101.

1502. Tice H, Barnes PD, Goumnerova L, Scott RM, Tarbell NJ (1993). Pediatric and adolescent oligodendrogliomas. *AJNR Am J Neuroradiol* 14: 1293-1300.

1503. Tohma Y, Gratas C, Van Meir EG, Desbaillets I, Tenan M, Tachibana O, Kleihues P, Ohgaki H (1998). Necrogenesis and Fas/APO-1(CD95) expression in primary (*de novo*) and secondary glioblastomas. *J Neuropath Exp Neurol* 57: 239-245.

1504. Tohyama T, Lee VM, Rorke LB, Marvin M, McKay RD, Trojanowski JQ (1992). Nestin expression in embryonic human neuroepithelium and in human neuroepithelial tumor cells. *Lab Invest* 66: 303-313.

1505. Tominaga T, Kayama T, Kumabe T, Sonoda Y, Yoshimoto T (1995). Anaplastic ependymomas: clinical features and tumour suppressor gene p53 analysis. *Acta Neurochir Wien* 135: 163-170.

1506. Tomita T, Yasue M, Engelhard HH, McLone DG, Gonzalez C, Bauer KD (1988). Flow cytometric DNA analysis of medulloblastoma. Prognostic implication of aneuploidy. *Cancer* 61: 744-749.

1507. Tomlinson FH, Jenkins RB, Scheithauer BW, Keelan PA, Ritland S, Parisi JE, Cunningham J, Olsen KD (1994). Aggressive medulloblastoma with high-level N-myc amplification. *Mayo Clin Proc* 69: 359-365.

1508. Tomlinson FH, Scheithauer BW, Hayostek CJ, Parisi JE, Meyer FB, Shaw EG, Weiland TL, Katzmann JA, Jack CR, Jr. (1994). The significance of atypia and histologic malignancy in pilocytic astrocytoma of the cerebellum: a clinicopathologic and flow cytometric study. *J Child Neurol* 9: 301-310.

1509. Torp SH, Helseth E, Dalen A, Unsgaard G (1992). Relationships between Ki-67 labelling index, amplification of the epidermal growth factor receptor gene, and prognosis in human glioblastomas. *Acta Neurochir Wien* 117: 182-186.

1510. Torres CF, Korones DN, Pilcher W (1997). Multiple ependymomas in a patient with Turcot's syndrome. *Med Pediatr Oncol* 28: 59-61.

1511. Toyota B, Barr HW, Ramsay D (1993). Hemodynamic activity associated with a paraganglioma of the cauda equina. Case report. *J Neurosurg* 79: 451-455.

1512. Treip CS (1957). A congenital medulloepithelioma of the midbrain. *J Path Bact* 74: 357-363.

1513. Tresser N, Parveen T, Roessmann U (1993). Intracranial lipomas with teratomatous elements. *Arch Pathol Lab Med* 117: 918-920.

1514. Trofatter JA, MacCollin MM, Rutter JL, Murrell JR, Duyao MP, Parry DM, Eldridge R, Kley N, Menon AG, Pulaski K (1993). A novel moesin-, ezrin-, radixin-like gene is a candidate for the neurofibromatosis 2 tumor suppressor. *Cell* 72: 791-800.

1515. Trojanowski JQ, Tascos NA, Rorke LB (1982). Malignant pineocytoma with prominent papillary features. *Cancer* 50: 1789-1793.

1516. Trojanowski JQ, Tohyama T, Lee VM (1992). Medulloblastomas and related primitive neuroectodermal brain tumors of childhood recapitulate molecular milestones in the maturation of neuroblasts. *Mol Chem Neuropathol* 17: 121-135.

1517. Troost D, Jansen GH, Dingemans KP (1990). Cerebral medulloepithelioma—electron microscopy and immunohistochemistry. *Acta Neuropathol (Berl)* 80: 103-107.

1518. Truwit CL, Barkovich AJ (1990). Pathogenesis of intracranial lipoma: an MR study in 42 patients. *AJR Am J Roentgenol* 155: 855-864.

1519. Tsang RW, Laperriere NJ, Simpson WJ, Brierley J, Panzarella T, Smyth HS (1993). Glioma arising after radiation therapy for pituitary adenoma. A report of four patients and estimation of risk. *Cancer* 72: 2227-2233.

1520. Tsuchida T, Matsumoto M, Shirayama Y, Imahori T, Kasai H, Kawamoto K (1996). Neuronal and glial characteristics of central neurocytoma: electron microscopical analysis of two cases. *Acta Neuropathol* 91: 573-577.

1521. Tsuda T, Obara M, Hirano H, Gotoh S, Kubomura S, Higashi K, Kuroiwa A, Nakagawara A, Nagahara N, Shimizu K (1987). Analysis of N-myc amplification in relation to disease stage and histologic types in human neuroblastomas. *Cancer* 60: 820-826.

1522. Tsumanuma I, Sato M, Okazaki H, Tanaka R, Washiyama K, Kawasaki T, Kumanishi T (1995). The analysis of p53 tumor suppressor gene in pineal parenchymal tumors. *Noshuyo Byori* 12: 39-43.

1523. Tsunoda S, Sasaoka Y, Sakaki T,

Morimoto T, Hiramatsu K, Kawaguchi S, Ishida Y, Goda K (1993). Suprasellar embryonal carcinoma which developed ten years after local radiation therapy for pineal germinoma. *Surg Neurol* 40: 146-150.

1524. Turcot J, Despres JP, St (1959). Malignant tumors of the central nervous system associated with familial polyposis of the colon. *Dis Colon Rectum* 2: 465-468.

1525. Ueki K, Ono Y, Henson JW, Efird JT, von Deimling A, Louis DN (1996). CDKN2/p16 or RB alterations occur in the majority of glioblastomas and are inversely correlated. *Cancer Res* 56: 150-153.

1526. Uematsu Y, Tsuura Y, Miyamoto K, Itakura T, Hayashi S, Komai N (1992). The recurrence of primary intracranial germinomas. Special reference to germinoma with STGC (syncytiotrophoblastic giant cell). *J Neurooncol* 13: 247-256.

1527. Uematsu Y, Yukawa S, Yokote H, Itakura T, Hayashi S, Komai N (1992). Meningeal melanocytoma: magnetic resonance imaging characteristics and pathological features. Case report. *J Neurosurg* 76: 705-709.

1528. Uhm JH, Dooley NP, Villemure JG, Yong VW (1997). Mechanisms of glioma invasion: role of matrix metalloproteinases. *Can J Neurol Sci* 24: 3-15.

1529. Ullrich A, Coussens L, Hayflick JS, Dull TJ, Gray A, Tam AW, Lee J, Yarden Y, Libermann TA, Schlessinger J (1984). Human epidermal growth factor receptor cDNA sequence and aberrant expression of the amplified gene in A431 epidermoid carcinoma cells. *Nature* 309: 418-425.

1530. Unden AB, Holmberg E, Lundh R, Stahle B, Zaphiropoulos PG, Toftgard R, Vorechovsky I (1996). Mutations in the human homologue of Drosophila patched (PTCH) in basal cell carcinomas and the Gorlin syndrome: different in vivo mechanisms of PTCH inactivation. *Cancer Res* 56: 4562-4565.

1531. Vagner C, Zattara C, Gambarelli D, Gentet JC, Genitori L, Lena G, Graziani N, Raybaud C, Choux M, Grisoli F (1994). Detection of i(17q) chromosome by fluorescent in situ hybridization (FISH) with interphase nuclei in medulloblastoma. *Cancer Genet Cytogenet* 78: 1-6.

1532. Vajtai I, Varga Z, Aguzzi A (1996). MIB-1 immunoreactivity reveals different labelling in low-grade and in malignant epithelial neoplasms of the choroid plexus. *Histopathology* 29: 147-151.

1533. Valtz NL, Hayes TE, Norregaard T, Liu SM, McKay RD (1991). An embryonic origin for medulloblastoma. *New Biol* 3: 364-371.

1534. van der Drift P, Chan A, Laureys G, van Roy N, Sickmann G, den Dunnen J, Westerveld A, Speleman F, Versteeg R (1995). Balanced translocation in a neuroblastoma patient disrupts a cluster of small nuclear RNA U1 and tRNA genes in chromosomal band 1p36. *Genes Chromosomes Cancer* 14: 35-42.

1535. Van Meir EG, Kikuchi T, Tada M, Li H, Diserens AC, Wojcik BE, Huang HJ, Friedmann T, de Tribolet N, Cavenee WK (1994). Analysis of the p53 gene and its expression in human glioblastoma cells. *Cancer Res* 54: 649-652.

1536. Van Meir EG, Polverini PJ, Chazin VR, Su H, de Tribolet N, Cavenee WK (1994). Release of an inhibitor of angiogenesis upon induction of wild type *p53* expression in glioblastoma cells. *Nat Genet* 8: 171-176.

1537. Van Meir EG, Roemer K, Diserens AC, Kikuchi T, Rempel SA, Haas M, Huang HJ, Friedmann T, de Tribolet N, Cavenee WK (1995). Single cell monitoring of growth arrest and morphological changes induced by transfer of wild-type p53 alleles to glioblastoma cells. *Proc Natl Acad Sci USA* 92: 1008-1012.

1538. van Meyel DJ, Ramsay DA, Casson AG, Keeney M, Chambers AF, Cairncross JG (1994). p53 mutation, expression, and DNA ploidy in evolving gliomas: evidence for two pathways of progression. *J Natl Cancer Inst* 86: 1011-1017.

1539. VandenBerg SR (1991). Desmoplastic infantile ganglioglioma: a clinicopathologic review of sixteen cases. *Brain Tumor Pathol* 8: 25-31.

1540. VandenBerg SR (1992). Current diagnostic concepts of astrocytic tumors. *J Neuropathol Exp Neurol* 51: 644-657.

1541. VandenBerg SR (1993). Desmoplastic infantile ganglioglioma and desmoplastic cerebral astrocytoma of infancy. *Brain Pathol* 3: 275-281.

1542. VandenBerg SR, Herman MM, Rubinstein LJ (1987). Embryonal central neuroepithelial tumors: current concepts and future challenges. *Cancer Metastasis Rev* 5: 343-365.

1543. VandenBerg SR, May EE, Rubinstein LJ, Herman MM, Perentes E, Vinores SA, Collins VP, Park TS (1987). Desmoplastic supratentorial neuroepithelial tumors of infancy with divergent differentiation potential ("desmoplastic infantile gangliogliomas"). Report on 11 cases of a distinctive embryonal tumor with favorable prognosis. *J Neurosurg* 66: 58-71.

1544. Vandewalle G, Brucher JM, Michotte A (1995). Intracranial facial nerve rhabdomyoma. Case report. *J Neurosurg* 83: 919-922.

1545. Vaquero J, Coca S, Martinez R, Escandon J (1990). Papillary pineocytoma. Case report. *J Neurosurg* 73: 135-137.

1546. Vaquero J, Ramiro J, Martinez R, Bravo G (1992). Neurosurgical experience with tumours of the pineal region at Clinica Puerta de Hierro. *Acta Neurochir Wien* 116: 23-32.

1547. Varga Z, Vajtai I, Marino S, Schauble B, Yonekawa Y, Aguzzi A (1996). Tubular adenoma of the choroid plexus: evidence for glandular differentiation of the neuroepithelium. *Pathol Res Pract* 192: 840-844.

1548. Vartanian RK (1996). Olfactory neuroblastoma: an immunohistochemical, ultrastructural, and flow cytometric study. *Cancer* 77: 1957-1959.

1549. Venter DJ, Thomas DG (1991). Multiple sequential molecular abnormalities in the evolution of human gliomas. *Br J Cancer* 63: 753-757.

1550. Versari P, Talamonti G, D'Aliberti G, Fontana R, Colombo N, Casadei G (1994). Leptomeningeal dissemination of juvenile pilocytic astrocytoma: case report. *Surg Neurol* 41: 318-321.

1551. Vertosick FT, Jr., Selker RG, Grossman SJ, Joyce JM (1994). Correlation of thallium-201 single photon emission computed tomography and survival after treatment failure in patients with glioblastoma multiforme. *Neurosurgery* 34: 396-401.

1552. Vincent S, Turque N, Plaza S, Dhellemmes P, Hladky JP, Assaker R, Ruchuox MM, Saule S (1996). Differential expression between PAX-6 and on proteins in medulloblastoma. *Int J Oncol* 8: 901.

1553. Vinchon M, Blond S, Lejeune JP, Krivosik I, Fossati P, Assaker R, Christiaens JL (1994). Association of Lhermitte-Duclos and Cowden disease: report of a new case and review of the literature. *J Neurol Neurosurg Psychiatry* 57: 699-704.

1554. Virchow R (1863). *Die Krankhaften Geschwulste.* Hirschwald: Berlin.

1555. Viskochil D,Carey JC (1994). Alternate and related forms of the neurofibromatoses. In: *The Neurofibromatoses*, Huson SM (eds). Chapman and Hall Medical: London. pp. 445-474.

1556. Vital A, Vital C, Martin N, McGrogan G, Bioulac P, Trojani M, Loiseau H, Rougier A (1994). Lhermitte-Duclos type cerebellum hamartoma and Cowden disease. *Clin Neuropathol* 13: 229-231.

1557. Voges J, Sturm V, Lehrke R, Treuer H, Gauss C, Berthold F (1997). Cystic craniopharyngioma: long-term results after intracavitary irradiation with stereotactilly applied colloidal beta-emitting radioactive sources. *Neurosurgery* 35: 1001-1010.

1558. von Deimling A, Bender B, Jahnke R, Waha A, Kraus J, Albrecht S, Wellenreuther R, Fassbender F, Nagel J, Menon AG, Louis DN, Lenartz D, Schramm J, Wiestler OD (1994). Loci associated with malignant progression in astrocytomas: a candidate on chromosome 19q[1]. *Cancer Res* 54: 1397-1401.

1559. von Deimling A, Eibl RH, Ohgaki H, Louis DN, von Ammon K, Petersen I, Kleihues P, Chung RY, Wiestler OD, Seizinger BR (1992). p53 mutations are associated with 17p allelic loss in grade II and grade III astrocytoma. *Cancer Res* 52: 2987-2990.

1560. von Deimling A, Janzer R, Kleihues P, Wiestler OD (1990). Patterns of differentiation in central neurocytoma. An immunohistochemical study of eleven biopsies. *Acta Neuropathol (Berl)* 79: 473-479.

1561. von Deimling A, Kleihues P, Saremaslani P, Yasargil MG, Spoerri O, Sudhof TC, Wiestler OD (1991). Histogenesis and differentiation potential of central neurocytomas. *Lab Invest* 64: 585-591.

1562. von Deimling A, Kraus JA, Stangl AP, Wellenreuther R, Lenartz D, Schramm J, Louis DN, Ramesh V, Gusella JF, Wiestler OD (1995). Evidence for subarachnoid spread in the development of multiple meningiomas. *Brain Pathol* 5: 11-14.

1563. von Deimling A, Louis DN, Menon AG, von Ammon K, Petersen I, Ellison D, Wiestler OD, Seizinger BR (1993). Deletions on the long arm of chromosome 17 in pilocytic astrocytoma. *Acta Neuropathol (Berl)* 86: 81-85.

1564. von Deimling A, Louis DN, von Ammon K, Petersen I, Hoell T, Chung RY, Martuza RL, Schoenfeld DA, Yasargil MG, Wiestler OD, Seizinger BR (1992). Association of epidermal growth factor receptor gene amplification with loss of chromosome 10 in human glioblastoma multiforme. *J Neurosurg* 77: 295-301.

1565. von Deimling A, Louis DN, von Ammon K, Petersen I, Wiestler OD, Seizinger BR (1992). Evidence for a tumor suppressor gene on chromosome 19q associated with human astrocytomas, oligodendrogliomas, and mixed gliomas. *Cancer Res* 52: 4277-4279.

1566. von Deimling A, Louis DN, Wiestler OD (1995). Molecular pathways in the formation of gliomas. *Glia* 15: 328-338.

1567. von Deimling A, von Ammon K, Schoenfeld D, Wiestler OD, Seizinger BR, Louis DN (1993). Subsets of glioblastoma multiforme defined by molecular genetic analysis. *Brain Pathol* 3: 19-26.

1568. von Haken MS, White EC, Daneshvar S, Sih S, Choi E, Kalra R, Cogen PH (1996). Molecular genetic analysis of chromosome arm 17p and chromosome arm 22q DNA sequences in sporadic pediatric ependymomas. *Genes Chromosomes Cancer* 17: 37-44.

1569. von Hippel E (1904). Uber eine sehr seltene Erkrankung der Netzhaut. *Graefe's Arch* 59: 83-86.

1570. Vowels MR, Tobias V, Mameghan H (1991). Second intracranial neoplasms following treatment of childhood acute lymphoblastic leukemia. *J Paediatr Chil Health* 27: 43-46.

1571. Vuorinen V, Sallinen P, Haapasalo H, Visakorpi T, Kallio M, Jaaskelainen J (1996). Outcome of 31 intracranial hemangiopericytomas: poor predictive value of cell proliferation indices. *Acta Neurochir* 138: 1399-1408.

1572. Wacker MR, Cogen PH, Etzell JE, Daneshvar L, Davis RL, Prados MD (1992). Diffuse leptomeningeal involvement by a ganglioglioma in a child. Case report. *J Neurosurg* 77: 302-306.

1573. Wakai S, Segawa H, Kitahara S, Asano T, Sano K, Ogihara R, Tomita S (1980). Teratoma in the pineal region in two brothers. Case reports. *J Neurosurg* 53: 239-243.

1574. Wakimoto H, Aoyagi M, Nakayama T, Nagashima G, Yamamoto S, Tamaki M, Hirakawa K (1996). Prognostic significance of Ki-67 labeling indices obtained using MIB-1 monoclonal antibody in patients with supratentorial astrocytomas. *Cancer* 77: 373-380.

1575. Wales MM, Biel MA, El Deiry W, Nelkin BD, Issa JP, Cavenee WK, Kuerbitz SJ, Baylin SB (1995). p53 activates expression of HIC-1, a new candidate tumour suppressor gene on 17p13.3. *Nat Med* 1: 570-577.

1576. Walker AE, Robins M, Weinfeld FD (1985). Epidemiology of brain tumors: the national survey of intracranial neoplasms. *Neurology* 35: 219-226.

1577. Walton BJ, Morain WD, Baughman RD, Jordan A, Crichlow RW (1986). Cowden's disease: a further indication for prophylactic mastectomy. *Surgery* 99: 82-86.

1578. Wang JL, Zhang ZJ, Hartman M, Smits A, Westermark B, Muhr C, Nister M (1995). Detection of TP53 gene mutation in human meningiomas: a study using immunohistochemistry, polymerase chain reaction/ single- strand conformation polymorphism and DNA sequencing techniques on paraffin-embedded samples. *Int J Cancer* 64: 223-228.

1579. Warneford SG, Witton LJ, Townsend ML, Rowe PB, Reddel PR, Dalla P, Symonds G (1992). Germ-line splicing mutation of the *p53* gene in a cancer-prone family. *Cell Growth Differ* 3: 839-846.

1580. Warnick RE, Raisanen J, Adornato BT, Prados MD, Davis RL, Larson DA, Gutin PH (1993). Intracranial myxopapillary ependymoma: case report. *J Neurooncol* 15: 251-

256.

1581. Wasdahl DA, Scheithauer BW, Andrews BT, Jeffrey RA, Jr. (1994). Cerebellar pleomorphic xanthoastrocytoma: case report. *Neurosurgery* 35: 947-950.

1582. Washiyama K, Muragaki Y, Rorke LB, Lee VM, Feinstein SC, Radeke MJ, Blumberg D, Kaplan DR, Trojanowski JQ (1996). Neurotrophin and neurotrophin receptor proteins in medulloblastomas and other primitive neuroectodermal tumors of the pediatric central nervous system. *Am J Pathol* 148: 929-940.

1583. Watanabe K, Ando Y, Iwanaga H, Ochiai C, Nagai M, Okada K, Watanabe N (1995). Choroid plexus papilloma containing melanin pigment. *Clin Neuropathol* 14: 159-161.

1584. Watanabe K, Ogata N, von Ammon K, Yonekawa Y, Nagai M, Ohgaki H, Kleihues P (1996). Immunohistochemical assessments of P53 protein accumulation and tumor growth fraction during the progression of astrocytomas. In: *Brain Tumour Research and Therapy*, Nagai M (eds). Springer-Verlag: Tokyo. pp. 255-262.

1585. Watanabe K, Sato K, Biernat W, Tachibana O, von Ammon K, Ogata N, Yonekawa Y, Kleihues P, Ohgaki H (1997). Incidence and timing of *p53* mutations during astrocytoma progression in patients with multiple biopsies. *Clin Cancer Res* 3: 523-530.

1586. Watanabe K, Tachibana O, Sato K, Yonekawa Y, Kleihues P, Ohgaki H (1996). Overexpression of the EGF receptor and *p53* mutations are mutually exclusive in the evolution of primary and secondary glioblastomas. *Brain Pathol* 6: 217-224.

1587. Watanabe K, Tachibana O, Yonekawa Y, Kleihues P, Ohgaki H (1997). Role of gemistocytes in astrocytoma progression. *Lab Invest* 76: 277-284.

1588. Watanabe T, Makiyama Y, Nishimoto H, Matsumoto M, Kikuchi A, Tsubokawa T (1995). Metachronous ovarian dysgerminoma after a suprasellar germ-cell tumor treated by radiation therapy. Case report. *J Neurosurg* 83: 149-153.

1589. Weary PE, Gorlin RJ, Gentry WC, Jr., Comer JE, Greer KE (1972). Multiple hamartoma syndrome (Cowden's disease). *Arch Dermatol* 106: 682-690.

1590. Weber RG, Sabel M, Reifenberger J, Sommer C, Oberstrasse J, Reifenberger G, Kiessling M, Cremer T (1996). Characterization of genomic alterations associated with glioma progression by comparative genomic hybridization. *Oncogene* 13: 983-994.

1591. Wechsler W, Kleihues P, Matsumoto S, Zulch KJ, Ivankovic S, Preussmann R, Druckrey H (1969). Pathology of experimental neurogenic tumors chemically induced during prenatal and postnatal life. *Ann N Y Acad Sci* 159: 360-408.

1592. Weeks DA, Beckwith JB, Mierau GW, Luckey DW (1989). Rhabdoid tumor of kidney. A report of 111 cases from the National Wilms' Tumor Study Pathology Center. *Am J Surg Pathol* 13: 439-458.

1593. Weindel K, Moringlane JR, Marme D, Weich HA (1994). Detection and quantification of vascular endothelial growth factor/vascular permeability factor in brain tumor tissue and cyst fluid:The key to angiogenesis? *Neurosurgery* 35: 439-449.

1594. Weiner HL, Wisoff JH, Rosenberg ME, Kupersmith MJ, Cohen H, Zagzag D, Shiminski M, Flamm ES, Epstein FJ, Miller DC (1994). Craniopharyngiomas: a clinicopathological analysis of factors predictive of recurrence and functional outcome. *Neurosurgery* 35: 1001-1010.

1595. Weiner HL, Zagzag D, Babu R, Weinreb HJ, Ransohoff J (1993). Schwannoma of the fourth ventricle presenting with hemifacial spasm. A report of two cases. *J Neurooncol* 15: 37-43.

1596. Weinstein JN, Myers TG, O'Connor PM, Friend SH, Fornace AJ, Jr., Kohn KW, Fojo T, Bates SE, Rubinstein LV, Anderson NL, Buolamwini JK, van Osdol WW, Monks AP, Scudiero DA, Sausville EA, Zaharevitz DW, Bunow B, Viswanadhan VN, Johnson GS, Wittes RE, Paull KD (1997). An information-intensive approach to the molecular pharmacology of cancer. *Science* 275: 343-349.

1597. Weiss SW, Langloss JM, Enzinger FM (1983). Value of S-100 protein in the diagnosis of soft tissue tumors with particular reference to benign and malignant Schwann cell tumors. *Lab Invest* 49: 299-308.

1598. Weith A, Martinsson T, Cziepluch C, Bruderlein S, Amler LC, Berthold F, Schwab M (1989). Neuroblastoma consensus deletion maps to 1p36.1-2. *Genes Chromosomes Cancer* 1: 159-166.

1599. Weldon-Linne GM, Victor TA, Groothuis DR, Vick NA (1983). Pleomorphic xanthoastrocytoma: ultrastructural and immunohistochemical study of a case with a rapidly fatal outcome following surgery. *Cancer* 52: 2055-2063.

1600. Wellenreuther R, Kraus JA, Lenartz D, Menon AG, Schramm J, Louis DN, Ramesh V, Gusella JF, Wiestler OD, von Deimling A (1995). Analysis of the neurofibromatosis 2 gene reveals molecular variants of meningioma. *Am J Pathol* 146: 827-832.

1601. Weller M, Malipiero U, Aguzzi A, Reed JC, Fontana A (1995). Protooncogene *bcl-2* gene transfer abrogates Fas/APO-1 antibody-mediated apoptosis of human malignant glioma cells and confers resistance to chemotherapeutic drugs and therapeutic irradiation. *J Clin Invest* 95: 2633-2643.

1602. Weller M, Malipiero U, Rensing-Ehl A, Barr PJ, Fontana A (1995). Fas/APO-1 gene transfer for human malignant glioma. *Cancer Res* 55: 2936-2944.

1603. Weller RO (1990). *Nervous System, Muscle and Eyes.* 3rd ed, Churchill Livingstone: Edinburgh.

1604. Wells GB, Lasner TM, Yousem DM, Zager EL (1994). Lhermitte-Duclos disease and Cowden's syndrome in an adolescent patient. Case report. *J Neurosurg* 81: 133-136.

1605. Wen PY, Alexander E, Black PM, Fine HA, Riese N, Levin JM, Coleman CN, Loeffler JS (1994). Long term results of stereotactic brachytherapy used in the initial treatment of patients with glioblastomas. *Cancer* 73: 3029-3036.

1606. Wenzel A, Schwab M (1995). The mycN/max protein complex in neuroblastoma. Short review. *Eur J Cancer* 31A: 516-519.

1607. Werner MH, Phuphanich S, Lyman GH (1995). The increasing incidence of malignant gliomas and primary central nervous system lymphoma in the elderly. *Cancer* 76: 1634-1642.

1608. Wernicke C, Thiel G, Lozanova T, Vogel S, Kintzel D, Janisch W, Lehmann K, Witkowski R (1995). Involvement of chromosome 22 in ependymomas. *Cancer Genet Cytogenet* 79: 173-176.

1609. Wesseling P, Schlingemann RO, Rietveld FJ, Link M, Burger PC, Ruiter DJ (1995). Early and extensive contribution of pericytes/vascular smooth muscle cells to microvascular proliferation in glioblastoma multiforme: an immuno-light and immuno-electron microscopic study. *J Neuropathol Exp Neurol* 54: 304-310.

1610. West CR, Bruce DA, Duffner PK (1985). Ependymomas. Factors in clinical and diagnostic staging. *Cancer* 56: 1812-1816.

1611. Wester DJ, Falcone S, Green BA, Camp A, Quencer RM (1993). Paraganglioma of the filum: MR appearance. *J Comput Assist Tomogr* 17: 967-969.

1612. Westermark B, Heldin CH, Nister M (1995). Platelet-derived growth factor in human glioma. *Glia* 15: 257-263.

1613. Westphal M, Stavrou D, Nausch H, Valdueza JM, Herrmann HD (1994). Human neurocytoma cells in culture show characteristics of astroglial differentiation. *J Neurosci Res* 38: 698-704.

1614. Whitaker SJ, Bessell EM, Ashley SE, Bloom HJ, Bell BA, Brada M (1991). Postoperative radiotherapy in the management of spinal cord ependymoma. *J Neurosurg* 74: 720-728.

1615. White FV, Anthony DC, Yunis EJ, Tarbell NJ, Scott RM, Schofield DE (1995). Nonrandom chromosomal gains in pilocytic astrocytomas of childhood. *Hum Pathol* 26: 979-986.

1616. White W, Shiu MH, Rosenblum MK, Erlandson RA, Woodruff JM (1990). Cellular schwannoma. A clinicopathologic study of 57 patients and 58 tumors. *Cancer* 66: 1266-1275.

1617. Whittle IR, Gordon A, Misra BK, Shaw JF, Steers AJ (1989). Pleomorphic xanthoastrocytoma: report of four cases. *J Neurosurg* 70: 463-468.

1618. Wicking C, Shanley S, Smyth I, Gillies S, Negus K, Graham S, Suthers G, Haites N, Edwards M, Wainwright B, Chenevix T (1997). Most germ-line mutations in the nevoid basal cell carcinoma syndrome lead to a premature termination of the PATCHED protein, and no genotype-phenotype correlations are evident. *Am J Hum Genet* 60: 21-26.

1619. Wiestler OD, von Siebenthal K, Schmitt HP, Feiden W, Kleihues P (1989). Distribution and immunoreactivity of cerebral micro-hamartomas in bilateral acoustic neurofibromatosis (neurofibromatosis 2). *Acta Neuropathol (Berl)* 79: 137-143.

1621. Williard W, Borgen P, Bol R, Tiwari R, Osborne M (1992). Cowden's disease. A case report with analyses at the molecular level. *Cancer* 69: 2969-2974.

1622. Wilson NW, Symon L, Lantos PL (1987). Gliomatosis cerebri: report of a case presenting as a focal cerebral mass. *J Neurol* 234: 445-447.

1623. Wilson PJ, Ramesh V, Kristiansen A, Bove C, Jozwiak S, Kwiatkowski DJ, Short MP, Haines JL (1996). Novel mutations detected in the TSC2 gene from both sporadic and familial TSC patients. *Hum Mol Genet* 5: 249-256.

1624. Winek RR, Scheithauer BW, Wick MR (1989). Meningioma, meningeal hemangiopericytoma (angioblastic meningioma), peripheral hemangiopericytoma, and acoustic schwannoma. A comparative immunohistochemical study. *Am J Surg Pathol* 13: 251-261.

1625. Winger MJ, Macdonald DR, Cairncross JG (1989). Supratentorial anaplastic gliomas in adults. The prognostic importance of extent of resection and prior low-grade glioma. *J Neurosurg* 71: 487-493.

1626. Wisniewski T, Sisti M, Inhirami G, Knowles DM, Powers JM (1990). Intracerebral solitary plasmacytoma. *Neurosurgery* 27: 826-829.

1627. Wizigmann V, Breier G, Risau W, Plate KH (1995). Up-regulation of vascular endothelial growth factor and its receptors in von Hippel-Lindau disease-associated and sporadic hemangioblastomas. *Cancer Res* 55: 1358-1364.

1628. Wizigmann V, Plate KH (1996). Pathology, genetics and cell biology of hemangioblastomas. *Histol Histopathol* 11: 1049-1061.

1629. Wolf HK, Muller MB, Spanle M, Zentner J, Schramm J, Wiestler OD (1988). Ganglioglioma: a detailed histopathological and immunohistochemical analysis of 61 cases. *Acta Neuropathol (Berl)* 88: 166-173.

1630. Wolf HK, Normann S, Green AJ, von Bakel I, Blumcke I, Pietsch T, Wiestler OD, von Deimling A (1997). Tuberous sclerosis-like lesions in epileptogenic human neocortex lack allelic loss at the TSC1 and TSC2 regions. *Acta Neuropathol* 93: 93-96.

1631. Wolf HK, Wellmer J, Muller MB, Wiestler OD, Hufnagel A, Pietsch T (1995). Glioneuronal malformative lesions and dysembryoplastic neuroepithelial tumors in patients with chronic pharmacoresistant epilepsies. *J Neuropathol Exp Neurol* 54: 245-254.

1632. Wolf HK, Wiestler OD (1995). Surgical pathology of chronic epileptic seizure disorders. *Brain Pathol* 3: 371-380.

1633. Woloschak M, Yu A, Post KD (1997). Detection of polyomaviral DNA sequences in normal and adenomatous human pituitary tissues using the polymerase chain reaction. *Cancer* 76: 490-496.

1634. Wolter M, Reifenberger J, Sommer C, Ruzicka T, Reifenberger G (1997). Mutations in the human homologue of the Drosophila segment polarity gene patched (PTCH) in sporadic basal cell carcinomas of the skin and primitive neuroectodermal tumors of the central nervous system. *Cancer Res* 57: 2581-2585.

1635. Wondrusch E, Huemer M, Budka H (1991). Production of glial fibrillary acidic protein (GFAP) by neoplastic oligodendrocytes. Gliofibrillary oligodendroglioma and transitional astrocytoma revisited. *Brain Tumor Pathol* 8: 11-15.

1636. Wong AJ, Bigner SH, Bigner DD, Kinzler KW, Hamilton SR, Vogelstein B (1987). Increased expression of the epidermal growth factor receptor gene in malignant gliomas is invariably associated with gene amplification. *Proc Natl Acad Sci USA* 84: 6899-6903.

1637. Wong AJ, Ruppert JM, Bigner SH, Grzeschik CH, Humphrey PA, Bigner DS, Vogelstein B (1992). Structural alterations of the epidermal growth factor receptor gene in human gliomas. *Proc Natl Acad Sci USA* 89: 2965-2969.

1638. Wong TT, Ho DM, Chang TK, Yang DD,

Lee LS (1995). Familial neurofibromatosis 1 with germinoma involving the basal ganglion and thalamus. *Childs Nerv Syst* 11: 456-458.

1639. Wood JR, Green SB, Shapiro WR (1988). The prognostic importance of tumor size in malignant gliomas: a computed tomographic scan study by the Brain Tumor Cooperative Group. *J Clin Oncol* 6: 338-343.

1640. Woodruff JM (1996). Pathology of major peripheral nerve sheath tumors. In: *Soft Tissue Tumors (International Academy of Pathology Monograph)*, Weiss SW, Brooks JSJ (eds). Williams and Wilkins: Baltimore. pp. 129-161.

1641. Woodruff JM, Chernik NL, Smith MC, Millett WB, Foote FW, Jr. (1973). Peripheral nerve tumors with rhabdomyosarcomatous differentiation (malignant "Triton" tumors). *Cancer* 32: 426-439.

1642. Woodruff JM, Christensen WN (1993). Glandular peripheral nerve sheath tumors. *Cancer* 72: 3618-3628.

1643. Woodruff JM, Godwin TA, Erlandson RA, Susin M, Martini N (1981). Cellular schwannoma: a variety of schwannoma sometimes mistaken for a malignant tumor. *Am J Surg Pathol* 5: 733-744.

1644. Woodruff JM, Marshall ML, Godwin TA, Funkhouser JW, Thompson NJ, Erlandson RA (1983). Plexiform (multinodular) schwannoma. A tumor simulating the plexiform neurofibroma. *Am J Surg Pathol* 7: 691-697.

1645. Woodruff JM, Perino G (1994). Non-germ-cell or teratomatous malignant tumors showing additional rhabdomyoblastic differentiation, with emphasis on the malignant Triton tumor. *Semin Diagn Pathol* 11: 69-81.

1646. Woodruff JM, Selig AM, Crowley K, Allen PW (1994). Schwannoma (neurilemoma) with malignant transformation. A rare, distinctive peripheral nerve tumor. *Am J Surg Pathol* 18: 882-895.

1647. Wu JK, Folkerth RD, Ye Z, Darras BT (1993). Aggressive oligodendroglioma predicted by chromosome 10 restriction fragment length polymorphism analysis. Case study. *J Neurooncol* 15: 29-35.

1648. Wu R, Zhang J, Fryns JP, Cassiman JJ,Legius E (1969). Genetic heterogeneity in neurofibromatosis type 1. *FASEB Summer Research Conference On Neurofibromatosis, Snowmass, Co, USA*

1649. Xiao GH, Jin F, Yeung RS (1995). Identification of tuberous sclerosis 2 messenger RNA splice variants that are conserved and differentially expressed in rat and human tissues. *Cell Growth Differ* 6: 1185-1191.

1650. Yachnis AT, Rorke LB, Trojanowski JQ (1994). Cerebellar dysplasias in humans: development and possible relationship to glial and primitive neuroectodermal tumors of the cerebellar vermis. *J Neuropathol Exp Neurol* 53: 61-71.

1651. Yagishita S, Kawano N, Oka H, Kameya T (1996). Palisades in cerebral astrocytoma simulating the so-called polar spongioblastoma: a histological, immunohistochemical and electron microscopical study of an adult case. *Brain Tumor Pathol* 18: 21-25.

1652. Yahanda AM, Bruner JM, Donehower LA, Morrison RS (1995). Astrocytes derived from p53-deficient mice provide a multistep in vitro model for development of malignant gliomas. *Mol Cell Biol* 15: 4249-4259.

1653. Yamada H, Haratake J, Narasaki T, Oda T (1995). Embryonal craniopharyngioma. Case report of the morphogenesis of a craniopharyngioma. *Cancer* 75: 2971-2977.

1654. Yamamoto T, Komori T, Shibata N, Toyoda C, Kobayashi M (1996). Multifocal neurocytoma/gangliocytoma with extensive leptomeningeal dissemination in the brain and spinal cord. *Am J Surg Pathol* 20: 363-370.

1655. Yamashiro S, Nagahiro S, Mimata C, Kuratsu J, Ushio Y (1994). Malignant trigeminal schwannoma associated with xeroderma pigmentosum—case report. *Neurol Med Chir Tokyo* 34: 817-820.

1656. Yamashita T, Kuwabara T (1983). Estimation of rate of growth of malignant brain tumors by computed tomography scanning. *Surg Neurol* 20: 464-470.

1657. Yamashita Y, Handa H, Toyama M (1975). Medulloblastoma in two brothers. *Surg Neurol* 4: 225-227.

1658. Yang E, Korsmeyer SJ (1996). Molecular thanatopsis: a discourse on the BCL2 family and cell death. *Blood* 88: 386-401.

1659. Yarden Y, Schlessinger J (1987). Epidermal growth factor induces rapid, reversible aggregation of the purified epidermal growth factor receptor. *Biochemistry* 26: 1443-1451.

1660. Yasargil MG, Curcic M, Kis M, Siegenthaler G, Teddy PJ, Roth P (1990). Total removal of craniopharyngiomas. Approaches and long-term results in 144 patients. *J Neurosurg* 73: 3-11.

1661. Yasargil MG, von Ammon K, von Deimling A, Valavanis A, Wichmann W, Wiestler OD (1992). Central neurocytoma: histopathological variants and therapeutic approaches. *J Neurosurg* 76: 32-37.

1662. Yasue M, Tomita T, Engelhard H, Gonzalez C, McLone DG, Bauer KD (1989). Prognostic importance of DNA ploidy in medulloblastoma of childhood. *J Neurosurg* 70: 385-391.

1663. Yates AJ, Becker LE, Sachs LA (1979). Brain tumors in childhood. *Childs Brain* 5: 31-39.

1664. Yin C, Knudson CM, Korsmeyer SJ, Van Dyke T (1997). Bax suppresses tumorigenesis and stimulates apoptosis in vivo. *Nature* 385: 637-640.

1665. Yogo Y, Kitamura T, Sugimoto C, Ueki T, Aso Y, Hara K, Taguchi F (1990). Isolation of a possible archetypal JC virus DNA sequence from nonimmunocompromised individuals. *J Virol* 64: 3139-3143.

1666. Yoshino T, Kondo E, Cao L, Takahashi K, Hayashi K, Nomura S, Akagi T (1994). Inverse expression of bcl-2 protein and Fas antigen in lymphoblasts in peripheral lymph nodes and activated peripheral blood T and B lymphocytes. *Blood* 83: 1856-1861.

1667. Yu IT, Griffin CA, Phillips PC, Strauss LC, Perlman EJ (1995). Numerical sex chromosomal abnormalities in pineal teratomas by cytogenetic analysis and fluorescence in situ hybridization. *Lab Invest* 72: 419-423.

1668. Zagzag D, Friedlander DR, Miller DC, Dosik J, Cangiarella J, Kostianovsky M, Cohen H, Grumet M, Greco MA (1995). Tenascin expression in astrocytomas correlates with angiogenesis. *Cancer Res* 55: 907-914.

1669. Zagzag D, Miller DC, Sato Y, Rifkin DB, Burstein DE (1990). Immunohistochemical localization of basic fibroblast growth factor in astrocytomas. *Cancer Res* 50: 7393-7398.

1670. Zang KD (1982). Cytological and cytogenetical studies on human meningiomas. *Cancer Genet Cytogenet* 6: 249-274.

1671. Zankl H, Zang KD (1972). Cytological and cytogenetical studies on brain tumors. 4. Identification of the missing G chromosome in human meningiomas as no. 22 by fluorescence technique. *Humangenetik* 14: 167-169.

1672. Zauberman A, Flusberg D, Haupt Y, Barak Y, Oren M (1995). A functional p53-responsive intronic promoter is contained within the human mdm2 gene. *Nucleic Acids Res* 23: 2584-2592.

1673. Zbar B, Kishida T, Chen F, Schmidt L, Maher ER, Richards FM, Crossey PA, webster AR, Affara NA, Ferguson S, Brauch H, Glavac D, Neumann HP, Tischerman S, Mulvihill JJ, Gross DJ, Suhin T, Seizinger B, Kley N, Olschwang S, Boisson C, Richard S, Lips CHM, Linehan WM, Lerman M (1996). Germline mutations in the von Hippel-Lindau disease (VHL) gene in families from North America, Europe and Japan. *Hum Mutat* 8: 348-357.

1674. Zentner J, Peiffer J, Roggendorf W, Grote E, Hassler W (1992). Periventricular neurocytoma: a pathological entity. *Surg Neurol* 38: 38-42.

1675. Zerbini C, Gelber RD, Weinberg D, Sallan SE, Barnes P, Kupsky W, Scott RM, Tarbell NJ (1993). Prognostic factors in medulloblastoma, including DNA ploidy. *J Clin Oncol* 11: 616-622.

1676. Zhu J, Frosch MP, Busque L, Beggs AH, Dashner K, Gilliland DG, Black PM (1995). Analysis of meningiomas by methylation- and transcription-based clonality assays. *Cancer Res* 55: 3865-3872.

1677. Zhu J, Guy SZ, Beggs AH, Maruyama T, Santarius T, Dashner K, Olsen N, Wu JK, Black P (1996). Microsatellite instability analysis of primary human brain tumors. *Oncogene* 12: 1417-1423.

1678. Zimmerman RA, Bilaniuk LT, Pahlajani H (1978). Spectrum of medulloblastomas demonstrated by computed tomography. *Radiology* 126: 137-141.

1679. Zimmerman RA, Bilaniuk LT, Rebsamen S (1992). Magnetic resonance imaging of pediatric posterior fossa tumors. *Pediatr Neurosurg* 18: 58-64.

1680. Zorludemir S, Scheithauer BW, Hirose T, Van Houten C, Miller G, Meyer FB (1995). Clear cell meningioma. A clinicopathologic study of a potentially aggressive variant of meningioma. *Am J Surg Pathol* 19: 493-505.

1681. zu Rhein G, Varakis JN (1979). Perinatal induction of medulloblastomas in Syrian golden hamsters by a human polyoma virus (JC). *NCI Monogr* 51: 205-208.

1682. Zuccaro G, Taratuto AL, Monges J (1986). Intracranial neoplasms during the first year of life. *Surg Neurol* 26: 29-36.

1683. Zulch KJ (1941). Ein Medulloblastom mit glatten Muskelfasern. *Arch Psychiatr Nervenkr* 114: 349-352.

1684. Zulch KJ (1957). *Brain Tumours. Their Biology and Pathology.* 1st ed, Springer-Verlag: New York.

1685. Zulch KJ (1979). *Histological Typing of Tumours of the Central Nervous System.* World Health Organization: Geneva.

1686. Zulch KJ (1986). *Brain Tumors. Their Biology and Pathology.* 3rd ed, Springer Verlag: Berlin Heidelberg.

1687. Cerda-Nicolas M, Kepes JJ (1993). Gliofibromas (including malignant forms), and gliosarcomas: a comparative study and review of the literature. *Acta Neuropathol* 85: 349-361.

1688. Friede RL (1978). Gliofibroma: a peculiar neoplasia of collagen forming glia-like cells. *J Neuropath Exp Neurol* 38: 300-313.

1689. Prayson RA (1996). Gliofibroma: a distinct entity or a subtype of desmoplastic astrocytoma? *Hum Pathol* 27: 610-613.

1690. Roland B, Ambros IM, Dehner LP, Hata JI, Joshi VV, Shimada H (1996). A proposed international neuroblastoma pathology classification. *Med Pediatr Oncol* 27: 225-

1691. Reifenberger J, Reifenberger J, Ichimura K, Schmidt EE, Wechsler W, Collins VP (1996). Epidermal growth factor receptor expression in oligodendroglial tumors. *Am J Pathol* 149: 29-35.

1692. Hunter T, Pines J (1994). Cyclins and cancer II: cyclin D and CDK inhibitors come of age. *Cell* 79: 573-582.

1693. Biernat W, Tohma Y, Yonekawa Y, Kleihues P, Ohgaki H (1997). Alterations of cell cycle regulatory genes in primary (de novo) and secondary glioblastomas. *Acta Neuropathol* 94: 303-309.

1694. Nishikawa R, Ji XD, Harmon RC, Lazar CS, Gill GN, Cavenee WK, Huang HJ (1994). A mutant epidermal growth factor receptor common in human glioma confers enhanced tumorigenicity. *Proc Natl Acad Sci USA* 91: 7727-7731.

1695. Haas JE, Palmer NF, Weinberg AG, Beckwith JB (1981). Ultrastructure of malignant rhabdoid tumor of the kidney. A distinctive renal tumor of children. *Hum Pathol* 12: 646-657.

1696. Lopes MBS, Altermatt HJ, Scheithauer BW, VandenBerg SR (1996). Immunohistochemical characterization of subependymal giant cell astrocytomas. *Acta Neuropathol* 91: 368-375.

1697. Babu R, Lansen T, Chadburn A, Kasoff S (1997). Erdheim-Chester disease of the central nervous system. *J Neurosurg* 86: 888-892.

1698. Belen D, Colak A, Ozcan O (1996). CNS involvement of Langerhans cell histiocytosis. report of 23 surgically treated cases. *Neurosurg Rev* 19: 247-252.

1699. Ben-Ezra J, Bailey A, Azumi N, Delsol G, Stroup R, Sheibani K, Rappaport H (19991). Malignant histiocytosis X. A distinct clinicopathologic entity. *Cancer* 68: 1050-1060.

1700. Bergmann M, Yuan Y, Brück W, Palm KV, Rohkamm R (1997). Solitary Langerhans cell histiocytosis lesion of the parieto-occipital lobe: a case report and review of the literature. *Clin Neurol Neurosurg* 99: 50-55.

1702. Brück W, Sander U, Blanckenberg P, Friede RL (1991). Symptomatic xanthogranuloma of choroid plexus with unilateral hydrocephalus. Case report. *Lancet* 1: 208-209.

1703. Chou T, D'Angio GJ, Favara BE, Ladisch S, Nesbit M, Pritchard J (1987). Histiocytosis syndromes in children. Writing Group of the Histiocyte Society. *Lancet* 1: 208-209.

1704. Erlandson RA (1994). *Diagnostic Transmission Electron Microscopy of Tumors.* Raven Press: New York.

1705. Gray F, Adle-Biasette H, Bernier M, Bergemer AM, Wingertsmann L, Wechsler J (1997). Neuropathologic findings in two autopsy cases of Erdheim Chester disease (ECD). *J Neuropathol Exp Neurol* 56: 613-613.

1706. Grois N, Tsunematsu Y, Barkovich AJ, Favara BE (1994). Central nervous system disease in Langerhans cell histiocytosis. *Br J Cancer Suppl* 23: S24-S28.

1707. Haddad E, Sulis ML, Jabado N, Blanche S, Fischer A, Tardieu M (1997). Frequency and severity of central nervous system lesions in hemophagocytic lymphohistiocytosis. *Blood* 89: 794-800.

1708. Hage C, Willman CL, Favara BE, Isaacson PG (1993). Langerhans' cell histiocytosis (histiocytosis X): immunophenotype and growth fraction. *Hum Pathol* 24: 840-845.

1709. Hammond RR, Mackenzie IR (1995). Xanthoma disseminatum with massive intracranial involvement. *Clin Neuropathol* 14: 314-321.

1710. Hasle H, Brandt C, Kerndrup G, Kjeldsen E, Sorensen AG (1996). Haemophagocytic lymphohistiocytosis associated with constitutional inversion of chromosome 9. *Br J Haematol* 93: 808-809.

1711. Henter JI, Nennesmo I (1997). Neuropathologic findings and neurologic symptoms in twenty-three children with hemophagocytic lymphohistiocytosis. *J Pediatr* 130: 358-365.

1712. Hicks MJ, Albrecht S, Trask T, Byrne ME, Narayan RK, Goodman JC (1993). Symptomatic choroid plexus xanthogranuloma of the lateral ventricle. Case report and brief critical review of xanthogranulomatous lesions of the brain. *Clin Neuropathol* 12: 92-96.

1713. Hulette CM (1996). Microglioma, a histiocytic neoplasm of the central nervous system. *Mod Pathol* 9: 316-319.

1714. Jones RV, Colegial CH, Andriko JW (1997). Extranodal sinus histiocytosis with massive lymphadenopathy (Rosai-Dorfman disease) of the central nervous system. *J Neuropathol Exp Neurol* 56: 613.

1715. Kepes JJ (1979). Histiocytosis X. In: *Handbook of Clinical Neurology*, Vinken PJ, Bruyn GW (eds). North Holland Publishing Co.: New York.

1717. Kim M, Provias J, Bernstein M (1995). Rosai-Dorfman disease mimicking multiple meningioma: case report. *Neurosurgery* 36: 1185-1187.

1718. Kollias SS, Ball WSJ, Tzika AA, Harris RE (1994). Familial erythrophagocytic lymphohistiocytosis: neuroradiologic evaluation with pathologic correlation. *Radiology* 192: 743-754.

1719. Lichtenstein L (1953). Histiocytosis X. Integration of eosinophilic granuloma of bone, Letterer-Siwe disease and Schüller-Christian disease as related manifestations of a single nosological entity. *Arch Pathol* 56: 89-103.

1720. Mader I, Stock KW, Radue EW, Steinbrich W (1996). Langerhans cell histiocytosis in monocygote twins: case reports. *Neuroradiology* 38: 163-165.

1721. Mazal PR, Hainfellner JA, Preiser J, Czech T, Simonitsch I, Radaszkiewicz T, Budka H (1996). Langerhans cell histiocytosis of the hypothalamus: diagnostic value of immunohistochemistry. *Clin Neuropathol* 15: 87-91.

1722. McClain K, Jin H, Gresik V, Favara B (1994). Langerhans cell histiocytosis: lack of a viral etiology. *Am J Hematol* 47: 16-20.

1723. Montine TJ, Hollensead SC, Ellis WG, Martin JS, Moffat EJ, Burger PC (1994). Solitary eosinophilic granuloma of the temporal lobe: a case report and long-term follow-up of previously reported cases. *Clin Neuropathol* 13: 225-228.

1724. Muenchau A, Laas R (1997). Xanthogranuloma and xanthoma of the choroid plexus: evidence for different etiology and pathogenesis. *Clin Neuropathol* 16: 72-76.

1725. Odell WD, Doggett RS (1993). Xanthoma disseminatum, a rare cause of diabetes insipidus. *J Clin Endocrinol Metab* 76: 777-780.

1726. Owen G, Webb DK (1995). Evidence of clonality in a child with haemophagocytic lymphohistiocytosis. *Br J Haematol* 89: 681-682.

1727. Paulli M, Bergamaschi G, Tonon L, Viglio A, Rosso R, Facchetti F, Geerts ML, Magrini U, Cazzola M (1995). Evidence for a polyclonal nature of the cell infiltrate in sinus histiocytosis with massive lymphadenopathy (Rosai-Dorfman disease). *Br J Haematol* 91: 415-418.

1728. Paulus W, Kirchner T, Michaela M, Kuhl J, Warmuth-Metz M, Sorensen N, Muller-Hermelink HK, Roggendorf W (1992). Histiocytic tumor of Meckel's cave. An intracranial equivalent of juvenile xanthogranuloma of the skin. *Am J Surg Pathol* 16: 76-83.

1729. Poe LB, Dubowy RL, Hochhauser L, Collins GH, Crosley CJ, Kanzer MD, Oliphant M, Hodge CJ, Jr. (1994). Demyelinating and gliotic cerebellar lesions in Langerhans cell histiocytosis. *Am J Neuroradiol* 15: 1921-1928.

1730. Resnick DK, Johnson BL, Lovely TJ (1996). Rosai-Dorfman disease presenting with multiple orbital and intracranial masses. *Acta Neuropathol* 91: 554-557.

1731. Risdall RJ, Dehner LP, Duray P, Kobrinsky N, Robison L, Nesbit ME, Jr. (1983). Histiocytosis X (Langerhans' cell histiocytosis). Prognostic role of histopathology. *Arch Pathol Lab Med* 107: 59-63.

1732. Schmitt S, Wichmann W, Martin E, Zachmann M, Schoenle EJ (1993). Pituitary stalk thickening with diabetes insipidus preceding typical manifestations of Langerhans cell histiocytosis in children. *Eur J Pediatr* 152: 399-401.

1733. Thomas C, Donnadieu J, Emile JF, Brousse N (1996). Langerhans cell histiocytosis. *Arch Pediatr* 3: 63-69.

1734. Veyssier-Belot C, Cacoub P, Caparros-Lefebvre D, Wechsler J, Brun B, Remy M, Wallaert B, Petit H, Grimaldi A, Wechsler B, Godeau P (1996). Erdheim-Chester disease. Clinical and radiologic characteristics of 59 cases. *Medicine (Baltimore)* 75: 157-169.

1735. Willis B, Ablin A, Weinberg V, Zoger S, Wara WM, Matthay KK (1996). Disease course and late sequelae of Langerhans' cell histiocytosis: 25- year experience at the University of California, San Francisco. *J Clin Oncol* 14: 2073-2082.

1736. Willman CL, Busque L, Griffith BB, Favara BE, McClain KL, Duncan MH, Gilliland DG (1994). Langerhans'-cell histiocytosis (histiocytosis X)—a clonal proliferative disease. *N Engl J Med* 331: 154-160.

1737. Zelger BW, Sidoroff A, Orchard G, Cerio R (1996). Non-Langerhans cell histiocytoses. A new unifying concept. *Am J Dermatopathol* 18: 490-504.

1738. Glick R, Backer C, Husain S, Hays A, Hibshoosh H (1997). Primary melanocytomas of the spinal cord: a report of seven cases. *Clin Neuropathol* 16: 127-132.

1739. Brat DJ, Scheithauer BW, Staugaitis SM, Cortez SC, Brecher K, Burger PC (1998). Third ventricular chordoid glioma: a distinct clinicopathologic entity. *J Neuropathol Exp Neurol* 57: 283-290.

1740. Wanschitz J, Schmidbauer M, Maier H, Rossler K, Vorkapic P, Budka H (1995). Suprasellar meningioma with expression of glial fibrillary acidic protein: a peculiar variant. *Acta Neuropathol (Berl)* 90: 539-544.

1742. Kondo S, Ishizaka Y, Okada T, Kondo Y, Hitomi M, Tanaka Y, Haqqi T, Barnett GH, Barna BP (1998). FADD gene therapy for malignant gliomas in vitro and in vivo. *Hum Gene Ther* 9: 1599-1608.

1743. Glaser T, Wagenknecht B, Groscurth P, Krammer PH, Weller M (1999). Death ligand/receptor-independent caspase activation mediates drug-induced cell death in malignant glioma cells. *Oncogene* 18: 5044-5053.

1744. Iwadate Y, Tagawa M, Fujimoto S, Hirose M, Namba H, Sueyoshi K, Sakiyama S, Yamaura A (1998). Mutation of the p53 gene in human astrocytic tumours correlates with increased resistance to DNA-damaging agents but not to anti-microtubule anti-cancer agents. *Br J Cancer* 77: 547-551.

1745. Newcomb EW, Cohen H, Lee SR, Bhalla SK, Bloom J, Hayes RL, Miller DC (1998). Survival of patients with glioblastoma multiforme is not influenced by altered expression of p16, p53, EGFR, MDM2 or Bcl-2 genes. *Brain Pathol* 8: 655-667.

1746. Pohl U, Wagenknecht B, Naumann U, Weller M (1999). p53 Enhances BAK and CD95 Expression in Human Malignant Glioma Cells but Does Not Enhance CD95L-Induced Apoptosis. *Cell Physiol Biochem* 9: 29-37.

1747. Kondo S, Tanaka Y, Kondo Y, Ishizaka Y, Hitomi M, Haqqi T, Liu J, Barnett GH, Alnemri ES, Barna BP (1998). Retroviral transfer of CPP32b gene into malignant gliomas in vitro and in vivo. *Cancer Res* 58: 962-967.

1748. Krajewski S, Krajewska M, Ehrmann J, Chatten J, Reed JC (1997). Immunohistochemical analysis of Bcl-2, Bcl-X, Mcl-1, and Bax in tumors of central and peripheral nervous system origin. *Am J Pathol* 150: 805-814.

1749. Miyashita T, Krajewski S, Krajewska M, Wang HG, Lin HK, Liebermann DA, Hoffman B, Reed JC (1994). Tumor suppressor p53 is a regulator of bcl-2 and bax gene expression in vitro and in vivo. *Oncogene* 9: 1799-1805.

1750. Shinoura N (1998). Apoptosis by retrovirus- and adenovirus-mediated gene transfer of Fas ligand to glioma cells: implications for gene therapy. *Hum Gene Ther* 9: 1983-1993.

1751. Rieger J, Naumann U, Glaser T, Ashkenazi A, Weller M (1998). APO2 ligand: a novel lethal weapon against malignant glioma? *FEBS Lett* 427: 124-128.

1752. Rieger L, Weller M, Bornemann A, Schabet M, Dichgans J, Meyermann R (1998). BCL-2 family protein expression in human malignant glioma: a clinical- pathological correlative study. *J Neurol Sci* 155: 68-75.

1753. Weller M, Kleihues P, Dichgans J, Ohgaki H (1998). CD95 ligand: lethal weapon against malignant glioma? *Brain Pathol* 8: 285-293.

1754. Tohma Y, Gratas C, Biernat W, Peraud A, Fukuda M, Yonekawa Y, Kleihues P, Ohgaki H (1998). PTEN (MMAC1) mutations are frequent in primary glioblastomas (de novo) but not in secondary glioblastomas. *J Neuropathol Exp Neurol* 57: 684-689.

1755. Watanabe K, Peraud A, Gratas C, Wakai S, Kleihues P, Ohgaki H (1998). p53 and PTEN gene mutations in gemistocytic astrocytomas. *Acta Neuropathol (Berl)* 95: 559-564.

1757. Gratas C, Tohma Y, Van Meir EG, Klein M, Tenan M, Ishii N, Tachibana O, Kleihues P, Ohgaki H (1997). Fas ligand expression in glioblastoma cell lines and primary astrocytic brain tumors. *Brain Pathol* 7: 863-869.

1758. Sato K, Gratas C, Lampe J, Biernat W, Kleihues P, Yamasaki H, Ohgaki H (1997). Reduced expression of the P2 form of the gap junction protein connexin43 in malignant meningiomas. *J Neuropathol Exp Neurol* 56: 835-839.

1759. Wagenknecht B, Glaser T, Naumann U, Kugler S, Isenmann S, Bahr M, Korneluk R, Liston P, Weller M (1999). Expression and biological activity of X-linked inhibitor of apoptosis (XIAP) in human malignant glioma. *Cell Death Differ* 6: 370-376.

1760. Weller M, Rieger J, Grimmel C, Van Meir EG, de Tribolet N, Krajewski S, Reed JC, von Deimling A, Dichgans J (1998). Predicting chemoresistance in human malignant glioma cells: the role of molecular genetic analyses. *Int J Cancer* 79: 640-644.

1761. Trepel M, Groscurth P, Malipiero U, Gulbins E, Dichgans J, Weller M (1998). Chemosensitivity of human malignant glioma: modulation by p53 gene transfer. *J Neurooncol* 39: 19-32.

1762. Chan AS, Leung SY, Wong MP, Yuen ST, Cheung N, Fan YW, Chung LP (1998). Expression of vascular endothelial growth factor and its receptors in the anaplastic progression of astrocytoma, oligodendroglioma, and ependymoma. *Am J Surg Pathol* 22: 816-826.

1763. Hanahan D (1997). Signaling vascular morphogenesis and maintenance [comment]. *Science* 277: 48-50.

1764. Lauren J, Gunji Y, Alitalo K (1998). Is angiopoietin-2 necessary for the initiation of tumor angiogenesis? *Am J Pathol* 153: 1333-1339.

1765. MacHein MR, Kullmer J, Ronicke V, Machein U, Krieg M, Damert A, Breier G, Risau W, Plate KH (1999). Differential downregulation of vascular endothelial growth factor by dexamethasone in normoxic and hypoxic rat glioma cells. *Neuropathol Appl Neurobiol* 25: 104-112.

1766. MacHein MR, Risau W, Plate KH (1999). Antiangiogenic gene therapy in a rat glioma model using a dominant- negative vascular endothelial growth factor receptor 2. *Hum Gene Ther* 10: 1117-1128.

1767. Stratmann A, Risau W, Plate KH (1998). Cell type-specific expression of angiopoietin-1 and angiopoietin-2 suggests a role in glioblastoma angiogenesis. *Am J Pathol* 153: 1459-1466.

1768. Cheney IW, Johnson DE, Vaillancourt MT, Avanzini J, Morimoto A, Demers GW, Wills KN, Shabram PW, Bolen JB, Tavtigian

SV, Bookstein R (1998). Suppression of tumorigenicity of glioblastoma cells by adenovirus- mediated MMAC1/PTEN gene transfer. *Cancer Res* 58: 2331-2334.

1769. Eng C, Peacocke M (1998). PTEN and inherited hamartoma-cancer syndromes. *Nat Genet* 19: 223.

1770. Furnari FB, Huang HJ, Cavenee WK (1998). The phosphoinositol phosphatase activity of PTEN mediates a serum- sensitive G1 growth arrest in glioma cells. *Cancer Res* 58: 5002-5008.

1771. Furnari FB, Lin H, Huang HS, Cavenee WK (1997). Growth suppression of glioma cells by PTEN requires a functional phosphatase catalytic domain. *Proc Natl Acad Sci U S A* 94: 12479-12484.

1772. Li DM, Sun H (1998). PTEN/MMAC1/TEP1 suppresses the tumorigenicity and induces G1 cell cycle arrest in human glioblastoma cells. *Proc Natl Acad Sci U S A* 95: 15406-15411.

1773. Li DM, Sun H (1997). TEP1, encoded by a candidate tumor suppressor locus, is a novel protein tyrosine phosphatase regulated by transforming growth factor beta. *Cancer Res* 57: 2124-2129.

1774. Maehama T, Dixon JE (1998). The tumor suppressor, PTEN/MMAC1, dephosphorylates the lipid second messenger, phosphatidylinositol 3,4,5-trisphosphate. *J Biol Chem* 273: 13375-13378.

1775. Mollenhauer J, Wiemann S, Scheurlen W, Korn B, Hayashi Y, Wilgenbus KK, von Deimling A, Poustka A (1997). DMBT1, a new member of the SRCR superfamily, on chromosome 10q25.3-26.1 is deleted in malignant brain tumours. *Nat Genet* 17: 32-39.

1776. Myers MP, Pass I, Batty IH, Van der Kaay J, Stolarov JP, Hemmings BA, Wigler MH, Downes CP, Tonks NK (1998). The lipid phosphatase activity of PTEN is critical for its tumor supressor function. *Proc Natl Acad Sci U S A* 95: 13513-13518.

1777. Stambolic V, Suzuki A, de la Pompa JL, Brothers GM, Mirtsos C, Sasaki T, Ruland J, Penninger JM, Siderovski DP, Mak TW (1998). Negative regulation of PKB/Akt-dependent cell survival by the tumor suppressor PTEN. *Cell* 95: 29-39.

1778. Tamura M, Gu J, Matsumoto K, Aota S, Parsons R, Yamada KM (1998). Inhibition of cell migration, spreading, and focal adhesions by tumor suppressor PTEN. *Science* 280: 1614-1617.

1779. Teng DH, Hu R, Lin H, Davis T, Iliev D, Frye C, Swedlund B, Hansen KL, Vinson VL, Gumpper KL, Ellis L, El-Naggar A, Frazier M, Jasser S, Langford LA, Lee J, Mills GB, Pershouse MA, Pollack RE, Tornos C, Troncoso P, Yung WK, Fujii G, Berson A, Steck PA (1997). MMAC1/PTEN mutations in primary tumor specimens and tumor cell lines. *Cancer Res* 57: 5221-5225.

1780. Wang SI, Puc J, Li J, Bruce JN, Cairns P, Sidransky D, Parsons R (1997). Somatic mutations of PTEN in glioblastoma multiforme. *Cancer Res* 57: 4183-4186.

1781. Wechsler DS, Shelly CA, Petroff CA, Dang CV (1997). MXI1, a putative tumor suppressor gene, suppresses growth of human glioblastoma cells. *Cancer Res* 57: 4905-4912.

1782. Wu X, Senechal K, Neshat MS, Whang YE, Sawyers CL (1998). The PTEN/MMAC1 tumor suppressor phosphatase functions as a negative regulator of the phosphoinositide 3-kinase/Akt pathway. *Proc Natl Acad Sci U S A* 95: 15587-15591.

1783. Antonyak MA, Moscatello DK, Wong AJ (1998). Constitutive activation of c-Jun N-terminal kinase by a mutant epidermal growth factor receptor. *J Biol Chem* 273: 2817-2822.

1784. Arap W, Knudsen E, Sewell DA, Sidransky D, Wang JY, Huang HJ, Cavenee WK (1997). Functional analysis of wild-type and malignant glioma derived CDKN2Abeta alleles: evidence for an RB-independent growth suppressive pathway. *Oncogene* 15: 2013-2020.

1785. Chintala SK, Fueyo J, Gomez-Manzano C, Venkaiah B, Bjerkvig R, Yung WK, Sawaya R, Kyritsis AP, Rao JS (1997). Adenovirus-mediated p16/CDKN2 gene transfer suppresses glioma invasion in vitro. *Oncogene* 15: 2049-2057.

1786. de Stanchina E, McCurrach ME, Zindy F, Shieh SY, Ferbeyre G, Samuelson AV, Prives C, Roussel MF, Sherr CJ, Lowe SW (1998). E1A signaling to p53 involves the p19(ARF) tumor suppressor. *Genes Dev* 12: 2434-2442.

1787. Duro D, Bernard O, Della V, V, Berger R, Larsen CJ (1995). A new type of p16INK4/MTS1 gene transcript expressed in B-cell malignancies. *Oncogene* 11: 21-29.

1788. El-Obeid A, Bongcam-Rudloff E, Sorby M, Ostman A, Nister M, Westermark B (1997). Cell scattering and migration induced by autocrine transforming growth factor alpha in human glioma cells in vitro. *Cancer Res* 57: 5598-5604.

1789. Fueyo J, Gomez-Manzano C, Yung WK, Liu TJ, Alemany R, McDonnell TJ, Shi X, Rao JS, Levin VA, Kyritsis AP (1998). Overexpression of E2F-1 in glioma triggers apoptosis and suppresses tumor growth in vitro and in vivo. *Nat Med* 4: 685-690.

1790. Fueyo J, Gomez-Manzano C, Puduvalli VK, Martin-Duque P, Perez-Soler R, Levin VA, Yung WK, Kyritsis AP (1998). Adenovirus-mediated p16 transfer to glioma cells induces G1 arrest and protects from paclitaxel and topotecan: implications for therapy. *Int J Oncol* 12: 665-669.

1791. Gomez-Manzano C, Fueyo J, Alameda F, Kyritsis AP, Yung WK (1999). Gene therapy for gliomas: p53 and E2F-1 proteins and the target of apoptosis. *Int J Mol Med* 3: 81-85.

1792. Hama S, Heike Y, Naruse I, Takahashi M, Yoshioka H, Arita K, Kurisu K, Goldman CK, Curiel DT, Saijo N (1998). Adenovirus-mediated p16 gene transfer prevents drug-induced cell death through G1 arrest in human glioma cells. *Int J Cancer* 77: 47-54.

1793. Han Y, Caday CG, Nanda A, Cavenee WK, Huang HJ (1996). Tyrphostin AG 1478 preferentially inhibits human glioma cells expressing truncated rather than wild-type epidermal growth factor receptors. *Cancer Res* 56: 3859-3861.

1794. Holland EC, Hively WP, DePinho RA, Varmus HE (1998). A constitutively active epidermal growth factor receptor cooperates with disruption of G1 cell-cycle arrest pathways to induce glioma-like lesions in mice. *Genes Dev* 12: 3675-3685.

1795. Kamijo T, Bodner S, van de Kamp E, Randle DH, Sherr CJ (1999). Tumor spectrum in ARF-deficient mice. *Cancer Res* 59: 2217-2222.

1796. Kamijo T, Weber JD, Zambetti G, Zindy F, Roussel MF, Sherr CJ (1998). Functional and physical interactions of the ARF tumor suppressor with p53 and Mdm2. *Proc Natl Acad Sci U S A* 95: 8292-8297.

1797. Kamijo T, Zindy F, Roussel MF, Quelle DE, Downing JR, Ashmun RA, Grosveld G, Sherr CJ (1997). Tumor suppression at the mouse INK4a locus mediated by the alternative reading frame product p19ARF. *Cell* 91: 649-659.

1798. Liu W, James CD, Frederick L, Alderete BE, Jenkins RB (1997). PTEN/MMAC1 mutations and EGFR amplification in glioblastomas. *Cancer Res* 57: 5254-5257.

1799. Louis DN, Gusella JF (1995). A tiger behind many doors: multiple genetic pathways to malignant glioma. *Trends Genet* 11: 412-415.

1800. Mao L, Merlo A, Bedi G, Shapiro GI, Edwards CD, Rollins BJ, Sidransky D (1995). A novel p16INK4A transcript. *Cancer Res* 55: 2995-2997.

1801. Moscatello DK, Holgado-Madruga M, Emlet DR, Montgomery RB, Wong AJ (1998). Constitutive activation of phosphatidylinositol 3-kinase by a naturally occurring mutant epidermal growth factor receptor. *J Biol Chem* 273: 200-206.

1802. Moscatello DK, Ramirez G, Wong AJ (1997). A naturally occurring mutant human epidermal growth factor receptor as a target for peptide vaccine immunotherapy of tumors. *Cancer Res* 57: 1419-1424.

1803. Nagane M, Levitzki A, Gazit A, Cavenee WK, Huang HJ (1998). Drug resistance of human glioblastoma cells conferred by a tumor- specific mutant epidermal growth factor receptor through modulation of Bcl-XL and caspase-3-like proteases. *Proc Natl Acad Sci U S A* 95: 5724-5729.

1804. Nagane M, Coufal F, Lin H, Bogler O, Cavenee WK, Huang HJ (1996). A common mutant epidermal growth factor receptor confers enhanced tumorigenicity on human glioblastoma cells by increasing proliferation and reducing apoptosis. *Cancer Res* 56: 5079-5086.

1805. O'Rourke DM, Nute EJ, Davis JG, Wu C, Lee A, Murali R, Zhang HT, Qian X, Kao CC, Greene MI (1998). Inhibition of a naturally occurring EGFR oncoprotein by the p185neu ectodomain: implications for subdomain contributions to receptor assembly. *Oncogene* 16: 1197-1207.

1806. Pomerantz J, Schreiber-Agus N, Liegeois NJ, Silverman A, Alland L, Chin L, Potes J, Chen K, Orlow I, Lee HW, Cordon-Cardo C, DePinho RA (1998). The Ink4a tumor suppressor gene product, p19Arf, interacts with MDM2 and neutralizes MDM2's inhibition of p53. *Cell* 92: 713-723.

1807. Prigent SA, Nagane M, Lin H, Huvar I, Boss GR, Feramisco JR, Cavenee WK, Huang HS (1996). Enhanced tumorigenic behavior of glioblastoma cells expressing a truncated epidermal growth factor receptor is mediated through the Ras- Shc-Grb2 pathway. *J Biol Chem* 271: 25639-25645.

1808. Quelle DE, Cheng M, Ashmun RA, Sherr CJ (1997). Cancer-associated mutations at the INK4a locus cancel cell cycle arrest by p16INK4a but not by the alternative reading frame protein p19ARF. *Proc Natl Acad Sci U S A* 94: 669-673.

1809. Quelle DE, Zindy F, Ashmun RA, Sherr CJ (1995). Alternative reading frames of the INK4a tumor suppressor gene encode two unrelated proteins capable of inducing cell cycle arrest. *Cell* 83: 993-1000.

1810. Sherr CJ (1998). Tumor surveillance via the ARF-p53 pathway. *Genes Dev* 12: 2984-2991.

1811. Stone S, Jiang P, Dayananth P, Tavtigian SV, Katcher H, Parry D, Peters G, Kamb A (1995). Complex structure and regulation of the P16 (MTS1) locus. *Cancer Res* 55: 2988-2994.

1812. Stott FJ, Bates S, James MC, McConnell BB, Starborg M, Brookes S, Palmero I, Ryan K, Hara E, Vousden KH, Peters G (1998). The alternative product from the human CDKN2A locus, p14(ARF), participates in a regulatory feedback loop with p53 and MDM2. *EMBO J* 17: 5001-5014.

1813. Wikstrand CJ, McLendon RE, Friedman AH, Bigner DD (1997). Cell surface localization and density of the tumor-associated variant of the epidermal growth factor receptor, EGFRvIII. *Cancer Res* 57: 4130-4140.

1814. Zhang Y, Xiong Y, Yarbrough WG (1998). ARF promotes MDM2 degradation and stabilizes p53: ARF-INK4a locus deletion impairs both the Rb and p53 tumor suppression pathways. *Cell* 92: 725-734.

1815. Zindy F, Eischen CM, Randle DH, Kamijo T, Cleveland JL, Sherr CJ, Roussel MF (1998). Myc signaling via the ARF tumor suppressor regulates p53-dependent apoptosis and immortalization. *Genes Dev* 12: 2424-2433.

1816. Mishima K, Nagane M, Lin H, Cavenee WK,Huang HJS (1999). Expression of a specific mutant epidermal growth factor receptor mediates glioma cell invasion in vivo. *Proc Am Assoc Cancer Res* 519-519.

1817. Amberger VR, Hensel T, Ogata N, Schwab ME (1998). Spreading and migration of human glioma and rat C6 cells on central nervous system myelin in vitro is correlated with tumor malignancy and involves a metalloproteolytic activity. *Cancer Res* 58: 149-158.

1818. Carnemolla B, Castellani P, Ponassi M, Borsi L, Urbini S, Nicolo G, Dorcaratto A, Viale G, Winter G, Neri D, Zardi L (1999). Identification of a glioblastoma-associated tenascin-C isoform by a high affinity recombinant antibody. *Am J Pathol* 154: 1345-1352.

1819. Giese A, Loo MA, Norman SA, Treasurywala S, Berens ME (1996). Contrasting migratory response of astrocytoma cells to tenascin mediated by different integrins. *J Cell Sci* 109: 2161-2168.

1820. Giese A, Loo MA, Tran N, Haskett D, Coons SW, Berens ME (1996). Dichotomy of astrocytoma migration and proliferation. *Int J Cancer* 67: 275-282.

1821. Giese A, Westphal M (1996). Glioma invasion in the central nervous system. *Neurosurgery* 39: 235-250.

1822. Knott JC, Mahesparan R, Garcia-Cabrera I, Bolge TB, Edvardsen K, Ness GO, Mork S, Lund-Johansen M, Bjerkvig R (1998). Stimulation of extracellular matrix components in the normal brain by invading glioma cells. *Int J Cancer* 75: 864-872.

1823. Noble M, Mayer-Proschel M (1997). Growth factors, glia and gliomas. *J Neurooncol* 35: 193-209.

1824. St Croix B, Kerbel RS (1997). Cell adhesion and drug resistance in cancer. *Curr Opin Oncol* 9: 549-556.

1825. van der Valk P, Lindeman J, Kamphorst W (1997). Growth factor profiles of human gliomas. Do non-tumour cells contribute to tumour growth in glioma? *Ann Oncol* 8: 1023-1029.

1826. Haas-Kogan DA, Yount G, Haas M, Levi D, Kogan SS, Hu L, Vidair C, Deen DF, Dewey WC, Israel MA (1996). p53-dependent G1 arrest and p53-independent apoptosis influence the radiobiologic response of glioblastoma. *Int J Radiat Oncol Biol Phys* 36: 95-103.

1827. Shu HK, Kim MM, Chen P, Furman F, Julin CM, Israel MA (1998). The intrinsic radioresistance of glioblastoma-derived cell lines is associated with a failure of p53 to induce p21(BAX) expression. *Proc Natl Acad Sci U S A* 95: 14453-14458.

1828. Haslam RH, Lamborn KR, Becker LE, Israel MA (1998). Tumor cell apoptosis present at diagnosis may predict treatment outcome for patients with medulloblastoma. *J Pediatr Hematol Oncol* 20: 520-527.

1829. Dee S, Haas-Kogan DA, Israel MA (1995). Inactivation of p53 is associated with decreased levels of radiation-induced apoptosis in medulloblastoma cell lines. *Cell Death Differ* 2;267-275.

1830. Myers MP, Stolarov JP, Eng C, Li J, Wang SI, Wigler MH, Parsons R, Tonks NK (1997). P-TEN, the tumor suppressor from human chromosome 10q23, is a dual-specificity phosphatase. *Proc Natl Acad Sci U S A* 94: 9052-9057.

1831. Thiessen B, Finlay J, Kulkarni R, Rosenblum MK (1998). Astroblastoma: does histology predict biologic behavior? *J Neurooncol* 40: 59-65.

1832. Kim DG, Yang HJ, Park IA, Chi JG, Jung HW, Han DH, Choi KS, Cho BK (1998). Gliomatosis cerebri: clinical features, treatment, and prognosis. *Acta Neurochir (Wien)* 140: 755-762.

1833. Kattar MM, Kupsky WJ, Shimoyama RK, Vo TD, Olson MW, Bargar GR, Sarkar FH (1997). Clonal analysis of gliomas. *Hum Pathol* 28: 1166-1179.

1834. Yasha TC, Mohanty A, Radhesh S, Santosh V, Das S, Shankar SK (1998). Infratentorial dysembryoplastic neuroepithelial tumor (DNT) associated with Arnold-Chiari malformation. *Clin Neuropathol* 17: 305-310.

1835. Rosemberg S, Vieira GS (1998). [Dysembryoplastic neuroepithelial tumor. An epidemiological study from a single institution]. *Arq Neuropsiquiatr* 56: 232-236.

1836. Daumas-Duport C, Varlet P, Bacha S, Beuvon F, Cervera-Pierot P, Chodkiewicz JP (1999). Dysembryoplastic neuroepithelial tumors: nonspecific histological forms — a study of 40 cases. *J Neurooncol* 41: 267-280.

1837. Honavar M, Janota I, Polkey CE (1999). Histological heterogeneity of dysembryoplastic neuroepithelial tumour: identification and differential diagnosis in a series of 74 cases. *Histopathology* 34: 342-356.

1838. Wolf HK, Buslei R, Blumcke I, Wiestler OD, Pietsch T (1997). Neural antigens in oligodendrogliomas and dysembryoplastic neuroepithelial tumors. *Acta Neuropathol (Berl)* 94: 436-443.

1839. Wong K, Gyure KA, Prayson RA, Morrison AL, Le TQ, Armstrong RC (1999). Dysembryoplastic neuroepithelial tumor: in situ hybridization of proteolipid protein (PLP) messenger ribonucleic acid (mRNA). *J Neuropath Exp Neurol* 58;542-542.

1840. Komori T, Scheithauer BW, Anthony DC, Rosenblum MK, McLendon RE, Scott RM, Okazaki H, Kobayashi M (1998). Papillary glioneuronal tumor: a new variant of mixed neuronal-glial neoplasm. *Am J Surg Pathol* 22: 1171-1183.

1841. Kim DH, Suh YL (1997). Pseudopapillary neurocytoma of temporal lobe with glial differentiation. *Acta Neuropathol (Berl)* 94: 187-191.

1842. Komori T, Scheithauer BW, Anthony DC, Scott RM, Okazaki H, Kobayashi M (1996). Pseudopapillary ganaglioneurocytoma. *J Neuropathol Exp Neurol* 55;654-654.

1843. Mokry M, Kleinert R, Clarici G, Obermayer-Pietsch B (1998). Primary paraganglioma simulating pituitary macroadenoma: a case report and review of the literature. *Neuroradiology* 40: 233-237.

1844. Sambaziotis D, Kontogeorgos G, Kovacs K, Horvath E, Levedis A (1999). Intrasellar paraganglioma presenting as nonfunctioning pituitary adenoma. *Arch Pathol Lab Med* 123: 429-432.

1845. Bilbao JM, Horvath E, Kovacs K, Singer W, Hudson AR (1978). Intrasellar paraganglioma associated with hypopituitarism. *Arch Pathol Lab Med* 102: 95-98.

1846. Gaffney EF, Doorly T, Dinn JJ (1986). Aggressive oncocytic neuroendocrine tumour ('oncocytic paraganglioma') of the cauda equina. *Histopathology* 10: 311-319.

1847. Moran CA, Rush W, Mena H (1997). Primary spinal paragangliomas: a clinicopathological and immunohistochemical study of 30 cases. *Histopathology* 31: 167-173.

1848. Steel TR, Botterill P, Sheehy JP (1994). Paraganglioma of the cauda equina with associated syringomyelia: case report. *Surg Neurol* 42: 489-493.

1849. Faro SH, Turtz AR, Koenigsberg RA, Mohamed FB, Chen CY, Stein H (1997). Paraganglioma of the cauda equina with associated intramedullary cyst: MR findings. *AJNR Am J Neuroradiol* 18: 1588-1590.

1850. Chetty R (1999). Cytokeratin expression in cauda equina paragangliomas. *Am J Surg Pathol* 23: 491.

1851. van Schothorst EM, Beekman M, Torremans P, Kuipers-Dijkshoorn NJ, Wessels HW, Bardoel AF, van der Mey AG, van d, V, van Ommen GJ, Devilee P, Cornelisse CJ (1998). Paragangliomas of the head and neck region show complete loss of heterozygosity at 11q22-q23 in chief cells and the flow-sorted DNA aneuploid fraction. *Hum Pathol* 29: 1045-1049.

1852. Baysal BE, van Schothorst EM, Farr JE, Grashof P, Myssiorek D, Rubinstein WS, Taschner P, Cornelisse CJ, Devlin B, Devilee P, Richard CW (1999). Repositioning the hereditary paraganglioma critical region on chromosome band 11q23. *Hum Genet* 104: 219-225.

1853. Milunsky J, DeStefano AL, Huang XL, Baldwin CT, Michels VV, Jako G, Milunsky A (1997). Familial paragangliomas: linkage to chromosome 11q23 and clinical implications. *Am J Med Genet* 72: 66-70.

1854. Vargas MP, Zhuang Z, Wang C, Vortmeyer A, Linehan WM, Merino MJ (1997). Loss of heterozygosity on the short arm of chromosomes 1 and 3 in sporadic pheochromocytoma and extra-adrenal paraganglioma. *Hum Pathol* 28: 411-415.

1855. Clarke MR, Weyant RJ, Watson CG, Carty SE (1998). Prognostic markers in pheochromocytoma. *Hum Pathol* 29: 522-526.

1856. Emory TS, Scheithauer BW, Hirose T, Wood M, Onofrio BM, Jenkins RB (1995). Intraneural perineurioma. A clonal neoplasm associated with abnormalities of chromosome 22. *Am J Clin Pathol* 103: 696-704.

1857. Giannini C, Scheithauer BW, Steinberg J, Cosgrove TJ (1998). Intraventricular perineurioma: case report. *Neurosurgery* 43: 1478-1481.

1858. Hirose T, Scheithauer BW, Sano T (1998). Perineurial malignant peripheral nerve sheath tumor (MPNST): a clinicopathologic, immunohistochemical, and ultrastructural study of seven cases. *Am J Surg Pathol* 22: 1368-1378.

1861. Giannini C, Scheithauer BW, Jenkins RB, Erlandson RA, Perry A, Borell TJ, Hoda RS, Woodruff JM (1997). Soft-tissue perineurioma. Evidence for an abnormality of chromosome 22, criteria for diagnosis, and review of the literature. *Am J Surg Pathol* 21: 164-173.

1862. Hirose T, Scheithauer BW (1999). Sclerosing perineurioma: a distinct entity? *Int J Surg Pathol* 7: 133-140.

1863. Prayson RA (1999). Bcl-2 and Bcl-X expression in gangliogliomas. *Hum Pathol* 30: 701-705.

1864. Mittler MA, Walters BC, Fried AH, Sotomayor EA, Stopa EG (1999). Malignant glial tumor arising from the site of a previous hamartoma/ganglioglioma: coincidence or malignant transformation? *Pediatr Neurosurg* 30: 132-134.

1865. Araki M, Fan J, Haraoka S, Moritake T, Yoshii Y, Watanabe T (1999). Extracranial metastasis of anaplastic ganglioglioma through a ventriculoperitoneal shunt: a case report. *Pathol Int* 49: 258-263.

1866. Dash RC, Provenzale JM, McComb RD, Perry DA, Longee DC, McLendon RE (1999). Malignant supratentorial ganglioglioma (ganglion cell-giant cell glioblastoma): a case report and review of the literature. *Arch Pathol Lab Med* 123: 342-345.

1867. Prayson RA (1999). Composite ganglioglioma and dysembryoplastic neuroepithelial tumor. *Arch Pathol Lab Med* 123: 247-250.

1868. Rumana CS, Valadka AB, Contant CF (1999). Prognostic factors in supratentorial ganglioglioma. *Acta Neurochir (Wien)* 141: 63-68.

1869. Rumana CS, Valadka AB (1998). Radiation therapy and malignant degeneration of benign supratentorial gangliogliomas. *Neurosurgery* 42: 1038-1043.

1870. Quinn B (1998). Diagnosis of ganglioglioma. *J Neurosurg* 88: 935-937.

1871. Jay V, Squire J, Blaser S, Hoffman HJ, Hwang P (1997). Intracranial and spinal metastases from a ganglioglioma with unusual cytogenetic abnormalities in a patient with complex partial seizures. *Childs Nerv Syst* 13: 550-555.

1872. Zentner J, Hufnagel A, Wolf HK, Ostertun B, Behrens E, Campos MG, Elger CE, Wiestler OD, Schramm J (1997). Surgical treatment of neoplasms associated with medically intractable epilepsy. *Neurosurgery* 41: 378-386.

1873. Zhu JJ, Leon SP, Folkerth RD, Guo SZ, Wu JK, Black PM (1997). Evidence for clonal origin of neoplastic neuronal and glial cells in gangliogliomas. *Am J Pathol* 151: 565-571.

1874. Johnson JH, Hariharan S, Berman J, Sutton LN, Rorke LB, Molloy P, Phillips PC (1997). Clinical outcome of pediatric gangliogliomas: ninety-nine cases over 20 years. *Pediatr Neurosurg* 27: 203-207.

1875. Sawin PD, Theodore N, Rekate HL (1999). Spinal cord ganglioglioma in a child with neurofibromatosis type 2. Case report and literature review. *J Neurosurg* 90: 231-233.

1876. Zentner J, Hufnagel A, Wolf HK, Ostertun B, Behrens E, Campos MG, Solymosi L, Elger CE, Wiestler OD, Schramm J (1995). Surgical treatment of temporal lobe epilepsy: clinical, radiological, and histopathological findings in 178 patients. *J Neurol Neurosurg Psychiatry* 58: 666-673.

1877. Armstrong D, Rouah E, Zhu Z, Rutecki P, Mizrahi E, Grossman R (1988). The spectrum of histopathology of ganagliogliomas in patients with complex partial epilepsy. *J Neuropath Exp Neurol* 47;373-373.

1878. McLendon RE, Enterline DS, Tien RD, Thorstad WL, Bruner JM (1998). Tumours of Central Neuroepithelial Origin. In: *Russel and Rubinstein's Pathology of Tumors of the Nervous System*, Bigner DD, McLendon RE, Bruner JM (eds), 6th ed. Arnold: London. pp. 307-571.

1879. Amoaku WM, Willshaw HE, Parkes SE, Shah KJ, Mann JR (1996). Trilateral retinoblastoma. A report of five patients. *Cancer* 78: 858-863.

1880. Cho BK, Wang KC, Nam DH, Kim DG, Jung HW, Kim HJ, Han DH, Choi KS (1998). Pineal tumors: experience with 48 cases over 10 years. *Childs Nerv Syst* 14: 53-58.

1881. DeGirolami U, Zvaigzne O (1973). Modification of the Achucarro-Hortega pineal stain for paraffin- embedded formalin-fixed tissue. *Stain Technol* 48: 48-50.

1882. Fevre-Montange M, Jouvet A, Privat K, Korf HW, Champier J, Reboul A, Aguera M, Mottolese C (1998). Immunohistochemical, ultrastructural, biochemical and in vitro studies of a pineocytoma. *Acta Neuropathol (Berl)* 95: 532-539.

1883. Grimoldi N, Tomei G, Stankov B, Lucini V, Masini B, Caputo V, Repetti ML, Lazzarini G, Gaini SM, Lucarini C, Fraschini F, Villani R (1998). Neuroendocrine, immunohistochemical, and ultrastructural study of pineal region tumors. *J Pineal Res* 25: 147-158.

1884. Ikeda J, Sawamura Y, Van Meir EG (1998). Pineoblastoma presenting in familial adenomatous polyposis (FAP): random association, FAP variant or Turcot syndrome? *Br J Neurosurg* 12: 576-578.

1885. Kees UR, Spagnolo D, Hallam LA, Ford J, Ranford PR, Baker DL, Callen DF, Biegel JA (1998). A new pineoblastoma cell line, PER-480, with der(10)t(10;17), der(16)t(1;16), and enhanced MYC expression in the absence of gene amplification. *Cancer Genet Cytogenet* 100: 159-164.

1886. Marcus DM, Brooks SE, Leff G, McCormick R, Thompson T, Anfinson S, Lasudry J, Albert DM (1998). Trilateral retinoblastoma: insights into histogenesis and management. *Surv Ophthalmol* 43: 59-70.

1887. Schild SE, Scheithauer BW, Haddock MG, Wong WW, Lyons MK, Marks LB, Norman MG, Burger PC (1996). Histologically confirmed pineal tumors and other germ cell tumors of the brain. *Cancer* 78: 2564-2571.

1888. Sreekantaiah C, Hubert J, Brecher ML, Sandberg AA (1989). Interstitial deletion of chromosome 11q in a pineoblastoma. *Cancer Genet Cytogenet* 39: 125-131.

1889. Burnett ME, White EC, Sih S, von Haken MS, Cogen PH (1997). Chromosome arm 17p deletion analysis reveals molecular genetic heterogeneity in supratentorial and infratentorial primitive neuroectodermal tumors of the central nervous system. *Cancer Genet Cytogenet* 97: 25-31.

1890. McLendon RE, Bentley RC, Parisi JE, Tien RD, Harrison JC, Tarbell NJ, Billitt AL, Gualtieri RJ, Friedman HS (1997). Malignant supratentorial glial-neuronal neoplasms: report of two cases and review of the literature. *Arch Pathol Lab Med* 121: 485-492.

1891. Avet-Loiseau H, Venuat AM, Terrier-Lacombe MJ, Lellouch-Tubiana A, Zerah M, Vassal G (1999). Comparative genomic hybridization detects many recurrent imbalances in central nervous system primitive neuroectodermal tumours in children. *Br J Cancer* 79: 1843-1847.

1893. Benitez J, Osorio A, Barroso A, Arranz E, Diaz-Guillen MA, Robledo M, Rodriguez dC, Heine-Suner D (1997). A region of allelic imbalance in 1q31-32 in primary breast cancer coincides with a recombination hot spot. *Cancer Res* 57: 4217-4220.

1894. Brandes AA, Palmisano V, Monfardini S (1999). Medulloblastoma in adults: clinical characteristics and treatment. *Cancer Treat Rev* 25: 3-12.

1895. Chidambaram B, Santhosh V, Shankar SK (1998). Identical twins with medulloblastoma occurring in infancy. *Childs Nerv Syst* 14: 421-425.

1896. Dean M (1996). Polarity, proliferation and the hedgehog pathway. *Nat Genet* 14: 245-247.

1897. Giordana MT, Schiffer P, Lanotte M, Girardi P, Chio A (1999). Epidemiology of adult medulloblastoma. *Int J Cancer* 80: 689-692.

1898. Goodrich LV, Scott MP (1998). Hedgehog and patched in neural development and disease. *Neuron* 21: 1243-1257.

1899. Brown HG, Kepner JL, Perlman EJ, Friedman HS, Strother DR, Duffner PK, Kun LE, Goldthwaite PT, Burger PC (1999). "Large cell/anaplastic" medulloblastomas. A pediatric oncology group study. *J Neuropathol Clin Neurol* (in press).

1900. Giangaspero F, Perilongo G, Fondelli MP, Brisigotti M, Carollo C, Burnelli R, Burger PC, Garre ML (1999). Medulloblastoma with extensive nodularity: a variant with favorable prognosis. *J Neurosurg* 91: 971-977.

1901. Grotzer MA, Fung KM, Janss AJ, Rorke LB, Sutton LN, Cnaan A, Phillips PC, Lee VMY,Trojanowski JQ (1999). Expression of TrkC receptors in primitive neuroectodermal tumor/medulloblastoma correlates with the expression of neurofilament protein and is associated with a favorable prognosis. *J Neuropathol Exp Neurol* 58;544-544.

1903. Khalili K, Krynska B, Del Valle L, Katsetos CD, Croul S (1999). Medulloblastomas and the human neurotropic polyomavirus JC virus. *Lancet* 353: 1152-1153.

1904. Kim JY, Sutton ME, Lu DJ, Cho TA, Goumnerova LC, Goritchenko L, Kaufman JR, Lam KK, Billet AL, Tarbell NJ, Wu J, Allen JC, Stiles CD, Segal RA, Pomeroy SL (1999). Activation of neurotrophin-3 receptor TrkC induces apoptosis in medulloblastomas. *Cancer Res* 59: 711-719.

1905. Koch A, Tonn J, Kraus JA, Sorensen N, Albrecht NS, Wiestler OD, Pietsch T (1996). Molecular analysis of the lissencephaly gene 1 (LIS-1) in medulloblastomas. *Neuropathol Appl Neurobiol* 22: 233-242.

1906. Kraus JA, Koch A, Albrecht S, von Deimling A, Wiestler OD, Pietsch T (1996). Loss of heterozygosity at locus F13B on chromosome 1q in human medulloblastoma. *Int J Cancer* 67: 11-15.

1907. Lam CW, Xie J, To KF, Ng HK, Lee KC, Yuen NW, Lim PL, Chan LY, Tong SF, McCormick F (1999). A frequent activated smoothened mutation in sporadic basal cell carcinomas. *Oncogene* 18: 833-836.

1908. McLendon RE, Friedman HS, Fuchs HE, Kun LE, Bigner SH (1999). Diagnostic markers in paediatric medulloblastoma: a Paediatric Oncology Group Study. *Histopathology* 34: 154-162.

1909. Packer RJ (1999). Childhood medulloblastoma: progress and future challenges. *Brain Dev* 21: 75-81.

1910. Rasheed BK, Stenzel TT, McLendon RE, Parsons R, Friedman AH, Friedman HS, Bigner DD, Bigner SH (1997). PTEN gene mutations are seen in high-grade but not in low-grade gliomas. *Cancer Res* 57: 4187-4190.

1911. Reardon DA, Michalkiewicz E, Boyett JM, Sublett JE, Entrekin RE, Ragsdale ST, Valentine MB, Behm FG, Li H, Heideman RL, Kun LE, Shapiro DN, Look AT (1997). Extensive genomic abnormalities in childhood medulloblastoma by comparative genomic hybridization. *Cancer Res* 57: 4042-4047.

1912. Reifenberger J, Wolter M, Weber RG, Megahed M, Ruzicka T, Lichter P, Reifenberger G (1998). Missense mutations in SMOH in sporadic basal cell carcinomas of the skin and primitive neuroectodermal tumors of the central nervous system. *Cancer Res* 58: 1798-1803.

1913. Rostomily RC, Bermingham-McDonogh O, Berger MS, Tapscott SJ, Reh TA, Olson JM (1997). Expression of neurogenic basic helix-loop-helix genes in primitive neuroectodermal tumors. *Cancer Res* 57: 3526-3531.

1914. Scheurlen WG, Schwabe GC, Joos S, Mollenhauer J, Sorensen N, Kuhl J (1998). Molecular analysis of childhood primitive neuroectodermal tumors defines markers associated with poor outcome. *J Clin Oncol* 16: 2478-2485.

1916. Schiffer D, Bortolotto S, Bosone I, Cancelli I, Cavalla P, Schiffer P, Piva R (1999). Cell-cycle inhibitor p27/Kip-1 expression in non-astrocytic and non- oligodendrocytic human nervous system tumors. *Neurosci Lett* 264: 29-32.

1917. Seranski P, Heiss NS, Dhorne-Pollet S, Radelof U, Korn B, Hennig S, Backes E, Schmidt S, Wiemann S, Schwarz CE, Lehrach H, Poustka A (1999). Transcription mapping in a medulloblastoma breakpoint interval and Smith-Magenis syndrome candidate region: identification of 53 transcriptional units and new candidate genes. *Genomics* 56: 1-11.

1918. Smyth I, Narang MA, Evans T, Heimann C, Nakamura Y, Chenevix-Trench G, Pietsch T, Wicking C, Wainwright BJ (1999). Isolation and characterization of human patched 2 (PTCH2), a putative tumour suppressor gene inbasal cell carcinoma and medulloblastoma on chromosome 1p32. *Hum Mol Genet* 8: 291-297.

1919. Stevens MC, Cameron AH, Muir KR, Parkes SE, Reid H, Whitwell H (1991). Descriptive epidemiology of primary central nervous system tumours in children: a population-based study. *Clin Oncol (R Coll Radiol)* 3: 323-329.

1920. Sure U, Berghorn WJ, Bertalanffy H, Wakabayashi T, Yoshida J, Sugita K, Seeger W (1995). Staging, scoring and grading of medulloblastoma. A postoperative prognosis predicting system based on the cases of a single institute. *Acta Neurochir (Wien)* 132: 59-65.

1921. Tajima Y, Molina RPJ, Rorke LB, Kaplan DR, Radeke M, Feinstein SC, Lee VM, Trojanowski JQ (1998). Neurotrophins and neuronal versus glial differentiation in medulloblastomas and other pediatric brain tumors. *Acta Neuropathol (Berl)* 95: 325-332.

1922. Sommer A, Koch A, Tonn J, Sorensen N, Hurlin P, Luscher B, Pietsch T (1999). Analysis of the Max binding protein MNT in human medulloblastomas. *Int J Cancer* 82: 810-816.

1923. Vorechovsky I, Tingby O, Hartman M, Stromberg B, Nister M, Collins VP, Toftgard R (1997). Somatic mutations in the human homologue of Drosophila patched in primitive neuroectodermal tumours. *Oncogene* 15: 361-366.

1924. Wechsler-Reya RJ, Scott MP (1999). Control of neuronal precursor proliferation in the cerebellum by Sonic Hedgehog. *Neuron* 22: 103-114.

1925. Wicking C, Evans T, Henk B, Hayward N, Simms LA, Chenevix-Trench G, Pietsch T, Wainwright B (1998). No evidence for the H133Y mutation in SONIC HEDGEHOG in a collection of common tumour types. *Oncogene* 16: 1091-1093.

1926. Xie J, Murone M, Luoh SM, Ryan A, Gu Q, Zhang C, Bonifas JM, Lam CW, Hynes M, Goddard A, Rosenthal A, Epstein EHJ, de Sauvage FJ (1998). Activating Smoothened mutations in sporadic basal-cell carcinoma. *Nature* 391: 90-92.

1927. Yokota N, Aruga J, Takai S, Yamada K, Hamazaki M, Iwase T, Sugimura H, Mikoshiba K (1996). Predominant expression of human zic in cerebellar granule cell lineage and medulloblastoma. *Cancer Res* 56: 377-383.

1928. Zurawel RH, Chiappa SA, Allen C, Raffel C (1998). Sporadic medulloblastomas contain oncogenic beta-catenin mutations. *Cancer Res* 58: 896-899.

1929. Green WR, Iliff WJ, Trotter RR (1974). Malignant teratoid medulloepithelioma of the optic nerve. *Arch Ophthalmol* 91: 451-454.

1930. Sharma MC, Mahapatra AK, Gaikwad S, Jain AK, Sarkar C (1998). Pigmented medulloepithelioma: report of a case and review of the literature. *Childs Nerv Syst* 14: 74-78.

1932. Khoddami M, Becker LE (1997). Immunohistochemistry of medulloepithelioma and neural tube. *Pediatr Pathol Lab Med* 17: 913-925.

1933. Cruz-Sanchez FF, Rossi ML, Hughes JT, Moss TH (1991). Differentiation in embryonal neuroepithelial tumors of the central nervous system. *Cancer* 67: 965-976.

1934. Dorsay TA, Rovira MJ, Ho VB, Kelley J (1995). Ependymoblastoma: MR presentation. A case report and review of the literature. *Pediatr Radiol* 25: 433-435.

1935. Monteferrante ML, Shimkin PM, Fichtenbaum C, Kleinman GM, Lipow KI (1991). Tentorial traversal by ependymoblastoma. *AJNR Am J Neuroradiol* 12: 181.

1936. Murphy MN, Dhalla SS, Diocee M, Halliday W, Wiseman NE, deSa DJ (1987). Congenital ependymoblastoma presenting as a sacrococcygeal mass in a newborn: an immunohistochemical, light and electron microscopic study. *Clin Neuropathol* 6: 169-173.

1937. Parkkila AK, Herva R, Parkkila S, Rajaniemi H (1995). Immunohistochemical demonstration of human carbonic anhydrase isoenzyme II in brain tumours. *Histochem J* 27: 974-982.

1938. Robertson PL, Zeltzer PM, Boyett JM, Rorke LB, Allen JC, Geyer JR, Stanley P, Li H, Albright AL, McGuire-Cullen P, Finlay JL, Stevens KRJ, Milstein JM, Packer RJ, Wisoff J (1998). Survival and prognostic factors following radiation therapy and chemotherapy for ependymomas in children: a report of the Children's Cancer Group. *J Neurosurg* 88: 695-703.

1939. Rorke LB, Gilles FH, Davis RL, Becker LE (1985). Revision of the World Health Organization classification of brain tumors for childhood brain tumors. *Cancer* 56: 1869-1886.

1940. Wada C, Kurata A, Hirose R, Tazaki Y, Kan S, Ishihara Y, Kameya T (1986). Primary leptomeningeal ependymoblastoma. Case report. *J Neurosurg* 64: 968-973.

1942. McClain K, Jin H, Gresik V, Favara B (1994). Langerhans cell histiocytosis: lack of a viral etiology. *Am J Hematol* 47: 16-20.

1943. Montine TJ, Hollensead SC, Ellis WG, Martin JS, Moffat EJ, Burger PC (1994). Solitary eosinophilic granuloma of the temporal lobe: a case report and long-term follow-up of previously reported cases. *Clin Neuropathol* 13: 225-228.

1944. Muenchau A, Laas R (1997). Xanthogranuloma and xanthoma of the choroid plexus: evidence for different etiology and pathogenesis. *Clin Neuropathol* 16: 72-76.

1945. Odell WD, Doggett RS (1993). Xanthoma disseminatum, a rare cause of diabetes insipidus. *J Clin Endocrinol Metab* 76: 777-780.

1946. Owen G, Webb DK (1995). Evidence of clonality in a child with haemophagocytic lymphohistiocytosis. *Br J Haematol* 89: 681-682.

1947. Paulli M, Bergamaschi G, Tonon L, Viglio A, Rosso R, Facchetti F, Geerts ML, Magrini U, Cazzola M (1995). Evidence for a polyclonal nature of the cell infiltrate in sinus histiocytosis with massive lymphadenopathy (Rosai-Dorfman disease). *Br J Haematol* 91: 415-418.

1948. Paulus W, Kirchner T, Michaela M, Kuhl J, Warmuth-Metz M, Sorensen N, Muller-Hermelink HK, Roggendorf W (1992). Histiocytic tumor of Meckel's cave. An intracranial equivalent of juvenile xanthogranuloma of the skin. *Am J Surg Pathol* 16: 76-83.

1949. Poe LB, Dubowy RL, Hochhauser L, Collins GH, Crosley CJ, Kanzer MD, Oliphant M, Hodge CJJ (1994). Demyelinating and gliotic cerebellar lesions in Langerhans cell histiocytosis. *AJNR Am J Neuroradiol* 15: 1921-1928.

1950. Resnick DK, Johnson BL, Lovely TJ (1996). Rosai-Dorfman disease presenting with multiple orbital and intracranial masses. *Acta Neuropathol (Berl)* 91: 554-557.

1951. Risdall RJ, Dehner LP, Duray P, Kobrinsky N, Robison L, Nesbit MEJ (1983). Histiocytosis X (Langerhans' cell histiocytosis). Prognostic role of histopathology. *Arch Pathol Lab Med* 107: 59-63.

1952. Schmitt S, Wichmann W, Martin E, Zachmann M, Schoenle EJ (1993). Pituitary stalk thickening with diabetes insipidus preceding typical manifestations of Langerhans cell histiocytosis in children. *Eur J Pediatr* 152: 399-401.

1953. Thomas C, Donnadieu J, Emile JF, Brousse N (1996). [Langerhans cell histiocytosis]. *Arch Pediatr* 3: 63-69.

1955. Willis B, Ablin A, Weinberg V, Zoger S, Wara WM, Matthay KK (1996). Disease course and late sequelae of Langerhans' cell histiocytosis: 25- year experience at the University of California, San Francisco. *J Clin Oncol* 14: 2073-2082.

1957. Zelger BW, Sidoroff A, Orchard G, Cerio R (1996). Non-Langerhans cell histiocytoses. A new unifying concept. *Am J Dermatopathol* 18: 490-504.

1958. Glick R, Baker C, Husain S, Hays A, Hibshoosh H (1997). Primary melanocytomas of the spinal cord: a report of seven cases. *Clin Neuropathol* 16: 127-132.

1959. Argani P, Perez-Ordonez B, Xiao H, Caruana SM, Huvos AG, Ladanyi M (1998). Olfactory neuroblastoma is not related to the Ewing family of tumors: absence of EWS/FLI1 gene fusion and MIC2 expression. *Am J Surg Pathol* 22: 391-398.

1960. Chang KC, Jin YT, Chen RM, Su LJ (1997). Mixed olfactory neuroblastoma and craniopharyngioma: an unusual pathological finding. *Histopathology* 30: 378-382.

1961. Gul B, Kulacoglu S, Yuksel M, Dogan H, Okten AI (1997). Esthesioneuroblastoma in a young child. *Neurosurg Rev* 20: 59-61.

1962. Koka VN, Julieron M, Bourhis J, Janot F, Le Ridant AM, Marandas P, Luboinski B, Schwaab G (1998). Aesthesioneuroblastoma. *J Laryngol Otol* 112: 628-633.

1963. McElroy EAJ, Buckner JC, Lewis JE (1998). Chemotherapy for advanced esthesioneuroblastoma: the Mayo Clinic experience. *Neurosurgery* 42: 1023-1027.

1964. Polin RS, Sheehan JP, Chenelle AG, Munoz E, Larner J, Phillips CD, Cantrell RW, Laws ERJ, Newman SA, Levine PA, Jane JA (1998). The role of preoperative adjuvant treatment in the management of esthesioneuroblastoma: the University of Virginia experience. *Neurosurgery* 42: 1029-1037.

1965. Ramsay HA, Kairemo KJ, Jekunen AP (1996). Somatostatin receptor imaging of olfactory neuroblastoma. *J Laryngol Otol* 110: 1161-1163.

1966. Hyams VJ (1983). Olfactory Neuroblastoma. In: *Special Tumors of the Head and Neck*, Batsakis JG, Hyams VJ, Morales AR (eds). American Society of Clinical Pathologists: Chicago. pp. 24-29.

1967. Hyams VJ (1988). Tumors of the upper respiratory tract and ear. In: *Atlas of Tumor Pathology*, Hyams VJ, Batsakis JG, Michaels L (eds). Armed Forces Institute of Pathology: Washington. pp. 240-248.

1969. Kourea HP, Bilsky MH, Leung DH, Lewis JJ, Woodruff JM (1998). Subdiaphragmatic and intrathoracic paraspinal malignant peripheral nerve sheath tumors: a clinicopathologic study of 25 patients and 26 tumors. *Cancer* 82: 2191-2203.

1970. Leone PE, Bello MJ, Mendiola M, Kusak ME, de Campos JM, Vaquero J, Sarasa JL, Pestana A, Rey JA (1998). Allelic status of 1p, 14q, and 22q and NF2 gene mutations in sporadic schwannomas. *Int J Mol Med* 1: 889-892.

1971. Rao UN, Surti U, Hoffner L, Yaw K (1996). Cytogenetic and histologic correlation of peripheral nerve sheath tumors of soft tissue. *Cancer Genet Cytogenet* 88: 17-25.

1972. Sakaguchi N, Sano K, Ito M, Baba T, Fukuzawa M, Hotchi M (1996). A case of von Recklinghausen's disease with bilateral pheochromocytoma- malignant peripheral nerve sheath tumors of the adrenal and gastrointestinal autonomic nerve tumors. *Am J Surg Pathol* 20: 889-897.

1973. Serra E, Puig S, Otero D, Gaona A, Kruyer H, Ars E, Estivill X, Lazaro C (1997). Confirmation of a double-hit model for the NF1 gene in benign neurofibromas. *Am J Hum Genet* 61: 512-519.

1974. Kourea HP, Cordon-Cardo C, Dudas M, Leung D, Woodruff JM (1999). Expression of p27^{KIP} and other cell-cycle regulators in malignant peripheral nerve sheath tumors and neurofibromas. The emerging role of p27^{KIP} in malignant transformation of neurofibromas. *Am J Pathol* 155: 1885-1891.

1975. Kourea HP, Orlow I, Scheithauer BW, Cordon-Cardo C, Woodruff JM (1999). Deletions of the INK4A gene occur in malignant peripheral nerve sheath tumors but not in neurofibromas. *Am J Pathol* 155: 1855-1860.

1976. Nielsen GP, Stemmer-Rachmaninov AO, Ino Y, Moller MB, Rosenberg AE, Louis DN (1999). Malignant transformation of neurofibromas in neurofibromatosis 1 is associated with CDKN2A/p16 inactivation. *Am J Pathol* 155: 1879-1884.

1977. Scheithauer BW, Woodruff JM, Erlandson RA (1999). *Tumors of the Peripheral Nervous System*. Armed Forces Institute of Pathology: Washington, D.C.

1978. Memoli VA, Brown EF, Gould VE (1984). Glial fibrillary acidic protein (GFAP) immunoreactivity in peripheral nerve sheath tumors. *Ultrastruct Pathol* 7: 269-275.

1979. Schwechheimer K, Braus DF, Schwarzkopf G, Feller AC, Volk B, Muller-Hermelink HK (1994). Polymorphous high-grade B cell lymphoma is the predominant type of spontaneous primary cerebral malignant lymphomas. Histological and immunomorphological evaluation of computed tomography-guided stereotactic brain biopsies. *Am J Surg Pathol* 18: 931-937.

1980. Antinori A, De Rossi G, Ammassari A, Cingolani A, Murri R, Di Giuda D, De Luca A, Pierconti F, Tartaglione T, Scerrati M, Larocca LM, Ortona L (1999). Value of combined approach with thallium-201 single-photon emission computed tomography and Epstein-Barr virus DNA polymerase chain reaction in CSF for the diagnosis of AIDS-related primary CNS lymphoma. *J Clin Oncol* 17: 554-560.

1981. Antinori A, Larocca LM, Fassone L, Cattani P, Capello D, Cingolani A, Saglio G, Fadda G, Gaidano G, Ortona L (1999). HHV-8/KSHV is not associated with AIDS-related primary central nervous system lymphoma. *Brain Pathol* 9: 199-208.

1982. Bakshi R, Mazziotta JC, Mischel PS, Jahan R, Seligson DB, Vinters HV (1999). Lymphomatosis cerebri presenting as a rapidly progressive dementia: clinical, neuroimaging and pathologic findings. *Dement Geriatr Cogn Disord* 10: 152-157.

1983. Cingolani A, De Luca A, Larocca LM, Ammassari A, Scerrati M, Antinori A, Ortona L (1998). Minimally invasive diagnosis of acquired immunodeficiency syndrome- related primary central nervous system lymphoma. *J Natl Cancer Inst* 90: 364-369.

1984. Cobbers JM, Wolter M, Reifenberger J, Ring GU, Jessen F, An HX, Niederacher D, Schmidt EE, Ichimura K, Floeth F, Kirsch L, Borchard F, Louis DN, Collins VP, Reifenberger G (1998). Frequent inactivation of CDKN2A and rare mutation of TP53 in PCNSL. *Brain Pathol* 8: 263-276.

1985. Corn BW, Marcus SM, Topham A, Hauck W, Curran WJ, Jr. (1997). Will primary central nervous system lymphoma be the most frequent brain tumor diagnosed in the year 2000? *Cancer* 79: 2409-2413.

1986. Deckert-Schluter M, Rang A, Wiestler OD (1998). Apoptosis and apoptosis-related gene products in primary non-Hodgkin's lymphoma of the central nervous system. *Acta Neuropathol (Berl)* 96: 157-162.

1987. Finn WG, Peterson LC, James C, Goolsby CL (1998). Enhanced detection of malignant lymphoma in cerebrospinal fluid by multiparameter flow cytometry. *Am J Clin Pathol* 110: 341-346.

1988. Hao D, DiFrancesco LM, Brasher PM, deMetz C, Fulton DS, DeAngelis LM, Forsyth PA (1999). Is primary CNS lymphoma really becoming more common? A population-based study of incidence, clinicopathological features and outcomes in Alberta from 1975 to 1996. *Ann Oncol* 10: 65-70.

1989. Julien S, Radosavljevic M, Labouret N, Camilleri-Broet S, Davi F, Raphael M, Martin T, Pasquali JL (1999). AIDS primary central nervous system lymphoma: molecular analysis of the expressed VH genes and possible implications for lymphomagenesis. *J Immunol* 162: 1551-1558.

1990. Kambham N, Chang Y, Matsushima AY (1998). Primary low-grade B-cell lymphoma of mucosa-associated lymphoid tissue (MALT) arising in dura. *Clin Neuropathol* 17: 311-317.

1991. Klein R, Mullges W, Bendszus M, Woydt M, Kreipe H, Roggendorf W (1999). Primary intracerebral Hodgkin's disease: report of a case with Epstein- Barr virus association and review of the literature. *Am J Surg Pathol* 23: 477-481.

1992. Kumar S, Kumar D, Kaldjian EP, Bauserman S, Raffeld M, Jaffe ES (1997). Primary low-grade B-cell lymphoma of the dura: a mucosa associated lymphoid tissue-type lymphoma. *Am J Surg Pathol* 21: 81-87.

1993. Larocca LM, Capello D, Rinelli A, Nori S, Antinori A, Gloghini A, Cingolani A, Migliazza A, Saglio G, Cammilleri-Broet S, Raphael M, Carbone A, Gaidano G (1998). The molecular and phenotypic profile of primary central nervous system lymphoma identifies distinct categories of the disease and is consistent with histogenetic derivation from germinal center-related B cells. *Blood* 92: 1011-1019.

1995. Nozaki M, Tada M, Matsumoto R, Sawamura Y, Abe H, Iggo RD (1998). Rare occurrence of inactivating p53 gene mutations in primary non- astrocytic tumors of the central nervous system: reappraisal by yeast functional assay. *Acta Neuropathol (Berl)* 95: 291-296.

1996. Vieren M, Sciot R, Robberecht W (1999). Intravascular lymphomatosis of the brain: a diagnostic problem. *Clin Neurol Neurosurg* 101: 33-36.

1997. Zhang SJ, Endo S, Ichikawa T, Washiyama K, Kumanishi T (1998). Frequent deletion and 5' CpG island methylation of the p16 gene in primary malignant lymphoma of the brain. *Cancer Res* 58: 1231-1237.

1998. Mason DY, Harris NL (1999). *Human Lymphoma: Clinical Implications of the REAL Classification*. Springer: Berlin.

1999. Bigelow DC, Eisen MD, Smith PG, Yousem DM, Levine RS, Jackler RK, Kennedy DW, Kotapka MJ (1998). Lipomas of the internal auditory canal and cerebellopontine angle. *Laryngoscope* 108: 1459-1469.

2000. Brown HG, Burger PC, Olivi A, Sills AK, Barditch-Crovo PA, Lee RR (1999). Intracranial leiomyosarcoma in a patient with AIDS. *Neuroradiology* 41: 35-39.

2001. Busam KJ, Fletcher CD (1997). The clinical role of molecular genetics in soft tissue tumor pathology. *Cancer Metastasis Rev* 16: 207-227.

2002. Buttner A, Marquart KH, Mehraein P, Weis S (1997). Kaposi's sarcoma in the cerebellum of a patient with AIDS. *Clin Neuropathol* 16: 185-189.

2003. Cannon TC, Bane BL, Kistler D, Schoenhals GW, Hahn M, Leech RW, Brumback RA (1998). Primary intracerebellar osteosarcoma arising within an epidermoid cyst. *Arch Pathol Lab Med* 122: 737-739.

2004. Chitoku S, Kawai S, Watabe Y, Nishitani M, Fujimoto K, Otsuka H, Fushimi H, Kotoh K, Fuji T (1998). Intradural spinal hibernoma: case report. *Surg Neurol* 49: 509-512.

2005. Korten AG, ter Berg HJ, Spincemaille GH, van der Laan RT, Van de Wel AM (1998). Intracranial chondrosarcoma: review of the literature and report of 15 cases. *J Neurol Neurosurg Psychiatry* 65: 88-92.

2006. Nishio S, Morioka T, Inamura T, Takeshita I, Fukui M, Sasaki M, Nakamura K, Wakisaka S (1998). Radiation-induced brain tumours: potential late complications of radiation therapy for brain tumours. *Acta Neurochir (Wien)* 140: 763-770.

2007. Pirotte B, Krischek B, Levivier M, Bolyn S, Brucher JM, Brotchi J (1998). Diagnostic and microsurgical presentation of intracranial angiolipomas. Case report and review of the literature. *J Neurosurg* 88: 129-132.

2008. Sinson G, Gennarelli TA, Wells GB (1998). Suprasellar osteolipoma: case report. *Surg Neurol* 50: 457-460.

2009. Bastin KT, Mehta MP (1992). Meningeal hemangiopericytoma: defining the role for radiation therapy. *J Neurooncol* 14: 277-287.

2010. Coffey RJ, Cascino TL, Shaw EG (1993). Radiosurgical treatment of recurrent hemangiopericytomas of the meninges: preliminary results. *J Neurosurg* 78: 903-908.

2011. Dufour H, Bouillot P, Figarella-Branger D, Ndoye N, Regis J, Bugha TN, Grisoli F (1998). [Meningeal hemangiopericytomas. A retrospective review of 20 cases]. *Neurochirurgie* 44: 5-18.

2012. Galanis E, Buckner JC, Scheithauer BW, Kimmel DW, Schomberg PJ, Piepgras

DG (1998). Management of recurrent meningeal hemangiopericytoma. *Cancer* 82: 1915-1920.

2013. Middleton LP, Duray PH, Merino MJ (1998). The histological spectrum of hemangiopericytoma: application of immunohistochemical analysis including proliferative markers to facilitate diagnosis and predict prognosis. *Hum Pathol* 29: 636-640.

2014. Miettinen MM, el Rifai W, Sarlomo-Rikala M, Andersson LC, Knuutila S (1997). Tumor size-related DNA copy number changes occur in solitary fibrous tumors but not in hemangiopericytomas. *Mod Pathol* 10: 1194-1200.

2015. Perry A, Scheithauer BW, Nascimento AG (1997). The immunophenotypic spectrum of meningeal hemangiopericytoma: a comparison with fibrous meningioma and solitary fibrous tumor of meninges. *Am J Surg Pathol* 21: 1354-1360.

2016. Probst-Cousin S, Bergmann M, Schroder R, Kuchelmeister K, Schmid KW, Ernestus RJ, Janus J (1996). Ki-67 and biological behaviour in meningeal haemangiopericytomas. *Histopathology* 29: 57-61.

2017. Clarke DB, Leblanc R, Bertrand G, Quartey GR, Snipes GJ (1998). Meningeal melanocytoma. Report of a case and a historical comparison. *J Neurosurg* 88: 116-121.

2018. Diaz-Insa S, Pineda M, Bestue M, Espada F, Alvarez-Fernandez E (1998). [Neurocutaneous melanosis]. *Rev Neurol* 26: 769-771.

2020. Hirose T, Horiguchi H, Kaneko F, Kusaka K, Morizumi H, Seki K, Sano T (1997). Melanocytoma of the foramen magnum. *Pathol Int* 47: 155-160.

2021. Matsumoto S, Kang Y, Sato S, Kawakami Y, Oda Y, Araki M, Kawamura J, Uchida H (1998). Spinal meningeal melanocytoma presenting with superficial siderosis of the central nervous system. Case report and review of the literature. *J Neurosurg* 88: 890-894.

2022. Kimura H, Itoyama Y, Fujioka S, Ushio Y (1997). Neurocutaneous melanosis with intracranial malignant melanoma in an adult: a case report. *No Shinkei Geka* 25: 819-822.

2023. McLendon RE,Tien RD (1998). Tumors and tumor-like lesions of maldevelopmental origin. In: *Russel's and Rubinstein's Pathology of Tumors of the Nervous System*, Bigner DD, McLendon RE, Bruner JM (eds), 6th ed. Arnold: London-Sidney-Auckland. pp. 297-302.

2024. Greenlee JE, Narayan O, Johnson RT, Herndon RM (1977). Induction of brain tumors in hamsters with BK virus, a human papovavirus. *Lab Invest* 36: 636-641.

2025. Kepes JJ, Collins J (1999). Choroid plexus epithelium (normal and neoplastic) expresses synaptophysin. A potentially useful aid in differentiating carcinoma of the choroid plexus from metastatic papillary carcinomas. *J Neuropathol Exp Neurol* 58: 398-401.

2026. Kubo S, Ogino S, Fukushima T, Maruno M, Yoshimine T, Hasegawa H (1999). Immunocytochemical detection of insulin-like growth factor II (IGF-II) in choroid plexus papilloma: a possible marker for differential diagnosis. *Clin Neuropathol* 18: 74-79.

2027. Martini F, Lazzarin L, Iaccheri L, Corallini A, Gerosa M, Trabanelli C, Calza N, Barbanti-Brodano G, Tognon M (1998). Simian virus 40 footprints in normal human tissues, brain and bone tumours of different histotypes. *Dev Biol Stand* 94:55-66: 55-66.

2028. Nagashima K, Yasui K, Kimura J, Washizu M, Yamaguchi K, Mori W (1984). Induction of brain tumors by a newly isolated JC virus (Tokyo-1 strain). *Am J Pathol* 116: 455-463.

2030. Vital A, Bringuier PP, Huang H, San Galli F, Rivel J, Ansoborlo S, Cazauran JM, Taillandier L, Kleihues P, Ohgaki H (1998). Astrocytomas and choroid plexus tumors in two families with identical p53 germline mutations. *J Neuropathol Exp Neurol* 57: 1061-1069.

2031. Van Meir EG, Oosterhuis JW,Looijenga LHJ (1998). Genesis and genetics of intracranial germ cell tumors. In: *Intracranial Germ Cell Tumors*, Sawamura Y, Shirato H, de Tribolet N (eds). Springer Verlag: Wien New York. pp. 45-76.

2032. al Sarraj ST, Parmar D, Dean AF, Phookun G, Bridges LR (1998). Clinicopathological study of seven cases of spinal cord teratoma: a possible germ cell origin. *Histopathology* 32: 51-56.

2033. Bhattacharjee MB, Armstrong DD, Vogel H, Cooley LD (1997). Cytogenetic analysis of 120 primary pediatric brain tumors and literature review. *Cancer Genet Cytogenet* 97: 39-53.

2034. Dal Cin P, Dei Tos AP, Qi H, Giannini C, Furlanetto A, Longatti PL, Marynen P, Van den BH (1998). Immature teratoma of the pineal gland with isochromosome 12p. *Acta Neuropathol (Berl)* 95: 107-110.

2035. Fujimaki T, Matsutani M, Funada N, Kirino T, Takakura K, Nakamura O, Tamura A, Sano K (1994). CT and MRI features of intracranial germ cell tumors. *J Neurooncol* 19: 217-226.

2036. Fujita T, Yamada K, Saitoh H, Itoh S, Nakai O (1992). Intracranial germinoma and Down's syndrome—case report. *Neurol Med Chir (Tokyo)* 32: 163-165.

2037. Hasle H, Mellemgaard A, Nielsen J, Hansen J (1995). Cancer incidence in men with Klinefelter syndrome. *Br J Cancer* 71: 416-420.

2038. Lemos JA, Barbieri-Neto J, Casartelli C (1998). Primary intracranial germ cell tumors without an isochromosome 12p. *Cancer Genet Cytogenet* 100: 124-128.

2039. Losi L, Polito P, Hagemeijer A, Buonamici L, Van den BH, Dal Cin P (1998). Intracranial germ cell tumour (embryonal carcinoma with teratoma) with complex karyotype including isochromosome 12p. *Virchows Arch* 433: 571-574.

2040. O'Callaghan AM, Katapodis O, Ellison DW, Theaker JM, Mead GM (1997). The growing teratoma syndrome in a nongerminomatous germ cell tumor of the pineal gland: a case report and review. *Cancer* 80: 942-947.

2041. Sano K (1999). Pathogenesis of intracranial germ cell tumors reconsidered. *J Neurosurg* 90: 258-264.

2042. Sainati L, Bolcato S, Montaldi A, Celli P, Stella M, Leszl A, Silvestro L, Perilongo G, Cordero dM, Basso G (1996). Cytogenetics of pediatric central nervous system tumors. *Cancer Genet Cytogenet* 91: 13-27.

2043. Satge D, Sasco AJ, Cure H, Leduc B, Sommelet D, Vekemans MJ (1997). An excess of testicular germ cell tumors in Down's syndrome: three case reports and a review of the literature. *Cancer* 80: 929-935.

2044. Suijkerbuijk RF, Looijenga L, de Jong B, Oosterhuis JW, Cassiman JJ, Geurts vK (1992). Verification of isochromosome 12p and identification of other chromosome 12 aberrations in gonadal and extragonadal human germ cell tumors by bicolor double fluorescence in situ hybridization. *Cancer Genet Cytogenet* 63: 8-16.

2045. Matsutani M, Ushio Y, Abe H, Yamashita J, Shibui S, Fujimaki T, Takakura K, Nomura KI, Tanaka R, Fukui M, Yoshimoto T, Hayakawa T, Nagashima T, Kurisu K, Kayama T, Japanese Pediatric Brain Tumor Study Group (1998). Combined chemotherapy and radiation therapy for central nervous system germ cell tumors: preliminary results of a phase II study of the Japanese Pediatric Brain Tumor Study Group. *Neurosurg Focus* 5: 1-5.

2046. Adle-Biassette H, Chetritt J, Bergemer-Fouquet AM, Wechsler J, Mussini JM, Gray F (1997). Pathology of the central nervous system in Chester-Erdheim disease: report of three cases. *J Neuropathol Exp Neurol* 56: 1207-1216.

2047. Dufourcq-Lagelouse R, Jabado N, Le Deist F, Stephan JL, Souillet G, Bruin M, Vilmer E, Schneider M, Janka G, Fischer A, de Saint BG (1999). Linkage of familial hemophagocytic lymphohistiocytosis to 10q21-22 and evidence for heterogeneity. *Am J Hum Genet* 64: 172-179.

2048. Favara BE, Feller AC, Pauli M, Jaffe ES, Weiss LM, Arico M, Bucsky P, Egeler RM, Elinder G, Gadner H, Gresik M, Henter JI, Imashuku S, Janka-Schaub G, Jaffe R, Ladisch S, Nezelof C, Pritchard J (1997). Contemporary classification of histiocytic disorders. The WHO Committee On Histiocytic/Reticulum Cell Proliferations. Reclassification Working Group of the Histiocyte Society. *Med Pediatr Oncol* 29: 157-166.

2049. Weintraub M, Bhatia KG, Chandra RS, Magrath IT, Ladisch S (1998). p53 expression in Langerhans cell histiocytosis. *J Pediatr Hematol Oncol* 20: 12-17.

2050. Wright RA, Hermann RC, Parisi JE (1999). Neurological manifestations of Erdheim-Chester disease. *J Neurol Neurosurg Psychiatry* 66: 72-75.

2051. Grois N, Broadbent V, Favara BE, D'Angio G (1997). Report of the Histiocyte Society workshop on "Central nervous system (CNS) disease in Langerhans cell histiocytosis (LCH)". *Med Pediatr Oncol* 29: 73-78.

2052. Xu W, Mulligan LM, Ponder MA, Liu L, Smith BA, Mathew CG, Ponder BA (1992). Loss of NF1 alleles in phaeochromocytomas from patients with type I neurofibromatosis. *Genes Chromosomes Cancer* 4: 337-342.

2053. Brannan CI, Perkins AS, Vogel KS, Ratner N, Nordlund ML, Reid SW, Buchberg AM, Jenkins NA, Parada LF, Copeland NG (1994). Targeted disruption of the neurofibromatosis type-1 gene leads to developmental abnormalities in heart and various neural crest-derived tissues [published erratum appears in Genes Dev 1994 Nov 15;8(22):2792]. *Genes Dev* 8: 1019-1029.

2054. Jacks T, Shih TS, Schmitt EM, Bronson RT, Bernards A, Weinberg RA (1994). Tumour predisposition in mice heterozygous for a targeted mutation in Nf1. *Nat Genet* 7: 353-361.

2055. Lazaro C, Gaona A, Lynch M, Kruyer H, Ravella A, Estivill X (1995). Molecular characterization of the breakpoints of a 12-kb deletion in the NF1 gene in a family showing germ-line mosaicism. *Am J Hum Genet* 57: 1044-1049.

2056. Colman SD, Rasmussen SA, Ho VT, Abernathy CR, Wallace MR (1996). Somatic mosaicism in a patient with neurofibromatosis type 1. *Am J Hum Genet* 58: 484-490.

2057. Kim HA, Ling B, Ratner N (1997). Nf1-deficient mouse Schwann cells are angiogenic and invasive and can be induced to hyperproliferate: reversion of some phenotypes by an inhibitor of farnesyl protein transferase. *Mol Cell Biol* 17: 862-872.

2058. Silva AJ, Frankland PW, Marowitz Z, Friedman E, Lazlo G, Cioffi D, Jacks T, Bourtchuladze R (1997). A mouse model for the learning and memory deficits associated with neurofibromatosis type I. *Nat Genet* 15: 281-284.

2059. Ainsworth PJ, Chakraborty PK, Weksberg R (1997). Example of somatic mosaicism in a series of de novo neurofibromatosis type 1 cases due to a maternally derived deletion. *Hum Mutat* 9: 452-457.

2060. Side L, Taylor B, Cayouette M, Conner E, Thompson P, Luce M, Shannon K (1997). Homozygous inactivation of the NF1 gene in bone marrow cells from children with neurofibromatosis type 1 and malignant myeloid disorders. *N Engl J Med* 336: 1713-1720.

2061. Klesse LJ, Parada LF (1998). p21 ras and phosphatidylinositol-3 kinase are required for survival of wild-type and NF1 mutant sensory neurons. *J Neurosci* 18: 10420-10428.

2062. Lakkis MM, Epstein JA (1998). Neurofibromin modulation of ras activity is required for normal endocardial-mesenchymal transformation in the developing heart. *Development* 125: 4359-4367.

2063. Zhang YY, Vik TA, Ryder JW, Srour EF, Jacks T, Shannon K, Clapp DW (1998). Nf1 regulates hematopoietic progenitor cell growth and ras signaling in response to multiple cytokines. *J Exp Med* 187: 1893-1902.

2064. Kluwe L, Friedrich R, Mautner V (1999). Loss of NF1 allele in schwann cells but not in fibroblasts derived from a NF1-associated neurofibroma. *Genes Chromosomes Cancer* 24: 283-285.

2065. Antinheimo J, Haapasalo H, Haltia M, Tatagiba M, Thomas S, Brandis A, Sainio M, Carpen O, Samii M, Jaaskelainen J (1997). Proliferation potential and histological features in neurofibromatosis 2-associated and sporadic meningiomas. *J Neurosurg* 87: 610-614.

2066. Jacoby LB, Jones D, Davis K, Kronn D, Short MP, Gusella J, MacCollin M (1997). Molecular analysis of the NF2 tumor-suppressor gene in schwannomatosis. *Am J Hum Genet* 61: 1293-1302.

2067. Evans DG, Wallace AJ, Wu CL, Trueman L, Ramsden RT, Strachan T (1998). Somatic mosaicism: a common cause of classic disease in tumor-prone syndromes? Lessons from type 2 neurofibromatosis. *Am J Hum Genet* 63: 727-736.

2068. Kluwe L, Mautner VF (1998). Mosaicism in sporadic neurofibromatosis 2 patients. *Hum Mol Genet* 7: 2051-2055.

2069. Kluwe L, MacCollin M, Tatagiba M, Thomas S, Hazim W, Haase W, Mautner VF (1998). Phenotypic variability associated with 14 splice-site mutations in the NF2 gene. *Am J Med Genet* 77: 228-233.

2070. Murthy A, Gonzalez-Agosti C, Cordero E, Pinney D, Candia C, Solomon F, Gusella J, Ramesh V (1998). NHE-RF, a regulatory co-factor for Na(+)-H+ exchange, is a common interactor for merlin and ERM (MERM) proteins. *J Biol Chem* 273: 1273-1276.

2071. Gusella JF, Ramesh V, MacCollin M, Jacoby LB (1999). Merlin: the neurofibromatosis 2 tumor suppressor. *Biochim Biophys Acta* 1423: M29-M36.

2072. Xu HM, Gutmann DH (1998). Merlin differentially associates with the microtubule and actin cytoskeleton. *J Neurosci Res* 51: 403-415.

2073. Stemmer-Rachamimov AO, Gonzalez-Agosti C, Xu L, Burwick JA, Beauchamp R, Pinney D, Louis DN, Ramesh V (1997). Expression of NF2-encoded merlin and related ERM family proteins in the human central nervous system. *J Neuropathol Exp Neurol* 56: 735-742.

2074. Stemmer-Rachamimov AO, Ino Y, Lim ZY, Jacoby LB, MacCollin M, Gusella JF, Ramesh V, Louis DN (1998). Loss of the NF2 gene and merlin occur by the tumorlet stage of schwannoma development in neurofibromatosis 2. *J Neuropathol Exp Neurol* 57: 1164-1167.

2075. Giannini C, Scheithauer BW, Burger PC, Christensen MR, Wollan PC, Sebo TJ, Forsyth PA, Hayostek CJ (1999). Cellular proliferation in pilocytic and diffuse astrocytomas. *J Neuropathol Exp Neurol* 58: 46-53.

2076. Ilgren EB, Kinnier-Wilson LM, Stiller CA (1985). Gliomas in neurofibromatosis: a series of 89 cases with evidence for enhanced malignancy in associated cerebellar astrocytomas. *Pathol Annu* 20: 331-358.

2077. Perilongo G, Carollo C, Salviati L, Murgia A, Pillon M, Basso G, Gardiman M, Laverda AM (1997). Diencephalic syndromoe and disseminated juvenile pilocytic astrocytomas of the hypothalamic-optic chiasm region. *Cancer* 80: 142-146.

2078. Tihan T, Burger PC (1998). A variant of "pilocytic astrocytoma" - a possible distinct clinicopathological entity with a less favorable outcome. *J Neuropath Exp Neurol* 57: 500-500.

2079. Atuk NO, Stolle C, Owen JA, Carpenter JT, Vance ML (1998). Pheochromocytoma in von Hippel-Lindau disease: clinical presentation and mutation analysis in a large multigenerational kindred. *J Clin Endocrinol Metab* 83: 117-120.

2080. Flamme I, Krieg M, Plate KH (1998). Upregulation of vascular endothelial growth factorin stromal cells is correlated with upregulation of the transcription factor HRF/HIF-2a. *Am J Pathol* 153: 25-29.

2081. Krieg M, Marti HH, Plate KH (1998). Coexpression of erythropoietin and vascular endothelial growth factor in nervous system tumors associated with von Hippel-Lindau tumor suppressor gene loss of function. *Blood* 92: 3388-3393.

2082. Neumann HPH, Bender BU (1998). Genotype-phenotype correlations in von Hippel-Lindau disease. *J Intern Med* 243: 541-545.

2083. Manski TJ, Heffner DK, Glenn GM, Patronas NJ, Pikus AT, Katz D, Lebovics R, Sledjeski K, Choyke PL, Zbar B, Linehan M, Oldfield EH (1997). Endolymphatric sac tumors. A source of morbid hearing loss in von Hippel-Lindau disease. *JAMA* 277: 1461-1466.

2084. Olschwang S, Richard S, Boisson S, Giraud S, Laurent-Puig P, Resche F, Thomas G (1998). Germline mutation profile of the VHL gene in von Hippel-Lindau disease and in sporadic hemangioblastomas. *Hum Mutat* 12: 424-430.

2085. Stolle C, Glenn G, Zbar B, Humphrey JS, Choyke P, Walther M, Pack S, Hurley K, Andrey C, Klausner R, Linehan WM (1998). Improved detection of germline mutations in the von Hippel-Lindau disease tumor suppressor gene. *Hum Mutat* 12: 417-423.

2086. Orlandi A, Marino B, Brunori M, Greco R, Spagnoli LG (1997). Lipomatous medulloblastoma. *Clin,Neuropathol* 16: 175-179.

2087. Uro-Coste A, Garnier A, Lagarrigue J, Bousquet P, Verdie JC, Delisle MB (1999). Cerebellar adult medulloblastomas: a clinicopathological study. *Neuropathol Appl Neurobiol* 25: 97-98.

2088. Montagna N, Vaz LCA, Castro MAR (1999). Meduloblastoma cerebelar em adulto com areas lipomatosas. *J Bras Patol* 35: 49-49.

2089. Wren D, Wolswijk G, Noble M (1992). In vitro analysis of origin and maintenance of O-2A adult progenitor cells. *J Cell Biol* 116: 167-176.

2090. Albrecht S, Goodman JC, Rajagopolan S, Levy M, Cech DA, Cooley LD (1994). Malignant meningioma in Gorlin's syndrome: cytogenetic and p53 gene analysis. Case report. *J Neurosurg* 81: 466-471.

2091. Alcedo J, Noll M (1997). Hedgehog and its patched-smoothened receptor complex: a novel signalling mechanism at the cell surface. *Biol Chem* 378: 583-590.

2092. Aszterbaum M, Rothman A, Johnson RL, Fischer M, Xie J, Bonifas JM, Zhang X, Scott MP, Epstein EH, Jr. (1998). Identification of mutations in the human *PATCHED* gene in sporadic basal cell carcinomas and in patients with the basal cell nevus syndrome. *J Invest Dermatol* 110: 885-888.

2093. Gorlin RJ (1987). Nevoid basal cell carcinoma syndrome. *Medicine* 66: 98-113.

2094. Hasenpusch-Theil K, Bataille V, Laehdetie J, Obermaye F, Sampson JR, Frischauf AM (1998). Gorlin syndrome: identification of 4 novel germ-line mutations of the human *patched* (*PTCH*) gene. *Hum Mutat* 11: 480-480.

2095. Ingham PW (1998). The *patched* gene in development and cancer. *Curr Opin Genet Dev* 8: 88-94.

2096. Kimonis VE, Goldstein AM, Pastakia B, Yang ML, Kase R, DiGiovanna JJ, Bale A, Bale SJ (1997). Clinical manifestations in 105 persons with nevoid basal cell carcinoma syndrome. *Am J Med Genet* 69: 299-308.

2097. Lench NJ, Telford EAR, High AS, Markham AF, Wicking C, Wainwright BJ (1997). Characterisation of human *patched* germ line mutations in naevoid basal cell carcinoma syndrome. *Hum Genet* 100: 497-502.

2098. Maesawa C, Tamura G, Iwaya T, Ogasawara S, Ishida K, Sato N, Nishizuka S, Suzuki Y, Ikeda K, Aoki K, Saito K, Satodate R (1998). Mutations in the human homologue of the *Drosophila patched* gene in esophageal squamous cell carcinoma. *Genes Chromosomes Cancer* 21: 276-279.

2099. McGarvey TW, Maruta Y, Tomaszewski JE, Linnenbach AJ, Malkowicz SB (1998). *PTCH* gene mutations in invasive transitional cell carcinoma of the bladder. *Oncogene* 17: 1167-1172.

2100. Ming JE, Kaupas ME, Roessler E, Brunner HG, Nance WE, Stratton RF, Sujanski E, Bale SJ, Muenke M (1998). Mutations of *PATCHED* in holoprosencephaly. *Am J Hum Genet* 63: A140-A140.

2101. O'Malley S, Weitman D, Olding M, Sekhar L (1994). Multiple neoplasms following craniospinal irradiation for medulloblastoma in a patient with nevoid basal cell carcinoma syndrome. Case report. *J Neurosurg* 86: 286-288.

2102. Vorechovsky I, Unden AB, Sandstedt B, Toftgard R, Stahle-Backdahl M (1997). Trichoepitheliomas contain somatic mutations in the overexpressed *PTCH* gene: support for a gatekeeper mechanism in skin tumorigenesis. *Cancer Res* 57: 4677-4681.

2103. Wicking C, Gillies S, Smyth I, Shanley S, Fowles L, Ratcliffe J, Wainwright B, Chenevix-Trench G (1997). De novo mutations of the *patched* gene in nevoid basal cell carcinoma syndrome help to define phenotype. *Am J Med Genet* 73: 304-307.

2104. Zaphiropoulos PG, Unden AB, Rahnama F, Hollingsworth RE, Toftgard R (1999). *PTCH2*, a novel human patched gene, undergoing alternative splicing and upregulated in basal cell carcinomas. *Cancer Res* 59: 787-792.

2105. Fukushima Y, Oshika Y, Tsuchida T, Tokunaga T, Hatanaka H, Kijima H, Yamazaki H, Ueyama Y, Tamaoki N, Nakamura M (1998). Brain-specific angiogenesis inhibitor 1 expression is inversely correlated with vascularity and distant metastasis of colorectal cancer. *Int J Oncol* 13: 967-970.

2106. Guo XZ, Friess H, Di Mola FF, Heinicke JM, Abou-Shady M, Graber HU, Baer HU, Zimmermann A, Korc M, Buchler MW (1998). KAI1, a new metastasis suppressor gene, is reduced in metastatic hepatocellular carcinoma. *Hepatology* 28: 1481-1488.

2107. Lloyd BH, Platt-Higgins A, Rudland PS, Barraclough R (1998). Human S100A4 (p9Ka) induces the metastatic phenotype upon benign tumour cells. *Oncogene* 17: 465-473.

2108. Mashimo T, Watabe M, Hirota S, Hosobe S, Miura K, Tegtmeyer PJ, Rinker-Shaeffer CW, Watabe K (1998). The expression of the KAI1 gene, a tumor metastasis suppressor, is directly activated by p53. *Proc Natl Acad Sci U S A* 95: 11307-11311.

2109. Roetger A, Merschjann A, Dittmar T, Jackisch C, Barnekow A, Brandt B (1998). Selection of potentially metastatic subpopulations expressing c-erbB-2 from breast cancer tissue by use of an extravasation model. *Am J Pathol* 153: 1797-1806.

2110. Saegusa M, Hashimura M, Hara A, Okayasu I (1999). Loss of expression of the gene deleted in colon carcinoma (DCC) is closely related to histologic differentiation and lymph node metastasis in endometrial carcinoma. *Cancer* 85: 453-464.

2111. Sun Y, Wicha M, Leopold WR (1999). Regulation of metastasis-related gene expression by p53: a potential clinical implication. *Mol Carcinog* 24: 25-28.

2112. Peraud A, Watanabe K, Schwechheimer K, Yonekawa Y, Kleihues P, Ohgaki H (1999). Genetic profile of the giant cell glioblastoma. *Lab Invest* 79: 123-129.

2113. Perry JR, Ang LC, Bilbao JM, Muller PJ (1995). Clinicopathologic features of primary and postirradiation cerebral gliosarcoma. *Cancer* 75: 2910-2918.

2114. Galanis E, Buckner JC, Dinapoli RP, Scheithauer BW, Jenkins RB, Wang CH, O'Fallon JR, Farr G, Jr. (1998). Clinical outcome of gliosarcoma compared with glioblastoma multiforme: North Central Cancer Treatment Group results. *J Neurosurg* 89: 425-430.

2115. Shintaku M, Miyaji K, Adachi Y (1998). Gliosarcoma with angiosarcomatous features: a case report. *Brain Tumor Pathol* 15: 101-105.

2116. Malone JC, Brown KZ, Parker JC, Jr. (1999). Pathologic quiz case. Gliosarcoma containing malignant fibrohistiocytic, osseous, and chondroid elements. *Arch Pathol Lab Med* 123: 358-360.

2117. Sousa O, Honavar M, Fernandes T, Vieira E, Lopes C (1998). [Gliosarcomas]. *Acta Med Port* 11: 573-576.

2118. Horiguchi H, Hirose T, Kannuki S, Nagahiro S, Sano T (1998). Gliosarcoma: an immunohistochemical, ultrastructural and fluorescence in situ hybridization study. *Pathol Int* 48: 595-602.

2119. Katano H, Kamiya K, Matsumoto T, Kanai H, Masago A, Misawa I, Kubota T, Yamada K (1998). Clinical-pathological varieties of gliosarcoma: report of two cases. *Acta Neurol Belg* 98: 209-214.

2120. Sasaki H, Yoshida K, Ikeda E, Asou H, Inaba M, Otani M, Kawase T (1998). Expression of the neural cell adhesion molecule in astrocytic tumors: an inverse correlation with malignancy. *Cancer* 82: 1921-1931.

2121. Probst-Cousin S, Rickert CH, Gullotta F (1998). Factor XIIIa-immunoreactivity in tumors of the central nervous system. *Clin Neuropathol* 17: 79-84.

2122. Classen J, Hoffmann W, Kortmann RD, Lehr A, Meyermann R, Palmbach M, Bamberg M (1997). Gliosarcoma - case report and review of the literature. *Acta Oncol* 36: 771-774.

2123. Asano K, Sekiya T, Shimamura N, Tanaka M, Takemura A, Suzuki S, Kubo O (1997). [A case of giant cell-rich gliosarcoma]. *No To Shinkei* 49: 938-944.

2124. Sarkar C, Sharma MC, Sudha K, Gaikwad S, Varma A (1997). A clinico-pathological study of 29 cases of gliosarcoma with special reference to two unique variants. *Indian J Med Res* 106: 229-235.

2125. Kattar MM, Kupsky WJ, Shimoyama RK, Vo TD, Olson MW, Bargar GR, Sarkar FH (1997). Clonal analysis of gliomas. *Hum Pathol* 28: 1166-1179.

2126. Sreenan JJ, Prayson RA (1997). Gliosarcoma. A study of 13 tumors, including p53 and CD34 immunohistochemistry. *Arch Pathol Lab Med* 121: 129-133.

2127. Ang LC, Perry JR, Bilbao JM, Ozane W, Peschke E, Young B, Nelson N (1996). Postirradiated and nonirradiated gliosarcoma: immunophenotypical profile. *Can J Neurol Sci* 23: 251-256.

2128. Kepes JJ, Bastian FO, Weber ED (1996). Gliosarcoma developing from an irradiated ependymoma. *Acta Neuropathol (Berl)* 92: 515-519.

2129. Reifenberger J, Janssen G, Weber RG, Bostrom J, Engelbrecht V, Lichter P, Borchard F, Gobel U, Lenard HG, Reifenberger G (1998). Primitive neuroectodermal tumors of the cerebral hemisheres in two siblings with *TP53* germline mutation. *J Neuropathol Exp Neurol* 57: 179-187.

2130. Reis RM, Konu-Lebleblicioglu D, Lopes JM, Kleihues P, Ohgaki H (2000). Genetic profile of the gliosarcoma. *Am J Pathol* (in press).

2131. Stebbins CE, Kaelin WG, Jr., Pavletich NP (1999). Structure of the VHL-ElonginC-ElonginB complex: implications for VHL tumor suppressor function. *Science* 284: 455-461.

2132. Maxwell PH, Wiesener MS, Chang G-W, Clifford SC, Vaux EC, Cockman ME, Wykoff CC, Pugh CW, Maher ER, Ratcliffe PJ (1999). The tumor suppressor gene VHL targets hypoxia-inducible factors for oxygen-dependent proteolysis. *Nature* 399: 271-275.

2133. Dal Cin P, Van den BH, Buonamici L, Losi L, Roncaroli F, Calbucci F (1999). Cytogenetic investigation in subependymoma. *Cancer Genet Cytogenet* 108: 84.

2134. Hirato J, Nakazato Y, Iijima M, Yokoo H, Sasaki A, Yokota M, Ono N, Hirato M, Inoue H (1997). An unusual variant of ependymoma with extensive tumor cell vacuolization. *Acta Neuropathol (Berl)* 93: 310-316.

2135. Horn B, Heideman R, Geyer R, Pollack I, Packer R, Goldwein J, Tomita T, Schomberg P, Ater J, Luchtman-Jones L, Rivlin K, Lamborn K, Prados M, Bollen A, Berger M, Dahl G, McNeil E, Patterson K, Shaw D, Kubalik M, Russo C (1999). A multi-institutional retrospective study of intracranial ependymoma in children: identification of risk factors. *J Pediatr Hematol Oncol* 21: 203-211.

2136. Kramer DL, Parmiter AH, Rorke LB, Sutton LN, Biegel JA (1998). Molecular cytogenetic studies of pediatric ependymomas. *J Neurooncol* 37: 25-33.

2137. Merchant TE, Haida T, Wang MH, Finlay JL, Leibel SA (1997). Anaplastic ependymoma: treatment of pediatric patients with or without craniospinal radiation therapy. *J Neurosurg* 86: 943-949.

2138. Min KW, Scheithauer BW (1997). Clear cell ependymoma: a mimic of oligodendroglioma: clinicopathologic and ultrastructural considerations. *Am J Surg Pathol* 21: 820-826.

2139. Prayson RA (1998). Cyclin D1 and MIB-1 immunohistochemistry in ependymomas: a study of 41 cases. *Am J Clin Pathol* 110: 629-634.

2140. Prayson RA (1997). Myxopapillary ependymomas: a clinicopathologic study of 14 cases including MIB-1 and p53 immunoreactivity. *Mod Pathol* 10: 304-310.

2141. Rawlings CE, III, Giangaspero F, Burger PC, Bullard DE (1988). Ependymomas: a clinicopathologic study. *Surg Neurol* 29: 271-281.

2142. Rhodes CH, Call KM, Budarf ML, Barnoski BL, Bell CJ, Emanuel BS, Bigner SH, Park JP, Mohandas TK (1997). Molecular studies of an ependymoma-associated constitutional t(1;22)(p22;q11.2). *Cytogenet Cell Genet* 78: 247-252.

2143. Ritter AM, Hess KR, McLendon RE, Langford LA (1998). Ependymomas: MIB-1 proliferation index and survival. *J Neurooncol* 40: 51-57.

2144. Robertson PL, Zeltzer PM, Boyett JM, Rorke LB, Allen JC, Geyer JR, Stanley P, Li H, Albright AL, McGuire-Cullen P, Finlay JL, Stevens KR, Jr., Milstein JM, Packer RJ, Wisoff J (1998). Survival and prognostic factors following radiation therapy and chemotherapy for ependymomas in children: a report of the Children's Cancer Group. *J Neurosurg* 88: 695-703.

2145. Rosenblum MK (1998). Ependymal tumors: A review of their diagnostic surgical pathology. *Pediatr Neurosurg* 28: 160-165.

2146. Nijssen PC, Deprez RH, Tijssen CC, Hagemeijer A, Arnoldus EP, Teepen JL, Holl R, Niermeyer MF (1994). Familial anaplastic ependymoma: evidence of loss of chromosome 22 in tumour cells. *J Neurol Neurosurg Psychiatry* 57: 1245-1248.

2147. Ruchoux MM, Kepes JJ, Dhellemmes P, Hamon M, Maurage CA, Lecomte M, Gall CM, Chilton J (1998). Lipomatous differentiation in ependymomas: a report of three cases and comparison with similar changes reported in other central nervous system neoplasms of neuroectodermal origin. *Am J Surg Pathol* 22: 338-346.

2148. Schiffer D, Giordana MT (1998). Prognosis of ependymoma. *Childs Nerv Syst* 14: 357-361.

2149. Schiffer D, Chio A, Giordana MT, Pezzulo T, Vigliani MC (1993). Proliferating cell nuclear antigen expression in brain tumors, and its prognostic role in ependymomas: an immunohistochemical study. *Acta Neuropathol (Berl)* 85: 495-502.

2150. Zec N, De Girolami U, Schofield DE, Scott RM, Anthony DC (1996). Giant cell ependymoma of the filum terminale. A report of two cases. *Am J Surg Pathol* 20: 1091-1101.

2151. Prayson RA (1999). Clinicopathologic study of 61 patients with ependymoma including MIB-1 immunohistochemistry. *Ann Diagn Pathol* 3: 11-18.

2152. Ebert C, von Haken M, Meyer-Puttlitz B, Wiestler OD, Reifenberger G, Pietsch T, von Deimling A (1999). Molecular genetic analysis of ependymal tumors: *NF2* mutations and chromosome 22q loss occur preferentially in intramedullary spinal ependymomas. *Am J Pathol* 155: 627-632.

2153. Weggen S, Bayer TA, von Deimling A, Reifenberger G, Wiestler OD, Pietsch T (1999). Low frequency of SV40, JC and BK polyoma virus sequences in human medulloblastomas, meningiomas and ependymomas. *Brain Pathol* 10:85-92.

2154. Scheinker IM (1945). Subependymoma (a newly recognized tumor of subependymal derivation). *J Neurosurg* 2: 232-240.

2155. Duerr EM, Rollbrocker B, Hayashi Y, Peters N, Meyer-Puttlitz B, Louis DN, Schramm J, Wiestler OD, Parsons R, Eng C, von Deimling A (1998). PTEN mutations in gliomas and glioneuronal tumors. *Oncogene* 16: 2259-2264.

2156. Eng C, Ji H (1998). Molecular classification of the inherited hamartoma polyposis syndromes: clearing the muddied waters. *Am J Hum Genet* 62: 1020-1022.

2157. Marsh DJ, Dahia PL, Zheng Z, Liaw D, Parsons R, Gorlin RJ, Eng C (1997). Germline mutations in PTEN are present in Bannayan-Zonana syndrome. *Nat Genet* 16: 333-334.

2158. Shepherd PR, Withers DJ, Siddle K (1998). Phosphoinositide 3-kinase: the key switch mechanism in insulin signalling. *Biochem J* 333: 471-490.

2159. Giannini C, Scheithauer BW, Burger PC, Brat DJ, Wollan PC, Lach B, O'Neill BP (1999). Pleomorphic xanthoastrocytoma: what do we really know about it? *Cancer* 85: 2033-2045.

2160. MacKenzie JM (1987). Pleomorphic xanthoastrocytoma in a 62-year-old male. *Neuropathol Appl Neurobiol* 13: 481-487.

2161. Palma L, Maleci A, Di Lorenzo N, Lauro GM (1985). Pleomorphic xanthoastrocytoma with 18-year survival. Case report. *J Neurosurg* 63: 808-810.

2162. Prayson RA, Morris HH, III (1998). Anaplastic pleomorphic xanthoastrocytoma. *Arch Pathol Lab Med* 122: 1082-1086.

2163. Zarate JO, Sampaolesi R (1999). Pleomorphic xanthoastrocytoma of the retina. *Am J Surg Pathol* 23: 79-81.

2164. McLean CA, Jellinek DA, Gonzales MF (1998). Diffuse leptomeningeal spread of pleomorphic xanthoastrocytoma. *J Clin Neurosci* 5: 230-233.

2165. Perry A, Scheithauer BW, Stafford SL, Lohse CM, Wollan PC (1999). "Malignancy" in meningiomas: a clinicopathologic study of 116 patients, with grading implications. *Cancer* 85: 2046-2056.

2166. Perry A, Stafford SL, Scheithauer BW, Suman VJ, Lohse CM (1997). Meningioma grading: an analysis of histologic parameters. *Am J Surg Pathol* 21: 1455-1465.

2167. Kepes JJ, Moral LA, Wilkinson SB, Abdullah A, Llena JF (1998). Rhabdoid transformation of tumor cells in meningiomas: a histologic indication of increased proliferative activity: report of four cases. *Am J Surg Pathol* 22: 231-238.

2168. Perry A, Scheithauer BW, Stafford SL, Abell-Aleff PC, Meyer FB (1998). "Rhabdoid" meningioma: an aggressive variant. *Am J Surg Pathol* 22: 1482-1490.

2169. Paulus W, Meixensberger J, Hofmann E, Roggendorf W (1993). Effect of embolisation of meningioma on Ki-67 proliferation index. *J Clin Pathol* 46: 876-877.

2170. Weber RG, Bostrom J, Wolter M, Baudis M, Collins VP, Reifenberger G, Lichter P (1997). Analysis of genomic alterations in benign, atypical, and anaplastic meningiomas: toward a genetic model of meningioma progression. *Proc Natl Acad Sci U S A* 94: 14719-14724.

2171. Carlson KM, Bruder C, Nordenskjold M, Dumanski JP (1997). 1p and 3p deletions in meningiomas without detectable aberrations of chromosome 22 identified by comparative genomic hybridization. *Genes Chromosomes Cancer* 20: 419-424.

2172. Kepes JJ (1975). The fine structure of hyaline inclusions (pseudopsammoma bodies) in meningiomas. *J Neuropathol Exp Neurol* 34: 282-294.

2173. Kepes JJ (1982). *Meningiomas. Biology, Pathology, and Differential Diagnosis.* Masson Publishing: New York.

2174. Ashraf R, Bentley RC, Awan AN, McLendon RE, Ragozzino MW (1997). Implantation metastasis of primary malignant rhabdoid tumor of the brain in an adult (one case report). *Med Pediatr Oncol* 28: 223-227.

2175. Biegel JA, Zhou JY, Rorke LB, Stenstrom C, Wainwright LM, Fogelgren B (1999). Germ-line and acquired mutations of INI1 in atypical teratoid and rhabdoid tumors. *Cancer Res* 59: 74-79.

2176. Burger PC, Yu IT, Tihan T, Friedman HS, Strother DR, Kepner JL, Duffner PK, Kun LE, Perlman EJ (1998). Atypical teratoid/rhabdoid tumor of the central nervous system: a highly malignant tumor of infancy and childhood frequently mistaken for medulloblastoma: a Pediatric Oncology Group study. *Am J Surg Pathol* 22: 1083-1092.

2177. Weiss E, Behring B, Behnke J, Christen HJ, Pekrun A, Hess CF (1998). Treatment of primary malignant rhabdoid tumor of the brain: report of three cases and review of the literature. *Int J Radiat Oncol Biol Phys* 41: 1013-1019.

2178. Sawyer JR, Goosen LS, Swanson CM, Tomita T, de Leon GA (1998). A new reciprocal translocation (12;22)(q24.3;q11.2-12) in a malignant rhabdoid tumor of the brain. *Cancer Genet Cytogenet* 101: 62-67.

2179. Vajtai I, Varga Z (1998). [Teratoid/rhabdoid tumor of the central nervous system]. *Orv Hetil* 139: 29-34.

2180. Bergmann M, Spaar HJ, Ebhard G, Masini T, Edel G, Gullotta F, Meyer H (1997). Primary malignant rhabdoid tumours of the central nervous system: an immunohistochemical and ultrastructural study. *Acta Neurochir (Wien)* 139: 961-968.

2181. Howlett DC, King AP, Jarosz JM, Stewart RA, al Sarraj ST, Bingham JB, Cox TC (1997). Imaging and pathological features of primary malignant rhabdoid tumours of the brain and spine. *Neuroradiology* 39: 719-723.

2182. Martinez-Lage JF, Nieto A, Sola J, Domingo R, Costa TR, Poza M (1997). Primary malignant rhabdoid tumor of the cerebellum. *Childs Nerv Syst* 13: 418-421.

2183. Bhattacharjee M, Hicks J, Langford L, Dauser R, Strother D, Chintagumpala M, Horowitz M, Cooley L, Vogel H (1997). Central nervous system atypical teratoid/rhabdoid tumors of infancy and childhood. *Ultrastruct Pathol* 21: 369-378.

2184. Klopfenstein K, Soukup S, Blough R, Mazewski C, Ballard E, Gotwals B, Lampkin B (1997). Chromosome analyses in a rhabdoid tumor of the brain. *Cancer Genet Cytogenet* 93: 152-156.

2185. Morizane A, Nakahara I, Takahashi JA, Ishikawa M, Kikuchi H (1997). [A malignant rhabdoid tumor appearing simultaneously in the kidney and the brain of an infant: case report]. *No Shinkei Geka* 25: 665-669.

2187. Kalpana GV, Marmon S, Wang W, Crabtree GR, Goff SP (1994). Binding and stimulation of HIV-1 integrase by a human homolog of yeast transcription factor SNF5. *Science* 266: 2002-2006.

2188. Kingston RE, Bunker CA, Imbalzano AN (1996). Repression and activation by multiprotein complexes that alter chromatin structure. *Genes Dev* 10: 905-920.

2189. Versteege I, Sevenet N, Lange J, Rousseau-Merck MF, Ambros P, Handgretinger R, Aurias A, Delattre O (1998). Truncating mutations of hSNF5/INI1 in aggressive paediatric cancer. *Nature* 394: 203-206.

2190. Burnett ME, White EC, Sih S, von Haken MS, Cogen PH (1997). Chromosome arm 17p deletion analysis reveals molecular genetic heterogeneity in supratentorial and infratentorial primitive neuroectodermal tumors of the central nervous system. *Cancer Genet Cytogenet* 97: 25-31.

2191. Rorke LB (1997). Atypical teratoid/rhabdoid tumours. In: *Pathology and Genetics - Tumours of the Nervous System*, Kleihues P, Cavenee WK (eds). IARC: Lyon. pp. 110-111.

2192. Rubio A (1997). March 1997 - 4 year old girl with ring chromosome 22 and brain tumor. *Brain Pathol* 7: 1027-1028.

2193. Biegel JA (1999). Neuro-oncology [serial on line], Doc. 98-30. *URL<neuro-oncology mc duke edu>*

2194. Moriuchi S, Shimizu K, Miyao Y, Hayakawa T (1996). An immunohistochemical analysis of medulloblastoma and PNET with emphasis on N-myc protein expression. *Anticancer Res* 16: 2687-2692.

2195. Rostomily RC, Bermingham-McDonogh O, Berger MS, Tapscott SJ, Reh TA, Olson JM (1997). Expression of neurogenic basic helix-loop-helix genes in primitive neuroectodermal tumors. *Cancer Res* 57: 3526-3531.

2196. Rao MS, Noble M, Mayer-Proschel M (1998). A tripotential glial precursor cell is present in the developing spinal cord. *Proc Natl Acad Sci U S A* 95: 3996-4001.

2197. Mayer-Proschel M, Kalyani AJ, Mujtaba T, Rao MS (1997). Isolation of lineage-restricted neuronal precursors from multipotent neuroepithelial stem cells. *Neuron* 19: 773-785.

2198. Alvarez-Buylla A, Temple S (1998). Stem cells in the developing and adult nervous system. *J Neurobiol* 36: 105-110.

2199. Rajan P, McKay RD (1998). Multiple routes to astrocytic differentiation in the CNS. *J Neurosci* 18: 3620-3629.

2200. Mi H, Barres BA (1999). Purification and characterization of astrocyte precursor cells in the developing rat optic nerve. *J Neurosci* 19: 1049-1061.

2201. Coffin CM, Swanson PE, Wick MR, Dehner LP (1993). An immunohistochemical comparison of chordoma with renal cell carcinoma, colorectal adenocarcinoma, and myxopapillary ependymoma: a potential diagnostic dilemma in the diminutive biopsy. *Mod Pathol* 6: 531-538.

2202. Ilhan I, Berberoglu S, Kutluay L, Maden HA (1998). Subcutaneous sacrococcygeal myxopapillary ependymoma. *Med Pediatr Oncol* 30: 81-84.

2203. Ross DA, McKeever PE, Sandler HM, Muraszko KM (1993). Myxopapillary ependymoma. Results of nucleolar organizing region staining. *Cancer* 71: 3114-3118.

2204. Sawyer JR, Miller JP, Ellison DA (1998). Clonal telomeric fusions and chromosome instability in a subcutaneous sacrococcygeal myxopapillary ependymoma. *Cancer Genet Cytogenet* 100: 169-175.

2205. Sawyer JR, Crowson ML, Roloson GJ, Chadduck WM (1991). Involvement of the short arm of chromosome 1 in a myxopapillary ependymoma. *Cancer Genet Cytogenet* 54: 55-60.

2206. Kernohan JW (1931). Primary tumors of the spinal cord and intradural filum terminale. In: *Cytology and Cellular Pathology of the Nervous System*, Penfield W (eds). Hoeber: New York. pp. 993.

2207. Woesler B, Moskopp D, Kuchelmeister K, Schul C, Wassmann H (1998). Intradural metastasis of a spinal myxopapillary ependymoma. A case report. *Neurosurg Rev* 21: 62-65.

2208. Johnson MW, Emelin JK, Park SH, Vinters HV (1999). Co-localization of TSC1 and TSC2 gene products in tubers of patients with tuberous sclerosis. *Brain Pathol* 9: 45-54.

2209. Plank TL, Logginidou H, Klein-Szanto A, Henske EP (1999). The expression of hamartin, the product of the TSC1 gene, in normal human tissues and in TSC1- and TSC2-linked angiomyolipomas. *Mod Pathol* 12: 539-545.

2210. Plank TL, Yeung RS, Henske EP (1998). Hamartin, the product of the tuberous sclerosis 1 (TSC1) gene, interacts with tuberin and appears to be localized to cytoplasmic vesicles. *Cancer Res* 58: 4766-4770.

2211. van Slegtenhorst M, Verhoef S, Tempelaars A, Bakker L, Wang Q, Wessels M, Bakker R, Nellist M, Lindhout D, Halley D, van den OA (1999). Mutational spectrum of the TSC1 gene in a cohort of 225 tuberous sclerosis complex patients: no evidence for genotype-phenotype correlation. *J Med Genet* 36: 285-289.

2212. van Slegtenhorst M, Nellist M, Nagelkerken B, Cheadle J, Snell R, van den OA, Reuser A, Sampson J, Halley D, van der SP (1998). Interaction between hamartin and tuberin, the TSC1 and TSC2 gene products. *Hum Mol Genet* 7: 1053-1057.

2213. van Slegtenhorst M, de Hoogt R, Hermans C, Nellist M, Janssen B, Verhoef S, Lindhout D, van den OA, Halley D, Young J, Burley M, Jeremiah S, Woodward K, Nahmias J, Fox M, Ekong R, Osborne J, Wolfe J, Povey S, Snell RG, Cheadle JP, Jones AC, Tachataki M, Ravine D, Kwiatkowski DJ (1997). Identification of the tuberous sclerosis gene TSC1 on chromosome 9q34. *Science* 277: 805-808.

2214. Nagib MG, Haines SJ, Erickson DL, Mastri AR (1984). Tuberous sclerosis: a review for the neurosurgeon. *Neurosurgery* 14: 93-98.

2215. Blumcke I, Lobach M, Wolf HK, Wiestler OD (1999). Evidence for developmental precursor lesions in epilepsy-associated glioneuronal tumors. *Micros Res Techn* 46: 53-58.

2216. Park K, Yoo J, Cho H, Cho W, Park S (1998). Desmoplastic cerebral astrocytoma of infancy: a case report. *J Korean Med Sci* 13: 440-444.

2217. Olas E, Kordek R, Biernat W, Liberski PP, Zakrzewski K, Alwasiak J, Polis L (1998). Desmoplastic cerebral astrocytoma of infancy: a case report. *Folia Neuropathol* 36: 45-51.

2218. Chacko G, Chandi SM, Chandy MJ (1995). Desmoplastic low grade astrocytoma: a case report and review of literature. *Clin Neurol Neurosurg* 97: 32-35.

2219. Torres LF, Reis Filho JS, Netto MR, de Noronha L, Alessio AB, de Carvalho NA (1998). [Infantile desmoplastic ganglioglioma: a clinical, histopathological and epidemiological study of five cases]. *Arq Neuropsiquiatr* 56: 443-448.

2220. Woesler B, Kuwert T, Kurlemann G, Morgenroth C, Probst-Cousin S, Lerch H, Gullotta F, Wassmann H, Schober O (1998). High amino acid uptake in a low-grade desmoplastic infantile ganglioglioma in a 14-year-old patient. *Neurosurg Rev* 21: 31-35.

2221. Rothman S, Sharon N, Shiffer J, Toren A, Pollak L, Mandel M, Kenet G, Neumann Y, Nass D (1997). Desmoplastic infantile ganglioglioma. *Acta Oncol* 36: 655-657.

2222. Galatioto S, Gullotta F (1996). Desmoplastic non-infantile ganglioglioma. *J Neurosurg Sci* 40: 235-238.

2223. Setty SN, Miller DC, Camras L, Charbel F, Schmidt ML (1997). Desmoplastic infantile astrocytoma with metastases at presentation. *Mod Pathol* 10: 945-951.

2224. Chan AS, Leung SY, Wong MP, Yuen ST, Cheung N, Fan YW, Chung LP (1998). Expression of vascular endothelial growth factor and its receptors in the anaplastic progression of astrocytoma, oligodendroglioma, and ependymoma. *Am J Surg Pathol* 22: 816-826.

2225. Maier D, Comparone D, Taylor E, Zhang Z, Gratzl O, Van Meir EG, Scott RJ, Merlo A (1997). New deletion in low-grade oligodendroglioma at the glioblastoma suppressor locus on chromosome 10q25-26. *Oncogene* 15: 997-1000.

2226. Cairncross JG, Ueki K, Zlatescu MC, Lisle DK, Finkelstein DM, Hammond RR, Silver JS, Stark PC, Macdonald DR, Ino Y, Ramsay DA, Louis DN (1998). Specific genetic predictors of chemotherapeutic response and survival in patients with anaplastic oligodendrogliomas. *J Natl Cancer Inst* 90: 1473-1479.

2227. Christov C, Adle-Biassette H, Le Guerinel C, Natchev S, Gherardi RK (1998). Immunohistochemical detection of vascular endothelial growth factor (VEGF) in the vasculature of oligodendrogliomas. *Neuropathol Appl Neurobiol* 24: 29-35.

2228. Coons SW, Johnson PC, Pearl DK (1997). The prognostic significance of Ki-67 labeling indices for oligodendrogliomas. *Neurosurgery* 41: 878-884.

2229. Dehghani F, Schachenmayr W, Laun A, Korf HW (1998). Prognostic implication of histopathological, immunohistochemical and clinical features of oligodendrogliomas: a study of 89 cases. *Acta Neuropathol (Berl)* 95: 493-504.

2230. Herbarth B, Meissner H, Westphal M, Wegner M (1998). Absence of polyomavirus JC in glial brain tumors and glioma-derived cell lines. *Glia* 22: 415-420.

2231. Huang H, Reis R, Yonekawa Y, Lopes JM, Kleihues P, Ohgaki H (1999). Identification in human brain tumors of DNA sequences specific for SV40 large T antigen. *Brain Pathol* 9: 33-42.

2232. Kaghad M, Bonnet H, Yang A, Creancier L, Biscan JC, Valent A, Minty A, Chalon P, Lelias JM, Dumont X, Ferrara P, McKeon F, Caput D (1997). Monoallelically expressed gene related to p53 at 1p36, a region frequently deleted in neuroblastoma and other human cancers. *Cell* 90: 809-819.

2233. Mai M, Huang H, Reed C, Qian C, Smith JS, Alderete B, Jenkins R, Smith DI, Liu W (1998). Genomic organization and mutation analysis of p73 in oligodendrogliomas with chromosome 1 p-arm deletions. *Genomics* 51: 359-363.

2234. Miettinen H, Kononen J, Sallinen P, Alho H, Helen P, Helin H, Kalimo H, Paljarvi L, Isola J, Haapasalo H (1999). CDKN2/p16 predicts survival in oligodendrogliomas: comparison with astrocytomas. *J Neurooncol* 41: 205-211.

2235. Nishikawa R, Cheng SY, Nagashima R, Huang HJ, Cavenee WK, Matsutani M (1998). Expression of vascular endothelial growth factor in human brain tumors. *Acta Neuropathol (Berl)* 96: 453-462.

2236. Pietsch T, Valter MM, Wolf HK, von Deimling A, Huang HJ, Cavenee WK, Wiestler OD (1997). Expression and distribution of vascular endothelial growth factor protein in human brain tumors. *Acta Neuropathol (Berl)* 93: 109-117.

2237. Di Rocco F, Carroll RS, Zhang J, Black PM (1998). Platelet-derived growth factor and its receptor expression in human oligodendrogliomas. *Neurosurgery* 42: 341-346.

2238. Taylor MD, Perry J, Zlatescu MC, Stemmer-Rachamimov AO, Ang LC, Ino Y, Schwartz M, Becker LE, Louis DN, Cairncross JG (1999). The hPMS2 exon 5 mutation and malignant glioma. Case report. *J Neurosurg* 90: 946-950.

2239. van den Bent MJ, Kros JM, Heimans JJ, Pronk LC, van Groeningen CJ, Krouwer HG, Taphoorn MJ, Zonnenberg BA, Tijssen CC, Twijnstra A, Punt CJ, Boogerd W (1998). Response rate and prognostic factors of recurrent oligodendroglioma treated with procarbazine, CCNU, and vincristine chemotherapy. Dutch Neuro-oncology Group. *Neurology* 51: 1140-1145.

2240. Wharton SB, Chan KK, Hamilton FA, Anderson JR (1998). Expression of neuronal markers in oligodendrogliomas: an immunohistochemical study. *Neuropathol Appl Neurobiol* 24: 302-308.

2241. Zhu JJ, Santarius T, Wu X, Tsong J, Guha A, Wu JK, Hudson TJ, Black PM (1998). Screening for loss of heterozygosity and microsatellite instability in oligodendrogliomas. *Genes Chromosomes Cancer* 21: 207-216.

2242. Wharton SB, Hamilton FA, Chan WK, Chan KK, Anderson JR (1998). Proliferation and cell death in oligodendrogliomas. *Neuropathol Appl Neurobiol* 24: 21-28.

2243. Bigner SH, Rasheed BK, Wiltshire R, McLendon RE (1999). Morphologic and molecular genetic aspects of oligodendroglial neoplasms. *Neuro-Oncology* 1: 52-60.

2244. Husemann K, Wolter M, Buschges R, Bostrom J, Sabel M, Reifenberger G (1999). Identification of two distinct deleted regions on the short arm of chromosome 1 and rare mutation of the *CDKN2C* gene from 1p32 in oligodendroglial tumors. *J Neuropathol Exp Neurol* 58: 1041-1050.

2245. Kros JM, van Run PRWA, Alers JC, Beverloo HB, van den Bent MJ, Avezaat CJJ, van Dekken H (1999). Genetic aberrations in oligodendroglial tumours: an analysis using comparative genomic hybridization (CGH). *J Pathol* 188: 282-288.

2246. Pohl U, Cairncross JG, Louis DN (1999). Homozygous deletions of the *CDKN2C/p18^{INK4C}* gene on the short arm of chromosome 1 in anaplastic oligodendrogliomas. *Brain Pathol* 9: 639-643.

2247. Smith JS, Alderete B, Minn Y, Borell TJ, Perry A, Mohapatra G, Smith SM, Kimmel D, Fallon JO, Tates A, Feuerstein BG, Burger PC, Scheithauer BW, Jenkins RB (1999). Localization of common deletion regions on 1p and 19q in human gliomas and their association with histological subtype. *Oncogene* 18: 4144-4152.

2248. Jeuken JW, Sprenger SH, Wesseling P, Macville MV, von Deimling A, Teepen HL, van Overbeeke JJ, Boerman RH (1999). Identification of subgroups of high-grade oligodendroglial tumors by comparative genomic hybridization. *J Neuropathol Exp Neurol* 58: 606-612.

2249. Beckmann MJ, Prayson RA (1997). A clinicopathologic study of 30 cases of oligoastrocytoma including p53 immunohistochemistry. *Pathology* 29: 159-164.

2250. Donahue B, Scott CB, Nelson JS, Rotman M, Murray KJ, Nelson DF, Banker

FL, Earle JD, Fischbach JA, Asbell SO, Gaspar LE, Markoe AM, Curran W (1997). Influence of an oligodendroglial component on the survival of patients with anaplastic astrocytomas: a report of Radiation Therapy Oncology Group 83-02. *Int J Radiat Oncol Biol Phys* 38: 911-914.

2251. Luider TM, Kros JM, Sillevis Smitt PA, van den Bent MJ, Vecht CJ (1999). Glial fibrillary acidic protein and its fragments discriminate astrocytoma from oligodendroglioma. *Electrophoresis* 20: 1087-1091.

2252. Uzal D, Ozyar E, Tukul A, Genc M, Soylemezoglu F, Atahan IL, Onol B (1996). Familial glioma in two siblings. *Radiat Med* 14: 43-47.

2253. Wang Y, Hagel C, Hamel W, Muller S, Kluwe L, Westphal M (1998). Trk A, B, and C are commonly expressed in human astrocytes and astrocytic gliomas but not by human oligodendrocytes and oligodendroglioma. *Acta Neuropathol (Berl)* 96: 357-364.

2254. Stephan CL, Kepes JJ, Arnold P, Green KD, Chamberlin F (1999). Neurocytoma of the cauda equina. Case report. *J Neurosurg* 90: 247-251.

2255. Mackenzie IR (1999). Central neurocytoma: histologic atypia, proliferation potential, and clinical outcome. *Cancer* 85: 1606-1610.

2256. Jay V, Edwards V, Hoving E, Rutka J, Becker L, Zielenska M, Teshima I (1999). Central neurocytoma: morphological, flow cytometric, polymerase chain reaction, fluorescence in situ hybridization, and karyotypic analyses. Case report. *J Neurosurg* 90: 348-354.

2257. Lee MC, Nam JH, Choi C, Park CS, Juhng SW, Yang KH, Yang BS, Suh CH, Kim SU (1997). Ultrastructural characteristics of central neurocytoma in cell culture. *Ultrastruct Pathol* 21: 393-404.

2258. Tomura N, Hirano H, Watanabe O, Watarai J, Itoh Y, Mineura K, Kowada M (1997). Central neurocytoma with clinically malignant behavior. *AJNR Am J Neuroradiol* 18: 1175-1178.

2259. Kim DG, Paek SH, Kim IH, Chi JG, Jung HW, Han DH, Choi KS, Cho BK (1997). Central neurocytoma: the role of radiation therapy and long term outcome. *Cancer* 79: 1995-2002.

2260. Schild SE, Scheithauer BW, Haddock MG, Schiff D, Burger PC, Wong WW, Lyons MK (1997). Central neurocytomas. *Cancer* 79: 790-795.

2261. Ishiuchi S, Nakazato Y, Iino M, Ozawa S, Tamura M, Ohye C (1998). In vitro neuronal and glial production and differentiation of human central neurocytoma cells. *J Neurosci Res* 51: 526-535.

2262. Gultekin SH, Dalmau J, Graus Y, Posner JB, Rosenblum MK (1998). Anti-Hu immunolabeling as an index of neuronal differentiation in human brain tumors: a study of 112 central neuroepithelial neoplasms. *Am J Surg Pathol* 22: 195-200.

2263. Quinn B (1998). Synaptophysin staining in normal brain: importance for diagnosis of ganglioglioma. *Am J Surg Pathol* 22: 550-556.

2264. Leung SY, Chan TL, Chung LP, Chan AS, Fan YW, Hung KN, Kwong WK, Ho JW, Yuen ST (1998). Microsatellite instability and mutation of DNA mismatch repair genes in gliomas. *Am J Pathol* 153: 1181-1188.

2265. Miyaki M, Nishio J, Konishi M, Kikuchi-Yanoshita R, Tanaka K, Muraoka M, Nagato M, Chong JM, Koike M, Terada T, Kawahara Y, Fukutome A, Tomiyama J, Chuganji Y, Momoi M, Utsunomiya J (1997). Drastic genetic instability of tumors and normal tissues in Turcot syndrome. *Oncogene* 15: 2877-2881.

2266. Wei Q, Bondy ML, Mao L, Gaun Y, Cheng L, Cunningham J, Fan Y, Bruner JM, Yung WK, Levin VA, Kyritsis AP (1997). Reduced expression of mismatch repair genes measured by multiplex reverse transcription-polymerase chain reaction in human gliomas. *Cancer Res* 57: 1673-1677.

2267. Van Meir EG (1998). "Turcot's syndrome": phenotype of brain tumors, survival and mode of inheritance. *Int J Cancer* 75: 162-164.

2268. Van Meir E, de Tribolet N (1995). Microsatellite instability in human brain tumors. *Neurosurgery* 37: 1231-1232.

2269. Amler LC, Schwab M (1989). Amplified N-myc in human neuroblastoma cells is often arranged as clustered tandem repeats of differently recombined DNA. *Mol Cell Biol* 9: 4903-4913.

2270. Berthold F, Sahin K, Hero B, Christiansen H, Gehring M, Harms D, Horz S, Lampert F, Schwab M, Terpe J (1997). The current contribution of molecular factors to risk estimation in neuroblastoma patients. *Eur J Cancer* 33: 2092-2097.

2271. Bordow SB, Norris MD, Haber PS, Marshall GM, Haber M (1998). Prognostic significance of MYCN oncogene expression in childhood neuroblastoma. *J Clin Oncol* 16: 3286-3294.

2272. Borrello MG, Bongarzone I, Pierotti MA, Luksch R, Gasparini M, Collini P, Pilotti S, Rizzetti MG, Mondellini P, De Bernardi B (1993). trk and ret proto-oncogene expression in human neuroblastoma specimens: high frequency of trk expression in non-advanced stages. *Int J Cancer* 54: 540-545.

2273. Bown N, Cotterill S, Lastowska M, O'Neill S, Pearson AD, Plantaz D, Meddeb M, Danglot G, Brinkschmidt C, Christiansen H, Laureys G, Speleman F (1999). Gain of chromosome arm 17q and adverse outcome in patients with neuroblastoma. *N Engl J Med* 340: 1954-1961.

2274. Bown NP, Pearson AD, Reid MM (1993). High incidence of constitutional balanced translocations in neuroblastoma. *Cancer Genet Cytogenet* 69: 166-167.

2275. Breit S, Schwab M (1989). Suppression of MYC by high expression of NMYC in human neuroblastoma cells. *J Neurosci Res* 24: 21-28.

2276. Brinkschmidt C, Christiansen H, Terpe HJ, Simon R, Boecker W, Lampert F, Stoerkel S (1997). Comparative genomic hybridization (CGH) analysis of neuroblastomas—an important methodological approach in paediatric tumour pathology. *J Pathol* 181: 394-400.

2277. Brodeur GM, Maris JM, Yamashiro DJ, Hogarty MD, White PS (1997). Biology and genetics of human neuroblastomas. *J Pediatr Hematol Oncol* 19: 93-101.

2278. Brodeur GM, Seeger RC, Schwab M, Varmus HE, Bishop JM (1984). Amplification of N-myc in untreated human neuroblastomas correlates with advanced disease stage. *Science* 224: 1121-1124.

2279. Brodeur GM, Azar C, Brother M, Hiemstra J, Kaufman B, Marshall H, Moley J, Nakagawara A, Saylors R, Scavarda N (1992). Neuroblastoma. Effect of genetic factors on prognosis and treatment. *Cancer* 70: 1685-1694.

2280. Bunin GR, Ward E, Kramer S, Rhee CA, Meadows AT (1990). Neuroblastoma and parental occupation. *Am J Epidemiol* 131: 776-780.

2281. Caron H, Peter M, van Sluis P, Speleman F, de Kraker J, Laureys G, Michon J, Brugieres L, Voute PA, Westerveld A (1995). Evidence for two tumour suppressor loci on chromosomal bands 1p35-36 involved in neuroblastoma: one probably imprinted, another associated with N-myc amplification. *Hum Mol Genet* 4: 535-539.

2282. Chan HS, Gallie BL, DeBoer G, Haddad G, Ikegaki N, Dimitroulakos J, Yeger H, Ling V (1997). MYCN protein expression as a predictor of neuroblastoma prognosis. *Clin Cancer Res* 3: 1699-1706.

2283. Cohn SL, Salwen H, Quasney MW, Ikegaki N, Cowan JM, Herst CV, Kennett RH, Rosen ST, DiGiuseppe JA, Brodeur GM (1990). Prolonged N-myc protein half-life in a neuroblastoma cell line lacking N-myc amplification. *Oncogene* 5: 1821-1827.

2284. Combaret V, Lasset C, Frappaz D, Bouvier R, Thiesse P, Rebillard AC, Philip T, Favrot MC (1995). Evaluation of CD44 prognostic value in neuroblastoma: comparison with the other prognostic factors. *Eur J Cancer* 31A: 545-549.

2285. Corvi R, Savelyeva L, Amler L, Handgretinger R, Schwab M (1995). Cytogenetic evolution of MYCN and MDM2 amplification in the neuroblastoma LS tumour and its cell line. *Eur J Cancer* 31A: 520-523.

2286. Fulda S, Lutz W, Schwab M, Debatin KM (1999). MycN sensitizes neuroblastoma cells for drug-induced apoptosis. *Oncogene* 18: 1479-1486.

2287. Heling KS, Chaoui R, Hartung J, Kirchmair F, Bollmann R (1999). Prenatal diagnosis of congenital neuroblastoma. Analysis of 4 cases and review of the literature. *Fetal Diagn Ther* 14: 47-52.

2288. Hughes M, Marsden HB, Palmer MK (1974). Histologic patterns of neuroblastoma related to prognosis and clinical staging. *Cancer* 34: 1706-1711.

2289. Jakobovits A, Schwab M, Bishop JM, Martin GR (1985). Expression of N-myc in teratocarcinoma stem cells and mouse embryos. *Nature* 318: 188-191.

2290. Jinbo T, Iwamura Y, Kaneko M, Sawaguchi S (1989). Coamplification of the L-myc and N-myc oncogenes in a neuroblastoma cell line. *Jpn J Cancer Res* 80: 299-301.

2291. Lastowska M, Nacheva E, McGuckin A, Curtis A, Grace C, Pearson A, Bown N (1997). Comparative genomic hybridization study of primary neuroblastoma tumors. United Kingdom Children's Cancer Study Group. *Genes Chromosomes Cancer* 18: 162-169.

2292. Lauder I, Aherne W (1972). The significance of lymphocytic infiltration in neuroblastoma. *Br J Cancer* 26: 321-330.

2293. Lutz W, Fulda S, Jeremias I, Debatin KM, Schwab M (1998). MycN and IFNgamma cooperate in apoptosis of human neuroblastoma cells. *Oncogene* 17: 339-346.

2294. Makinen J (1972). Microscopic patterns as a guide to prognosis of neuroblastoma in childhood. *Cancer* 29: 1637-1646.

2295. Maris JM, Kyemba SM, Rebbeck TR, White PS, Sulman EP, Jensen SJ, Allen C, Biegel JA, Yanofsky RA, Feldman GL, Brodeur GM (1996). Familial predisposition to neuroblastoma does not map to chromosome band 1p36. *Cancer Res* 56: 3421-3425.

2296. Martinsson T, Sjoberg RM, Hedborg F, Kogner P (1995). Deletion of chromosome 1p loci and microsatellite instability in neuroblastomas analyzed with short-tandem repeat polymorphisms. *Cancer Res* 55: 5681-5686.

2297. Meddeb M, Danglot G, Chudoba I, Venuat AM, Benard J, Avet-Loiseau H, Vasseur B, Le Paslier D, Terrier-Lacombe MJ, Hartmann O, Bernheim A (1996). Additional copies of a 25 Mb chromosomal region originating from 17q23.1-17qter are present in 90% of high-grade neuroblastomas. *Genes Chromosomes Cancer* 17: 156-165.

2298. Nakagawara A, Azar CG, Scavarda NJ, Brodeur GM (1994). Expression and function of TRK-B and BDNF in human neuroblastomas. *Mol Cell Biol* 14: 759-767.

2299. Nakagawara A, Arima M, Azar CG, Scavarda NJ, Brodeur GM (1992). Inverse relationship between trk expression and N-myc amplification in human neuroblastomas. *Cancer Res* 52: 1364-1368.

2300. Nisen PD, Waber PG, Rich MA, Pierce S, Garvin JR, Jr., Gilbert F, Lanzkowsky P (1988). N-myc oncogene RNA expression in neuroblastoma. *J Natl Cancer Inst* 80: 1633-1637.

2301. Plantaz D, Mohapatra G, Matthay KK, Pellarin M, Seeger RC, Feuerstein BG (1997). Gain of chromosome 17 is the most frequent abnormality detected in neuroblastoma by comparative genomic hybridization. *Am J Pathol* 150: 81-89.

2302. Rubie H, Hartmann O, Michon J, Frappaz D, Coze C, Chastagner P, Baranzelli MC, Plantaz D, Avet-Loiseau H, Benard J, Delattre O, Favrot M, Peyroulet MC, Thyss A, Perel Y, Bergeron C, Courbon-Collet B, Vannier JP, Lemerle J, Sommelet D (1997). N-Myc gene amplification is a major prognostic factor in localized neuroblastoma: results of the French NBL 90 study. Neuroblastoma Study Group of the Societe Francaise d'Oncologie Pediatrique. *J Clin Oncol* 15: 1171-1182.

2303. Ryden M, Sehgal R, Dominici C, Schilling FH, Ibanez CF, Kogner P (1996). Expression of mRNA for the neurotrophin receptor trkC in neuroblastomas with favourable tumour stage and good prognosis. *Br J Cancer* 74: 773-779.

2304. Sandstedt B, Jereb B, Eklund G (1983). Prognostic factors in neuroblastomas. *Acta Pathol Microbiol Immunol Scand [A]* 91: 365-371.

2305. Schmidt ML, Salwen HR, Chagnovich D, Bauer KD, Crawford SE, Cohn SL (1993). Evidence for molecular heterogeneity in human ganglioneuroblastoma. *Pediatr Pathol* 13: 787-796.

2306. Schwab M, Ellison J, Busch M, Rosenau W, Varmus HE, Bishop JM (1984). Enhanced expression of the human gene N-myc consequent to amplification of DNA may contribute to malignant progression of neuroblastoma. *Proc Natl Acad Sci U S A* 81: 4940-4944.

2307. Schwab M (1998). Amplification of oncogenes in human cancer cells. *Bioessays* 20: 473-479.

2308. Schweigerer L, Breit S, Wenzel A, Tsunamoto K, Ludwig R, Schwab M (1990). Augmented MYCN expression advances the malignant phenotype of human neuroblastoma cells: evidence for induction of autocrine growth factor activity. *Cancer Res* 50: 4411-4416.

2309. Seeger RC, Brodeur GM, Sather H, Dalton A, Siegel SE, Wong KY, Hammond D (1985). Association of multiple copies of the N-myc oncogene with rapid progression of neuroblastomas. *N Engl J Med* 313: 1111-1116.

2310. Shiloh Y, Shipley J, Brodeur GM, Bruns G, Korf B, Donlon T, Schreck RR, Seeger R, Sakai K, Latt SA (1985). Differential amplification, assembly, and relocation of multiple DNA sequences in human neuroblastomas and neuroblastoma cell lines. *Proc Natl Acad Sci U S A* 82: 3761-3765.

2311. Slavc I, Ellenbogen R, Jung WH, Vawter GF, Kretschmar C, Grier H, Korf BR (1990). myc gene amplification and expression in primary human neuroblastoma. *Cancer Res* 50: 1459-1463.

2312. Srivatsan ES, Ying KL, Seeger RC (1993). Deletion of chromosome 11 and of 14q sequences in neuroblastoma. *Genes Chromosomes Cancer* 7: 32-37.

2313. Suzuki T, Yokota J, Mugishima H, Okabe I, Ookuni M, Sugimura T, Terada M (1989). Frequent loss of heterozygosity on chromosome 14q in neuroblastoma. *Cancer Res* 49: 1095-1098.

2314. Suzuki T, Bogenmann E, Shimada H, Stram D, Seeger RC (1993). Lack of high-affinity nerve growth factor receptors in aggressive neuroblastomas. *J Natl Cancer Inst* 85: 377-384.

2315. Takayama H, Suzuki T, Mugishima H, Fujisawa T, Ookuni M, Schwab M, Gehring M, Nakamura Y, Sugimura T, Terada M (1992). Deletion mapping of chromosomes 14q and 1p in human neuroblastoma. *Oncogene* 7: 1185-1189.

2316. Takita J, Hayashi Y, Kohno T, Shiseki M, Yamaguchi N, Hanada R, Yamamoto K, Yokota J (1995). Allelotype of neuroblastoma. *Oncogene* 11: 1829-1834.

2317. van Roy N, Forus A, Myklebost O, Cheng NC, Versteeg R, Speleman F (1995). Identification of two distinct chromosome 12-derived amplification units in neuroblastoma cell line NGP. *Cancer Genet Cytogenet* 82: 151-154.

2318. van Roy N, Laureys G, Cheng NC, Willem P, Opdenakker G, Versteeg R, Speleman F (1994). 1;17 translocations and other chromosome 17 rearrangements in human primary neuroblastoma tumors and cell lines. *Genes Chromosomes Cancer* 10: 103-114.

2319. Vandesompele J, van Roy N, Van Gele M, Laureys G, Ambros P, Heimann P, Devalck C, Schuuring E, Brock P, Otten J, Gyselinck J, De Paepe A, Speleman F (1998). Genetic heterogeneity of neuroblastoma studied by comparative genomic hybridization. *Genes Chromosomes Cancer* 23: 141-152.

2320. Wenzel A, Cziepluch C, Hamann U, Schurmann J, Schwab M (1991). The N-Myc oncoprotein is associated in vivo with the phosphoprotein Max(p20/22) in human neuroblastoma cells. *EMBO J* 10: 3703-3712.

2321. White PS, Maris JM, Beltinger C, Sulman E, Marshall HN, Fujimori M, Kaufman BA, Biegel JA, Allen C, Hilliard C (1995). A region of consistent deletion in neuroblastoma maps within human chromosome 1p36.2-36.3. *Proc Natl Acad Sci U S A* 92: 5520-5524.

2322. Yamashiro DJ, Nakagawara A, Ikegaki N, Liu XG, Brodeur GM (1996). Expression of TrkC in favorable human neuroblastomas. *Oncogene* 12: 37-41.

2323. Hogarty MH,Brodeur GM (1999). Oncogene amplification. In: *Genetic Basis of Human Cancer*, Vogelstein B, Kinzler K (eds), 8th ed. McGraw Hill: New York.

2324. Maris JM, White PS, Hogarty MD, Thompson PM, Stram DO, Matthay KK, Seeger RS, Brodeur GM (1999). Chromosome 11q22 allelic deletion is common in neuroblastomas. *Eur J Cancer* (in press).

2325. Maris JM, Weiss M, Guo C, White PS, Hogarty MD, Resende I, Shusterman S, Urbanek M, Spielman R, Rebbeck T, Brodeur GM (1999). Evidence for a familial neuroblastoma predisposition locus at 16p12-13. (*submitted*).

2326. Roald B, Ambros I, Dehner LP, Hata JI, Joshi V, Shimada H (1996). A proposed international neuroblastoma pathology classification. *Med Pediatr Oncol* 27: 225.

2327. Shimada H, Ambros IM, Dehner LP, Hata J, Joshi VV, Roald B (1999). Terminology and morphologic criteria of neuroblastic tumors: recommendations by the International Neuroblastoma Pathology Committee. *Cancer* 86: 349-363.

2328. Shimada H, Wang H, Wu HW, Peters J, Lukens J, Matthay KK,Seeger RC (1999). TrkA expression, MYCN amplification and histopathology in neuroblastomas. *Mod Pathol* 12;5P.

2329. Shimada H, Ambros IM, Dehner LP, Hata J-I, Joshi VV, Roald B, Stram DO, Gerbing RB, Lukens JN, Matthay KK, Castleberry RP (1999). Establishment of the International Neuroblastoma Pathology Classification (Shimada system). *Cancer* 86: 364-372.

2330. Thompson PM, Kyemba SK, Jensen SJ, Guo C, Maris JM, Brodeur GM, Stram DO, Matthay KK, Seeger RC, White PS (1999). Loss of heterozygosity (LOH) for chromosome 14q in neuroblastoma. *Eur J Cancer* (in press).

2331. Al-Sarraj ST, Bridges LR (1996). Desmoplastic cerebral glioblastoma of infancy. *Br J Neurosurg* 10: 215-219.

2332. Guerrieri C, Jarlsfelt I (1993). Ependymoma of the ovary. A case report with immunohistochemical, ultrastructural, and DNA cytometric findings, as well as histogenetic considerations. *Am J Surg Pathol* 17: 623-632.

2333. Carlsson B, Havel G, Kindblom LG, Knutson F, Mark J (1989). Ependymoma of the ovary. A clinico-pathologic, ultrastructural and immunohistochemical investigation. A case report. *APMIS* 97: 1007-1012.

2334. Kleinman GM, Young RH, Scully RE (1984). Ependymoma of the ovary: report of three cases. *Hum Pathol* 15: 632-638.

2335. Gonzalez-Campora R, Weller RO (1998). Lipidized mature neuroectodermal tumour of the cerebellum with myoid differentiation. *Neuropathol Appl Neurobiol* 24: 397-402.

2336. Baylac F, Martinoli A, Marie B, Bracard S, Marchal JC, Sommelet D, Hassoun J, Plenat F (1997). Une variete exceptionelle de medulloblastome: le medulloblastome melanotique. *Ann Pathol* 17: 403-405.

2337. Agosti RM, Leuthold M, Gullick WJ, Yasargil MG, Wiestler OD (1992). Expression of the epidermal growth factor receptor in astrocytic tumours is specifically associated with glioblastoma multiforme. *Virchows Arch A Pathol Anat Histopathol* 420: 321-325.

2338. Baxendine-Jones J, Campbell I, Ellison D (1997). p53 status has no prognostic significance in glioblastomas treated with radiotherapy. *Clin Neuropathol* 16: 332-336.

2339. Bostrom J, Cobbers JM, Wolter M, Tabatabai G, Weber RG, Lichter P, Collins VP, Reifenberger G (1998). Mutation of the PTEN (MMAC1) tumor suppressor gene in a subset of glioblastomas but not in meningiomas with loss of chromosome arm 10q. *Cancer Res* 58: 29-33.

2340. Burns KL, Ueki K, Jhung SL, Koh J, Louis DN (1998). Molecular genetic correlates of p16, cdk4, and pRb immunohistochemistry in glioblastomas. *J Neuropathol Exp Neurol* 57: 122-130.

2341. Cheng Y, Ng HK, Ding M, Zhang SF, Pang JC, Lo KW (1999). Molecular analysis of microdissected de novo glioblastomas and paired astrocytic tumors. *J Neuropathol Exp Neurol* 58: 120-128.

2342. Chiariello E, Roz L, Albarosa R, Magnani I, Finocchiaro G (1998). PTEN/MMAC1 mutations in primary glioblastomas and short-term cultures of malignant gliomas. *Oncogene* 16: 541-545.

2343. Dreyling MH, Bohlander SK, Adeyanju MO, Olopade OI (1995). Detection of CDKN2 deletions in tumor cell lines and primary glioma by interphase fluorescence in situ hybridization. *Cancer Res* 55: 984-988.

2344. Hamel W, Westphal M, Shepard HM (1993). Loss in expression of the retinoblastoma gene product in human gliomas is associated with advanced disease. *J Neurooncol* 16: 159-165.

2345. Petronio J, He J, Fults D, Pedone C, James CD, Allen JR (1996). Common alternative gene alterations in adult malignant astrocytomas, but not in childhood primitive neuroectodermal tumors: P 16ink4 homozygous deletions and CDK4 gene amplifications. *J Neurosurg* 84: 1020-1023.

2346. He J, Olson JJ, James CD (1995). Lack of p16INK4 or retinoblastoma protein (pRb), or amplification- associated overexpression of cdk4 is observed in distinct subsets of malignant glial tumors and cell lines. *Cancer Res* 55: 4833-4836.

2347. He J, Allen JR, Collins VP, Allalunis-Turner MJ, Godbout R, Day RS, III, James CD (1994). CDK4 amplification is an alternative mechanism to p16 gene homozygous deletion in glioma cell lines. *Cancer Res* 54: 5804-5807.

2348. Hunter SB, Abbott K, Varma VA, Olson JJ, Barnett DW, James CD (1995). Reliability of differential PCR for the detection of EGFR and MDM2 gene amplification in DNA extracted from FFPE glioma tissue. *J Neuropathol Exp Neurol* 54: 57-64.

2349. Koga H, Zhang S, Kumanishi T, Washiyama K, Ichikawa T, Tanaka R, Mukawa J (1994). Analysis of p53 gene mutations in low- and high-grade astrocytomas by polymerase chain reaction-assisted single-strand conformation polymorphism and immunohistochemistry. *Acta Neuropathol (Berl)* 87: 225-232.

2350. Kordek R, Biernat W, Alwasiak J, Maculewicz R, Yanagihara R, Liberski PP (1995). p53 protein and epidermal growth factor receptor expression in human astrocytomas. *J Neurooncol* 26: 11-16.

2351. Korkolopoulou P, Christodoulou P, Kouzelis K, Hadjiyannakis M, Priftis A, Stamoulis G, Seretis A, Thomas-Tsagli E (1997). MDM2 and p53 expression in gliomas: a multivariate survival analysis including proliferation markers and epidermal growth factor receptor. *Br J Cancer* 75: 1269-1278.

2352. Kyritsis AP, Xu R, Bondy ML, Levin VA, Bruner JM (1996). Correlation of p53 immunoreactivity and sequencing in patients with glioma. *Mol Carcinog* 15: 1-4.

2353. Leenstra S, Oskam NT, Bijleveld EH, Bosch DA, Troost D, Hulsebos TJ (1998). Genetic sub-types of human malignant astrocytoma correlate with survival. *Int J Cancer* 79: 159-165.

2354. Leenstra S, Bijlsma EK, Troost D, Oosting J, Westerveld A, Bosch DA, Hulsebos TJ (1994). Allele loss on chromosomes 10 and 17p and epidermal growth factor receptor gene amplification in human malignant astrocytoma related to prognosis. *Br J Cancer* 70: 684-689.

2355. Li Y, Millikan RC, Carozza S, Newman B, Liu E, Davis R, Miike R, Wrensch M (1998). p53 mutations in malignant gliomas. *Cancer Epidemiol Biomarkers Prev* 7: 303-308.

2356. Li YJ, Hoang-Xuan K, Delattre JY, Poisson M, Thomas G, Hamelin R (1995). Frequent loss of heterozygosity on chromosome 9, and low incidence of mutations of cyclin-dependent kinase inhibitors p15 (MTS2) and p16 (MTS1) genes in gliomas. *Oncogene* 11: 597-600.

2357. Lin H, Bondy ML, Langford LA, Hess KR, Delclos GL, Wu X, Chan W, Pershouse MA, Yung WK, Steck PA (1998). Allelic deletion analyses of MMAC/PTEN and DMBT1 loci in gliomas: relationship to prognostic significance. *Clin Cancer Res* 4: 2447-2454.

2358. Maier D, Zhang Z, Taylor E, Hamou MF, Gratzl O, Van Meir EG, Scott RJ, Merlo A (1998). Somatic deletion mapping on chromosome 10 and sequence analysis of PTEN/MMAC1 point to the 10q25-26 region as the primary target in low- grade and high-grade gliomas. *Oncogene* 16: 3331-3335.

2359. Moulton T, Samara G, Chung WY, Yuan L, Desai R, Sisti M, Bruce J, Tycko B (1995). MTS1/p16/CDKN2 lesions in primary glioblastoma multiforme. *Am J Pathol* 146: 613-619.

2360. Muller MB, Schmidt MC, Schmidt O, Hayashi Y, Rollbrocker B, Waha A, Fimmers R, Volk B, Warnke P, Ostertag CB, Wiestler OD, von Deimling A (1999). Molecular genetic analysis as a tool for evaluating stereotactic biopsies of glioma specimens. *J Neuropathol Exp Neurol* 58: 40-45.

2361. Olson JJ, James CD, Krisht A, Barnett D, Hunter S (1995). Analysis of epidermal growth factor receptor gene amplification and alteration in stereotactic biopsies of brain tumors. *Neurosurgery* 36: 740-746.

2362. Rainov NG, Dobberstein KU, Fittkau M, Bahn H, Holzhausen HJ, Gantchev L, Burkert W (1995). Absence of p53 autoantibodies in sera from glioma patients. *Clin Cancer Res* 1: 775-781.

2363. Rainov NG, Dobberstein KU, Bahn H, Holzhausen HJ, Lautenschlager C, Heidecke V, Burkert W (1997). Prognostic factors in malignant glioma: influence of the overexpression of oncogene and tumor-suppressor gene products on survival. *J Neurooncol* 35: 13-28.

2364. Rollbrocker B, Waha A, Louis DN, Wiestler OD, von Deimling A (1996). Amplification of the cyclin-dependent kinase 4 (CDK4) gene is associated with high cdk4 protein levels in glioblastoma multiforme. *Acta Neuropathol (Berl)* 92: 70-74.

2365. Saxena A, Shriml LM, Dean M, Ali IU (1999). Comparative molecular genetic profiles of anaplastic astrocytomas/glioblastomas multiforme and their subsequent recurrences. *Oncogene* 18: 1385-1390.

2366. Saxena A, Clark WC, Robertson JT, Ikejiri B, Oldfield EH, Ali IU (1992). Evidence for the involvement of a potential second tumor suppressor gene on chromosome 17 distinct from p53 in malignant astrocytomas. *Cancer Res* 52: 6716-6721.

2367. Schlegel J, Merdes A, Stumm G, Albert FK, Forsting M, Hynes N, Kiessling M (1994). Amplification of the epidermal-growth-factor-receptor gene correlates with different growth behaviour in human glioblastoma. *Int J Cancer* 56: 72-77.

2368. Somerville RP, Shoshan Y, Eng C, Barnett G, Miller D, Cowell JK (1998). Molecular analysis of two putative tumour suppressor genes, PTEN and DMBT, which have been implicated in glioblastoma multiforme disease progression. *Oncogene* 17: 1755-1757.

2369. Sonoda Y, Yoshimoto T, Sekiya T (1995). Homozygous deletion of the MTS1/p16 and MTS2/p15 genes and amplification of the CDK4 gene in glioma. *Oncogene* 11: 2145-2149.

2370. Tenan M, Colombo BM, Pollo B, Cajola L, Broggi G, Finocchiaro G (1994). p53 mutations and microsatellite analysis of loss of heterozygosity in malignant gliomas. *Cancer Genet Cytogenet* 74: 139-143.

2371. Tsuzuki T, Tsunoda S, Sakaki T, Konishi N, Hiasa Y, Nakamura M (1996). Alterations of retinoblastoma, p53, p16(CDKN2), and p15 genes in human astrocytomas. *Cancer* 78: 287-293.

2372. Ueki K, Rubio MP, Ramesh V, Correa KM, Rutter JL, von Deimling A, Buckler AJ, Gusella JF, Louis DN (1994). MTS1/CDKN2 gene mutations are rare in primary human astrocytomas with allelic loss of chromosome 9p. *Hum Mol Genet* 3: 1841-1845.

2373. Venter DJ, Bevan KL, Ludwig RL, Riley TE, Jat PS, Thomas DG, Noble MD (1991). Retinoblastoma gene deletions in human glioblastomas. *Oncogene* 6: 445-448.

2374. Waha A, Baumann A, Wolf HK, Fimmers R, Neumann J, Kindermann D, Astrahantseff K, Blumcke I, von Deimling A, Schlegel U (1996). Lack of prognostic relevance of alterations in the epidermal growth factor receptor-transforming growth factor-alpha pathway in human astrocytic gliomas. *J Neurosurg* 85: 634-641.

2375. Wang SI, Puc J, Li J, Bruce JN, Cairns P, Sidransky D, Parsons R (1997). Somatic mutations of PTEN in glioblastoma multiforme. *Cancer Res* 57: 4183-4186.

2376. Wu JK, Ye Z, Darras BT (1993). Frequency of p53 tumor suppressor gene mutations in human primary brain tumors. *Neurosurgery* 33: 824-830.

2377. Zhou XP, Li YJ, Hoang-Xuan K, Laurent-Puig P, Mokhtari K, Longy M, Sanson M, Delattre JY, Thomas G, Hamelin R (1999). Mutational analysis of the PTEN gene in gliomas: molecular and pathological correlations. *Int J Cancer* 84: 150-154.

2378. Zhu A, Shaeffer J, Leslie S, Kolm P, El Mahdi AM (1996). Epidermal growth factor receptor: an independent predictor of survival in astrocytic tumors given definitive irradiation. *Int J Radiat Oncol Biol Phys* 34: 809-815.

2379. Bhattacharjee MB, Bruner JM (1997). p53 protein in pediatric malignant astrocytomas: a study of 21 patients. *J Neurooncol* 32: 225-233.

2380. Chozick BS, Weicker ME, Pezzullo JC, Jackson CL, Finkelstein SD, Ambler MW, Epstein MH, Finch PW (1994). Pattern of mutant p53 expression in human astrocytomas suggests the existence of alternate pathways of tumorigenesis. *Cancer* 73: 406-415.

2381. Chung R, Whaley J, Kley N, Anderson K, Louis D, Menon A, Hettlich C, Freiman R, Hedley-Whyte ET, Martuza R (1991). TP53 gene mutations and 17p deletions in human astrocytomas. *Genes Chromosomes Cancer* 3: 323-331.

2382. Drach LM, Kammermeier M, Neirich U, Jacobi G, Kornhuber B, Lorenz R, Schlote W (1996). Accumulation of nuclear p53 protein and prognosis of astrocytomas in childhood and adolescence. *Clin Neuropathol* 15: 67-73.

2383. Felix CA, Slavc I, Dunn M, Strauss EA, Phillips PC, Rorke LB, Sutton L, Bunin GR, Biegel JA (1995). p53 gene mutations in pediatric brain tumors. *Med Pediatr Oncol* 25: 431-436.

2384. Hunter SB, Bandea C, Swan D, Abbott K, Varma VA (1993). Mutations in the p53 gene in human astrocytomas: detection by single- strand conformation polymorphism analysis and direct DNA sequencing. *Mod Pathol* 6: 442-445.

2385. Litofsky NS, Hinton D, Raffel C (1994). The lack of a role for p53 in astrocytomas in pediatric patients. *Neurosurgery* 34: 967-972.

2386. Louis DN, von Deimling A, Chung RY, Rubio MP, Whaley JM, Eibl RH, Ohgaki H, Wiestler OD, Thor AD, Seizinger BR (1993). Comparative study of p53 gene and protein alterations in human astrocytic tumors. *J Neuropathol Exp Neurol* 52: 31-38.

2387. Ono Y, Tamiya T, Ichikawa T, Matsumoto K, Furuta T, Ohmoto T, Akiyama K, Seki S, Ueki K, Louis DN (1997). Accumulation of wild-type p53 in astrocytomas is associated with increased p21 expression. *Acta Neuropathol (Berl)* 94: 21-27.

2388. Ono Y, Tamiya T, Ichikawa T, Kunishio K, Matsumoto K, Furuta T, Ohmoto T, Ueki K, Louis DN (1996). Malignant astrocytomas with homozygous CDKN2/p16 gene deletions have higher Ki-67 proliferation indices. *J Neuropathol Exp Neurol* 55: 1026-1031.

2389. Orellana C, Hernandez-Marti M, Martinez F, Castel V, Millan JM, Alvarez-Garijo JA, Prieto F, Badia L (1998). Pediatric brain tumors: loss of heterozygosity at 17p and TP53 gene mutations. *Cancer Genet Cytogenet* 102: 93-99.

2390. Pollack IF, Hamilton RL, Finkelstein SD, Campbell JW, Martinez AJ, Sherwin RN, Bozik ME, Gollin SM (1997). The relationship between TP53 mutations and overexpression of p53 and prognosis in malignant gliomas of childhood. *Cancer Res* 57: 304-309.

2391. Schiffer D, Cavalla P, Di Sapio A, Giordana MT, Mauro A (1995). Mutations and immunohistochemistry of p53 and proliferation markers in astrocytic tumors of childhood. *Childs Nerv Syst* 11: 517-522.

2392. Sure U, Ruedi D, Tachibana O, Yonekawa Y, Ohgaki H, Kleihues P, Hegi ME (1997). Determination of p53 mutations, EGFR overexpression, and loss of p16 expression in pediatric glioblastomas. *J Neuropathol Exp Neurol* 56: 782-789.

2393. Tada M, Iggo RD, Waridel F, Nozaki M, Matsumoto R, Sawamura Y, Shinohe Y, Ikeda J, Abe H (1997). Reappraisal of p53 mutations in human malignant astrocytic neoplasms by p53 functional assay: comparison with conventional structural analyses. *Mol Carcinog* 18: 171-176.

2394. Walker DG, Duan W, Popovic EA, Kaye AH, Tomlinson FH, Lavin M (1995). Homozygous deletions of the multiple tumor suppressor gene 1 in the progression of human astrocytomas. *Cancer Res* 55: 20-23.

2395. Wasson JC, Saylors RL, III, Zeltzer P, Friedman HS, Bigner SH, Burger PC, Bigner DD, Look AT, Douglass EC, Brodeur GM (1990). Oncogene amplification in pediatric brain tumors. *Cancer Res* 50: 2987-2990.

2396. Ye Z, Qu JK, Darras BT (1993). Loss of heterozygosity for alleles on chromosome 10 in human brain tumours. *Neurol Res* 15: 59-62.

2397. Zhang S, Feng X, Koga H, Ichikawa T, Abe S, Kumanishi T (1993). p53 gene mutations in pontine gliomas of juvenile onset. *Biochem Biophys Res Commun* 196: 851-857.

2398. Nakamura M, Konishi N, Hiasa Y, Tsunoda S, Fukushima Y, Tsuzuki T, Takemura K, Aoki H, Kobitsu K, Sakaki T (1996). Immunohistochemical detection of CDKN2, retinoblastoma and p53 gene products in primary astrocytic tumors. *Int J Oncol* 8: 889-893.

2399. Newcomb EW, Alonso M, Sung T,Miller DC (1999). Inactivation of the INK4a-ARF pathway by co-deletion of the p16INK4a and p14ARF genes in high grade astrocytomas. *Proc Am Assoc Cancer Res* 40;280.

2400. Rao L, Miller DC, Newcomb EW (1997). Correlative immunohistochemistry and molecular genetic study of the inactivation of the p16INK4 genes in astrocytomas. *Diagn Mol Pathol* 6: 115-122.

2401. Cheng Y, Ng HK, Zhang SF, Ding M, Pang JCS, Zheng J (1999). Alterations of p53, PTEN, EGFR, chromosome 9p21 and microsatellite instability in pediatric high-grade astrocytomas. *Hum Pathol* 30: 1284-1290.

2402. Vortmeyer AO, Stavrou T, Selby D, Li G, Weil RJ, Park WS, Moon YW, Chandra R, Goldstein AM, Zhuang Z (1999). Deletion analysis of the adenomatous polyposis coli and *PTCH* gene loci in patients with sporadic and nevoid basal cell acrcinoma syndrome-associated medulloblastoma. *Cancer* 85: 2662-2667.

2403. Paulino AC, Melian E (1999). Medulloblastoma and supratentorial primitive neuroectodermal tumors. An institutional experience. *Cancer* 86: 142-148.

2404. Alleyne CH, Jr., Hunter S, Olson JJ, Barrow DL (1998). Lipomatous glioneurocytoma of the posterior fossa with divergent differentiation: case report. *Neurosurgery* 42: 639-643.

2405. Mazzone D, Magro G, Lucenti A, Grasso S (1995). Report of a case of congenital glioblastoma multiforme: an immunohistochemical study. *Childs Nerv Syst* 11: 311-313.

2406. Lee DY, Kim YM, Yoo SJ, Cho BK, Chi JG, Kim IO, Wang KC (1999). Congenital glioblastoma diagnosed by fetal sonography. *Childs Nerv Syst* 15: 197-201.

2407. Sylvestre G, Sherer DM (1998). Prenatal sonographic findings associated with malignant astrocytoma following normal early third-trimester ultrasonography. *Am J Perinatol* 15: 581-584.

2408. Doren M, Tercanli S, Gullotta F, Holzgreve W (1997). Prenatal diagnosis of a highly undifferentiated brain tumour—a case report and review of the literature. *Prenat Diagn* 17: 967-971.

2409. Lee TT, Manzano GR (1997). Third ventricular glioblastoma multiforme: case report. *Neurosurg Rev* 20: 291-294.

2410. Buetow PC, Smirniotopoulos JG, Done S (1990). Congenital brain tumors: a review of 45 cases. *AJR Am J Roentgenol* 155: 587-593.

2411. Nagashima G, Suzuki R, Hokaku H, Takahashi M, Miyo T, Asai J, Nakagawa N, Fujimoto T (1999). Graphic analysis of microscopic tumor cell infiltration, proliferative potential, and vascular endothelial growth factor expression in an autopsy brain with glioblastoma. *Surg Neurol* 51: 292-299.

2412. Cheng SY, Nagane M, Huang HS, Cavenee WK (1997). Intracerebral tumor-associated hemorrhage caused by overexpression of the vascular endothelial growth factor isoforms VEGF121 and VEGF165 but not VEGF189. *Proc Natl Acad Sci U S A* 94: 12081-12087.

2413. Buhl R, Barth H, Hugo HH, Hutzelmann A, Mehdorn HM (1998). Spinal drop metastases in recurrent glioblastoma multiforme. *Acta Neurochir (Wien)* 140: 1001-1005.

2414. Fecteau AH, Penn I, Hanto DW (1998). Peritoneal metastasis of intracranial glioblastoma via a ventriculoperitoneal shunt preventing organ retrieval: case report and review of the literature. *Clin Transplant* 12: 348-350.

2415. Salvati M, Oppido PA, Artizzu S, Fiorenza F, Puzzilli F, Orlando ER (1991). Multicentric gliomas. Report of seven cases. *Tumori* 77: 518-522.

2416. Shafqat S, Hedley-Whyte ET, Henson JW (1999). Age-dependent rate of anaplastic transformation in low-grade astrocytoma. *Neurology* 52: 867-869.

2417. Dropcho EJ, Soong SJ (1996). The prognostic impact of prior low grade histology in patients with anaplastic gliomas: a case-control study. *Neurology* 47: 684-690.

2418. Teo JG, Gultekin SH, Bilsky M, Gutin P, Rosenblum MK (1999). A distinctive glioneuronal tumor of the adult cerebrum with neuropil-like (including "rosetted") islands: report of 4 cases. *Am J Surg Pathol* 23: 502-510.

2419. Berens ME, Giese A (1999). "...those left behind." Biology and oncology of invasive glioma cells. *Neoplasia* (in press).

2420. Boch AL, van Effenterre R, Kujas M (1997). Craniopharyngiomas in two consanguineous siblings: case report. *Neurosurgery* 41: 1185-1187.

2421. Bunin GR, Surawicz TS, Witman PA, Preston-Martin S, Davis F, Bruner JM (1998).

The descriptive epidemiology of craniopharyngioma. *J Neurosurg* 89: 547-551.

2422. Kuratsu J, Ushio Y (1996). Epidemiological study of primary intracranial tumors in childhood. A population-based survey in Kumamoto Prefecture, Japan. *Pediatr Neurosurg* 25: 240-246.

2423. Nishi T, Kuratsu JI, Takeshima H, Saito Y, Kochi M, Ushio Y (1999). Prognostic significance of the MIB-1 labeling index for patient with craniopharyngioma. *Int J Mol Med* 3: 157-161.

2424. Paulus W, Stockel C, Krauss J, Sorensen N, Roggendorf W (1997). Odontogenic classification of craniopharyngiomas: a clinicopathological study of 54 cases. *Histopathology* 30: 172-176.

2425. Paulus W, Honegger J, Keyvani K, Fahlbusch R (1999). Xanthogranuloma of the sellar region: a clinicopathological entity different from adamantinomatous craniopharyngioma. *Acta Neuropathol (Berl)* 97: 377-382.

2426. Sartoretti-Schefer S, Wichmann W, Aguzzi A, Valavanis A (1997). MR differentiation of adamantinous and squamous-papillary craniopharyngiomas. *AJNR Am J Neuroradiol* 18: 77-87.

2427. Dickey T, Raghaven R, Rushing E (1999). MIB-1 (Ki-67) immunoreactivity as predictor of the risk of recurrence of craniopharyngiomas. *J Neuropath Exp Neurol* 58: 567-567.

2428. Russell DS,Rubinstein LJ (1989). Craniopharyngiomas and suprasellar epidermoid cysts. In: *Pathology of Tumours of the Nervous System*, Russell DS, Rubinstein LJ (eds), 5th ed. Edward Arnold: London. pp. 695-702.

2429. Thapar K,Kovacs K (1998). Neoplasms of the sellar region. In: *Russell and Rubinstein's Pathology of Tumours of the Nervous System*, Bigner DD, McLendon RE, Bruner J (eds), 6th ed. Arnold: London, Sydney, Auckland. pp. 561-677.

2430. Thomas C, Kristopaitis T, Petruzelli G, Lee J (1999). Malignant craniopharyngioma. *J Neuropath Exp Neurol* 58: 567-567.

2431. Brat DJ, James CD, Jedlicka AE, Connolly DC, Chang E, Castellani RJ, Schmid M, Schiller M, Carson DA, Burger PC (1999). Molecular genetic alterations in radiation-induced astrocytomas. *Am J Pathol* 154: 1431-1438.

2432. Rickert CH, Dockhorn-Dworniczak B, Simon R, Paulus W (1999). Chromosomal imbalances in primary lymphomas of the central nervous system. *Am J Pathol* 155: 1445-1451.

2434. Kleihues P, Ohgaki H (1999). Primary and secondary glioblastoma: from concept to clinical diagnosis. *Neuro-Oncology* 1: 44-51.

2435. Strojnik T, Kos J, Zidanik B, Golouh R, Lah T (1999). Cathepsin B immunohistochemical staining in tumor and endothelial cells is a new prognostic factor for survival in patients with brain tumors. *Clin Cancer Res* 5: 559-567.

2436. Sano T, Lin H, Chen X, Langford LA, Koul D, Bondy ML, Hess KR, Myers JN, Hong YK, Yung WK, Steck PA (1999). Differential expression of MMAC/PTEN in glioblastoma multiforme: relationship to localization and prognosis. *Cancer Res* 59: 1820-1824.

2437. Bouvier-Labit C, Chinot O, Ochi C, Gambarelli D, Dufour H, Figarella-Branger D (1998). Prognostic significance of Ki67, p53 and epidermal growth factor receptor immunostaining in human glioblastomas. *Neuropathol Appl Neurobiol* 24: 381-388.

2438. Scott JN, Rewcastle NB, Brasher PM, Fulton D, Hagen NA, MacKinnon JA, Sutherland G, Cairncross JG, Forsyth P (1998). Long-term glioblastoma multiforme survivors: a population-based study. *Can J Neurol Sci* 25: 197-201.

2439. Pierallini A, Bonamini M, Pantano P, Palmeggiani F, Raguso M, Osti MF, Anaveri G, Bozzao L (1998). Radiological assessment of necrosis in glioblastoma: variability and prognostic value. *Neuroradiology* 40: 150-153.

2440. Sharpless NE, DePinho RA (1999). The INK4A/ARF locus and its two gene products. *Curr Opin Genet Dev* 9: 22-30.

2441. Badie B, Schartner J, Klaver J, Vorpahl J (1999). In vitro modulation of microglia motility by glioma cells is mediated by hepatocyte growth factor/scatter factor. *Neurosurgery* 44: 1077-1082.

2442. Moriyama T, Kataoka H, Koono M, Wakisaka S (1999). Expression of hepatocyte growth factor/scatter factor and its receptor c-Met in brain tumors: evidence for a role in progression of astrocytic tumors (Review). *Int J Mol Med* 3: 531-536.

2443. Hegi ME, zur HA, Ruedi D, Malin G, Kleihues P (1997). Hemizygous or homozygous deletion of the chromosomal region containing the p16INK4a gene is associated with amplification of the EGF receptor gene in glioblastomas. *Int J Cancer* 73: 57-63.

2444. Tao W, Levine AJ (1999). P19(ARF) stabilizes p53 by blocking nucleo-cytoplasmic shuttling of Mdm2. *Proc Natl Acad Sci U S A* 96: 6937-6941.

2445. Kraus A, Neff F, Behn M, Schuermann M, Muenkel K, Schlegel J (1999). Expression of alternatively spliced mdm2 transcripts correlates with stabilized wild-type p53 protein in human glioblastoma cells. *Int J Cancer* 80: 930-934.

2446. Rieger J, Ohgaki H, Kleihues P, Weller M (1999). Human astrocytic brain tumors express AP02L/TRAIL. *Acta Neuropathol (Berl)* 97: 1-4.

2447. Laws ER, Jr., Goldberg WJ, Bernstein JJ (1993). Migration of human malignant astrocytoma cells in the mammalian brain: Scherer revisited. *Int J Dev Neurosci* 11: 691-697.

2448. Ohgaki H, Watanabe K, Peraud A, Biernat W, von Deimling A, Yasargil MG, Yonekawa Y, Kleihues P (1999). A case history of glioma progression. *Acta Neuropathol (Berl)* 97: 525-532.

2449. McCormack BM, Miller DC, Budzilovich GN, Voorhees GJ, Ransohoff J (1992). Treatment and survival of low-grade astrocytoma in adults—1977-1988. *Neurosurgery* 31: 636-642.

2450. Vertosick FT, Jr., Selker RG, Arena VC (1991). Survival of patients with well-differentiated astrocytomas diagnosed in the era of computed tomography. *Neurosurgery* 28: 496-501.

2451. Koochekpour S, Jeffers M, Rulong S, Taylor G, Klineberg E, Hudson EA, Resau JH, Vande Woude GF (1997). Met and hepatocyte growth factor/scatter factor expression in human gliomas. *Cancer Res* 57: 5391-5398.

2452. Huang RP, Hossain MZ, Sehgal A, Boynton AL (1999). Reduced connexin43 expression in high-grade human brain glioma cells. *J Surg Oncol* 70: 21-24.

2453. Huang RP, Fan Y, Hossain MZ, Peng A, Zeng ZL, Boynton AL (1998). Reversion of the neoplastic phenotype of human glioblastoma cells by connexin 43 (cx43). *Cancer Res* 58: 5089-5096.

2454. Meyerhardt JA, Caca K, Eckstrand BC, Hu G, Lengauer C, Banavali S, Look AT, Fearon ER (1999). Netrin-1: interaction with deleted in colorectal cancer (DCC) and alterations in brain tumors and neuroblastomas. *Cell Growth Differ* 10: 35-42.

2455. Fujisawa H, Kurrer M, Reis RM, Yonekawa Y, Kleihues P, Ohgaki H (1999). Acqusition of the glioblastoma phenotype during astrocytoma progression is associated with LOH on 10q25-qter. *Am J Pathol* 155: 387-394.

2456. Fujisawa H, Reis RM, Nakamura M, Colella S, Yonekawa Y, Kleihues P, Ohgaki H (2000). Loss of heterozygosity on chromosome 10 is more extensive in primary (*de novo*) than in secondary glioblastomas. *Lab Invest* 80: 1-8.

2457. Mollenhauer J, Holmskov U, Wiemann S, Krebs I, Herbertz S, Madsen J, Kioschis P, Coy JF, Poustka A (1999). The genomic structure of the *DMBT1* gene: evidence for a region with susceptibility to genomic instability. *Oncogene* 18: 6233-6240.

2458. Fults D, Pedone C (1993). Deletion mapping of the long arm of chromosome 10 in glioblastoma multiforme. *Genes Chromosomes Cancer* 7: 173-177.

2459. Matsumoto R, Tada M, Nozaki M, Zhang CL, Sawamura Y, Abe H (1998). Short alternative splice transcriprts of the mdm2 oncogene correlate to malignancy in human astrocytic neoplasms. *Cancer Res* 58: 609-613.

2460. Nigro JM, Baker SJ, Preisinger AC, Jessup JM, Hostetter R, Cleary K, Bigner SH, Davidson N, Baylin S, Devilee P (1989). Mutations in the p53 gene occur in diverse human tumour types. *Nature* 342: 705-708.

2461. von Deimling A, Nagel J, Bender B, Lenartz D, Schramm J, Louis DN, Wiestler OD (1994). Deletion mapping of chromosome 19 in human gliomas. *Int J Cancer* 57: 676-680.

2462. Hjalmars U, Kulldorff M, Wahlqvist Y, Lannering B (1999). Increased incidence rates but no space-time clustering of childhood astrocytoma in Sweden, 1973-1992: a population-based study of pediatric brain tumors. *Cancer* 85: 2077-2090.

2463. Hilton DA, Love S, Barber R, Ellison D, Sandeman DR (1998). Accumulation of p53 and Ki-67 expression do not predict survival in patients with fibrillary astrocytomas or the response of these tumors to radiotherapy. *Neurosurgery* 42: 724-729.

2464. Swensen AR, Bushhouse SA (1998). Childhood cancer incidence and trends in Minnesota, 1988-1994. *Minn Med* 81: 27-32.

2465. Hemminki K, Kyyronen P, Vaittinen P (1999). Parental age as a risk factor of childhood leukemia and brain cancer in offspring. *Epidemiology* 10: 271-275.

2466. Peraud A, Ansari H, Bise K, Reulen HJ (1998). Clinical outcome of supratentorial astrocytoma WHO grade II. *Acta Neurochir (Wien)* 140: 1213-1222.

2467. Roelcke U, von Ammon K, Hausmann O, Kaech DL, Vanloffeld W, Landolt H, Rem JA, Gratzl O, Radu EW, Leenders KL (1999). Operated low grade astrocytomas: a long term PET study on the effect of radiotherapy. *J Neurol Neurosurg Psychiatry* 66: 644-647.

2469. Frappaz D, Ricci AC, Kohler R, Bret P, Mottolese C (1999). Diffuse brain stem tumor in an adolescent with multiple enchondromatosis (Ollier's disease). *Childs Nerv Syst* 15: 222-225.

2470. Schrock E, Blume C, Meffert MC, du MS, Bersch W, Kiessling M, Lozanowa T, Thiel G, Witkowski R, Ried T, Cremer T (1996). Recurrent gain of chromosome arm 7q in low-grade astrocytic tumors studied by comparative genomic hybridization. *Genes Chromosomes Cancer* 15: 199-205.

2471. Nishizaki T, Ozaki S, Harada K, Ito H, Arai H, Beppu T, Sasaki K (1998). Investigation of genetic alterations associated with the grade of astrocytic tumor by comparative genomic hybridization. *Genes Chromosomes Cancer* 21: 340-346.

2473. Kinzler KW, Vogelstein B (1998). Landscaping the cancer terrain. *Science* 280: 1036-1037.

2474. Hofman S, Heeg M, Klein JP, Krikke AP (1998). Simultaneous occurrence of a supra- and an infratentorial glioma in a patient with Ollier's disease: more evidence for non-mesodermal tumor predisposition in multiple enchondromatosis. *Skeletal Radiol* 27: 688-691.

2475. Prayson RA, Estes ML (1996). MIB1 and p53 immunoreactivity in protoplasmic astrocytomas. *Pathol Int* 46: 862-866.

2476. Shinoda J, Sakai N, Nakatani K, Funakoshi T (1998). Prognostic factors in supratentorial WHO grade II astrocytoma in adults. *Br J Neurosurg* 12: 318-324.

2477. Davis FG,Preston-Martin S (1998). Epidemiology. Incidence and survival. In: *Russell and Rubinstein's Pathology of Tumors of the Nervous System*, Bigner DD, McLendon RE, Bruner JM (eds), 6th ed. Arnold: London. pp. 5-45.

2478. Nakamura M, Yang F, Fujisawa H, Yonekawa Y, Kleihues P, Ohgaki H (1999). Loss of heterozygosity on chromosome 19 in secondary glioblastomas. (*submitted*).

2479. Ishii N, Maier D, Merlo A, Tada M, Sawamura Y, Diserens AC, Van Meir E (1999). Frequent co-alterations of *TP53*, *p16/CDKN2A*, *p14^{ARF}*, *PTEN* tumor suppressor genes in human glioma cell lines. *Brain Pathol* 9: 469-479.

2480. Hayes VM, Dirven CM, Dam A, Verlind E, Molenaar WM, Jakob J, Hofstra RMW, Buys CHCM (1999). High frequency of *TP53* mutations in juvenile pilocytic astrocytomas indicates role of *TP53* in the development of these tumors. *Brain Pathol* 9: 463-467.

2481. Buschges R, Weber RG, Actor B, Lichter P, Collins VP, Reifenberger G (1999). Amplification and expression of cyclin D genes (*CCND1*, *CCND2* and *CCND3*) in human malignant gliomas. *Brain Pathol* 9: 435-443.

2482. Holash J, Maisonpierre PC, Compton D, Boland P, Alexander CR, Zagzag D, Yancopoulos GD, Wiegand SJ (1999). Vessel cooption, regression, and growth in tumors mediated by angiopoetins and VEGF. *Science* 284: 1994-1998.

2483. Grover WD, Rorke LB (1968). Invasive craniopharyngioma. *J Neurol Neurosurg Psychiatry* 31: 580-582.

2484. Ichimura K, Schmidt EE, Miyakawa A, Goike HM, Collins VP (1998). Distinct patterns of deletion on 10p and 10q suggest involvement of multiple tumor suppressor genes in the development of astrocytic gliomas of different malignancy grades. *Genes Chromosomes Cancer* 22: 9-15.

2485. Blumcke I, Giencke K, Wardelmann E, Beyenburg S, Kral T, Sarioglu N, Pietsch T, Wolf HK, Schramm J, Elger CE, Wiestler OD (1999). The CD34 epitope is expressed in neoplastic and malformative lesions associated with chronic, focal epilepsia. *Acta Neuropathol* 97: 481-490.

2486. Kuchelmeister K, Steinhauser A, Korf B, Wagner D, Prey N, Schachenmayr W (1996). Anaplastic desmoplastic infantile ganglioglioma: a case report. *Clin Neuropathol* 15: 280-280.

2487. Kuchelmeister K, Schonmeyr R, Albani M, Schachenmayr W (1998). Anaplastic desmoplastic infantile ganglioglioma. *Clin Neuropathol* 17: 269-269.

2488. Lamszus K, Kluwe L, Matschke J, Meissner H, Laas R, Westphal M (1999). Allelic losses at 1p, 9q, 10q, 14q, and 22q in the progression of aggressive meningiomas and undifferentiated meningeal sarcomas. *Cancer Genet Cytogenet* 110: 103-110.

2489. Gläsker S, Bender BU, Apel TW, Natt E, van Velthoven V, Scheremet R, Zentner J, Neumann HPH (1999). The impact of molecular genetic analysis of the VHL gene in patients with hemangioblastomas of the central nervous system. *J Neurol Neurosurg Psychiatry*. 67: 758-762.

2490. Ali JBM, Sepp T, Ward S, Green AJ, Yates JRW (1998). Mutations in the TSC1 gene account for a minority of patients with sclerosis. *J Med Genet* 35: 969-972.

2491. Daumas-Duport C, Tucker ML, Kolles H, Cervera P, Beuvon F, Varlet P, Udo N, Koziak M, Chodkiewicz JP (1997). Oligodendrogliomas. Part II: A new grading system based on morphological and imaging criteria. *J Neurooncol* 34: 61-78.

2492. Schiffer D, Bosone I, Dutto A, Di Vito N, Chio A (1999). The prognostic role of vessel productive changes and vessel density in oligodendroglioma. *J Neurooncol* 44: 99-107.

2494. Schiffer D, Dutto A, Cavalla P, Chio A, Migheli A, Piva R (1997). Role of apoptosis in the prognosis of oligodendrogliomas. *Neurochem Int* 31: 245-250.

2495. Bruggers CS, Welsh CT, Boyer RS, Byrne JL, Pysher TJ (1999). Successful therapy in a child with a congenital peripheral medulloepithelioma and disruption of hindquarter development. *J Pediatr Hematol Oncol* 21: 161-164.

2496. Figarella-Branger D, Gambarelli D, Perez-Castillo M, Gentet JC, Grisoli F, Pellissier JF (1992). Ectopic intrapelvic medulloepithelioma: case report. *Neuropathol Appl Neurobiol* 18: 408-414.

2497. Morrison AL, Mena H, Jones RV, Gyure KA, Bratthauer GL (1998). Central neurocytomas express photoreceptor differentiation. *J Neuropath Exp Neurol* 57;519-519.

2498. Brown DF, Chason DP, Schwartz LF, Coimbra CP, Rushing EJ (1998). Supratentorial giant cell ependymoma: a case report. *Mod Pathol* 11: 398-403.

2499. Ernestus RI, Schroder R, Stutzer H, Klug N (1997). The clinical and prognostic relevance of grading in intracranial ependymomas. *Br J Neurosurg* 11: 421-428.

2500. Ernestus RI, Schroder R, Stutzer H, Klug N (1996). Prognostic relevance of localization and grading in intracranial ependymomas of childhood. *Childs Nerv Syst* 12: 522-526.

2501. Rosenblum MK, Erlandson RA, Aleksic SN, Budzilovich GN (1990). Melanotic ependymoma and subependymoma. *Am J Surg Pathol* 14: 729-736.

2502. Zuppan CW, Mierau GW, Weeks DA (1994). Ependymoma with signet-ring cells. *Ultrastruct Pathol* 18: 43-46.

2503. Friede RL, Pollak A (1978). The cytogenetic basis for classifying ependymomas. *J Neuropathol Exp Neurol* 37: 103-118.

2504. Afra D, Muller W, Slowik F, Wilcke O, Budka H, Turoczy L (1983). Supratentorial lobar ependymomas: reports on the grading and survival periods in 80 cases, including 46 recurrences. *Acta Neurochir (Wien)* 69: 243-251.

2505. Figarella-Branger D, Gambarelli D, Dollo C, Devictor B, Perez-Castillo AM, Genitori L, Lena G, Choux M, Pellissier JF (1991). Infratentorial ependymomas of childhood. Correlation between histological features, immunohistological phenotype, silver nucleolar organizer region staining values and post-operative survival in 16 cases. *Acta Neuropathol (Berl)* 82: 208-216.

2506. Ho KL (1990). Microtubular aggregates within rough endoplasmic reticulum in myxopapillary ependymoma of the filum terminale. *Arch Pathol Lab Med* 114: 956-960.

2507. Lombardi D, Scheithauer BW, Meyer FB, Forbes GS, Shaw EG, Gibney DJ, Katzmann JA (1991). Symptomatic subependymoma: a clinicopathological and flow cytometric study. *J Neurosurg* 75: 583-588.

2508. Tomlinson FH, Scheithauer BW, Kelly PJ, Forbes GS (1991). Subependymoma with rhabdomyosarcomatous differentiation: report of a case and literature review. *Neurosurgery* 28: 761-768.

2509. Louis DN, Hedley-Whyte ET, Martuza RL (1989). Sarcomatous proliferation of the vasculature in a subependymoma. *Acta Neuropathol (Berl)* 78: 332-335.

2510. Perry A, Giannini C, Scheithauer BW, Rojiani AM, Yachnis AT, Seo IS, Johnson PC, Kho J, Shapiro S (1997). Composite pleomorphic xanthoastrocytoma and ganglioglioma: report of four cases and review of the literature. *Am J Surg Pathol* 21: 763-771.

2511. D'Addario V, Pinto V, Meo F, Resta M (1998). The specificity of ultrasound in the detection of fetal intracranial tumors. *J Perinat Med* 26: 480-485.

2512. Pencalet P, Sainte-Rose C, Lellouch-Tubiana A, Kalifa C, Brunelle F, Sgouros S, Meyer P, Cinalli G, Zerah M, Pierre-Kahn A, Renier D (1998). Papillomas and carcinomas of the choroid plexus in children. *J Neurosurg* 88: 521-528.

2513. Donovan MJ, Yunis EJ, DeGirolami U, Fletcher JA, Schofield DE (1994). Chromosome aberrations in choroid plexus papillomas. *Genes Chromosomes Cancer* 11: 267-270.

2514. Norman MG, Harrison KJ, Poskitt KJ, Kalousek DK (1995). Duplication of 9P and hyperplasia of the choroid plexus: a pathologic, radiologic, and molecular cytogenetics study. *Pediatr Pathol Lab Med* 15: 109-120.

2515. Li YS, Fan YS, Armstrong RF (1996). Endoreduplication and telomeric association in a choroid plexus carcinoma. *Cancer Genet Cytogenet* 87: 7-10.

2516. Sommer A, Bousset K, Kremmer E, Austen M, Luscher B (1998). Identification and characterization of specific DNA-binding complexes containing members of the Myc/Max/Mad network of transcriptional regulators. *J Biol Chem* 273: 6632-6642.

2517. Huang MC, Kubo O, Tajika Y, Takakura K (1996). A clinico-immunohistochemical study of giant cell glioblastoma. *Noshuyo Byori* 13: 11-16.

2518. Klein R, Molenkamp G, Sorensen N, Roggendorf W (1998). Favorable outcome of giant cell glioblastoma in a child. Report of an 11-year survival period. *Childs Nerv Syst* 14: 288-291.

2519. Sung T, Miller DC, Hayes RL, Alonso M, Yee H, Newcomb EW (1999). Preferential inactivation of the p53 tumour suppressor pathway and lack of EGFR receptor amplification distinguished de novo high grade pediatric astrocytomas from de novo adult astrocytomas. *Brain Pathol* (in press).

2520. Newcomb EW, Alonso M, Sung T, Miller DC (2000). Incidence of p14ARF gene deletion in high grade adult and pediatric astrocytomas. *Hum Pathol* 31: 115-119.

2521. Wagenknecht B, Hermisson M, Eitel K, Weller M (1999). Proteasome Inhibitors Induce p53/p21-Independent Apoptosis in Human Glioma Cells. *Cell Physiol Biochem* 9: 117-125.

2522. Kleihues P, Aguzzi A, Ohgaki H (1995). Genetic and environmental factors in the etiology of human brain tumors. *Toxicol Lett* 82-83:601-5: 601-605.

2523. van Nielen KM, de Jong BM (1999). A case of Ollier's disease associated with two intracerebral low-grade gliomas. *Clin Neurol Neurosurg* 101: 106-110.

2524. Kokunai T, Tamaki N (1999). Relationship between expression of p21WAF1/CIP1 and radioresistance in human gliomas. *Jpn J Cancer Res* 90: 638-646.

2525. Li YJ, Hoang-Xuan K, Zhou XP, Sanson M, Mokhtari K, Faillot T, Cornu P, Poisson M, Thomas G, Hamelin R (1998). Analysis of the p21 gene in gliomas. *J Neurooncol* 40: 107-111.

2526. Chen YQ, Hsieh JT, Yao F, Fang B, Pong RC, Cipriano SC, Krepulat F (1999). Induction of apoptosis and G2/M cell cycle arrest by DCC. *Oncogene* 18: 2747-2754.

2527. Mellon CD, Carter JE, Owen DB (1988). Ollier's disease and Maffucci's syndrome: distinct entities or a continuum. Case report: enchondromatosis complicated by an intracranial glioma. *J Neurol* 235: 376-378.

2528. Gander M, Leyvraz S, Decosterd L, Bonfanti M, Marzolini C, Shen F, Lienard D, Perey L, Colella G, Biollaz J, Lejeune F, Yarosh D, Belanich M, D'Incalci M (1999). Sequential administration of temozolomide and fotemustine: depletion of O6-alkyl guanine-DNA transferase in blood lymphocytes and in tumours. *Ann Oncol* 10: 831-838.

2529. D'Incalci M, Bonfanti M, Pifferi A, Mascellani E, Tagliabue G, Berger D, Fiebig HH (1998). The antitumour activity of alkylating agents is not correlated with the levels of glutathione, glutathione transferase and O6-alkylguanine-DNA- alkyltransferase of human tumour xenografts. EORTC SPG and PAMM Groups. *Eur J Cancer* 34: 1749-1755.

2530. Friedman HS, Kokkinakis DM, Pluda J, Friedman AH, Cokgor I, Haglund MM, Ashley DM, Rich J, Dolan ME, Pegg AE, Moschel RC, McLendon RE, Kerby T, Herndon JE, Bigner DD, Schold SC, Jr. (1998). Phase I trial of O6-benzylguanine for patients undergoing surgery for malignant glioma. *J Clin Oncol* 16: 3570-3575.

2531. Dolan ME, Pegg AE (1997). O6-benzylguanine and its role in chemotherapy. *Clin Cancer Res* 3: 837-847.

2532. Martini F, Iaccheri L, Lazzarin L, Carinci P, Corallini A, Gerosa M, Iuzzolino P, Barbanti-Brodano G, Tognon M (1996). SV40 early region and large T antigen in human brain tumors, peripheral blood cells, and sperm fluids from healthy individuals. *Cancer Res* 56: 4820-4825.

2533. Naumann U, Weit S, Rieger L, Meyermann R, Weller M (1999). p27 modulates cell cycle progression and chemosensitivity in human malignant glioma. *Biochem Biophys Res Commun* 261: 890-896.

2534. Piva R, Cavalla P, Bortolotto S, Cordera S, Richiardi P, Schiffer D (1997). p27/kip1 expression in human astrocytic gliomas. *Neurosci Lett* 234: 127-130.

2535. Piva R, Cancelli I, Cavalla P, Bortolotto S, Dominguez J, Draetta GF, Schiffer D (1999). Proteasome-dependent degradation of p27/kip1 in gliomas. *J Neuropathol Exp Neurol* 58: 691-696.

2536. Butel JS, Lednicky JA (1999). Cell and molecular biology of simian virus 40: implications for human infections and disease. *J Natl Cancer Inst* 91: 119-134.

2537. Ino Y, Silver JS, Blazejewski L, Nishikawa R, Matsutani M, von Deimling A, Louis DN (1999). Common regions of deletion on chromosome 22q12.3-q13.1 and 22q13.2 in human astrocytomas appear related to malignancy grade. *J Neuropathol Exp Neurol* 58: 881-885.

2538. Ohh M, Kaelin WG, Jr. (1999). The von Hippel-Lindau tumour suppressor protein: new perspectives. *Mol Med Today* 5: 257-263.

2539. Sakashita N, Takeya M, Kishida T, Stackhouse TM, Zbar B, Takahashi K (1999). Expression of von Hippel-Lindau protein in normal and pathological human tissues. *Histochem J* 31: 133-144.

2540. Corless CL, Kibel AS, Iliopoulos O, Kaelin WG, Jr. (1997). Immunostaining of the von Hippel-Lindau gene product in normal and neoplastic human tissues. *Hum Pathol* 28: 459-464.

2541. Nagashima Y, Miyagi Y, Udagawa K, Taki A, Misugi K, Sakai N, Kondo K, Kaneko S, Yao M, Shuin T (1996). Von Hippel-Lindau tumour suppressor gene. Localization of expression by in situ hybridization. *J Pathol* 180: 271-274.

2542. Miyakawa A, Ichimura K, Schmidt EE, Varmeh-Ziaie S, Collins PV (1999). Multiple deleted regions on the long arm of chromosome 6 in astrocytic tumours. *Br J Cancer* (in press).

2543. Pal L, Santosh V, Gayathri N, Das S, Das BS, Jayakumar PN, Shankar SK (1998). Neurocytoma/rhabdomyoma (myoneurocytoma) of the cerebellum. *Acta Neuropathol (Berl)* 95: 318-323.

2544. Reifenberger G, Weber T, Weber RG, Wolter M, Brandis A, Kuchelmeister K, Pilz P, Reusche E, Lichter P, Wiestler OD (1999). Chordoid glioma of the third ventricle: immunohistochemical and molecular genetic characterization of a novel tumor entity.

Brain Pathol 9: 617-626.

2546. Giannini C, Lopes MBS, Scheithauer BW, Hirose T, VandenBerg SR,Kros M (1998). Immunophenotype of pleomorphic xanthoastrocytoma. *J Neuropathol Exp Neurol* 57;501.

2547. Kleihues P, Cavenee WK (1997). *Pathology and Genetics of Tumours of the Nervous System.* International Agency for Research on Cancer: Lyon.

2548. Shimoji K, Yasuma Y, Mori K, Eguchi M, Maeda M (1999). Unique Radiological Appearance of a Microcystic Meningioma. *Acta Neurochir (Wien)* 141: 1119-1121.

2549. Onda K, Davis RL, Edwards MS (1996). Comparison of bromodeoxyuridine uptake and MIB 1 immunoreactivity in medulloblastomas determined with single and double immunohistochemical staining methods. *J Neurooncol* 29: 129-136.

2550. Krynska B, Del Valle L, Croul S, Gordon J, Katsetos CD, Carbone M, Giordano A, Khalili K (1999). Detection of human neurotropic JC virus DNA sequence and expression of the viral oncogenic protein in pediatric medulloblastomas. *Proc Natl Acad Sci U S A* 96: 11519-11524.

2551. Zurawel RH, Allen C, Chiappa S, Cato W, Biegel J, Cogen P, de Sauvage F, Raffel C (2000). Analysis of PTCH/SMO/SHH pathway genes in medulloblastoma. *Genes Chromosomes Cancer* 27: 44-51.

2552. Huang H, Mahler-Araujo BM, Sankila A, Chimelli L, Yonekawa Y, Kleihues P, Ohgaki H (2000). APC mutations in sporadic medulloblastomas. *Am J Pathol* (in press).

2553. Groden J, Thliveris A, Samowitz W, Carlson M, Gelbert L, Albertsen H, Joslyn G, Stevens J, Spirio L, Robertson M (1991). Identification and characterization of the familial adenomatous polyposis coli gene. *Cell* 66: 589-600.

2554. Barth AI, Nathke IS, Nelson WJ (1997). Cadherins, catenins and APC protein: interplay between cytoskeletal complexes and signaling pathways. *Curr Opin Cell Biol* 9: 683-690.

2555. Behrens J, von Kries JP, Kuhl M, Bruhn L, Wedlich D, Grosschedl R, Birchmeier W (1996). Functional interaction of beta-catenin with the transcription factor LEF-1. *Nature* 382: 638-642.

2556. Hirohashi S (1998). Inactivation of the E-cadherin-mediated cell adhesion system in human cancers. *Am J Pathol* 153: 333-339.

2557. Miyoshi Y, Nagase H, Ando H, Horii A, Ichii S, Nakatsuru S, Aoki T, Miki Y, Mori T, Nakamura Y (1992). Somatic mutations of the APC gene in colorectal tumors: mutation cluster region in the APC gene. *Hum Mol Genet* 1: 229-233.

2558. Sparks AB, Morin PJ, Vogelstein B, Kinzler KW (1998). Mutational analysis of the APC/beta-catenin/Tcf pathway in colorectal cancer. *Cancer Res* 58: 1130-1134.

2559. Munemitsu S, Albert I, Souza B, Rubinfeld B, Polakis P (1995). Regulation of intracellular beta-catenin levels by the adenomatous polyposis coli (APC) tumor-suppressor protein. *Proc Natl Acad Sci U S A* 92: 3046-3050.

2560. Yong WH, Raffel C, von Deimling A, Louis DN (1995). The APC gene in Turcot's syndrome. *N Engl J Med* 333: 524.

2561. Shuangshoti S, Chantra K, Navalitloha Y, Charoonwatanalaoha S, Shuangshoti S (1998). Atypical granular cell tumor of the neurohypophysis: a case report with review of the literature. *J Med Assoc Thai* 81: 641-646.

2562. Becker DH, Wilson CB (1981). Symptomatic parasellar granular cell tumors. *Neurosurgery* 8: 173-180.

2563. Boecher-Schwarz HG, Fries G, Bornemann A, Ludwig B, Perneczky A (1992). Suprasellar granular cell tumor. *Neurosurgery* 31: 751-754.

2564. Schaller B, Kirsch E, Tolnay M, Mindermann T (1998). Symptomatic granular cell tumor of the pituitary gland: case report and review of the literature. *Neurosurgery* 42: 166-170.

2565. Barrande G, Kujas M, Gancel A, Turpin G, Bruckert E, Kuhn JM, Luton JP (1995). [Granular cell tumors. Rare tumors of the neurohypophysis]. *Presse Med* 24: 1376-1380.

2566. Luse SA, Kernohan JW (1955). Granullar-cell tumors of the stalk and posterior lobe of the pituitary gland. *Cancer* 8: 816-822.

2567. Shanklin WM (1953). The origin, histology and senescence of tumorettes in the human neurohypophysis. *Acta Anat (Basel)* 18: 1-20.

2568. Vogelgesang S, Junge MH, Pahnke J, Gaab MR, Wasdahl DA (2000). 59 year old woman with a sellar/suprasellar mass. *Brain Pathol* (in press).

2570. Ohgaki H, Hernandez T, Kleihues P,Hainaut P (1999). p53 Germline mutations and the molecular basis of Li-Fraumeni syndrome. In: *Molecular Biology in Cancer Medicine*, Kurzrock R, Talpaz M (eds), 2nd ed. Martin Dunitz: London. pp. 477-492.

2571. Weber T, Weber RG, Kaulich K, Actor B, Meyer-Puttlitz B, Lampel S, Buschges R, Weigel R, Deckert-Schluter M, Schmiedek P, Reifenberger G, Lichter P (2000). Characteristic chromosomal imbalances in primary central nervous system lymphomas of the diffuse large B-cell type. *Brain Pathol* 10: 73-84.

2572. von Deimling A, Larson J, Wellenreuther R, Stangl AP, van V, V, Warnick R, Tew J, Jr., Balko G, Menon AG (1999). Clonal origin of recurrent meningiomas. *Brain Pathol* 9: 645-650.

2573. Birch JM, Hartley AL, Tricker KJ, Prosser J, Condie A, Kelsey AM, Harris M, Jones PH, Binchy A, Crowther D (1994). Prevalence and diversity of constitutional mutations in the p53 gene among 21 Li-Fraumeni families. *Cancer Res* 54: 1298-1304.

2574. Boddy MN, Russell P (1999). DNA replication checkpoint control. *Front Biosci* 4: D841-D848.

2575. Eng C, Schneider K, Fraumeni JF, Jr., Li FP (1997). Third international workshop on collaborative interdisciplinary studies of p53 and other predisposing genes in Li-Fraumeni syndrome. *Cancer Epidemiol Biomarkers Prev* 6: 379-383.

2576. Bell DW, Varley JM, Szydlo TE, Kang DH, Wahrer DC, Shannon KE, Lubratovich M, Verselis SJ, Isselbacher KJ, Fraumeni JF, Birch JM, Li FP, Garber JE, Haber DA (1999). Heterozygous germ line hCHK2 mutations in Li-Fraumeni syndrome. *Science* 286: 2528-2531.

2577. Szymas J, Wolf G, Petersen S, Schluens K, Nowak S, Petersen I (2000). Comparative genomic hybridisation indicates two distinct subgroups of pilocytic astrocytomas. *J Neurosurg* (in press).

2578. Russo C, Pellarin M, Tingby O, Bollen AW, Lamborn KR, Mohapatra G, Collins VP, Feuerstein BG (1999). Comparative genomic hybridization in patients with supratentorial and infratentorial primitive neuroectodermal tumors. *Cancer* 86: 331-339.

2579. Petersen I, Hidalgo A, Petersen S, Schluens K, Schewe C, Pacyna-Gengelbach M, Goeze A, Krebber B, Knosel T, Kaufmann O, Szymas J, von Deimling A (2000). Chromosomal imbalances in brain metastases of solid tumors. *Brain Pathol* (in press).

2580. Marcus VA, Madlensky L, Gryfe R, Kim H, So K, Millar A, Temple LK, Hsieh E, Hiruki T, Narod S, Bapat BV, Gallinger S, Redston M (1999). Immunohistochemistry for hMLH1 and hMSH2: a practical test for DNA mismatch repair-deficient tumors. *Am J Surg Pathol* 23: 1248-1255.

2581. Wolf HK, Zentner J, Hufnagel A, Campos MG, Schramm J, Elger CE, Wiestler OD (1994). [Morphological findings in temporal lobe epilepsy: experience with 216 consecutive surgical specimens]. *Verh Dtsch Ges Pathol* 78:438-42: 438-442.

2582. Paulus W, Brandner S (1999). Synaptophysin in choroid plexus epithelial cells: no useful aid in differential diagnosis. *J Neuropath Exp Neurol* 58: 1111-1112.

2583. Geddes JF, Swash M (1999). Hugh Cairns, Dorothy Russell and the first pleomorphic xanthoastrocytoma? *Br J Neurosurg* 13: 174-177.

2584. Hagel C, Krog B, Laas R, Stavrou DK (1999). Prognostic relevance of TP53 mutations, p53 protein, Ki-67 index and conventional histological grading in oligodendrogliomas. *J Exp Clin Cancer Res* 18: 305-309.

2585. Kaelin WG, Jr. (1999). Cancer. Many vessels, faulty gene. *Nature* 399: 203-204.

2586. Kamura T, Koepp DM, Conrad MN, Skowyra D, Moreland RJ, Iliopoulos O, Lane WS, Kaelin WG, Jr., Elledge SJ, Conaway RC, Harper JW, Conaway JW (1999). Rbx1, a component of the VHL tumor suppressor complex and SCF ubiquitin ligase. *Science* 284: 657-661.

2587. Pack SD, Zbar B, Pak E, Ault DO, Humphrey JS, Pham T, Hurley K, Weil RJ, Park WS, Kuzmin I, Stolle C, Glenn G, Liotta LA, Lerman MI, Klausner RD, Linehan WM, Zhuang Z (1999). Constitutional von Hippel-Lindau (VHL) gene deletions detected in VHL families by fluorescence in situ hybridization. *Cancer Res* 59: 5560-5564.

2588. Ohh M, Takagi Y, Aso T, Stebbins CE, Pavletich NP, Zbar B, Conaway RC, Conaway JW, Kaelin WG, Jr. (1999). Synthetic peptides define critical contacts between elongin C, elongin B, and the von Hippel-Lindau protein. *J Clin Invest* 104: 1583-1591.

2589. Koochekpour S, Jeffers M, Wang PH, Gong C, Taylor GA, Roessler LM, Stearman R, Vasselli JR, Stetler-Stevenson WG, Kaelin WG, Jr., Linehan WM, Klausner RD, Gnarra JR, Vande Woude GF (1999). The von Hippel-Lindau tumor suppressor gene inhibits hepatocyte growth factor/scatter factor-induced invasion and branching morphogenesis in renal carcinoma cells. *Mol Cell Biol* 19: 5902-5912.

2590. Pagni CA, Canavero S, Gaidolfi E (1991). Intramedullary "holocord" oligodendroglioma: case report. *Acta Neurochir (Wien)* 113: 96-99.

2591. Pause A, Peterson B, Schaffar G, Stearman R, Klausner RD (1999). Studying interactions of four proteins in the yeast two-hybrid system: structural resemblance of the pVHL/elongin BC/hCUL-2 complex with the ubiquitin ligase complex SKP1/cullin/F-box protein. *Proc Natl Acad Sci U S A* 96: 9533-9538.

2592. Pause A, Lee S, Lonergan KM, Klausner RD (1998). The von Hippel-Lindau tumor suppressor gene is required for cell cycle exit upon serum withdrawal. *Proc Natl Acad Sci U S A* 95: 993-998.

2593. Lonergan KM, Iliopoulos O, Ohh M, Kamura T, Conaway RC, Conaway JW, Kaelin WG, Jr. (1998). Regulation of hypoxia-inducible mRNAs by the von Hippel-Lindau tumor suppressor protein requires binding to complexes containing elongins B/C and Cul2. *Mol Cell Biol* 18: 732-741.

2594. Iwai K, Yamanaka K, Kamura T, Minato N, Conaway RC, Conaway JW, Klausner RD, Pause A (1999). Identification of the von Hippel-lindau tumor-suppressor protein as part of an active E3 ubiquitin ligase complex [see comments]. *Proc Natl Acad Sci U S A* 96: 12436-12441.

2595. Brat DJ, Cohen KJ, Sanders JM, Feuerstein BG, Burger PC (1999). Clinicopathologic features of astroblastoma. *J Neuropath Exp Neurol* 58: 509-509.

2596. Cummings TJ, Hulette CM, Longee DC, Bottom KS, McLendon RE, Chu CT (1999). Gliomatosis cerebri: cytologic and autopsy findings in a case involving the entire neuraxis. *Clin Neuropathol* 18: 190-197.

2597. Ohh M, Yauch RL, Lonergan KM, Whaley JM, Stemmer-Rachamimov AO, Louis DN, Gavin BJ, Kley N, Kaelin WG, Jr., Iliopoulos O (1998). The von Hippel-Lindau tumor suppressor protein is required for proper assembly of an extracellular fibronectin matrix. *Mol Cell* 1: 959-968.

2598. Ivanov SV, Kuzmin I, Wei MH, Pack S, Geil L, Johnson BE, Stanbridge EJ, Lerman MI (1998). Down-regulation of transmembrane carbonic anhydrases in renal cell carcinoma cell lines by wild-type von Hippel-Lindau transgenes. *Proc Natl Acad Sci U S A* 95: 12596-12601.

2599. Montesinos-Rongen M, Küppers R, Schlüter D, Spieker T, Van Roost D, Schaller C, Reifenberger G, Wiestler OD, Deckert-Schlüter M (1999). Primary central nervous system lymphomas are derived from germinal-center B cells and show a preferential usage of the V4-34 gene segment. *Am J Pathol* 155: 2077-2086.

2600. Stepp SE, Dufourcq-Lagelouse R, Le Deist F, Bhawan S, Certain S, Mathew PA, Henter JI, Bennett M, Fischer A, de Saint Basile G, Kumar V (1999). Perforin gene defects in familial hemophagocytic lymphohistocytosis. *Science* 286: 1957-1959.

Subject index

D

E

F

G

H

I

J

K

L

M

N

T

U

V

W

X

Y

Z